Genetic Eye Diseases

Retinitis Pigmentosa and Other Inherited Eye Disorders

RECENT TITLES PUBLISHED BY ALAN R. LISS, INC.
FOR MARCH OF DIMES BIRTH DEFECTS FOUNDATION

Birth Defects Compendium, Second Edition, Daniel Bergsma, *Editor*

BIRTH DEFECTS: ORIGINAL ARTICLE SERIES

1981 — Volume XVII

No. 1 **Annual Review of Birth Defects, 1980, The Fetus and the Newborn,** Proceedings of the 1980 New York City Birth Defects Conference, Arthur D. Bloom and L. Stanley James, *Editors*

No. 2 **Morphogenesis and Malformation of the Skin,** Richard J. Blandau, *Editor*

No. 3 **Pregnancy and Childbearing During Adolescence: Research Priorities for the 1980s,** Elizabeth R. McAnarney and Gabriel Stickle, *Editors*

No. 4 **Reproductive Pasts, Reproductive Futures: Genetic Counseling and Its Effectiveness,** James R. Sorenson, Judith P. Swazey, and Norman A. Scotch

No. 6 **Perinatal Parental Behavior: Nursing Research and Implications for Newborn Health,** Regina Placzek Lederman, *Conference Coordinator–Consulting Editor,* and Beverly S. Raff, *Editor*

1982 — Volume 18

No. 1 **Craniofacial Anomalies: New Perspectives,** Carlos F. Salinas, *Editor*

No. 3A **Annual Review of Birth Defects, 1981, Prenatal Diagnosis and Mechanisms of Teratogenesis,** William L. Nyhan and Kenneth Lyons Jones, *Editors*

No. 3B **Annual Review of Birth Defects, 1981, Dysmorphology,** William L. Nyhan and Kenneth Lyons Jones, *Editors*

No. 4 **Children With Sex Chromosome Aneuploidy,** Donald A. Stewart, *Editor*

No. 5 **Cumulative Index: Birth Defects: Original Article Series Volumes I (1965)–XVI (1980),** Natalie W. Paul, *Editor*

No. 6 **Genetic Eye Diseases: Retinitis Pigmentosa and Other Inherited Eye Disorders,** Edward Cotlier, Irene H. Maumenee, and Elaine R. Berman, *Editors*

See pages following the index for previous titles in this series published by Alan R. Liss, Inc.

March of Dimes Birth Defects Foundation
Birth Defects: Original Article Series, Volume 18, Number 6, 1982

Genetic Eye Diseases

Retinitis Pigmentosa and Other Inherited Eye Disorders

Proceedings of the International Symposium on Genetics and Ophthalmology Held in Jerusalem, Israel September 1981

Editors

Edward Cotlier, MD
Department of Ophthalmology and Visual Sciences
Yale University School of Medicine
New Haven, Connecticut

Irene H. Maumenee, MD
The Wilmer Ophthalmological Institute
The Johns Hopkins University School of Medicine
The Johns Hopkins Hospital
Baltimore, Maryland

Elaine R. Berman, PhD
Ophthalmic Biochemistry Unit
Department of Ophthalmology
Hadassah Medical Organization
Hadassah University Hospital
Jerusalem, Israel

ALAN R. LISS, INC., NEW YORK

To enhance medical communication in the birth defects field, the March of Dimes Birth Defects Foundation publishes the *Birth Defects Compendium (Second Edition)*, an *Original Article Series, Syndrome Identification,* a *Reprint Series,* and provides a series of films and related brochures.

Further information can be obtained from:

Professional Education Department
March of Dimes Birth Defects Foundation
1275 Mamaroneck Avenue
White Plains, New York 10605

Published by:
Alan R. Liss, Inc.
150 Fifth Avenue
New York, New York 10011

Library of Congress Cataloging in Publication Data

International Symposium on Genetics and Ophthalmology
(1981 : Jerusalem)
Genetic eye diseases.

(Birth defects original article series ; v. 18, no. 6)
Includes index.
1. Eye—Diseases and defects—Genetic aspects—Congresses. 2. Retinitis pigmentosa—Genetic aspects—Congresses. I. Cotlier, Edward. II. Maumenee, Irene H. III. Berman, Elaine R. IV. Title. V. Series.
RE48.I58 1981 617.7'042 82-13049
ISBN 0-8451-1050-0

Printed in the United States of America.

The **March of Dimes Birth Defects Foundation** is dedicated to the goals of preventing birth defects and ameliorating their consequences for patients, families, and society.

As part of our efforts to achieve these goals, we sponsor, or participate in, a variety of scientific meetings where all questions relating to birth defects are freely discussed. Through our professional education program we speed the dissemination of information by publishing the proceedings of these and other meetings. From time to time, we also reprint pertinent journal articles to help achieve our goal. Now and then, in the course of these articles or discussions, individual viewpoints may be expressed which go beyond the purely scientific and into controversial matters. It should be noted, therefore, that personal viewpoints about such matters will not be censored but this does not constitute an endorsement of them by the **March of Dimes Birth Defects Foundation.**

Contents

Contributors

H. Abulafia, Departments of Ophthalmology and Pediatrics, Hadassah University Hospital, Jerusalem, Israel **[571]**

Gregory Acland, University of Pennsylvania School of Medicine, Philadelphia, Pennsylvania 19104 **[119]**

Gustavo Aguirre, University of Pennsylvania School of Veterinary Medicine, Philadelphia, Pennsylvania 19104 **[119]**

D.M. Albert, Massachusetts Eye and Ear Infirmary, Eye Research Institute of the Retina Foundation and Howe Laboratory of Ophthalmology, Harvard Medical School, Boston, Massachusetts 02114 **[411]**

William F. Benedict, Clayton Ocular Oncology Center and Division of Hematology-Oncology, Children's Hospital of Los Angeles, Los Angeles, California 90054 **[681]**

D. BenEzra, Departments of Ophthalmology and Pediatrics, Hadassah University Hospital, Jerusalem, Israel **[571]**

K. Berg, Institute of Human Genetics, University of Oslo, Oslo, Norway **[669]**

Elaine R. Berman, Ophthalmic Biochemistry Unit, Hadassah University Hospital, Jerusalem, Israel **[135]**

Eliot L. Berson, Berman-Gund Laboratory for the Study of Retinal Degenerations, Harvard Medical School, Massachusetts Eye and Ear Infirmary, Boston, Massachusetts 02114 **[209]**

W.S. Blaner, College of Physicians and Surgeons, Columbia University, New York, New York 10032 **[53]**

L.K. Borysiewicz, The Royal Postgraduate Medical School, London, United Kingdom **[433]**

Joann A. Boughman, Department of Human Genetics, Medical College of Virginia, Richmond, Virginia 23298 **[151, 161, 669]**

M.E. Boulton, Polytechnic of Central London, London, United Kingdom **[101]**

T.A.S. Boyd, Department of Ophthalmology, University of Alberta, Edmonton, Alberta, Canada **[561]**

George Bresnick, Department of Ophthalmology, University of Wisconsin, Madison, Wisconsin 53792 **[281]**

J.H. Bryars, Department of Ophthalmology, Royal Victoria Hospital, Belfast, Northern Ireland **[729]**

Robert M. Bumsted, University of Iowa, Iowa City, Iowa 52242 **[539]**

Gerald Chader, Laboratory of Vision Research, National Eye Institute, National Institutes of Health, Bethesda, Maryland 20205 **[119]**

Gerhard W. Cibis, Children's Mercy Hospital, Kansas City, Missouri 64108 and University of Kansas Medical School, Kansas City, Kansas 66103 **[359, 629]**

The boldface number in brackets following each contributor's affiliation is the opening page number of that contributor's article.

L.A. Corey, Medical College of Virginia, Richmond, Virginia 23298 **[669]**

G. Cornu, Department of Biochemistry, ICP, Brussels, Belgium **[327]**

Edward Cotlier, Department of Ophthalmology and Visual Sciences, Yale University Medical School, New Haven, Connecticut 06510 **[xix, 27]**

Donnell Creel, Veterans Administration Hospital, Salt Lake City, Utah 84148 **[299]**

D.J.D'Amico, Massachusetts Eye and Ear Infirmary, Eye Research Institute of the Retina Foundation and Howe Laboratory of Ophthalmology, Harvard Medical School, Boston, Massachusetts 02114 **[411]**

Monte A. Del Monte, The Wilmer Ophthalmological Institute, The Johns Hopkins University Medical School, Baltimore, Maryland 21205 **[67]**

P. Dhermy, Service d'Ophtalmologie, Hôpital St-Pierre, 322 rue Haute, B-1000 Brussels, Belgium **[327]**

Daniel R. Doiron, Clayton Ocular Oncology Center, Children's Hospital of Los Angeles, Los Angeles, California 90054 **[681]**

J.L. Dufier, Service d'Ophtalmologie, Hôpital St-Pierre, Brussels, Belgium **[327]**

Ross B. Edwards, Berman-Gund Laboratory for the Study of Retinal Degenerations, Harvard Medical School, Massachusetts Eye and Ear Infirmary, Boston, Massachusetts 02114 **[95]**

V. Feiler-Ofry, Departments of Ophthalmology and Genetics, Ichilov Hospital and Sheba Medical Center, Tel Aviv University Medical School, Tel Aviv, Israel **[581]**

Daniel Finkelstein, The Wilmer Ophthalmological Institute, The Johns Hopkins University Medical School, Baltimore, Maryland 21205 **[161, 197]**

M.T. Flood, College of Physicians and Surgeons, Columbia University, New York, New York 10032 **[53]**

Albert T. Franceschetti, Unité de Diagnostic et d'Urgence Opthalmologiques, Hôpital de la Tour, Geneva, Switzerland **[29]**

Jules François, Ophthalmological Clinic of the University of Ghent, Ghent, Belgium **[xxi, 3, 595]**

Brenda L. Gallie, Department of Ophthalmology, University of Toronto and the Ontario Cancer Institute, Toronto, Ontario, Canada **[689]**

M. Gheiler, Department of Ophthalmology, Kaplan Hospital, Rehovot, Israel **[577]**

Egil Gjone, Department of Medicine, University Hospital, Rikshospitalet, Oslo, Norway **[423]**

Victor Godel, Department of Ophthalmology, Ichilov Hospital, Tel Aviv University Medical School, Tel Aviv, Israel **[263, 577, 581, 587, 621]**

Hans H. Goebel, Department of Neuropathology, University of Göttingen, Göttingen, Federal Republic of Germany **[241]**

Charles J. Gomer, Clayton Ocular Oncology Center and Division of Hematology-Oncology, Children's Hospital of Los Angeles, Los Angeles, California 90054 **[681]**

Richard M. Goodman, Department of Genetics, Sheba Medical Center, Tel Hashomer, Israel **[587, 621]**

P. Gouras, College of Physicians and Surgeons, Columbia University, New York, New York 10032 **[53]**

V. Goya, Department of Ophthalmology, Sheba Medical Center, Tel Hashomer, Israel **[621]**

R.W. Guillery, University of Chicago, Chicago, Illinois 60637 **[299]**

J.E. Haley, College of Physicians and Surgeons, Columbia University, New York, New York 10032 **[53]**

J.E. Hanna, Department of Medical Genetics, The Queen's University of Belfast, Belfast, Northern Ireland **[729]**

L. Hanninen, Massachusetts Eye and Ear Infirmary, Eye Research Institute of the Retina Foundation and Howe Laboratory of Ophthalmology, Harvard Medical School, Boston, Massachusetts 02214 **[411]**

Arthur H. Hanson III, Berman-Gund Laboratory for the Study of Retinal Degenerations, Harvard Medical School, Massachusetts Eye and Ear Infirmary, Boston, Massachusetts 02214 **[209]**

James W. Hanson, University of Iowa, Iowa City, Iowa 52242 **[539]**

David J. Harris, Children's Mercy Hospital, Kansas City, Missouri 64108 **[359, 629]**

John R. Heckenlively, Jules Stein Eye Institute and the Department of Ophthalmology, UCLA School of Medicine, Los Angeles, California 90024 **[193]**

Vernon Hermsen, University of Iowa, Iowa City, Iowa 52242 **[539]**

A. Hillis, The Wilmer Ophthalmological Institute, The Johns Hopkins University Hospital, Baltimore, Maryland 21205 **[197]**

Tatsuo Hirose, Retina Associates and The Eye Research Institute of the Retina Foundation, Boston, Massachusetts 02114 **[525]**

Rufus O. Howard, Department of Ophthalmology and Visual Sciences, Yale University School of Medicine, New Haven, Connecticut 06510 and Department of Surgery, University of Connecticut Medical School, Farmington, Connecticut 06032 **[703]**

Dan-Ning Hu, The Wilmer Ophthalmological Institute, The Johns Hopkins University Medical School, Baltimore, Maryland 21205 **[67]**

Barrie Jay, Moorfields Eye Hospital, London, United Kingdom **[299, 319]**

Marcelle Jay, Moorfields Eye Hospital, London, United Kingdom **[167]**

S.S. Johnston, Department of Ophthalmology, Royal Victoria Hospital, Belfast, Northern Ireland **[729]**

H. Kashima, Department of Otolaryngology, The Johns Hopkins University Hospital, Baltimore, Maryland 21205 **[197]**

C.G. Keith, Royal Children's Hospital, Parville, Victoria, Australia **[269]**

Nancy G. Kennaway, Oregon Health Sciences University, Portland, Oregon 97201 **[219]**

Kenneth R. Kenyon, Pediatric Service and Cornea Service of the Massachusetts Eye and Ear Infirmary, Harvard Medical School, Boston, Massachusetts 02114 **[381, 411]**

N.M.K. Ng Ying Kin, Montreal Neurological Institute and Hospital, Montreal, Quebec, Canada **[233]**

Richard A. King, Department of Medicine, School of Medicine, University of Minnesota, Minneapolis, Minnesota 55455 **[319]**

Ronald Klein, Department of Ophthalmology, University of Wisconsin, Madison, Wisconsin 53792 **[281]**

Gordon K. Klintworth, Duke University Medical Center, Durham, North Carolina 27710 **[463]**

Bernd Köhnecke, Department of Neuropathology, University of Göttingen, Göttingen, Federal Republic of Germany **[241]**

Nils Koppang, National Veterinary Institute, Oslo, Norway **[241]**

Jay Krachmer, University of Iowa, Iowa City, Iowa 52242 **[479]**

B.D. Lake, Department of Histopathology, Hospital for Sick Children and Institute of Child Health, London, United Kingdom **[391]**

Moshe Lazar, Department of Ophthalmology, Ichilov Hospital, Tel Aviv University Medical School, Tel Aviv, Israel **[263, 581]**

Ruth M. Liberfarb, Retina Associates and The Eye Research Institute of the Retina Foundation, Boston, Massachusetts 02114 **[525]**

J. Libert, Service d'Ophtalmologie, Hôpital St-Pierre, Brussels, Belgium **[327, 347]**

Sammy Liu, The Wilmer Ophthalmological Institute, The Johns Hopkins University Medical School, Baltimore, Maryland 21205 **[67]**

Gilles Lyon, Service de Neurologie Pédiatrique, Université de Louvain, Brussels, Belgium **[255]**

William G. Macrae, Department of Ophthalmology, University of Toronto and Hospital for Sick Children, Toronto, Canada **[175]**

G. Maftzir, Departments of Ophthalmology and Pediatrics, Hadassah University Hospital, Jerusalem, Israel **[571]**

P. Magnus, Institute of Human Genetics, Oslo, Norway **[669]**

J. Marshall, Institute of Ophthalmology, London, United Kingdom **[101]**

Robert W. Massof, The Wilmer Ophthalmological Institute, The Johns Hopkins University Medical School, Baltimore, Maryland 21205 **[161, 197]**

Irene H. Maumenee, The Wilmer Ophthalmological Institute, The Johns Hopkins University Medical School, Baltimore, Maryland 21205 **[67, 515]**

J. Mellerio, Polytechnic of Central London, London, United Kingdom **[101]**

Saul Merin, Department of Ophthalmology, Hadassah University Hospital, Jerusalem, Israel **[135, 187]**

Jean Michiels, Service d'Ophtalmologie, Université de Louvain, Brussels, Belgium **[255]**

P.J. Milla, Department of Child Health, Institute of Child Health, London, United Kingdom **[391]**

A. Linn Murphree, Clayton Ocular Oncology Center and Division of Ophthalmology, Children's Hospital of Los Angeles, Los Angeles, California 90054 **[681]**

W.E. Nance, Medical College of Virginia, Richmond, Virginia 23298 **[669]**

Pinhas Nemet, Department of Ophthalmology, Ichilov Hospital, Tel Aviv University Medical School, Tel Aviv, Israel **[263]**

N.C. Nevin, Department of Medical Genetics, The Queens University of Belfast, Belfast, Northern Ireland **[729]**

David Newsome, Clinical Branch, National Eye Institute, National Institutes of Health, Bethesda, Maryland 20205 **[81, 479]**

Magnus Odland, Department of Ophthalmology, Haukeland Hospital, University of Bergen, Bergen, Norway **[657]**

William H. Olin, University of Iowa, Iowa City, Iowa 52242 **[539]**

M. Oliver, Department of Ophthalmology, Kaplan Hospital, Rehovot, Israel **[577]**

R.S. Ombres, Department of Ophthalmology, University of Alberta, Edmonton, Alberta, Canada **[561]**

J. Paez, Departments of Ophthalmology and Pediatrics, Hadassah University Hospital, Jerusalem, Israel **[571]**

W.G. Pearce, Department of Ophthalmology, University of Alberta, Edmonton, Alberta, Canada **[561]**

Bo T. Philipson, Department of Ophthalmology, Karolinska Hospital, Stockholm, Sweden **[441]**

Robert A. Phillips, Department of Medical Biophysics, University of Toronto and the Ontario Cancer Institute, Toronto, Ontario, Canada **[689]**

S. Photiou, Department of Ophthalmology, Hadassah University Hospital, Jerusalem, Israel **[135]**

A. Pollack, Department of Ophthalmology, Kaplan Hospital, Rehovot, Israel **[577]**

D. Proctor, Department of Otolaryngology, The Johns Hopkins University Hospital, Baltimore, Maryland 21205 **[197]**

L. Regenbogen, Department of Ophthalmology, Sheba Medical Center, Tel Hashomer, Israel **[581, 621]**

M. Reissig, The Johns Hopkins School of Hygiene and Public Health, Baltimore, Maryland 21205 **[197]**

Merlyn M. Rodrigues, Clinical Branch, National Eye Institute, National Institutes of Health, Bethesda, Maryland 20205 **[81, 479]**

Louis J. Rosenbaum, Veterans Administration Hospital, St. Luke's Hospital Medical Center, Phoenix, Arizona 85012 **[645]**

Bernard Rosner, Berman-Gund Laboratory for the Study of Retinal Degenerations, Harvard Medical School, Massachusetts Eye and Ear Infirmary, Boston, Massachusetts 02114 **[209]**

A.B. Salter, Department of Ophthalmology, University of Alberta, Edmonton, Alberta, Canada **[561]**

N. Segal, Department of Ophthalmology, Hadassah University Hospital, Jerusalem, Israel **[135]**

Vivian E. Shih, Berman-Gund Laboratory for the Study of Retinal Degenerations, Harvard Medical School, Massachusetts Eye and Ear Infirmary, Boston, Massachusetts 02114 **[209]**

Bianca Stanescu, Service d'Ophtalmologie, Université de Louvain, Brussels, Belgium **[255]**

Kerstin Strömland, Department of Ophthalmology, Sahlgrens Hospital, Göteborg, Sweden **[651]**

Tung-tien Sun, The Johns Hopkins Medical School, Baltimore, Maryland 21205 **[479]**

D.S.I. Taylor, Department of Ophthalmology, Hospital for Sick Children, London, United Kingdom **[391]**

D. Toussaint, Université Libre de Bruxelles, Brussels, Belgium **[347]**

Brenda Tripathi, University of Chicago, Chicago, Illinois 60637 **[629]**

Ramesh C. Tripathi, University of Chicago, Chicago, Illinois 60637 **[359, 629]**

D. Uchenik, Department of Ophthalmology, Kaplan Hospital, Rehovot, Israel **[577]**

F. Van Hoof, Department of Biochemistry, ICP, Brussels, Belgium **[327]**

Mette Warburg, Eye Clinic for the Multiple Handicapped, Gentofte Hospital, Gentofte, Denmark **[31]**

George O. Waring, Emory University Clinic, Atlanta, Georgia 30322 **[493]**

A.F. Winder, Institute of Ophthalmology and Moorfields Eye Hospital, London, United Kingdom **[433, 449]**

Thomas A. Weingeist, University of Iowa, Iowa City, Iowa 52242 **[539]**

Stuart L. Weinstein, University of Iowa, Iowa City, Iowa 52242 **[539]**

Richard G. Weleber, Oregon Health Sciences University, Portland, Oregon 97201 **[219]**

James G. White, University of Minnesota, Health Sciences Unit, Minneapolis, Minnesota 55455 **[493]**

Mary K. Wirtz, Oregon Health Sciences University, Portland, Oregon 97201 **[219]**

Carl J. Witkop, Jr., Department of Oral Pathology and Genetics, University of Minnesota, Minneapolis, Minnesota 55455 **[299, 319, 493]**

Leonhard S. Wolfe, Montreal Neurological Institute and Hospital, Montreal, Quebec, Canada **[233, 405]**

H.T. Wyatt, Department of Ophthalmology, University of Alberta, Edmonton, Alberta, Canada **[561]**

S. Yatziv, Departments of Ophthalmology and Pediatrics, Hadassah University Hospital, Jerusalem, Israel **[571]**

Elisabeth P. Young, Department of Chemical Pathology, Institute of Child Health, London, United Kingdom **[391]**

A. Zelikovitch, Departments of Ophthalmology and Pediatrics, Hadassah University Hospital, Jerusalem, Israel **[571]**

Johan Zwaan, Department of Ophthalmology, Harvard Medical School, and Morphology Unit and Cornea Research Department of the Eye Research Institute of the Retina Foundation, Boston, Massachusetts 02114 **[381]**

Opening Remarks

Loss of sight is one of the events most feared by all members of the human race. It is also a major deprivation to children and those who are born with visual problems. That is why we are here today, to put together our brains, our experiments and our plans for the future to conquer the many blinding diseases of birth and childhood. That goal has been one of the major objectives of one of the sponsoring organizations, the March of Dimes Birth Defects Foundation. This organization has an unsurpassed track record for generating public interest in genetic diseases and transforming it into knowledge and prevention of inherited diseases. We are happy to acknowledge their support. In 1975 the March of Dimes Birth Defects Foundation supported the gathering at Oxford, England for the subject "The Eye and Inborn Errors of Metabolism", a pioneering landmark for those involved in genetic eye research. At that time our host was Mr. Anthony Bron who made that meeting a great scientific success. We are at this time also indebted to the Retinitis Pigmentosa Foundation for financial and moral support. This grass roots organization is an example of the relentless force generated by those affected by a crippling visual disease. During the last 10 years the Retinitis Pigmentosa Foundation has generated more basic research on hereditary retinal degenerations than ever before in the history of ophthalmology. The research to be presented here may be crucial to the conquest of retinitis pigmentosa. For the Retinitis Pigmentosa Foundation every experiment counts and every effort is a step closer to the prevention or cure of retinitis pigmentosa.

Israel was the host country for The International Congress of Human Genetics which has just finished their deliberations. Israel is in the forefront of human genetic research and Israeli ophthalmologists and scientists have already made fundamental contributions to eye research in general and to genetic eye diseases in particular. That is why it is a pleasure to acknowledge the support of the Israeli Academy of Sciences, the Israeli Ophthalmological Society, and the American-Israeli Ophthalmological group. Ideas and concepts grow in fertile soil and the intellectual climate of Israel is optimum for our gathering.

The International Society for Genetic Eye Diseases is a true international group binding clinicians and basic scientists with interest in the devastating genetic disorders of the eye. We are a small group but full of enthusiasm and hope for the future. Ideas and fruitful concepts may originate in the papers and discussions of the next four days. It is comforting to know that we are not alone; all of our patients, all of those children affected by inherited eye problems are with us. They are a constant reminder of the need for more research to alleviate their problems. In the name of the Board of ISGED and my co-chairperson, Dr. Irene Maumenee, I would like to wish all of the participants a stimulating, productive, and enjoyable meeting.

Edward Cotlier
Jerusalem, 1981

Inaugural Speech

It is my great pleasure to greet you very cordially on behalf of the International Council of Ophthalmology and of the International Federation of Ophthalmological Societies, as well as in my own name, and to wish you all a fruitful, pleasant and interesting meeting. I hope that during this symposium, science will gain as much as friendship, and that we will move closer to each other in heart and mind for the greatest benefit of humanity, peace, and knowledge.

I would like to congratulate and to thank very warmly the organizing committee and particularly Professor Merin, Dr. Cotlier and Dr. Irene Maumenee for having so beautifully arranged this meeting in this wonderful and historical place. I am sure that thanks to their efforts, this symposium will be a great success.

Geneticists and ophthalmologists are brought here together not only to discuss their common problems, but also to learn what is happening in the other discipline. We hope that from these discussions many problems may be solved or at least better understood. We are indeed very happy to have so many speakers who will present the conclusions of their research work. Thanks to them, this meeting will be able to fulfill its purpose, namely an interchange of ideas which can provide a better understanding and elucidation of the many complex problems in modern ophthalmic genetics. This will be achieved through the addition of new information and by the discussion of current viewpoints and interpretations.

Let me say that we have the greatest admiration for the Israeli people, admiration for what you have accomplished, admiration for your struggle for life, admiration for what you, the ophthalmologists of Israel, are realizing. We all hope from the bottom of our heart that peace will very soon be your recompense. I am very happy to be once more in Jerusalem and in Israel, where I have so many good friends. I will always remember one of my dearest friends, Professor Richard Stein, a unique personality who passed away recently and for whom I had the greatest admiration and deepest affection. I am also very happy that this symposium will remember Professor Adolphe Franceschetti, a very close friend, who was truly a pioneer in ophthalmic genetics.

I am sure that this symposium will leave in your mind the happiest of memories and stimulate you to continue research in ophthalmic genetics, which is so important both from the etiological as well as the counseling point of view. Therefore, on behalf of all of you and in my own name, I should like to present to Professor Merin, to Dr. Cotlier, and to Dr. Irene Maumenee our warmest congratulations and our very sincere gratitude.

As Blaise Pascal, one of the most famous French philosophers and scientists, said: "Your symposium will concentrate in its unity all the diversity of the forces of thinking and feeling, which are bestowed on humanity, in order to ask the heart to appeal to the spirit and the intelligence to appeal to love and affection."

Jules François
Jerusalem, 1981

Genetic Research in Ophthalmology

THE SIGNIFICANCE OF GENETIC RESEARCH IN OPHTHALMOLOGY

Jules Francois

Ophthalmological Clinic of the University of Ghent
Ghent, Belgium

The importance of genetics in ophthalmology is illustrated by the fact that 50% of blindness before the age of 6 is inherited, and of the entire blind population up to the age of 100, about 33% of the cases have a genetic basis.

The study of heredity in ophthalmology is of capital importance not only because there are so many hereditary ocular diseases, but particularly because the least malformative anomaly of the eye can be identified. Moreover ocular manifestations associated with systemic genetic diseases are being recognized with increasing frequency. In addition, when the manifestations are specific, they permit the establishment of a diagnosis with certainty. This is, for example, the case when a child is suspected of presenting Lowe's oculocerebrorenal syndrome. Cataract is pathognomonic for this disorder and in the absence of this anomaly, the diagnosis cannot be confirmed.

The study of heredity in ophthalmology no longer consists solely of establishing genealogical trees, since they only serve to confirm the mode of transmission of a given disease. This study must now have a triple objective: (1) detailed knowledge of the ocular malformations or of the ocular manifestations of general genetic diseases, (2) elucidation of the pathogenesis of the ocular symptoms, and (3) devising curative or palliative therapy.

Finally, a distinction must be made between classical mendelian heredity and the more recently discovered chromosomal heredity. As it is not possible to review all known

Birth Defects: Original Article Series, Volume 18, Number 6, pages 3–25

genetic problems in a single lecture, I shall content myself by citing two personal examples of mendelian heredity, Fabry's disease and macular dystrophy of the cornea, and two very recent examples of chromosomal aberrations, retinoblastoma and the "aniridia-Wilms' tumor" syndrome.

I. MENDELIAN HEREDITY

1. Fabry's Disease

In 1905, Fleischer described a verticillate dystrophy of the cornea characterized by a fine stippling of the epithelium and of Bowman's membrane (Fig. 1). These opaque

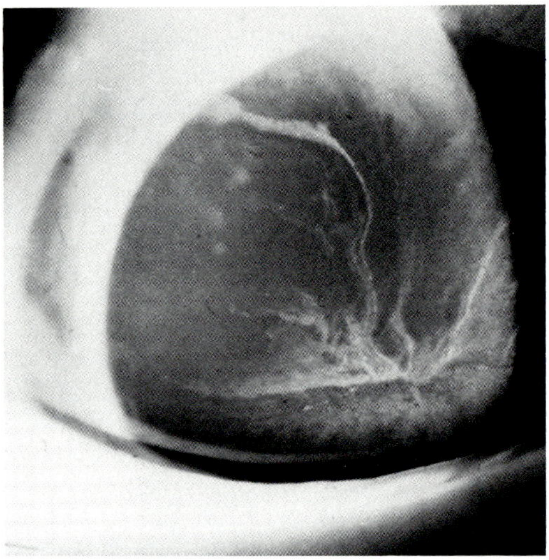

Figure 1. Cornea verticillata

and brownish stipples were disposed in incurvated lines converging to an infero-internal paracentral point, like the lines of force of a magnetic field. Some family cases (Lutz, 1930, Gruber, 1946; Denden, 1963, 1966) indicated that Fleischer's corneal dystrophy was hereditary and, in fact, was autosomal dominant (Fig. 2) in transmission. It is under this name and with this mode of heredity that the disease was described in all the early classifications of corneal degenerations.

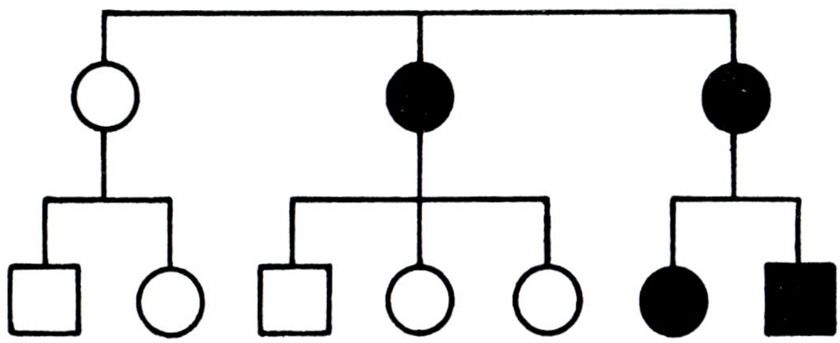

Figure 2. Fleischer's cornea verticillata with apparent autosomal dominant inheritance (from Gruber, 1946)

In studying this disease and in reflecting on the verticillate dystrophy of Fleischer, I was impressed by certain facts (Francois, 1966): (1) The four families mentioned in the literature did not justify the conclusion of dominant transmission because only two generations were cited and there was no father-to-son transmission (2) As an alternative, X-linked heredity was considered because more than 75% of the cases of Fleischer's corneal dystrophy were present in females (there were 16 females to only 5 males). (3) For these reasons, I concluded that Fleischer's dystrophy was not an isolated clinical entity, but that it was probably a manifestation of Fabry's disease, the affected females being heterozygotes and the affected males hemizygotes whose general state of health was still good. (4) Finally, in the publications of Fleischer's dystrophy, no mention was made of the general state of either the patients or their relatives. However, the affected males were young, so that the systemic manifestations were not yet apparent and the cutaneous lesions were either rather rare or unnoticed.

My conclusion was all the more plausible not only because the morphological aspect of Fleischer's dystrophy was identical to that of the keratopathy of Fabry's disease but also because the mode of inheritance appeared to be the same, namely X-linked (Fig. 3).

Upon reexamining the families of Gruber and Denden, my conclusion turned out to be correct. They were indeed patients with Fabry's disease, a sphingoglycolipidosis characterized by cutaneous angiokeratomas (Fig. 4), renal insuf-

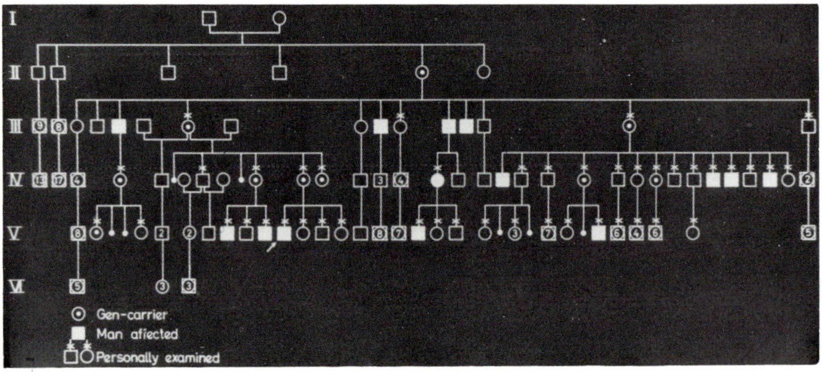

Figure 3. Intermediary sex-linked inheritance of Fabry's disease (from Opitz et al, 1965)

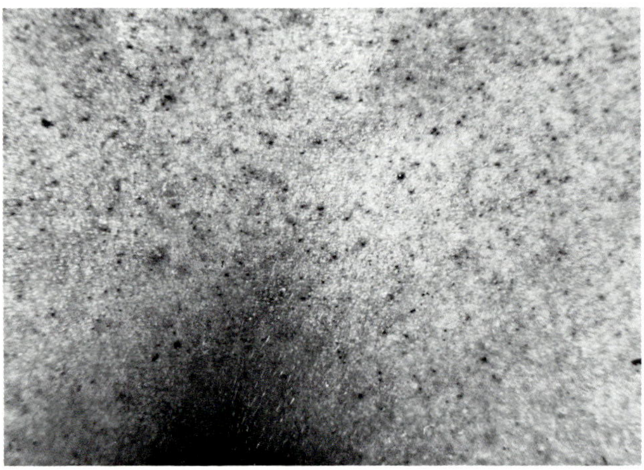

Figure 4. Cutaneous angiokeratomas in Fabry's disease

ficiency, and verticillate dystrophy of the cornea. Thus Fleischer's dystrophy is no longer included in the group of idiopathic corneal degenerations.

2. <u>Macular Dystrophy of the Cornea</u>

Macular dystrophy of the cornea, with onset during the first decade of life, is characterized by opacities of the corneal stroma; they first appear in the central and anterior layers, and subsequently become more numerous in the periphery and in the deeper layers (Fig. 5). The disease is transmitted as an autosomal recessive trait. Consanguinity of the parents is frequent (Fig. 6); only siblings are affected, the disease is not found in other generations, and about 25% of the siblings in a family inherit the disorder.

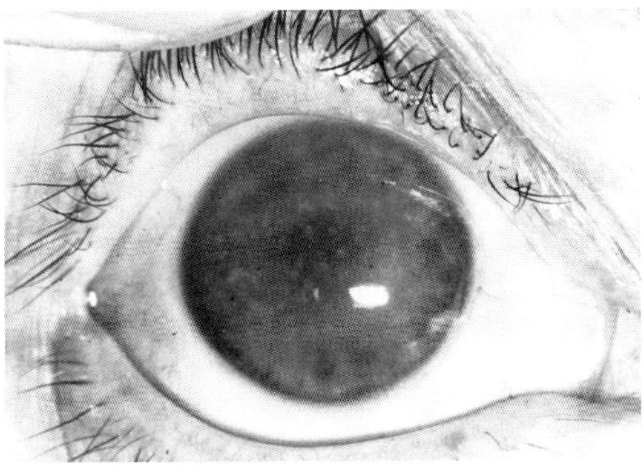

Figure 5. Macular dystrophy of the cornea

The histochemical studies of macular dystrophy, particularly staining by colloidal iron and Alcian blue, show that the intracytoplasmic granules in the keratocytes and the interlamellar deposits of the stroma consist of sulfated glycosaminoglycans (mucopolysaccharides) having the characteristics of keratan sulfate.

We were the first to demonstrate that the stored glycosaminoglycan is in fact keratan sulfate, as shown by fluorescence microscopy after Saunders-staining with acridine orange. It appears to be a true storage disease, the interlamellar deposits being granules of keratocytes released after the rupture of the cell. Furthermore, the stored granules within the keratocytes are secondary lysosomes because, in addition to the accumulated glycosaminoglycans, they also contain acid phosphatase. This is demonstrated by the positivity of the Takeuchi and Tanoue staining with β-glycerophosphate and with ammoniacal silver nitrate, which may also indicate other enzymes of the lysosomal pool. Moreover, the interlamellar deposits contain the same elements

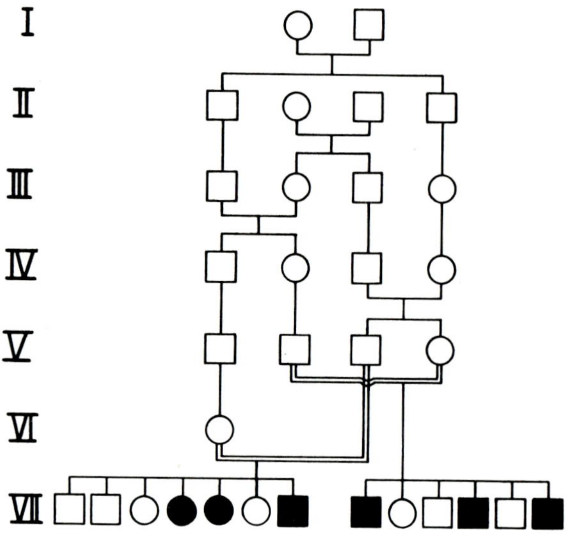

Figure 6. Macular dystrophy of the cornea. Autosomal recessive inheritance with consanguinity of the parents (from Blum, 1945)

as those found within the cells, the origin of which must be identical, as is demonstrated by the presence of acid phosphatase. The lesions of the corneal lamellae show, in addition, progressive stages of destruction due to the catabolic action of lysosomal enzymes originating from the ruptured keratocytes.

Four stages in the development of the intracellular storage in the keratocytes can be distinguished:

In stage I, only a few glycosaminoglycan granules are found in the cytoplasm (Fig. 7). In stage II, the accumulation of these granules becomes progressively greater, and the cells take on a globular shape (Fig. 8). In stage III, the nucleus becomes pycnotic, and the cell membrane ruptures (Fig. 9). In stage IV, the nucleus has disappeared, and only an interlamellar deposit remains (Fig. 10).

Electron microscopy (Fig. 11) confirms histochemical examination with the light microscope. The keratocytes

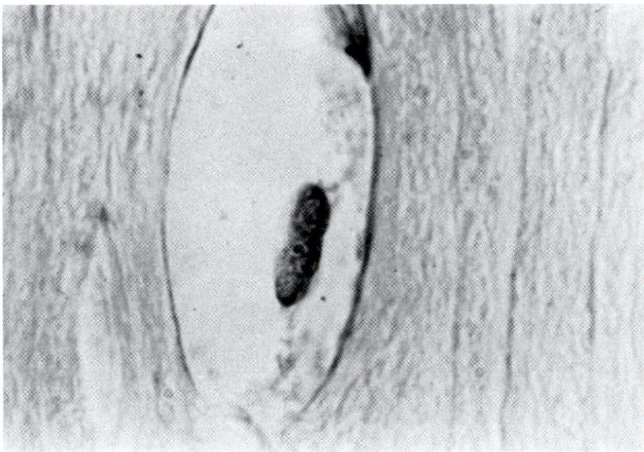

Figure 7. Macular dystrophy of the cornea. Stage I. Cytoplasm positive for Alcian blue pH 1

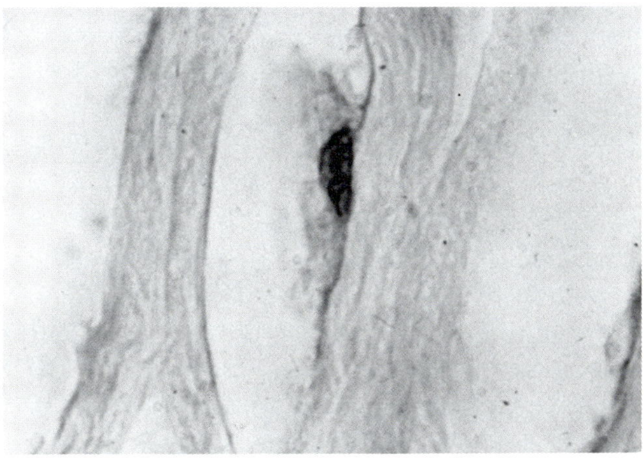

Figure 8. Macular dystrophy of the cornea. Stage II. Nucleus becomes smaller. The keratan sulfate increases

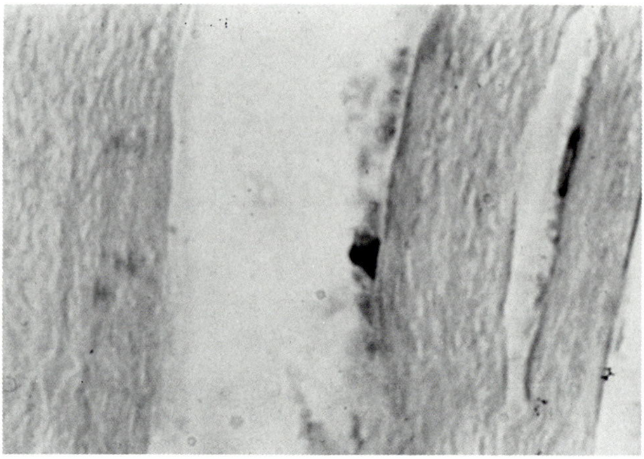

Figure 9. Macular dystrophy of the cornea. Stage III. Pycnotic nucleus and rupture of the cell membrane

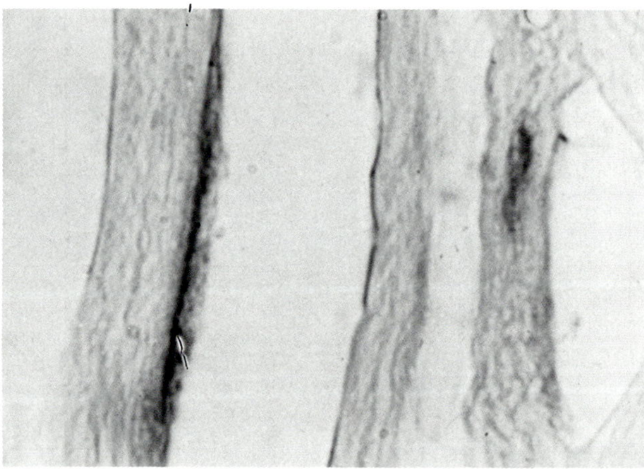

Figure 10. Macular dystrophy of the cornea. Stage IV. Disappearance of the nucleus and rupture of the cell

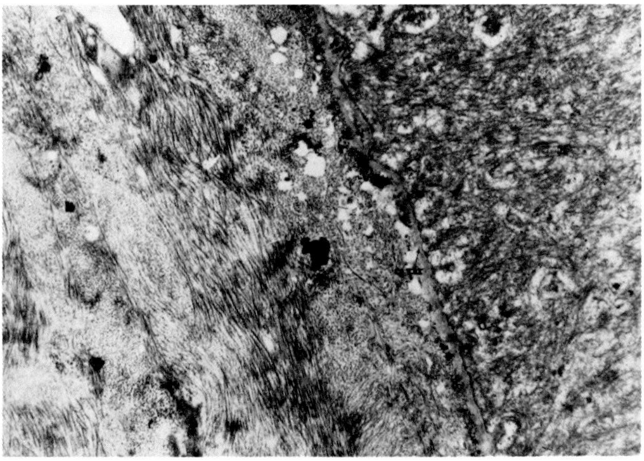

Figure 11. Macular dystrophy of the cornea. Electronmicroscopy. Rupture of the base membrane of the epithelium and destruction of the Bowman's membrane

contain numerous particles of the lysosomal type, large dilated cisternae and vacuoles, either empty or filled with various substances, which progressively accumulate until the cell ruptures. The material released acts upon the neighboring stroma which subsequently degenerates. There is a close relationship between the changes in the stroma and those in the keratocytes. Indeed, an area of degenerated stroma always contains a degenerated keratocyte.

We were able to culture corneal stroma obtained from patients with macular dystrophy (Fig. 12). These tissue cultures show the same anomalies as the corneal stroma in situ. We also saw the keratocytes rupturing, releasing cytoplasmic granules highly positive for glycosaminoglycans and acid phosphatase staining. The histochemical study, in conjunction with phase-contrast microscopy in vivo, both of the implanted specimen and of monolayers, demonstrates the accelerated pathological process of macular dystrophy. It is also obvious here that the lesions of the corneal stroma are due to cytolytic phenomena, accompanied by the release of lysosomal enzymes which digest the neighboring tissue, because all the lesions are positive for acid phosphatase, an enzyme specific for the lysosome.

Furthermore, studies of lysosomal enzymes in cultures of keratocytes obtained from macular dystrophy show the absence of β-glucuronidase, which is present in cultures of normal keratocytes (Fig. 13).

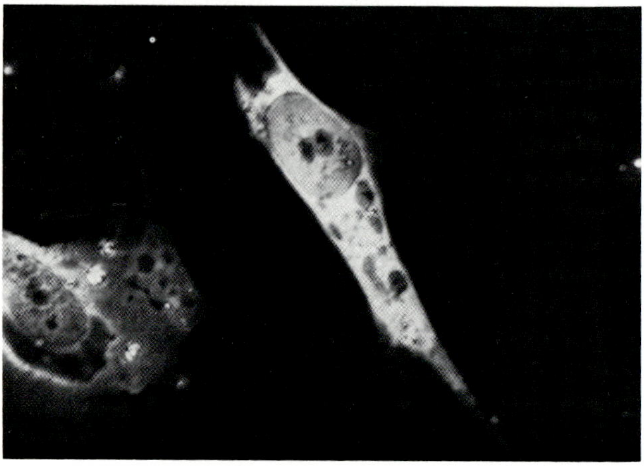

Figure 12. Macular dystrophy of the cornea. Tissue culture. Numerous vacuoles in the cytoplasm. Polarization microscope

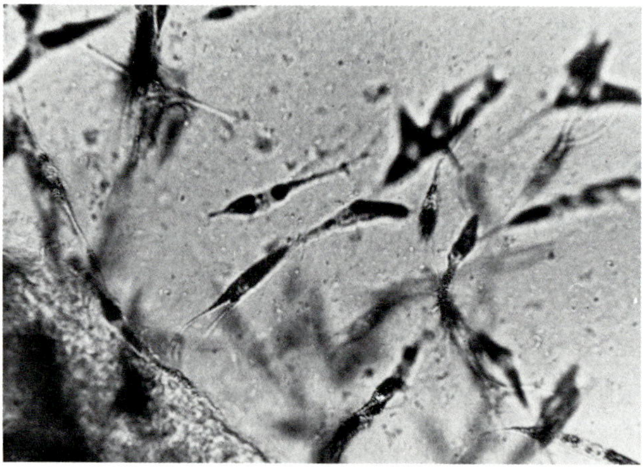

Figure 13. Beta-glucuronidase in normal keratocytes

Vital staining with acridine orange shows, moreover, hypertrophy of the lysosomal system of the pathological keratocytes, as if this system were attempting to compensate the enzymatic deficiency, but was unable to accomplish it. Indeed, the lysosomes show a very wide variety of forms, from the normal up to the giant form, which occupies a whole pole of the cell (Fig. 14). Most of the lysosomes have, in any case, large dimensions, measuring from 2 to 5 μm. We know that they contain enzymes capable of catabolizing glycosaminoglycans, proteins, certain lipids and hydrocarbons. The accumulation of glycosaminoglycans in macular dystrophy may be due not only to a defect in their catabolism resulting from the absence of β-glucuronidase, but also perhaps to an excess production. The later cannot be excluded in view of the hypertrophy of the Golgi apparatus and to a deterioration of the mitochondria which supply the energy for essential metabolic process.

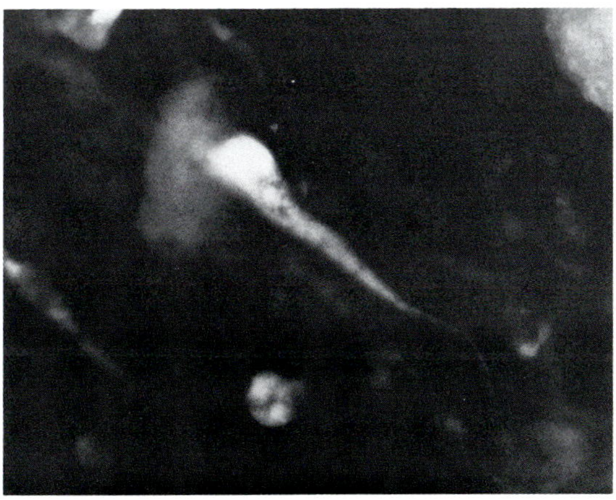

Figure 14. Macular dystrophy of the cornea. Abnormal lysosomes. Giant lysosome. Vital staining with acridine orange.

Tissue culture enabled us for the first time to observe the _in vivo_ behavior of keratocytes and to demonstrate an inborn error in the metabolism of keratan sulfate. From this it is possible to conclude that macular dystrophy of the cornea is really a primary storage disorder of the keratocytes, characterized by an accumulation of a specific sulfated glycosaminoglycan, keratan sulfate. The evolution of this process until the death of the cell can be observed. This disorder is, finally, a mucopolysaccharidosis localized to the cornea, possibly because this particular type of β-glucuronidase is found exclusively in the lysosomal membranes of this tissue.

We have also found an active biological substance capable of neutralizing the glycosaminoglycans, in particular the keratan sulfate, stored in macular dystrophy of the cornea. It must be an enzyme or an enzymatic complex. Staining with toluidine blue shows, indeed, that sections of macular dystrophy treated with a culture homogenate of normal keratocytes or normal corneal stroma are stained orthochromatically, whereas those treated only with potassium chloride, used as a hypotonic solvent, are stained metachromatically. Similarly, staining with colloidal iron and Alcian blue is negative in sections treated with homogenates of normal corneas (Fig. 15), whereas they remain positive in sections treated with the solvent alone. The active substance must, therefore, originate from the cell; it is probably enzymatic in nature because it is obtained by adding a hypotonic solvent which breaks down the lysosomal membranes.

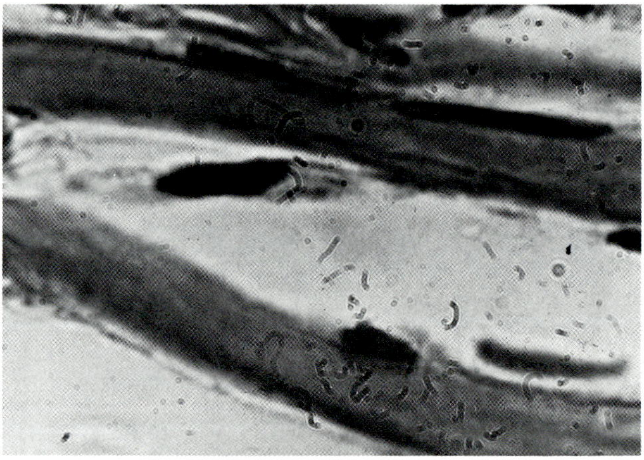

Figure 15. Macular dystrophy of the cornea. Treatment by a homogenate of normal keratocytes. The Alcian blue staining becomes negative

There is no medical treatment for macular dystrophy of the cornea. It seems possible that enzyme therapy at an early stage might be of value since the deposits of keratan sulfate are sensitive to the catabolic enzymes present in normal keratocytes. It might nevertheless happen that these enzymes, acting over a prolonged period of time, could also change the normal glycosaminoglycan structure of the stroma.

In conclusion, macular dystrophy of the cornea is an inborn error of glycosaminoglycan (mucopolysaccharide) metabolism. The disease, localized to the cornea, is the result of a deficiency of β-glucuronidase. It is autosomal recessive as are most of the known inborn errors of metabolism.

II. CHROMOSOMAL HEREDITY

1. Retinoblastoma

Retinoblastoma can be both hereditary and sporadic or non-hereditary. It is hereditary in approximately 40% of the cases. The mode of inheritance is autosomal dominant and sometimes irregular with incomplete penetrance which, nonetheless, ranges between about 75 and 95%. The tumor can be unilateral as well as bilateral. Bilateral cases are always hereditary, while only 10 to 15% of the unilateral cases are inherited.

Recently, two hypotheses have been put forward, both of which suggested that fundamentally there is no etiological difference between hereditary and non-hereditary retinoblastoma: 1) the premutation or "delayed" mutation theory (Herrman, 1976); 2) the multiphase mutation theory (Knudson, 1971).

a. Premutation theory. This model postulates a 2-phase mutation acting on a specific locus. By a process called premutation, the normal allele is changed into an unstable form which, in turn, can change into a completely mutated allele by a second mutation (telomutation). The phenotype caused by the premutated allele is still normal. The premutated allele is hereditary, and both the premutation and the telomutation can take place during meiotic (germinal mutation) or mitotic (somatic mutation) cell division.

Sporadic unilateral retinoblastoma cases are generally the result of exclusive mitotic mutation and thus non-hereditary. The cases of hereditary retinoblastoma are caused either by an exclusive meiotic mutation or by a meiotic premutation followed by a mitotic telomutation.

b. Multiple mutation theory. This model postulates that all retinoblastomas, hereditary as well as non-hereditary, are also caused by at least two mutations, both of which are necessary to transform a normal retinal cell into a tumor cell. After the first mutation, the cell is not yet carcinogenic. In the hereditary cases, the first step is already present prezygotically, while the following mutation would occur in a somatic retinal cell. In the non-hereditary cases, the two mutations take place in the same somatic retinal cell and the retinoblastoma is unilateral. This explains why, in the hereditary cases, the affected persons may develop tumors in either one or both eyes and why, too, the hereditary retinoblastomas appear at an earlier age.

All new germinal mutations are hereditary. The resulting retinoblastomas are unilateral in one-third of the cases and bilateral in two-thirds of the cases. The bilateral retinoblastomas (one-third of all the cases as a whole), are always hereditary. According to Knudson, the first mutation occurs during gametogenesis and is present in the fertilizing gamete. This mutation will be present postzygotically in all the somatic cells, but the tumor growth only starts after a somatic mutational event has taken place in one of the "initiated" retinal cells. If this second mutational event does not take place, the person remains an unaffected carrier who can, nevertheless, transmit the mutation to his offspring.

Both models are based on a 2-phase mutation process, but they differ in clinical prognosis. The premutational model implies that the bearer of the completely mutated gene will always develop retinoblastoma, while in the second model, a somatic mutation is always necessary for retinoblastoma to develop.

c. Deletion of the long arm of chromosome 13. Recent karyotyping with banding techniques, which have been in existence for only about 10 years, and particularly high resolution trypsin-Giemsa banding of prometaphase chromosomes, have led to a veritable revolution in the study of chromosome genetics. Thus, in more than 35 cases of retinoblastoma, which were bilateral for the great majority and among which was a personal case, a deletion of the long arm of chromosome 13 was revealed (Fig. 16). When applying the banding

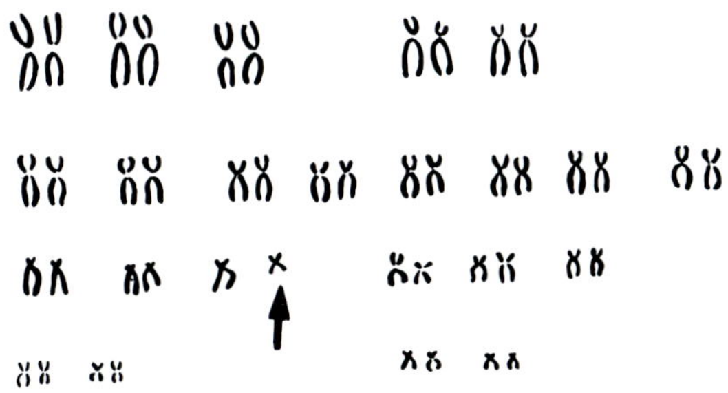

Figure 16. Retinoblastoma. Deletion of the long arms of chromosome 13 (personal observation)

technique, an interstitial deletion of 13q14 was always found.

Several of these retinoblastoma patients with a small deletion manifested only minimal somatic deviations and only mild mental retardation, and some (about 50%) even manifested no congenital anomalies. The possibility exists, therefore, that very small deletions of chromosome 13 are present in more retinoblastoma patients, deletions that cannot or only with great difficulty be identified even with modern banding techniques because they are too small or are limited to a single locus. Thus, it is not ruled out that one of the mutations necessary for the development of a retinoblastoma is a minimal chromosomal deletion, all the more so because even in the presence of an apparently normal peripheral karyotype (blood cells), the tumor cell line may show a 13 deletion (Murphree, 1978). It is worth noting that there is an esterase deficiency in the lymphocytes of retinoblastoma patients when there is a deletion, visible or invisible, of chromosome 13 (Murphree et al, 1980; Sparkes et al, 1980). The esterase D gene is localized on band 14 of the long arm of chromosome 13, near or at the site of the retinoblastoma gene. In the case of retinoblastoma, the activity, which is normally 60-75 Units is reduced by 50% (30-35 Units). In the case of trisomy 13 the amount is increased to 150%. When there is a deletion above or below 13q14, but not involving 13q14, the amount is normal (100%).

On the other hand, none of the patients with deletion of the short arm of a D-chromosome had retinoblastoma. In at least 10 cases of deletion of chromosome 13 without involving the 13q14 band, no retinoblastomas were found. This 13q deletion syndrome without retinoblastoma is characterized by mental retardation, facial abnormalities, malformation of the fingers, anal atresia, genital anomalies, and congenital heart disease.

What role the deletion plays in the development of the retinoblastoma is not yet clear. It is possible that the removal of a normal allele might facilitate the expression of a mutated gene on the intact homologue. It is, nevertheless, difficult to reconcile this suggestion with the dominant mode of inheritance of bilateral retinoblastoma. Possibly, too, the loss of 13q14 gives rise to faulty development and differentiation of the retina, which predisposes the retinal cell to uncontrolled growth. This may happen after a second mutational event.

2. Aniridia-Nephroblastoma Syndrome

The frequency of aniridia in the general population is 1/50,000 to 1/100,000. Two-thirds of the cases are manifestly due to a dominant autosomal gene with high penetrance and expressivity. The frequency of nephroblastoma or Wilms' tumor in the general population is only 1/250,000 in subjects 15 years of age or younger. Wilms' tumor is hereditary in 40% of the cases, and follows an autosomal dominant mode of inheritance. The familial cases are characterized by precocious development before the age of 3 years and by a high percentage of bilateral cases (21%). The sporadic tumors develop later, between the ages of 4 and 6 years.

Aniridia and nephroblastoma are sometimes associated in the same infant. This is the "aniridia-Wilms' tumor" syndrome and, apparently, it is not hereditary. Currently, there are more than 60 known cases, 2 of them being personal ones. This syndrome is characterized essentially by: (1) sporadic congenital aniridia, and (2) nephroblastoma that develops early in life, usually before the age of 2 or 3.

In 75% of the cases, the syndrome is accompanied by other anomalies (Fig. 17): pronounced mental retardation, genito-urinary abnormalities (e.g. hypospadias or cryptorchidism in boys*) and cranio-facial dysmorphism characterized by a long and narrow face, a flat boxer's nose, poorly lobed and low-set ears, ptosis of the upper eyelids, narrow palpebral fissures, and sometimes microcephaly.

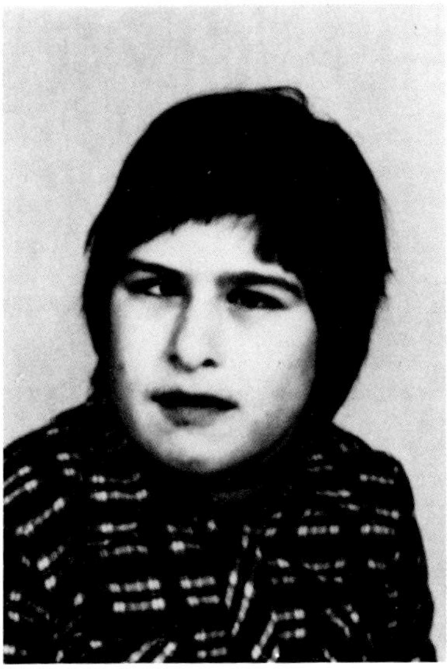

Fig. 17. Aniridia-Wilms' tumor syndrome (personal observation)

The syndrome is genetic, but before we can decide whether it is mendelian or chromosomal, certain facts must be considered. Until now, all the cases of aniridia-nephroblastoma syndrome have been sporadic. Miller (1966) and Di George (1965) found 8 cases of aniridia among 469 cases of Wilms' tumor, i.e. 1:58 or 1.72%. On the other hand, Fraumeni and Glass)1969) found 7 Wilms' tumors among 28 cases of sporadic aniridia, i.e., in 25% of the cases. From these studies, one can conclude that a nephroblastoma develops in about a third of the cases of sporadic aniridia. This means that the incidence of nephroblastoma is higher in cases of sporadic

* The association of aniridia, genito-urinary anomalies, and mental retardation is designated by the term "ARG triad".

aniridia than in the general population, the difference being highly significant.

The Wilms' tumor is bilateral in more than 20% of the cases when it is associated with aniridia, but it is generally unilateral when it is not. Monozygotic twins are not always concordant. Three cases are known. Both had aniridia, but only one had a Wilms' tumor (Juberg et al, 1975; Cotlier et al, 1978; Maurer et al, 1979). There is no sex predominance in the aniridia-nephroblastoma syndrome. In this syndrome, the Wilms' tumor develops before the age of 3 years. In some cases of aniridia-Wilms' tumor, the karyotype is normal, while in others it is not. Applying chromosome band analysis in prophase, there is an interstitial deletion of the short arm of chromosome 11 (band 13) (del 11p13) in some cases of the aniridia-Wilms' tumor syndrome. Until now, this chromosomal anomaly has been observed in more than 10 cases, so that one may conclude that a deletion of band 13 of chromosome 11 is always associated with aniridia (Fig.18).

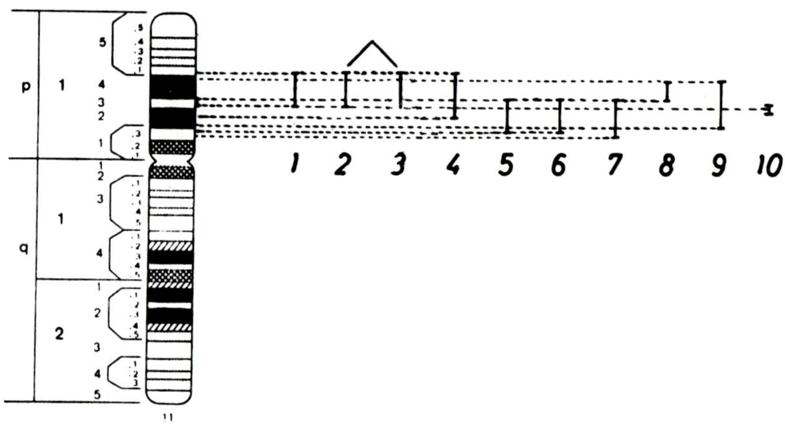

Figure 18. Interstitial deletions of 11 p. Cases 1, 4, 5 (Francke et al, 1977; Riccardi et al, 1978), cases 2 and 3 (identical twins) (Cotlier et al, 1978; Francke et al, 1978; Maurer et al, 1979), case 6 (Andersen et al, 1978), case 7 (Hittner et al, 1979), case 8 (Francke et al, 1979), case 9 (personal observation I) and case 10 (personal observation II)

In one of our cases an interstitial deletion involving bands 11p14 to 11p12 of the short arms of one of the chromosomes no. 11 was found in every cell (Fig. 19). In our

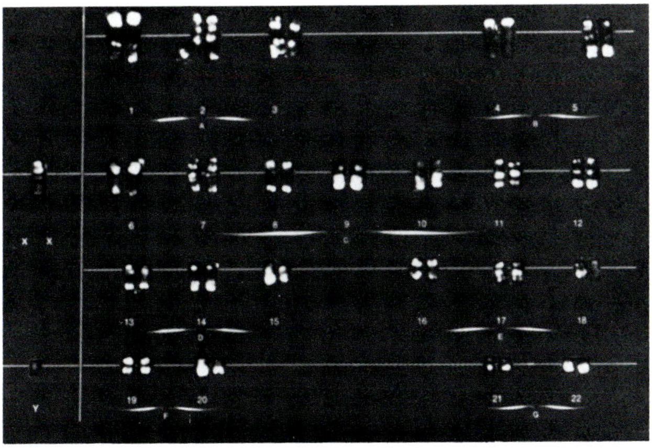

Figure 19. Deletion of bands 11p14 to 11p12 of the short arms of one of the chromosomes no. 11 in a case of aniridia-Wilms' tumor syndrome (personal observation)

second case, which was published in 1977, the karyotype seemed to be normal at first. But recently, applying high resolution trypsin-Giemsa banding of prophase chromosomes, we were able to demonstrate an interstitial deletion involving exclusively band 11p13 of the short arm of one of the chromosomes no. 11 (Fig. 20). This is the first time that a deletion of only one band has been demonstrated.

These observations support the view that the genes for aniridia and the Wilms' tumor are very near to one another on the short arm of chromosome 11, so that the deletion of this segment and more particularly of band 13 explains the association of the two anomalies. One may wonder if all the cases of aniridia-nephroblastoma syndrome are not due to a deletion. The cases in which this is not found can be accounted for if the deletion is too small to be visualized cytogenetically. The problem is precisely the same for retinoblastoma.

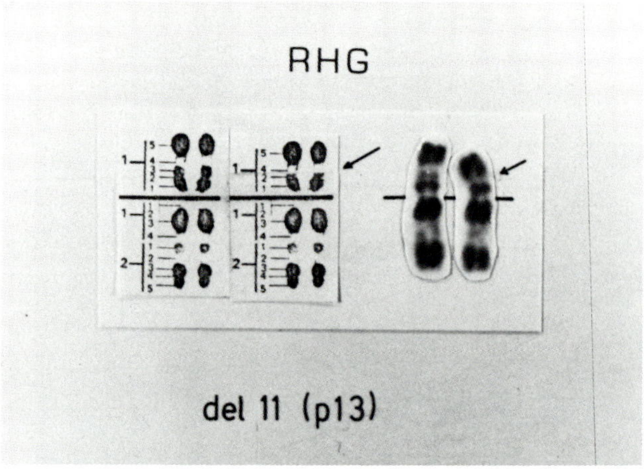

Figure 20. Deletion of band 11p13 of the short arms of one of the chromosomes no.11 in a case of aniridia-Wilms' tumor syndrome (personal observation)

According to Knudson (1971), a nephroblastoma, like a retinoblastoma, can only develop after two successive mutations. The first stage, which can be either a classic gene mutation or a chromosomal aberration by deletion, for example, would be the initiating stage that predisposes the cells to the action of a second mutational event that actually sets in motion the active proliferation of the cells. While the second event, which is probably an external factor, is the same for a hereditary or non-hereditary tumor, the first event takes place during gametogenesis for genetic tumors, and this germinal mutation will be present in the fertilizing gamete. In the case of nephroblastoma, this mutation is the cause of a defect in the development of the metanephrotic blastoma, which remains undifferentiated and will be present postzygotically in all the somatic cells. The tumor growth will not begin until after a somatic mutational event has occurred in one of the "initiated" renal cells. This mutation in two stages is the most plausible explanation for the Wilms' tumor and for retinoblastoma and it also explains the frequent discordance in monozygotic twins.

It should also be pointed out that there are other syndromes associated with aniridia, some of which manifest a deletion of the short arm of chromosome 11. In addition, the deletions that differ in dimension or localization can produce different phenotypes such as the AGR triad without a Wilms' tumor, the AGR triad with a Wilms' tumor, a Wilms' tumor without the AGR triad, or aniridia without a Wilms' tumor.

1. The "AGR triad" is characterized by the association of aniridia, genito-urinary anomalies or ambiguous genital organs, and mental retardation, but without a Wilms' tumor. At least 10 cases are known where the syndrome is accompanied by an interstitial deletion of the short arm of chromosome 11 and always of band 13.

2. There is a syndrome with aniridia, bilateral gonadoblastoma, and mental retardation, but without a Wilms' tumor. At least 6 cases are known, of which 2 had a deletion of band 13 of the short arm of chromosome 11 as in the "aniridia-Wilms' tumor" syndrome.

3. A syndrome characterized by aniridia, cerebellar ataxia, and mental retardation. We observed two sisters affected by this syndrome. Another affected sibship and a sporadic case are known. The karyotype is normal. The heredity is probably autosomal recessive.

4. As I have said, there are examples of aniridia with a deletion of band 13 of the short arm of chromosome 11 but without a Wilms' tumor. Among others, three pairs of monozygotic twins are known of which only one member had a nephroblastoma.

5. Francke and coworkers (1977) have observed a patient who presented an interstitial deletion of bands 11 and 12 of the short arm of chromosome 11. This patient had a lactose dehydrogenase A deficiency, facial anomalies, and some minor malformations, but no aniridia.

These observations show that aniridia is not always a simple, isolated malformation, but that it can be a part of several syndromes, can depend on a chromosomal aberration, and can have different etiologies. Apart from the syndromes I have mentioned, aniridia may sometimes be observed in Marfan's syndrome and in the Smith-Lemli-Opitz syndrome.

These are only but a few examples demonstrating the importance of genetics in ophthalmology, as much for the study of ocular diseases, of which more than half are hereditary, as for the diagnosis of systemic diseases. The importance is illustrated just as well by mendelian as by chromosomal heredity. While chromosomal aberrations generally produce generalized malformations, they can also produce isolated anomalies, such as retinoblastoma or the "aniridia-Wilms' tumor" syndrome

REFERENCES

Blum JD (1945). Relations entre les degenerescences heredofamiliales et les opacites congenitales de la corneee. Etude clinique et genealogique. Ophthalmologica, Basel, 109:123

Cotlier E, Rose M and Moel SA (1978). Aniridia, cataracts and Wilms' tumor in monozygous twins. Amer J Ophthal 86:129

Denden A (1963). Zur Frage der Dystrophia corneae verticillata, Typ Fleischer-Gruber. Ber dt Ophthal Ges 65:125

Denden A (1966). Ueber Erblichkeit der Dystrophia corneae verticillata. Graefes Arch klin exp Ophthal 169:264

Di george AM (1965). In Miller et al. Excessive concurrence of Wilms' tumor with aniridia, hemi-hypertrophy and anomalies. Amer J Dis Child 109:459

Fleischer B (1910). Ueber eine eigenartige, bisher nicht bekannte Hornhauttrubung (ein Hinweis auf die normale Struktur der Hornhaut?). Graefes Arch Ophthal 77:136

Francke U, George DL, Brown MG and Riccardi VM (1977). Gene dose effect. Intraband mapping of the LDHA locus using cells from four individuals with different interstitial deletions of 11 p. Cytogenet Cell Genet 19:197

Francois J (1966). Fleischer's vortex corneal dystrophy. Heredofamilial corneal dystrophies. Trans Ophthal Soc UK 86:367

Francois J and Victoria-Troncoso V (1980). The cornea in normal condition and in Groenouw's macular dystrophy. Ed. Dr. W. Junk, The Hague

Fraumeni JF and Glass AG (1969). Wilms' tumor and congenital aniridia. Amer J Cancer 19:289

Gruber M (1946). Cornea verticillata. Ophthalmologica, Basel, 111:120

Herrmann J (1976). Delayed mutation as a cause of retinoblastoma. Application to genetic counseling. Birth Def Orig Art Ser 121:79

Juberg RC, Martin EC and Hundley JL (1975). Familial occurrence of Wilms' tumor. Nephroblastoma in one of monozygous twins and in another sibling. Amer J Hum Genet 27:155

Knudson AG (1971). Mutation and cancer. Statistical study of retinoblastoma. Proc Nat Acad Sci, Washington, 68:820

Lutz A (1930). Ueber wirbelformige Trubung beider Hornhaute bei Mutter und Tochter (ein Beitrag zur Lehre von der normalen Saftestromung in der Kornea). Graefes Arch Ophthal 123:704

Maurer HS, Pendergrass TW, Borges W and Honig GR (1979). The role of genetic factors in the etiology of Wilms' tumor. Two pairs of monozygous twins with congenital abnormalities (aniridia, hemihypertrophy) and discordance for Wilms' tumor. Cancer, Philadelphia, 43:205

Miller RW (1966). Relation between cancer and congenital defects in man. New Engl J Med 275:87

Murphree L (1978). Personal communication

Murphree L, Sparkes RS and Benedict W (1980). Communication to the American Genetic Club of Ophthalmology, Chicago.

Murphree AL, Sparkes RS, Lingua RW and Benedict WF (1981). Importance of the esterase D locus in retinoblastoma. Intern Symp Genet Ophthal, Jerusalem (in press)

Opitz JM, Stiles FC, Wise D, Race RR, Sanger R, Gemmingen GR, Von Kierland RR, Crosse EG and De Groot WP (1965). The genetics of angiokeratoma corporis diffusum (Fabry's disease) and its linkage relations with the Xg locus. Amer J Hum Genet 17:325

Sparkes RS, Miller H, Klisak I and Abraham JA (1979). Retinoblastoma with 13q-chromosomal deletion associated with maternal paracentric inversion of 13q. Science 203:1027

Franceschetti Award

Professor E. Cotlier

Yale University

New Haven, Connecticut

Professor Adolphe Franceschetti was born in 1896 and died in 1968. He was Professor of Ophthalmology, Director of the Ophthalmological Clinic at the University of Geneva and one of the towering figures of XX century ophthalmology and human genetics. Professor Franceschetti, throughout his long and productive scientific career, was interested in all aspects of heredity. He wrote 454 papers including 85 on human and ophthalmological genetics. His studies included inborn errors of metabolism, malformation syndromes, connective tissue anomalies, chromosomal genetics and craniofacial abnormalities. Many such studies are classics in the field, such as those on mandibulo facial dysostosis. In ocular genetics Professor Franceschetti devoted a great deal of time to the tapeto retinal degenerations and was instrumental in the recognition of fundus flavimaculatus and its variations. He classified the hereditary corneal dystrophies as no one before him had done and thus allowed practicing ophthalmologists to recognize it and patients to receive proper genetic counseling. His studies included inheritance of retinoblastoma, of glaucoma, of disc anomalies, of color blindness, of phakomatoses, of myopia. His works represent a real treasury of intellectual and scientific curiosity by a most remarkable human being. Upon his death in 1968, his long time friend and collaborator, Professor Francois, wrote in Professor Franceschetti's obituary:

"Who could help being captivated by a personality as attractive as Franceschetti's? All who knew him were

Birth Defects: Original Article Series, Volume 18, Number 6, pages 27–28

impressed by his immense knowledge and vast erudition, but also, and perhaps even more, fascinated by the youthful vigor of his mind, his enthusiasm, his joviality, and what we may call his simplicity; in fact, we ask ourselves which we admired the more - his achievements as a scientist or his humanity. This master of genetics and ophthalmology would not have been so great had he not been so humane."

Professor Franceschetti organized the Institute of Medical Genetics attached to the Eye Clinic in Geneva and was the founder and editor of the Journal de Genetique Humaine. He served with distinction as president of the permanent committee of the International Congress of Human Genetics and as president of the International Association for the Prevention of Blindness. To honor his memory, the International Society for Genetic Eye Diseases together with the Foundation Franceschetti established, a lecture and award is to be presented by an outstanding scientist or physician. The Selection Committee is pleased to announce Dr. Mette Warburg of Copenhagen, Denmark as the 1st Franceschetti Lecturer.

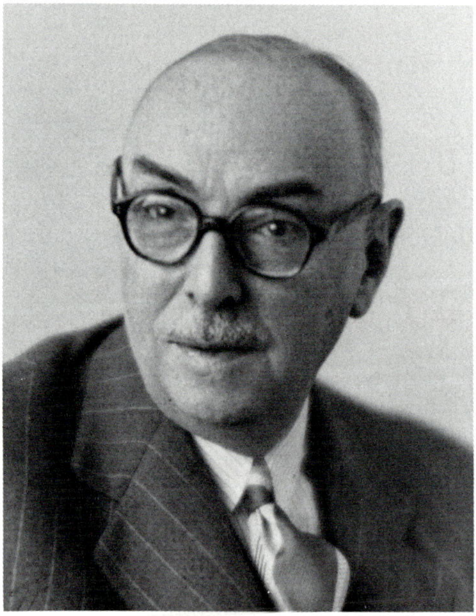

PRESENTATION OF THE FRANCESCHETTI AWARD TO DR. WARBURG

Albert T. Franceschetti, M.D.

Unité de Diagnostic et d'Urgence ophtalmologiques,
Hôpital de la Tour, 1-3, J.-D. Maillard,
1217 Meyrin, Geneva (Switzerland)

Ladies and Gentlemen,

Last year I was here for the inauguration of the Luigi Gedda Institute of Gemellology, on the Mount of Olives. Luigi Gedda was a close friend of my father and is a close friend of mine. It is a pleasure to be back in Jerusalem for another important event, in this city of peace. I come from Geneva, another city of peace, where I hope this group will convene in the future.

While Gedda was able to continue his activity, Professor Franceschetti died in 1968 of an aneurysm. I do remember that his last letter, written with a shaky hand, was for a geneticist to whom he had promised something.

I was very pleased when Ed wrote to me asking how I would feel about a Franceschetti award. Of course, I said yes. The International Society for Genetic Eye Diseases seemed to me the right authority for such an award. On the other hand, my father had been one of the first geneticists between the two wars.

In this connection, I would like to mention that in the classical german text-book of ophthalmology (Schieck and Brückner), the chapter on genetics was written by the young Oberarzt Franceschetti. This was certainly an honour and the beginning of a life-long passion for this science.

Birth Defects: Original Article Series, Volume 18, Number 6, pages 29–30

Mette Warburg, I first met you in Baltimore in 1969. It was the 29th of May, at the second Conference on the Clinical Delineation of Birth Defects. At this meeting, were also present Herman Burian, my former Chief at Iowa, Ed Maumenee, Jules François, David Klein, and many others.

I well remember that your presentation on Norrie's disease, dear Mette, opened with the picture of a rose : a charming introduction for such a terrible disease.

I believe, Mette, that you rightly deserve this award. In the first place, you have always shown a remarkable scientific activity in the field of ophthalmological genetics. This has been well illustrated by Professor Michaelson.

Secondly, this is the year of the disabled. You have devoted your activity to mentally handicapped persons, and I feel this should be acknowledged. As a member of the Swiss National Committee for the Mentally Handicapped, I am particularly happy that you have been chosen to receive this award.

Thirdly, since 1969 I have met you in various occasions, mainly in connection with the European Paediatric Ophthalmology group. It is a pleasure for me to give this award to a friend.

Ladies and Gentlemen, I would like to present the 1981 Franceschetti award to Mette Warburg on behalf of the Franceschetti Foundation in Geneva. The members of the Board and myself are pleased to honour both the late Professor Franceschetti and Doctor Mette Warburg.

DIAGNOSTIC PRECISION IN MICROPHTHALMOS AND COLOBOMA OF HETEROGENEOUS ORIGIN

Mette Warburg, M.D.

Gentofte Hospital: Eye Clinic for the Multiply Handicapped
Sognevej 40, DK-2820 Gentofte, Denmark

ABSTRACT

Heterogeneity of microphthalmos and coloboma is considerable and the clinical morphology is insufficient for etiological classification. A nosological classification has been performed in 86 cases of microphthalmos and coloboma occurring in mentally retarded individuals. Although nearly all were sporadic cases, a precise diagnosis could be established in 45 per cent of the cases. In 13 per cent, the phenotypes could not be assigned to any similar malformation syndrome described in the literature, and in 42 per cent the precision of the classification was low although the malformations had been repeatedly described before. An unknown number of the last-mentioned cases may have been environmentally induced, but little is known of environmentally induced ocular malformations and how to diagnose them after the first year of life.

INTRODUCTION

It is a great honor to have been chosen to give the first Franceschetti Memorial Lecture, an honor which would not be given to me unless I had such wonderful people working with me. Professor Franceschetti was interested in genetics from his early years, and already in 1930 he had written the section on heredity in Kurzes Handbuch der Ophthalmologie. This section greatly influenced the teaching and practice of ophthalmology in Europe. His original contributions comprised descriptions of immense numbers of rare dis-

Birth Defects: Original Article Series, Volume 18, Number 6, pages 31–50

eases, many of them new. His name is eponymically associated with the mandibulo-facial dysostosis. He was also a hard-working surgeon and was one of the first in Europe to perform corneal grafts. When he left his chair he had performed so many of these operations that he was able to classify all of the corneal dystrophies known at the time.

Emphasis on genetics was new paradigm in ophthalmology, and although there were other eminent geneticists in ophthalmology at his time, the firm establishment of the paradigm was mainly due to Franceschetti's charismatic personality, his diplomacy and perseverance. He established the Institute of Medical Genetics in Geneva and was instrumental in creating the first chair in medical genetics in Switzerland under Professor David Klein, his coworker for many years.

It was not only in Switzerland that Franceschetti spread the message of genetics in ophthalmology. He was a great traveller and missed few international meetings; he was always a dominating figure due to his knowledge, wisdom and common sense. At the social gatherings, his charm, humor and proverbial vitality - also at the dances - always made him the center of attraction. Franceschetti's publications had a lasting effect on research and development in ophthalmology, but this tribute to his memory would be incomplete if his humanitarian attitude was not stressed. This he proved not only in his relationship to his patients but also to his colleagues many of whom found refuge in Geneva during World War II.

In the 1970's the central interest of clinical genetic research was the delineation of heterogeneous entities. This problem was brought into focus by McKusick's presentation "On Lumpers and Splitters" in 1969 at the First Conference on the Clinical Delineation of Birth Defects, sponsored by The National Foundation.

A great number of identical phenotypes with dissimilar etiologies have been described since then, most of the information having appeared in casuistic reports. I shall here discuss the ophthalmological benefit of such insight, and in order to make the issue clear, shall concentrate on microphthalmos and coloboma. I shall begin by giving details of the application of present knowledge on a series of 86 patients with microphthalmos and coloboma, discuss the precision of nosological identification of the cases, and finally emphasize the class of cases with poor diagnostic precision because they present the problems for the 1980's.

The morphology of microphthalmos has been classified (Francois 1958, Duke-Elder 1964) into

1. Pure microphthalmos or nanophthalmos
2. Colobomatous microphthalmos
3. Complicated microphthalmos

However this classification tells us little about the etiology. Thus, the pedigree (Fig. 1) of an inbred Bedouin family shows that the same recessive trait may result in anophthalmos, microphthalmos, coloboma and congenital cystic eye.

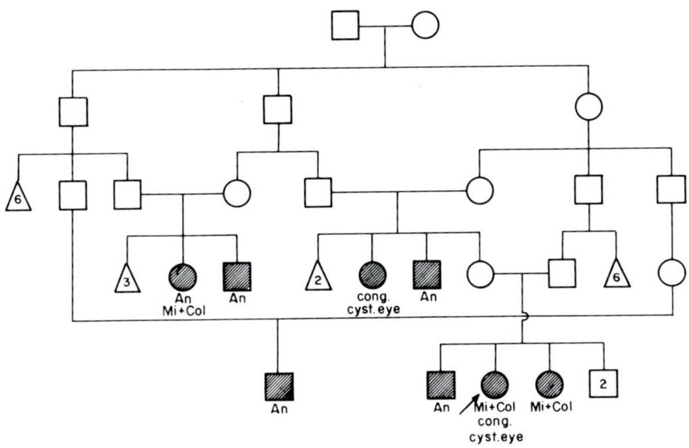

Fig. 1. This figure demonstrates the pleiotrophic expression of the autosomal recessive anophthalmos-microphthalmos-coloboma trait (After Mabrouk et al 1969/69).

Microphthalmos and coloboma may be due to a variety of genetic and environmental causes. The genetic causes are chromosomal or mendelian.

CAUSES OF MICROPHTHALMOS AND COLOBOMA

Genetic Causes

Chromosomal aberrations described with microphthalmos or coloboma are triploidies, trisomies of chromosomes 9, 13 and 18, partial trisomies of a great number of autosomes and various deletions and rings. The vast majority of the aberrations are trisomies of no. 13.

Mendelian Traits

I have found descriptions of 45 mendelian traits with microphthalmos in the literature. All modes of inheritance are represented, and there are at least 25 traits with coloboma, some of them identical to those leading to microphthalmos (Warburg 1981, Pagon 1981).

Prenatally acquired malformations with microphthalmos or coloboma have also been described. Rubella, toxoplasmosis and cytomegalic virus disease are well-known. Recently prenatal herpes infection has been added to the list (Webster and Smith 1977; von Herzen and Benirschke 1976) and varicella has been incriminated (Charles et al 1977). Microphthalmos and coloboma have also been described in cases where the fetus had been exposed to alcohol (van Biervliet 1977), LSD (Chan et al 1978) or trimethadione (Goldman and Yaffe 1978). We also have information of cases with an abnormal physical intra-uterine environment such as hyperthermia (Smith et al 1978) or amniotic bands (Higginbottom et al 1979). Manifest intra-uterine abnormalities have been produced by amniocentesis, and there is a single example of perforation of a fetal eye during this procedure (Merin and Beyth 1980).

MATERIAL

It was my problem to determine whether the available information on heterogeneity in microphthalmos and coloboma was of clinical value because the nosological entities described appeared to be so rare that cases to which the descriptions could be applied might be very few.

I had established a National register of 993 mentally retarded patients with visual impairment. Among these cases

86 had microphthalmos or coloboma, 59 were personally examined and the rest were seen by other ophthalmologists. All the patients had been repeatedly examined by pediatricians or internists. Of the cases, 78 were sporadic. Chromosomal examinations were done in 55 cases.

The disorders observed could be etiologically subdivided into six classes, i.e. prenatal infections, chromosomal aberrations, identified syndromes, private syndromes, provisionally identified syndromes and unidentified associations.

NOSOLOGICAL IDENTIFICATION

Prenatal Infections

Six patients had elevated titres for toxoplasmosis in infancy and two had chorioretinal scars in their microphthalmic eyes. Mothers of seven patients had identified rubella infections during the first trimester. In one case, microphthalmos, hearing defects and congenital cataract suggested that rubella might have been the etiology; the parents and siblings were normal.

Chromosomal Anomalies

Two patients had a deletion of the short arm of chromosome 4 (Wolf-Hirschhorn syndrome); one patient, with a female phenotype and gonadal dysgenesis, had a 46,XY karyotype; another woman had a de novo translocation between chromosomes 10 and 16, and a male patient had a mosaicism in which some cells carried a supernumerary chromosome 9. A female patient had a de novo duplication of the short arms of chromosome 8. Inversion of chromosome 9 (one case) was considered irrelevant for the ophthalmological malformations.

Identified Syndromes

In 14 cases it was possible to identify the syndrome with others previously described in the literature. The cases are presented in Table 1. Eleven of these were sporadic. In one case, the parents of a retarded man with microphthalmos without systemic anomalies, were consanguineous; thus he presumably had autosomal recessive microphthalmos.

TABLE 1. IDENTIFIED SYNDROMES

Case no.	Sex	Syndrome	Karyotype
260658	M	Aut. rec. mi. Consanguinity	
*201078	M	Cerebro-oculo-facio-skeletal syn. Consanguinity	46,XY
*081031	F	Focal dermal hypoplasia syn.	46,XX
*140869	F	Focal dermal hypoplasia syn.	46,XX
*280579	F	Focal dermal hypoplasia syn.	46,XX
*021170	M	Hydrocephaly and retinal non-attachment. Consanguinity	46,XY
*130664	M	Lowe syndrome	46,XY
*031273	M	Meckel syndrome	
*220845	F	Lacunar retinal depigmentation	
*061275	M	Lacunar retinal depigmentation, son of above	46,XY
*050377	M	Lacunar retinal depigmentation, brother of above	
*230474	F	Rieger anomaly	
190654	M	Goldenhar syndrome	46,XY
*211273	M	Mi., symblepharon and oblique facial cleft	46,XY

*Personally examined

Consanguinity was also present between the parents of a patient with the COFS syndrome and parents of a child with hydrocephaly and retinal non-attachment (Warburg 1978). Two brothers and their mother had lacunar retinal depigmentations (Fig. 2, next page), an autosomal dominant syndrome recently described (Alzial et al 1980). Altogether 12 patients had recognizable genetic syndromes, a young man had the Goldenhar syndrome which is probably not genetic in origin, and a small boy had an oblique facial cleft which is thought to be due to amniotic bands (Higginbottom et al 1979). Chromosomal examinations were performed in 9 cases and all were found to be normal.

Private Syndromes

Private genetic syndromes are those which have not been described in the literature, thus it is unknown whether or not a mutation has occurred in other patients. In this

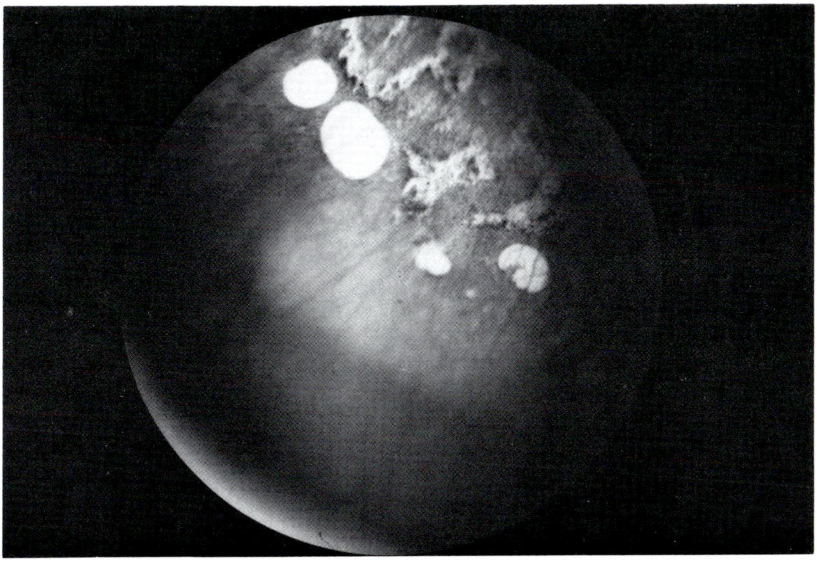

Fig. 2. Autosomal dominant lacunar retinal depigmentation syndrome. Fundus of case no. 061275, Table 1.

series I found a mother and one of her two sons having slight microcephaly, subnormal intelligence, microphthalmos and falciform folds of the retina. Microcephaly, microphthalmos and falciform folds have previously only been described as an autosomal recessive trait (Warburg 1979). The material also comprised a girl with retinal cystic lesions and microphthalmos, whose mother had had a large number of abortions (Plum et al 1978).

Provisionally Identified Syndromes

Provisionally identified syndromes are sporadic cases with phenotypes which resemble known genetic syndromes, or syndromes with a known environmental etiology. In spite of the resemblance, it was impossible in 36 cases to prove whether the etiology was identical with previously described cases. This class is presented in Table 2.

TABLE 2. PROVISIONALLY IDENTIFIED SYNDROMES

Case no.	Sex	Malformations	Karyotype
120931	F	Mi.	
*020562	M	Mi.	46,XY
*310312	M	Mi., col.	46,XY,q^+
060630	F	Mi., col., cat.	
*271054	M	Mi., col.	46,XY
*090567	F	Mi., col.	46,XX
221039	F	Col.	46,XX
261251	F	Col.	46,XX,$14s^+$
291251	F	Col.	46,XX
*300761	F	Col.	46,XX
*271164	M	Col.	46,XY
*220268	M	Col.	46,XY
070960	F	Col., polydactyl, cl., pal., malf. of the heart	46,XX
*280663	F	Col., ectopia of the lens, polydactyly, malf. of the heart	46,XX
*151169	F	Col. polysyndactyly, vestibular anus, VSD, pulm. hypertension	46,XX
310545	F	Mi., clinodactyly, malf. of the heart	46,XX
*270858	F	Col. of the optic nerve, VSD, atresia of bicuspid	46,XX
*061268	F	Mi., col., ectopia of the lens, PHPV, VSD	46,XX
*021177	M	Col., oesoph.-trach. fistula, malf. of central vessels	46,XY,inv9
190552	M	Col., Eisenmenger S., persistent foramen ovale, epilepsy	46,XY
*170780	M	Col., malformation of central vessels	46,XY
*260756	M	Mi., col., cl. lip & pal., VSD	46,XY
*311261	F	Col., Mi., syndactyly	46,XX
220153	F	Mi., col., cong. cat., cl. pal., hearing loss	46,XX
*020254	M	An., mi., microcephaly, choanal atresia	46,XY
*270866	M	Microcornea, microcephaly and falciform folds	
120720	M	Mi., cat.	

*Personally examined.

TABLE 2. (ctn.)

Case no.	Sex	Malformations	Karyotype
*310355	M	Mi., cat., optic atrophy	
*281149	M	Mi., cong. cat., normal teeth and fingers; mother subnormal with exc. myopia	46,XY
*180221	F	Microcornea; ectopia of the lens; col. of the optic nerve	46,XX
*230950	F	Mi., ectopia of the lens	46,XX
171032	M	Mi., cerebral palsy	
220634	F	Mi., col., spastic palsy	46,XX
*061142	F	Microcornea, spastic palsy	
310763	F	Col., spastic palsy, cortial cerebral atrophy	
*011268	F	Mi., col., cerebral palsy, cerebral atrophy	46,XX

*Personally examined.

Abbreviations: cat. cataract; cl. cleft; col. coloboma; cong. congenital; malf. malformation; mi. microphthalmos; oesop.-trach. oesophageal-tracheal; pal. palate; PHPV persistent hyperplastic primary vitreous; umbil. umbilical; VSD ventricular septal defect.

The first group comprised 13 patients with microphthalmos or coloboma without other congenital malformations. Ten of them had chromosomal examinations, all of which were normal. A majority of these patients probably have the autosomal recessive anophthalmos-microphthalmos-coloboma syndrome, which is often associated with mental retardation. However, the same phenotypes are also present in the autosomal dominant anophthalmos-microphthalmos-coloboma syndrome (Warburg 1981). Moreover the results of an adverse fetal environment cannot be excluded.

Microphthalmos and coloboma were associated with congenital malformations of the heart and central vessels in 10 patients, classifiable into two groups, i.e. one with malformations of the fingers and one without (Fig. 3). Thus four patients with microphthalmos or coloboma and congenital

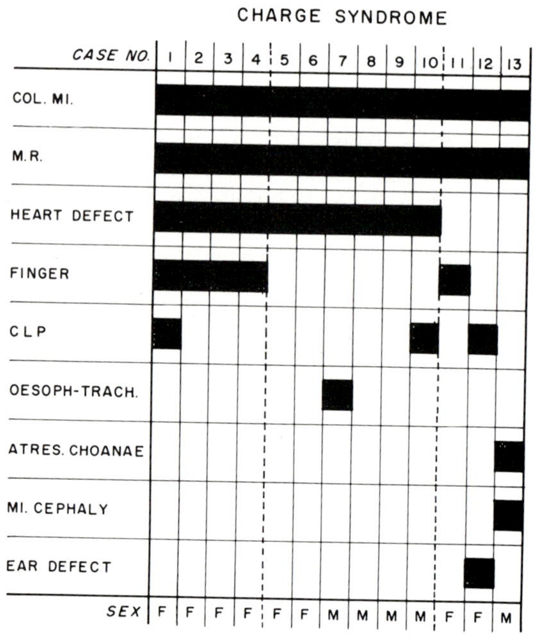

Fig. 3. Survey of 13 patients with microphthalmos, coloboma, mental retardation, heart malformations and additional congenital anomalies.

cardiac malformations had polydactyly and six had microphthalmos, coloboma and cardiac malformations without malformations of the fingers. Among the latter a male had an esophago-tracheal fistula (Lillquist et al 1980), and another had cleft lip-palate. Three patients had similar but not identical phenotypes, i.e. a girl with colobomatous microphthalmos and syndactyly without cardiac malformations, a young woman with coloboma, microphthalmos, cleft palate and hearing loss, and a young man with anophthalmos, microphthalmos, microcephaly and choanal atresia.

For each of these 13 patients, a similarly affected person can be found in the literature. Recently these patients have been described as having a non-random association of malformations (Ho et al 1975) which may be identified if the patients have a number of the malformations surveyed in Table 3. Pagon (1981) found indications of both autosomal

TABLE 3. CHARGE SYNDROME (PAGON 1981)

C oloboma-microphthalmos	CNS malformations
H eart malformations	Facial palsy
A tresia of the choanae	Cleft lip-palate
R etardation (mental, growth)	Micrognatia
G enital malformations	
E ar malformations, hearing loss	

Ho et al 1975, Hall 1979, Hittner et al 1979

dominant and recessive inheritance among 24 patients. The pattern of malformations obviously depends upon the ascertainment of the cases. Thus Hall (1979) described 17 patients with choanal atresia in whom coloboma was present in nine, and cardiac defects in 12. Hittner et at (1979) examined 10 patients with colobomatous microphthalmos, cardiac malformations, hearing loss and mental retardation. Of these, six had VIIth nerve paralysis. Transmission from a mother to her daughter was observed. It is unknown to what extent the malformations may be due to intrauterine environmental factors.

Among the provisionally identified syndromes, microcephaly, microphthalmos and falciform folds were observed in a boy with borderline mental retardation, and was clinically identical to the syndrome described by Gartner (1941) and Masuda (1962).

Microphthalmos and congenital cataract have been described both as autosomal dominant, autosomal recessive and X-linked traits, but in the two males from this series it was impossible to assess whether the malformations were prenatally acquired or genetic.

Microphthalmos, coloboma and ectopia of the lens were observed in two patients of the present series. This association was noted in two out of 128 patients with microphthalmos studied by Sjögren and Larsson (1949), in a member of a family with microphthalmos and in a sporadic case observed among 776 blind children by Fraser and Friedman (1967, H1,M35).

Five patients had microcornea, microphthalmos or coloboma and spastic palsy; all were sporadic, and birth history was not remarkable. This association was described by Sjögren and Larsson (1949) in 5 patients out of 58 with microphthalmos and mental retardation. The etiology is unknown.

Unidentified Syndromes

While it was possible to find cases in the literature comparable to the aforementioned patients, there were 11 patients who presented phenotypes previously apparently undescribed. These cases are summarized in Table 4.

TABLE 4. UNIDENTIFIED SYNDROMES

Case no.	Sex	Malformations	Karyotype
030414	F	Mi., microcephaly	46,XX
060635	M	Col., microcephaly	46,XY
160641	M	Mi., microcephaly, equinovarus, umbil. hernia, malf. of ears	
*291152	F	Mi., col., microcephaly	46,XX
*030854	M	Mi., col., microcephaly	
*090864	M	Col., optic atrophy, microcephaly	
021134	F	Col., optic atrophy, hydrocephaly	
090742	F	Mi., col., cong. cat., hydrocephaly	46,XX
*111163	M	Col., very low arylsulfatase	46,XY
300377	F	Mi., preauricular appendages	46,XX
210873	F	Col., double renal collecting system, umbil. hernia, hypoplastic alae of the nose	46,XX22s+

*Personally examined.

Six patients had microphthalmos or coloboma and microcephaly; major systemic malformations were absent. The karyotype was examined and found to be normal in three. It is unknown if genetic or environmental factors were causative in these cases. There were two patients with hydrocephaly and colobomata, one of whom had congenital cataract. The etiology was unknown. A presumably fortuitous association of very low arylsulfatase and coloboma was demonstrated in a young man whose parents had normal enzymatic activities. Preauricular appendages were noted in a girl with microphthalmos without other systemic malformations. A female had coloboma, a double collecting system of the kidneys, umbilical hernia, hypoplastic alae of the nose and a normal karyotype.

RESULTS

Diagnostic Precision

The results of the nosological delineation among the 86 patients with microphthalmos and coloboma are shown in Table 5; it appears that 19 per cent had prenatally acquired infections, seven per cent had chromosomal aberrations. In 16 per cent a syndrome with a fairly well understood etiology was present and three per cent had private genetic syndromes. Thus in 45 per cent the diagnostic precision was optimal.

TABLE 5. DIAGNOSTIC PRECISION IN THE PRESENT SERIES OF MICROPHTHALMOS AND COLOBOMAS

Diagnosis	No.	%
Infections	16	19
Chromosomal aberrations	6	7
Identified syndromes	14	16
Private syndromes	3	3
Provisionally identified	36	42
Unidentified associations	11	13
Total	86	100

In 36 sporadic cases (42 per cent), the malformations had been previously described, but since the sporadic cases were unclassifiable, the diagnostic precision was low.

In 13 per cent (11 cases) classification of the association of malformations observed was purely morphological.

DISCUSSION

The results of the present study show that 87 per cent of the patients surveyed had syndromes previously described, thus the malformation syndromes are not as rare as one might think. Is the delineation of heterogeneous malformations with microphthalmos and coloboma also of clinical value? If we assume that it is of clinical value to establish an etiological diagnosis, genetic or environmental as the case may be, valuable information has been obtained in 45 per cent of the cases.

Microphthalmos and Coloboma

Ophthalmology is well known for the precision with which morphological aberrations can be detected with noninvasive methods. Unfortunately correlations between morphology and nosology are rare in this specialty and there are only four reports in the ophthalmological literature with which the present study can be directly compared.

Sjögren and Larsson (1949) examined the records of 137 patients with microphthalmos and found three affected sibships, three families with X-linked inheritance (Norrie disease), four families with an autosomal dominant transmission and four patients whose parents were consanguineous. Prenatal rubella and toxoplasmosis could not be identified with certainty at the time of examination, and there was little knowledge of the heterogeneity of microphthalmos. Yet, Sjögren and Larsson suggested that microphthalmos, mental retardation and spastic palsy which they observed in five of 58 mentally retarded persons constituted a specific syndrome. Thus in 137 patients the mode of heredity was established in 30 (22%) and a provisional diagnosis was presented in five per cent.

Zeiter (1963) described four patients with autosomal dominant cataract and microphthalmos and gave a restrospective description of 44 microphthalmic patients from an outpatient clinic. Two had toxoplasmosis, two showed chorioretinitis and two patients were sisters. An etiological diagnosis was thus established in 9 out of 48 cases (19%).

Scouras, Catti and Cuendet (1970) gave a restrospective account of 70 patients with microphthalmos from an out-patient clinic. A chromosomal count was done in 17, and an etiological diagnosis was identified in 15 cases (21%).

Bleeker-Wagemakers (1981) studied 353 mentally retarded patients from a Dutch institution for the blind. There were 50 individuals with microphthalmos and coloboma among the patients, and the etiology was established in 78 per cent of them (Table 6).

TABLE 6. DIAGNOSTIC PRECISION IN 50 CASES OF MICROPHTHALMOS AND COLOBOMA. ADAPTED FROM BLEEKER-WAGEMAKERS (1981)

Diagnosis	No.	%
Toxoplasmosis	5	48
Rubella, prenatal	19	
Autosomal dominant	4	30
Autosomal recessive	9	
Goldenhar	1	
Hallerman-Streiff	1	
Provisional genetic	11	22
Total	50	100

In the present series 45 per cent of the patients had a precise etiology diagnosis. The publications of rare diseases and the interest in nosology which has been prevalent over the last 10 years thus has increased diagnostic precision considerably among patients with microphthalmos and/or coloboma.

Multiple Congenital Anomalies/Mental Retardation Syndrome

The diagnostic precision in the present series can also be compared with results from nosological studies among other patients with multiple congenital anomalies/mental retardation syndromes.

Diagnostic evaluations among severely mentally retarded individuals were first done on a large scale by Penrose (1938), and recent data have been presented by Opitz et al (1977), Laxova et al (1977), Gustavson et al (1977) and Bleeker-Wagemakers (1981). To be comparable with the present study, I have extracted from these reports data concerning disorders with a prenatal etiology, but without established metabolic disorders, since Opitz et al (1978) found that no metabolic defects were found among the malformation syndromes.

I have further deleted patients with Down's syndrome, since these were not represented in the present series. The results are shown in Table 7. Opitz, Laxova and Gustavson examined mentally retarded patients with a variety of additional malformations, Bleeker ascertained all her patients from a single institution for blind retarded individuals, and my cases derive from a National registration of visually impaired people who are mentally retarded. Opitz et al established an etiological diagnosis in 54 per cent, Laxova et al in 28 per cent, Gustavson et al in 51 per cent, Bleeker-Wagemakers in 78 per cent and in the present series it was 45 per cent.

TABLE 7. DIAGNOSTIC PRECISION AMONG PATIENTS WITH PRENATALLY INDICED MALFORMATIONS.
Adapted from 1. Bleeker-Wagemakers 1981; 2. Opitz et al 1978; 3. Laxova et al 1977; 4. Gustavson et al 1977.
Prenatally induced malformations and deformations have been extracted from the materials; cases with Down's syndrome and heritable metabolic disorders have also been deleted from the original data.

Etiology	Present series		1		2		3		4	
	No	%	No	%	No	%	No	%	No	%
Prenatal infections	16	19	39	20	47	13	1	1	12	27
Chromosomal excl. Down	6	7	8	4	54	15	1	1	5	11
Identified S.	14	16	102	52	77	22	13	15	6	13
Private S.	3	3	4	2	12	3	9	11		
Provisionally identified S.	36	42	26	13			9	11		
Unidentified S.	11	13	18	9	160	46	52	61	22	49
Total	86		197		350		85		45	

The diagnostic precision in the materials by Opitz et al, Laxova et al and Gustavson et al and the precision obtained in the present series are thus comparable. Bleeker-Wagemakers had greater precision in her material; moreover, provisionally identified syndromes were few among her patients.

The reason for this is probably that her patients were all living in the same place, she could get 5-generation pedigrees and thereby detect consanguinity, and finally she could perform clinical examinations of relatives when required.

It is interesting to note that syndromes previously undescribed were rare among the visually impaired patients, while among the cases ascertained among all types of mentally retarded individuals such cases were found in about one half of the total. This demonstrates the prevalent tradition of descriptive morphology in ophthalmology.

FUTURE RESEARCH

Nosological identification of genetic malformations of the eye has been carried far in the 1970's and is still in progress. Improved tissue culture techniques will add to the list of new chromosomal and metabolic lesions. Cell hybridization and copy DNA synthesis will allow us to follow a mutation within the generations of a family without having to understand the translational product or the pathologic biological metabolite.

Over the last years, emphasis on intra-uterine environmental lesions has increased, but in ophthalmology the study of prenatal environmental disorders has only just begun, although some phenocopies have been known for years. The present findings underline the importance of this aspect in future research.

For truly sporadic cases, however, it is still very difficult to differentiate between genetic and acquired conditions because our knowledge of the prenatally acquired lesions and the methods of diagnosing them after the first year of life is very limited. Improved understanding of prenatal environmental causes of ocular malformations, I believe, will be a central issue for the next ten years.

REFERENCES

Alzial C, Dufier JL, Aicardi J, de Grouchy J and Saraux H (1980). Ocular abnormalities of true microcephaly. Ophthalmologica 180:333-339.

Bleeker-Wagemakers EM (1981). On the causes of blindness in the mentally retarded. Bartimeus Foundation Ser. The Netherlands

Chan CC, Fishman M and Egbert PR (1978). Multiple ocular anomalies associated with maternal LSD ingestion. Arch Ophthal 96:282-284.

Charles NC, Bennett TW and Margolis S (1977). Ocular pathology of the congenital varicella syndrome. Arch Ophthal 95:2034-2037.

Duke-Elder, Sir S (1964). System of Ophthalmology. Vol. III. Kimpton London, p 488-494.

Francois J. L'Hérédité en Ophthalmologie. Masson et Cie, Paris, 1958, p 190.

Fraser GR and Friedman AI (1967). The Causes of Blindness in Childhood. The Johns Hopkins Press Baltimore.

Gartner S (1941). Congenital retinal folds and microcephaly. Arch Ophthal 25:93-100.

Goldman AS and Yaffe SJ (1978). Fetal trimethadione syndrome. Teratology 17:103-106.

Gustavson K-H, Hagberg B, Hagberg G and Sars K (1977). Severe mental retardation in a Swedish county II. Etiologic and pathogenetic aspects of children born 1959-1970. Neuropädiatrie 8:293-304.

Hall BD (1979). Choanal atresia and associated multiple anomalies. J Pediat 95:395-398.

Higginbottom MC, Jones KL, Hall BD and Smith DW (1979). The amniotic band disrupting complex: Timing of amniotic rupture and variable spectra of consequent defects. J Pediatr 95:544-549

Hittner HM, Hirsch NJ, Kreh GM and Rudolph AJ (1979). Colobomatous microphthalmos, heart disease, hearing loss, and mental retardation: - A syndrome. J Pediatr Ophthalm 16: 122-128.

Ho CK, Kaufman RL and Podos SM (1975). Ocular colobomata, cardiac defect and other anomalies: a study of seven cases including two sibs. J Med Genet 12:289-293.

Laxova R, Ridler MAC and Bowen-Bravery M (1977). An etiological survey of the severely retarded Hertfordshire children who were born between January 1, 1965 and December 31, 1967. Amer J Med Gen 1:75-86.

Lillquist K, Warburg M, Andersen SR and Hägerstrand I (1980). Colobomata of the iris, ciliary body and choroid in an infant with oesophago-tracheal fistula and congenital heart defects. An unknown malformation complex. Acta Paediatr Scand 69:427-430.

Mabrouk R, Chadli A, Djedidi H and Cheikh T-B (1968/1969). A propos de 4 cas de kyste orbito palpébral colobomateux. Bull Mém Soc Fr Ophtal 81:173-194.

Masuda Y (1962). Two cases of ablatio flaciformis congenita and two other cases of ocular congenital anomalies, which appeared in a pedigree with consanguineous marriages. J Clin Ophthalm, Tokyo 16:325.

McKusick VA (1969). On lumpers and splitters, or the nosology of genetic disease. Birth Def:Orig Art Ser 5/1:23-32.

Merin S and Beyth Y (1980). Uniocular congenital blindness as a complication of midtrimester amniocentesis. Am J Ophthal 89:299-301.

Opitz JM, Kaveggia EG, Durkin-Stamm MV and Pendleton E (1978). Diagnostic/genetic studies in severe mental retardation. Birth Def:Orig Art Ser 14/6B:1-38.

Pagon RA (1981). Ocular coloboma. Surv Ophthal 25:223-236.

Penrose LS (1938). A clinical and genetic study of 1280 cases of mental defect. London MRC Spec Rep Ser No 229, HMSO.

Plum CM, Warburg M and Danielsen J (1978). Defective maturation of granulocytes, retinal cysts and multiple skeletal malformations in a mentally retarded girl. Acta Haematologica 59:53-63

Scouras J, Catti A and Cuendet J-F (1970). Les microphtalmies congénitales. Ann Oculist, Paris, 203:953-970.

Sjögren T and Larsson T (1949). Microphthalmos and anophthalmos with and without coincident oligophrenia. Munksgaard Cph.

Smith DW, Clarren SK and Harvey MAS (1978). Hyperthermia as a possible teratogenic agent. J Pediatr 92:878-883.

Van Biervliet JP (1977). The foetal alcohol syndrome. Acta Paediatr Belg 30:113-116.

Von Herzen JL and Benirschke K (1976). Unexpected disseminated herpes simplex infection in a newborn. Obstet & Gynec 50:728-730.

Warburg M (1978). Hydrocephaly, congenital retinal non-attachment and congenital falciform fold. Amer J Ophthal 85:88-94.

Warburg M (1979). Retinal malformations: Aetiological heterogeneity and morphological similarity in congenital retinal non-attachment and falciform folds. Trans Ophthalm Soc U K 99/2:272-283.

Warburg M (1981). The heterogeneity of microphthalmos. Int Ophthal 4:45-65.

Webster MH and Smith CS (1977). Congenital abnormalities and maternal herpes zoster. Brit Med J ii 1193.
Zeiter HJ (1963). Congenital microphthalmos. A pedigree of four affected siblings and an additional report of forty-four sporadic cases. Am J Ophthal 55:910-922.

Retinal Pigment Epithelium and Experimental Retinal Degeneration

HUMAN RETINAL PIGMENT EPITHELIUM IN VITRO: ORGANIZATION, ULTRASTRUCTURE, AND BIOCHEMISTRY

M. T. Flood, P. Gouras, J. E. Haley and W. S. Blaner

College of Physicians & Surgeons, Columbia University

630 West 168 Street, New York, N.Y. 10032 U.S.A.

The functional and metabolic relationship between the retinal pigment epithelium (RPE) and photoreceptors (Bairati and Orzalesi, 1963; Young and Bok, 1970) and the many abnormalities of the retinal pigment epithelium found in various disease states of the eye have focused attention on the importance of this cell layer in the normal visual process. The post mortem viability of RPE cells from human donor eyes together with advances in tissue culture techniques have opened new avenues in studying these cells. Human RPE cells obtained from donor eyes up to 60 hours post mortem can be maintained in primary cultures and subcultured. Detailed reports on the monolayer organization of these cells in cultures, the in vitro growth patterns, and the ultrastructural characteristics of individual RPE cells in vitro have been published (Flood et al 1980, 1981). The present paper describes some aspects of Vitamin A metabolism and specific protein patterns that have been observed in these cells in vivo and in vitro. Studying aspects of Vitamin A metabolism suspected to be unique to the RPE and identifying specific protein patterns of RPE cells may serve to distinguish human RPE cells from other types and play a significant role in recognizing possible biochemical aberrations in RPE cells from donors with genetic diseases of the retina.

MATERIALS AND METHODS

Cell Cultures. Post mortem eyes, ranging in chronological age from 6 to 100 years, were received from the New York Eye Bank for Sight Restoration after the corneas were removed for corneal transplants. The cells were obtained by trypsin-dissociation and primary cultures were established and maintained according to methods pre-

Birth Defects: Original Article Series, Volume 18, Number 6, pages 53–66

viously described (Flood et al. 1980). Cells removed from post mortem eyes by trypsin-dissociation and not plated out are referred to as fresh cells. In vitro age was calculated as post mortem time plus time in culture. Subculturing was done when the primary cultures became confluent, generally 21 to 30 days after the primary culture was established. A solution of 0.05% trypsin and Versene (1:1000) in a 4:1 mixture was added to the petri dishes for 5 minutes at 37°C to release the cells. The cell suspension was split approximately 3:1 and cultures were plated out at 1.5-2.0x10^5 cells/ml. Experiments on the subcultures were done on the seventh to tenth day when the subcultures were confluent.

Vitamin A Studies. To determine the Vitamin A content of freshly isolated and cultured human RPE cells, the Vitamin A was extracted from the cells with hexane after saponification, concentrated under nitrogen, and separated chromatographically on an alumina column as described by Harrison et al (1979). Each fraction was assayed fluorometrically according to the method of Thompson and his colleagues (1971) with the modification of Muto et al (1972). Additional RPE cell cultures were supplemented with all-trans retinol (Hoffman-LaRoche) for 9 to 24 hours. Retinol, in concentrations of 0.1 to 50 μg/ml, was added to MEM which contained 500 μg/ml fatty acid free bovine serum albumen as the retinol carrier. In these studies the fetal calf serum was removed from the incubation medium before retinol was added. After the desired incubation time, the cultures were thoroughly washed with Hank's balanced salt solution, Ca^{++} and Mg^{++} free, and removed from the culture surface by mild trypsinization. Vitamin A content per cell in retinol-supplemented cultures was determined as described above. Retinyl palmitate hydrolase enzyme activity was assayed at pH 8.0 according to the method of Prystowsky et al (1981). The same procedure was used for the pH 5.0 assay; in this assay 50 mM Na Acetate (pH 5.0) containing 5% (w/v) fatty acid free bovine serum albumin was used as the buffer. The synthesis of retinyl-^{14}C-palmitate, which is used in the enzyme assay and not available commercially, has been published (Prystowsky et al 1981). The assay used to study esterification has been described by Berman et al 1980. High pressure liquid chromotography (HPLC) was used to analyze the complex mixtures of retinyl esters, aldehydes, and alcohols in freshly-isolated and cultured human RPE cells and to identify the fatty acid moiety of the retinyl esters synthesized in retinol-supplemented cultures. The HPLC analyses was carried out by C. David Bridges and his associates according to published methodology (Alvarez et al 1981).

2-Dimensional Protein Electrophoresis. For two-dimensional gel electrophoresis, 10^6 cells (approximately 1 mg protein) were partially delipidated with ether/ethanol to remove the residual salts. The cell pellet was dried under a stream of nitrogen and evaporated.. The dried residue was then solubilized by sonication in 2% buffered SDS and prepared for isoelectric focusing according to the method of Ames and Nikaiko (1976). Two-dimensional gel electrophoresis was performed as described by O'Farrell et al (1977). The gels were stained with Coomasie blue to visualize the protein patterns. To study protein synthesis, two-dimensional electrophoresis was performed on radioactively labeled cultures. In these studies, confluent primary and subcultures were washed with 2 ml of methionine-free Eagle's MEM (Flow Laboratories) containing 20% fetal calf serum. The medium was removed and replaced with fresh medium (2 ml) to which 40 µCi ^{35}S-l-methionine (NEN, 935.7 Ci/mM) was added. After 6 hours incubation the cells were washed with phosphate buffered saline (PBS), pH 7.4, and removed from the culture surface with a rubber policeman. The cells were centrifuged, washed again with PBS and processed for gel electrophoresis as described above. The dried slab gels containing 1×10^5 cpm of ^{35}S total protein radioactivity were exposed for 16 days to kodak no-screen film (NS-2T) for autoradiography.

RESULTS

Over 90% of the human RPE cells plated out adhered to the culture surface and remained viable. In some cultures the cells went into division and gave rise to confluent cultures; in others, the cells remained stationary, that is, there was no evidence of cell division. Figure 1 summarizes much of the information we have obtained from human RPE cells in vitro. The data show that approximately 28% of the cultures plated out remained stationary. The stationary cultures were primarily from donors over 50 years of age. All cultures established from donors less than 50 years of age went into division with the exception of those cultures that were plated out at cell concentration levels that approximated confluency. In over 80% of the cultures that went into division the onset of division occurred between day 7 and day 27. If the cultures were analyzed with respect to the chronological age of the donor, almost 60% of the cultures established from donors less than 50 years of age went into division between days 7 and 13; for the cultures established from donors over 50 years of age, the onset of division occurred between days 14 and

27 for 55% of the cultures. If the division did not occur by day 30, the cultures usually remained stationary.

In studying the in vitro growth properties of the retinal pigment epithelium we used two media; Eagle's minimum essential medium and Ham's F-10 medium both of which were supplemented with fetal calf serum and glucose. The onset of division occurred earlier in the cultures established from donors greater than 50 years of age that were maintained in Ham's F-10; the culture medium had no apparent effect on the onset of division in cultures established from donors less than 50 years of age. However, the cells maintained in MEM, regardless of donor age, were more epithelial-like in morphology.

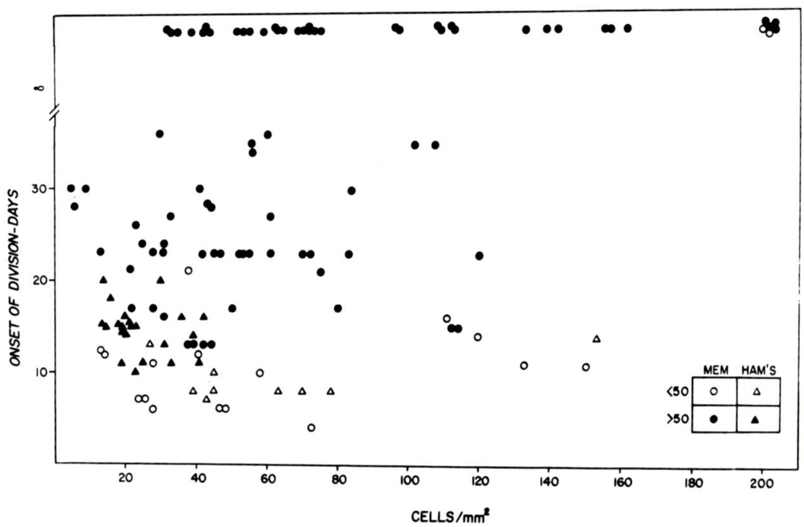

Fig. 1: Onset of division for human RPE cells cultured in MEM and Ham's F-10 medium.

The concentration of cells initially plated out had an interesting effect on the proliferative capacity of the RPE cell population. Initial attachment concentrations up to 140 cells/mm^2 did not interfere with the onset of division. If the cultures were plated out at concentrations approximating confluency, cell division was not evident. In high plating concentrations, the cells established a hexagonal monolayer similar to the pigment epithelial layer in vivo. Cells have been maintained as hexagonal monolayers for as long as 7 months without any evidence of cell division.

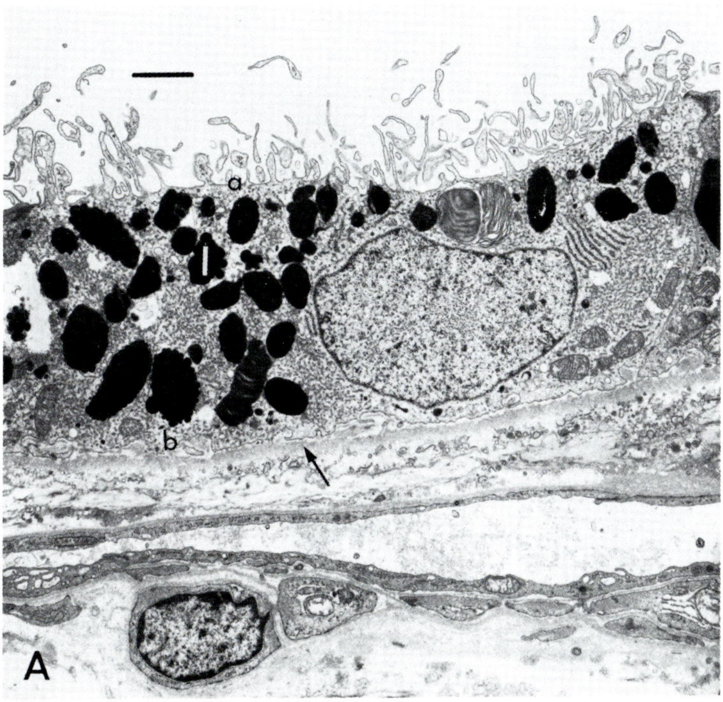

Fig. 2A - see legend on next page

Electron microscopy demonstrated that the human RPE cells in vitro maintain many of their in vivo characteristics (Fig. 2). Confluent primary cultures consisted of a monolayer of polarized cells. The apical surface had a number of slender cytoplasmic projections similar to the apical surface of RPE in vivo. Endocytotic vesicles were seen in various stages of formation and cytoplasmic transport and may also influence the movement of lipofuscin granules. The basal surface of the cells had thicker, more convoluted processes which make only occasional contact with the surface of the culture plate. Although varying amounts of electron dense extracellular material was observed there was no evidence of basal lamina formation. The usual cell

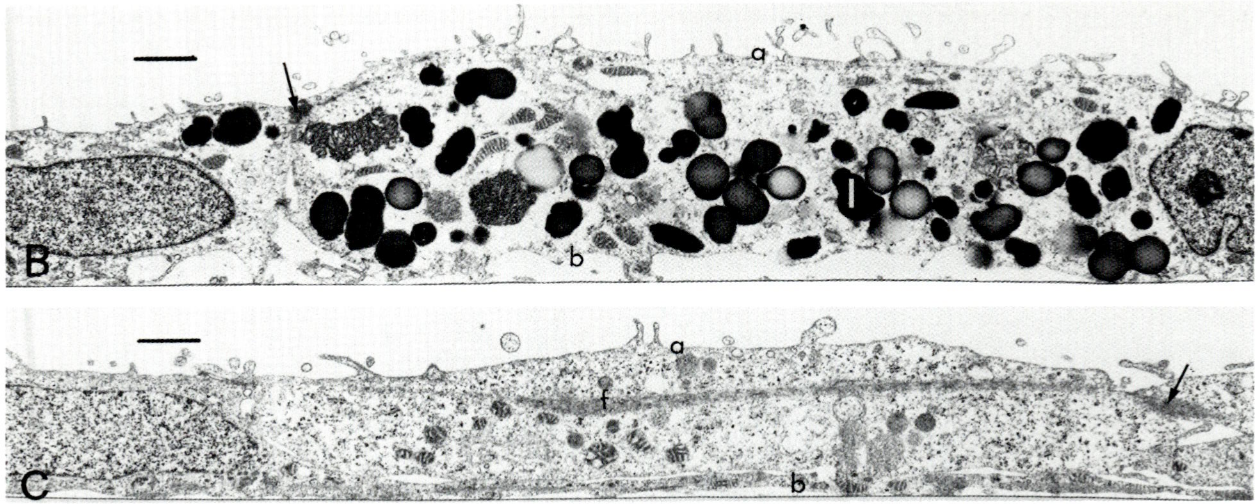

Fig. 2A: Electron micrograph of human RPE cell in post mortem donor eye. Note microvilli projections on apical surface (a), the infoldings of the basal surface (b), the lipofuscin granules (l), and Bruch's membrane (↑).

Fig. 2B: Electron micrograph of human RPE cell in primary culture. Note the apical (a) basal (b) surfaces, the lipofuscin granules (l) and the junctional complex (↑).

Fig. 2C: Electron micrograph of human RPE cell in subculture. Note apical (a) and basal (b) surfaces, the accumulation of filamentous material (f) and the junctional complex (↑).

* The bar represents 1μ.

organelles and ultrastructural features characteristic of epithelial cells – such as junctional complexes and tonofilaments converging on the junctions – were present. Varying amounts of melanin, lipofuscin, and melanolipofuscin granules were seen in the cytoplasm of these cells; occasionally, collections of these granules were found clustered together. The fusiform melanin granules were rare and cells undergoing active division had few, if any, melanin or melanolipofuscin granules.

Subcultured cells also retained the characteristic ultrastructural organization of RPE cells in vivo. In Figure 2C note the apical-basal polarity, the apical cytoplasmic projections, and the dense infoldings of the basal surface. The junctional complexes so prevalent in the cells of the primary culture are still well defined in these later subcultures. The cells, however, are practically devoid of pigmentation, have little endoplasmic reticulum, and have increased amounts of a filamentous material.

The data on total Vitamin A content in the human RPE cells is illustrated in Figure 3. The cells used in the Vitamin A determinations were obtained from 24 pairs of donor eyes that ranged from 14 to 79 years in chronological age. The Vitamin A content per cell for those cell populations obtained from donors with no known liver disease (closed circle data points) and which were analyzed in less than 4 days in vitro age generally ranged from 1–4 pg/cell. The freshest donor material used in this study was RPE cells from a 55 year old donor analyzed at 9 hours post mortem time. The retinol content of this cell population was 4.2 pg/cell, the highest value we obtained. The Vitamin A content in subcultured cells that ranged from 50–250 days in in vitro age was less than 0.02 pg/cell, 50 to 100 times less than the Vitamin A content in fresh cells and in cells in primary cultures.

The data was grouped into three categories according to the chronological age of the donor – less than 30, 30–50 and over 50 years of age – and Vitamin A content per cell was analyzed to identify trends (Table 1). It was interesting to note that while the individual values cover a broad range, an aging trend can be observed. As donor age increases, there is a tendency for the Vitamin A content per cell to increase. There is a 42% increase in the average Vitamin A content per cell in the cells obtained from donors over 50 years of age as compared with the cells obtained from donors less than 30 years old. However, the sampling size in the young group is small.

For 7 sets of cultures Vitamin A content per cell at an in vitro age of less than 4 days was compared with Vitamin A content per cell in the same cell population after approximately one week in culture (Table 2). In all cases Vitamin A content decreased with increasing in vitro age. At less than 4 days in vitro, the Vitamin A content in 7 cell populations studied averaged 2.12 pg/cell; 8-12 days later the Vitamin A level had fallen to an average of 0.34 pg/cell, an 84% decrease. The Vitamin A level in the subcultures is undetectable. Analyses of the fetal calf serum used to supplement the culture medium showed that it had a very low level of Vitamin A (0.13 μg/ml).

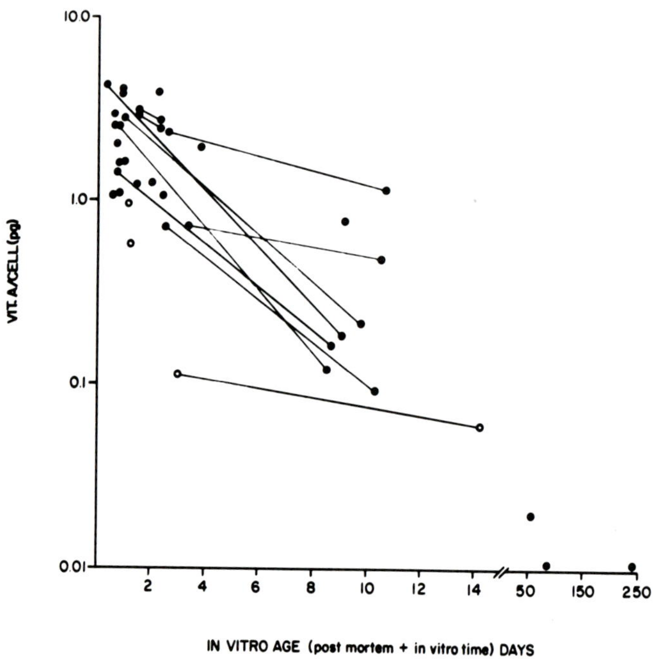

Fig. 3: Vitamin A content in human RPE cells with respect to in vitro age. Closed circles (●) represent cells from donors with no known liver disease; open circles (O) represent cells from donors with liver pathology. Data points connected by a line indicate cell populations from the same donor analyzed at different times in vitro.

DONOR AGE AND VITAMIN A CONTENT IN RETINAL EPITHELIAL CELLS

I

Donor Age (yrs.)	No. of Donors	Vit. A Content ± SEM (pg/cell)
< 30	2	1.31 ± 0.10
30-50	6	1.85 ± 0.45
> 50	12	2.29 ± 0.33

Retinyl palmitate hydrolase enzyme activity studied in fresh and subcultured cells is reported in Table 3. The only significant activity detected was in the fresh cells and this activity was maximum at pH 5.0. Preliminary studies on the esterifying enzyme activity in fresh RPE cells showed a significant level of activity at pH 8.0 (Fig. 4). The activity of the esterifying enzymes at pH 8.0 may mask the hydrolase activity at this pH. In these studies no exogenous palmitate or palmityl Co A were added for esterifying enzyme. High pressure liquid chromatography (HPLC) studies identified all-trans palmitate as the major ester in fresh cells. HPLC also confirmed the loss of Vitamin A derivatives in RPE cells with increasing in vitro age.

IN VITRO AGE AND VITAMIN A CONTENT IN RETINAL EPITHELIAL CELLS

II

In Vitro Age* (days)	No. of Cultures	Vit. A Content ± SEM (pg/cell)	Percent Decrease
< 4	7	2.12 ± 0.48	--
8-12	7	0.34 ± 0.14	84%
> 50	3 (subcultures)	0.01 ± 0.004	99%

*In Vitro Age = Post Mortem + In Vitro Time

Four sets of cultures from donors who ranged from 52 to 55 years of age were supplemented with varying concentrations of retinol from 0.1 to 50.0 μg/ml for 18 hours (Fig. 5). At retinol supplementation doses of 0.25-0.50 μg/ml the Vitamin A content/cell can be raised to the Vitamin A range observed in these cells at less than 4 days in vitro. At 2.5 μg/ml, the cells began to slough off the culture surface indicating that Vitamin A becomes toxic to these cells when presented in this concentration and in this manner. HPLC analyses of the retinol-supplemented cells (Table 4) showed that the cells in the primary cultures can take up all-trans retinol and synthesize it to palmitate, stearate, and oleate; palmitate ester is the major ester synthesized as in the in vivo situation. Subcultured cells also synthesize retinyl esters of palmitate, stearate, and oleate; however, the proportions of these esters differ from the original endogenous material. In subcultures, oleate is more prominant. The esters that were synthesized were all-trans; there was no evidence of cis-trans isomerization in the cultured RPE cells.

RETINYL PALMITATE HYDROLASE ACTIVITY *

Sample	Donor Age (yr)	In Vitro Age	RPH Activity nmol retinol/hr/mg protein
Fresh cells	22	16 hr	1.24
1st Subculture	65	84 days	0.50
1st Subculture	67	29 days	0.02
1st Subculture	65	40 days	0.03
2nd Subculture	65	35 days	0.03

III * 2 - 2 1/2 hr incubation 37°C, pH 5.0, 50 mM acetate, 5% BSA

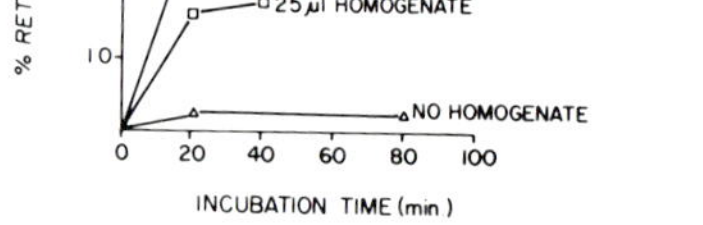

Fig. 4: Retinyl ester formation by homogenates of human RPE cells after removal by trypsinization from post mortem donor eye. The reaction was at 37°C and a retinol concentration of 50 µM. No exogenous palmitate or palmityl Co A were added.

The Coomasie blue-stained 2-dimensional polyacrylamide gels from fresh cells and cells from primary and subcultures showed approximately 25 major proteins common to all three cell populations (Fig. 6 a,b). Analyses of the gel patterns from the different cell populations demonstrated that there was a greater proportion of low molecular weight proteins (25 kDaltons) in fresh cells than in cultured cells. Primary and subcultures, on the other hand, had more acidic

PERCENT ESTERIFICATION IN RETINOL-SUPPLEMENTED CULTURES

Donor Age (yrs)	Culture	In Vitro Age (days)	Retinol Supplementation (hrs)	AT-Retinol Esters (nmol)	Percent Esterification		
					stearate	palmitate	oleate
48	Primary	11	--	--	--	--	--
48	Primary	11	18	0.73	38.2	47.7	13.7
71	Primary	11	--	--	--	--	--
71	Primary	11	24	0.32	36.3	45.0	18.1
30	Subculture	50	--	--	--	--	--
30	Subculture	50	9	0.30	29.6	39.7	25.0
30	Subculture	51	18	0.31	36.1	34.5	30.7
30	Subculture	51	24	0.33	33.0	38.2	29.1

Table 4

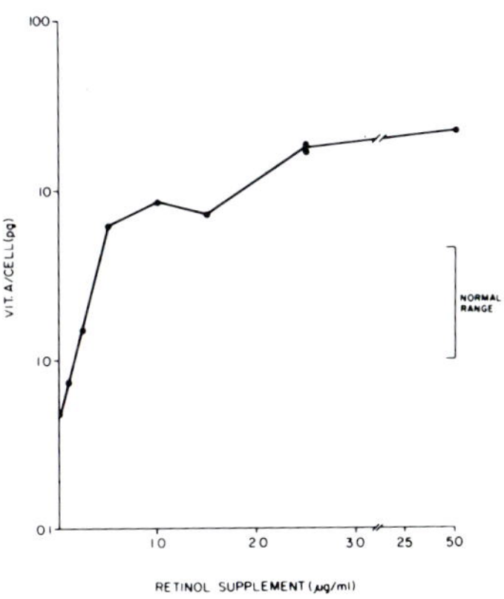

Fig. 5: Uptake at 37°C of all-trans retinal by human RPE cells in primary cultures.

proteins and showed a complex of several proteins with a molecular weight of about 43 kDaltons and isoelectric points of 5.6 to 5.9 characteristic of nonmuscle actin. The protein complex at 56 kDaltons appears to be tubulin. Autoradiographic studies with ^{35}S-l-methionine visualized about 60 major proteins and showed that the actin and tubulin-like materials were being actively synthesized. Identification of specific proteins is being pursued currently in our laboratory.

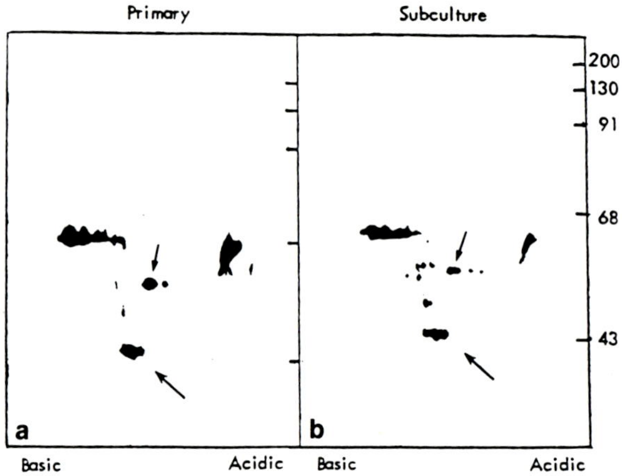

Fig. 6: Two-dimensional gel of human RPE cells in primary and subcultures. An actin-like protein has been identified at 43 kDal and a tubulin-like protein at 56 kDal (arrows).

DISCUSSION

Although human RPE cells from post mortem donor eyes retain much of their epithelial-like morphology, they do lose their pigmentation, one of their most identifying features, with continued cell division. In order to confirm the presence of a differentiated cell population in both primary and subcultures, we are trying to find specific identifying markers. The cell marker may be the retention of an RPE cell function as Vitamin A storage, transport, or metabolism or the presence of a particular protein pattern characteristic of RPE cells. While much of our data is preliminary and must be tested more extensively, certain important trends can be observed. First of all, Vitamin A enzyme systems and RPE cell protein patterns can be studied in RPE cells in vitro and compared to the in vivo situation. Secondly, contrary to the previous reports in the literature on human RPE (Maraini and Gozzeli, 1976) and bovine RPE (Chen and Heller, 1977),our studies showed that human RPE cells do take up retinol from the culture medium in the absence of retinol binding protein and metabolize it as was shown by the synthesis of retinal esters in retinol-supplemented primary and subcultures. Whether the residual Vitamin A binding protein present in bovine serum albumen is responsible for this difference must be considered. Although cis-trans isomerization, so crucial to the visual cycle, does not appear to occur in the cultured cells, this function appears to be absent also in RPE in vivo (Dowling, 1960; Daeman et al 1974). Our studies indicate that it is possible to do an enormous amount of experimentation on the RPE cell layer of the human retina through tissue culture techniques. However there are definite biochemical differences appearing in cultured human RPE cells that must be carefully controlled for comparison with mutant material.

REFERENCES

Alvarez R, Bridges CD, Fong S, (1981). High pressure liquid chromatography of fatty acid esters of retinol isomers. Invest Ophthal and Vis Sci 20:304.

Ames GF-L, Nikaido K, (1976). Two-dimensional gel electrophoresis of membrane proteins. Biochem 15:616.

Bairati A, Orzalesi N, (1963). The ultrastructure of the pigment epithelium of the photoreceptor - pigment epithelium junction in human retina. J Ultrastr Res 9:484.

Berman ER, Horowitz J, Segal N, Fisher S, Feeney-Burns L, (1980). Enzymatic esterification of vitamin A in the pigment epithelium of bovine retina. Biochim Biophys Acta 630:36.

Chen C, Heller J, (1977). Uptake of retinol and retinoic acid from serum retinol-binding protein by retinal pigment epithelial cells. J Biol Chem 252:5216.

Daemer FJM, Rotmans JP, Bonting SL, (1974). On the rhodopsin cycle. Exp Eye Res 18:97.

Dowling J, (1960). Chemistry of visual adaptation in the rat. Nature 188:114.

Flood MT, Gouras P, (1981). The organization of human retinal pigment epithelium in vitro. Vis Res 21:119.

Flood MT, Gouras P, Kjeldbye H, (1980). Growth characteristics and ultrastructure of human retinal pigment epithelium in vitro. Invest Ophthal and Vis Sci 19:1309.

Harrison EH, Smith JE, Goodman DS, (1979). Unusual properties of retinyl palmitate hydrolase activity in rat liver. J Lipid Res 20:760.

Maraini G, Gozzoli F, (1976). Normal interaction of plasma retinol binding protein from retinitis pigmentosa with bovine pigment epithelium. Invest Ophthal and Vis Sci 15:1020.

Muto Y, Smith JE, Milch PO, Goodman DS, (1972). Regulations of retinyl-binding protein metabolism by vitamin A status in the rat. J Biol Chem 247:2542.

O'Farrell P, (1975). High resolution two dimensional electrophorresis of proteins. J Biol Chem 250:4007.

Prystowsky JH, Smith JE, Goodman DS, (1981). Retinyl palmitate hydrolase activity in normal rat liver. J Biol Chem 256:4498.

Thompson JN, Erdody P, Brien R, Murray TK, (1971). Fluorometric determination of vitamin A in human blood and liver. Biochem Med 5:67.

Young R, Bok D, (1970). Autoradiographic studies on the metabolism of the retinal pigment epithelium. Invest Ophthal 9:524.

This research was supported by NIH Research Grant EY 03854 and a Center Grant from the National Retinitis Pigmentosa Foundation.

The authors thank Anne Leitch for secretarial services, Mary K. Bilek for assistance with the tissue culture studies and Hild Kjeldbye for assistance with the electron microscopy.

MORPHOLOGY, PHAGOCYTOSIS, AND VITAMIN A METABOLISM OF CULTURED HUMAN RETINAL PIGMENT EPITHELIUM

Dan-Ning Hu, M.D.
Monte A. Del Monte, M.D.
Sammy Liu, Ph.D.
Irene H. Maumenee, M.D.

The Johns Hopkins Hospital, Wilmer Institute
Baltimore, Maryland 21205

The retinal pigment epithelium (RPE) is one of the most important cell layers of the visual system, essential to the maintenance of normal retinal function. In recent years, at least five important RPE functions have been documented in experimental animals (Del Monte and Maumenee, 1980), including: 1. secretory and nutritive functions; 2. pigmentation, i.e. screening out stray light; 3. storage and possibly conversion of retinol to the biologically active 11-cis form, 4. phagocytosis of shedded photoreceptor outer segments; and 5. important morphogenic roles in the differentiation of the rod outer segments and choroid. Certainly, many examples of visual dysfunction may be secondary to pathology of one or more of these important RPE functions. Unfortunately, however, because of its relatively protected in vivo position in the eye, little direct study of human pigment epithelium has been possible. With the development of in vitro tissue culture techniques, RPE has been successfully cultured, and some investigators have begun to use cultured RPE to study cell biology and biochemistry. The majority of these studies have been performed on the retinal pigment epithelium from experimental animals. Only over the last two or three years has RPE from human eyes been successfully cultured in quantities adequate to gegin to study these important functions in man.

Uptake and storage of vitamin A as well as phagocytosis of shedded photoreceptor outer segments are two of the important functions of the retinal pigment epithelium which have been delineated through animal studies, both in vivo and in vitro tissue culture. Over the past year we have established in vitro cultures of the retinal pigment epithelium from over 30 pairs of normal human eyes. This report

Birth Defects: Original Article Series, Volume 18, Number 6, pages 67–79

documents our studies using these cultures to: 1. investigate the phagocytic activity of human RPE for polystyrene latex spheres; and 2. demonstrate the presence of a cytoplasmic retinol binding protein (RBP) in cultured human RPE.

MATERIALS AND METHODS

Eyeballs from 37 patients without known ocular disorders were obtained through the Maryland Eye Bank between July, 1980 and June, 1981. The age of these patients varied from 22 to 88 years with an average of 66.8 years. The post mortem time varied from 15 to 89 hours with an average of 50 hours. The retinal pigment epithelium was isolated for culture as previously described (Del Monte and Maumenee, 1981). Briefly, the anterior segment, vitreous, and neuroretina were removed and the remaining eye cup was filled with Hank's solution. The RPE cells were gently vacuumed free with a fire-blown Pasteur pipette under direct observation using a disecting microscope. The explanted cells were placed in 60 mm Falcon plastic tissue culture dishes containing 3.5 ml of Ham's F-12 medium supplemented with 16% fetal calf serum, 0.2 mM glutamine, and 100 u/ml penicillin, 100 ug/ml streptomycin. The cells were incubated at 37 degrees in a humidified 95% air, 5% CO_2 atmosphere. The media was changed after the third day and then every three days thereafter. After primary cultures were confluent, the cells were detached with 0.12% trypsin solution for routine subculture. Some of the cells were cryopreserved in DMSO-culture media at -60° C and later recultured for study after various times in storage. Human skin fibroblasts from normal donors were cultured in identical media for use as controls.

Morphological Studies

The cultures were observed daily with phase contrast microscopy. After various periods of culture, either primary cultures or subcultures were fixed, stained, and examined by light microscopy, as well as transmission and scanning electron microscopy. Giemsa staining was used for the light microscopy. Fixation and staining for electron microscopy was performed as previously described (Hu and Maumenee, in press).

Phagocytosis

Polystyrene latex spheres (Dow Chemical, Indianapolis, Indiana) 1.0 micron in diameter, were suspended in culture media and adjusted to a concentration of 2 x 10^8 particles per ml. This media latex suspension was then added to established cultures in the log phase of growth. For quantitation of phagocytosis, the latex spheres were removed after incubations of ½, 1, 2, 4, 12, and 24 hours, and the cells were rinsed thoroughly with phosphate buffered saline. The cells were then fixed and stained with Giemsa for light microscopy. The number of ingested latex spheres was counted under the light microscope in 50 cells per culture. In addition, portions of each culture were prepared for electron microscopy.

Retinol Binding Protein

The cells from several confluent flasks of subcultured human retinal pigment epithelium were harvested by treatment with trypsin and washed three times with normal saline. The resulting volume of packed cells (approximately 0.2 ml) was resuspended in 0.05 M TRIS buffer, pH 7.5, containing 0.2 M NaCl, and sonically disrupted. The resulting solution was centrifuged at 70,000 x G for 45 minutes at 4° C. The presence of retinol binding protein was determined by a modification of the method of Swanson et al (1976), using a 1.5 x 120 cm column containing Sephadex G-75 beads (Pharmancia Fine Chemicals, Inc., Piscatarway, N.J.) equilibrated in a similar TRIS NaCl buffer. A 1.0 ml aliquot of the supernatant was incubated with 3 µCi of H^3-retinol (5.0 µCi/mmole, New England Nuclear Corp., Boston, Mass.) for 20 minutes at 4° C. The radiolabled mixture was then applied to the column and eluted at a flow rate of 30 ml per hour. Fractions of 2.0 ml were collected and a 0.2 ml aliquot of each fraction was analyzed for radioactivity. Marker proteins of known molecular size including myoglobin, alphachymotrypsin, and bovine serum albumin were used to determine the approximate molecular weight of eluted peaks.

RESULTS

Morphology and Growth Characteristics

The culture success rate during this study, defined as the percentage of pairs of eyes which grow and become confluent in primary culture so that subculture can be performed, was 90.5%. As we have previously reported (Del Monte and Maumenee, 1980), there was no relationship between success rate and donor sex, age, or cause of death. Again, most eyes cultured within 72 hours of death produced successful cultures; however, later culture was associated with a significantly lower success rate. A double-blind comparison of F-12 medium with minimal essential medium revealed no significant differences in culture success or growth.

The plating efficiency in primary culture was less than 10%. The time needed for attachment varied from two to eight days with an average of 3.5 days. After an average lag phase of 8.4 days (range from 4 to 18 days) the attached cells began to show mitotic activity and proliferate. As a rule, cultures with shorter implantation and lag times grew to produce more vigorous cultures.

In primary culture two different morphologic patterns cound be identified, Fig. 1. The first type of cell

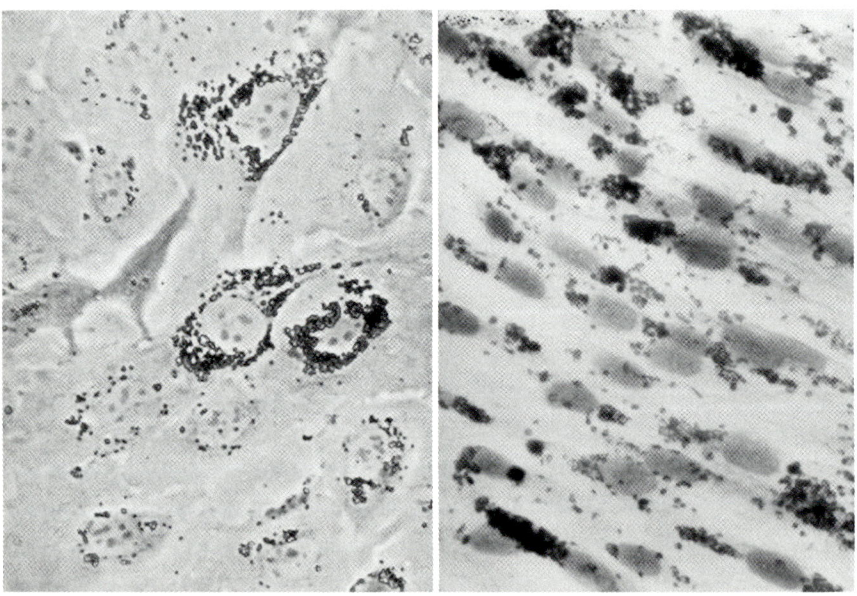

Fig. 1. Phase contrast microscopy of polygonal RPE cells (left) and spindle RPE cells (right) (X 200).

remained definitely epithelioid in morphology with a polygonal or ovoid shape, large openfaced nucleus, and many pigment granules clustered primarily in the nuclear region. The second type was smaller and appeared more spindle shaped, with a smaller nucleus, and pigment spread more generally throughout the cell. In primary culture, it sometimes appeared that colonies of primarily polygonal cells transformed into colonies of the more spindle-shaped type. After subculture, however, the cell morphology was very consistent, even after multiple passages. In 60 mm dishes, both morphological cell types reached confluence in an average of 24.8 days (range 15 to 48 days). However, the dishes containing spindle-shaped cells reached confluence more quickly than those containing polygonal ones. After subculture, the spindle-shaped cells also grew significantly faster. The generation time (time necessary for cell doubling) for the spindle-shaped cells varied between 2.5 and 4 days with an average of 3.2 days, while that of the polygonal shaped cells varied between 3 and 6 days with an average of 4.7 days.

Early in primary culture, both cell types were highly pigmented. Cell division, however, appeared to result in a gradual dilution of pigment with the faster dividing cells becoming depigmented more rapidly. There was no evidence of pigment synthesis in any of these cultures. After subculture, most cells contained very few pigment granules and after four to six subcultures, most of the cells were non-pigmented.

A third cell type, which has been previously recognized and called a stationary cell, was apparent in most cultures. These are large, polygonal or polyhedral in shape, very heavily pigmented, and show no evidence of cell division. They had been thought possibly of macrophage origin; however, histochemical staining for non-specific esterase was negative.

Transmission and scanning electron microscopy (Fig. 2) showed that the polygonal shaped cells in primary culture maintain many epithelioid characteristics, including apical/basal polarization, numerous long narrow microvilli, tight cell junctions, and basal infoldings. Numerous mitochondria, melanin granules, and lipofuscin were also apparent. In subculture these cells continued to demonstrate epithelioid characteristics, however, the melanin granules and lipofuscin became less prominent. Some of the spindle-shaped cells also had prominent, although fewer, microvilli, which were shorter and wider (Fig. 3).

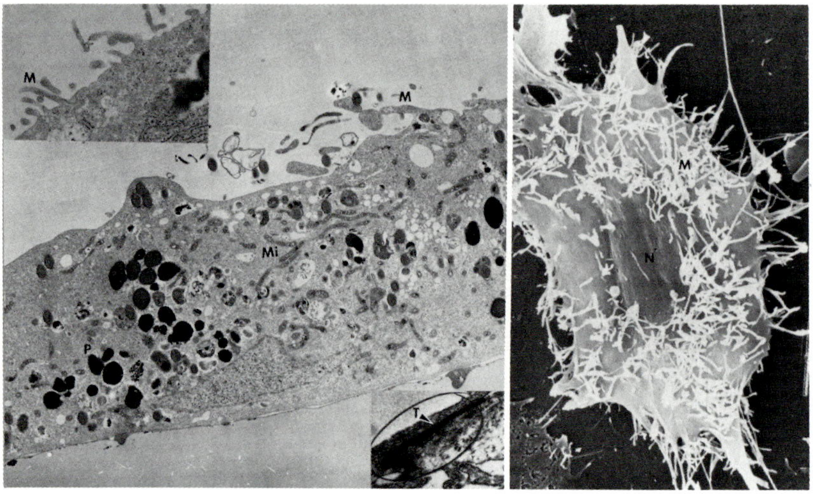

Fig. 2. Transmission (left) and scanning (right) EM of polygonal RPE cell showing numerous microvilli (M), mitochondria Mi, tight junction (T) pigment granules (P); and nucleus (N).

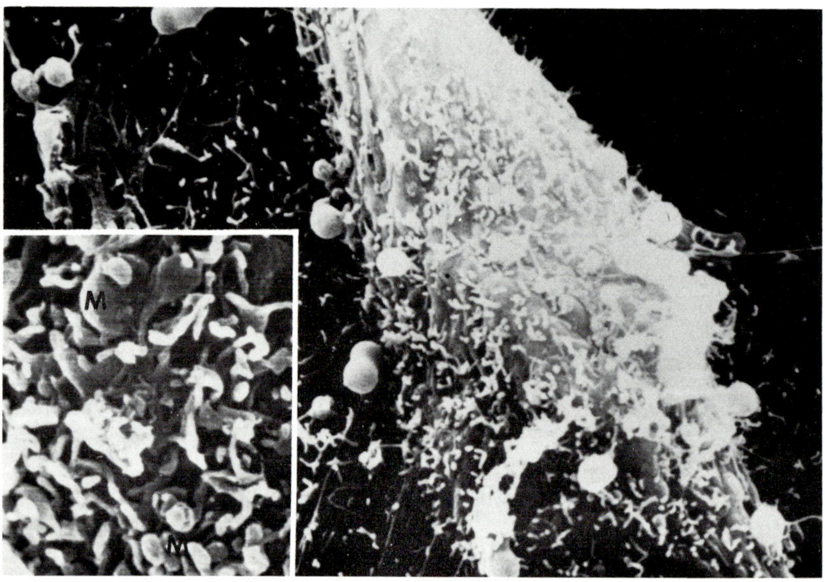

Fig. 3. Scanning EM of spindle RPE cell showing wide, short microvilli (M).

Hours	Number of Latex Spheres per Cell RPE (Polygonal)	RPE (Spindle)	Fibroblasts
½	10.3	7.1	0
1	44.2	18.6	0
2	111.4	78.3	2.2
4	203.3	142.7	5.1
6	305.1	215.8	16.1
8	427.3	285.4	27.8
12	667.9	416.4	46.6
24	820.0	624.6	101.3

Table 1. Quantitative phagocytosis of latex particles by cultured human RPE and skin fibroblasts.

Phagocytosis

Table 1 shows the quantitative phagocytic activity of cultured human RPE cells toward latex particles. Both the polygonal and spindle shaped cell types demonstrated active phagocytosis. Ingestion of latex spheres could be easily demonstrated within 30 minutes. Active phagocytosis continued throughout the first 24 hours as shown in Fig. 4. The

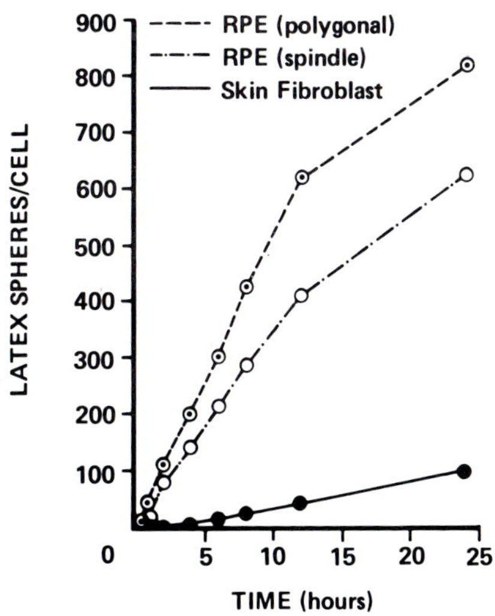

Fig. 4. Phagocytic activity of cultured human RPE and skin fibroblasts toward latex particles.

number of spheres per cell phagocytosed by the spindle shaped cells was apparently less than that phagocytosed by the polygonal cells throughout the first 24 hours. It must be remembered however, that the spindle shaped cells are somewhat smaller, and therefore, the phagocytic activity per cell surface of the two morphologic cell types appears quite similar. Fibroblasts also phagocytosed a few latex spheres after a prolonged latent periods but the number was always less than 15-20% of those phagocytosed by the RPE cells.

Light microscopy revealed latex spheres to be relatively randomly distributed throughout the entire cell cytoplasm (Fig. 5). Transmission and scanning (Fig. 5) electron microscopy nicely demonstrated the various phases of normal phagocytosis seen in animal studies, including adhesion to the

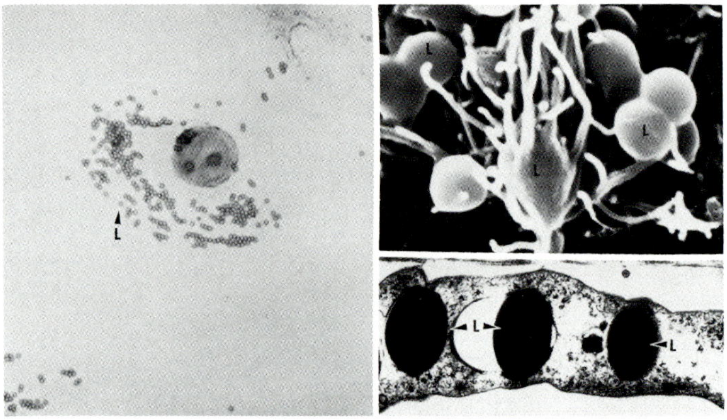

Fig. 5. Light microscopic photo of RPE cell after phagocytosis of latex spheres (L) (left); scanning EM showing engulfment of latex spheres (L) by microvilli of RPE cell (upper right); transmission EM showing phagocytosed latex particles (L) in single membrane bound phagosomes (lower right).

cell surface, engulfment by microvilli, and ingestion into single membrane bound phagosomes. Some phagosomes contained single spheres while others contained two to three. Fusion of lysosomes with phagosomes containing latex spheres was clearly evident.

Retinol Binding Protein

Fig. 6 shows the gel filtration elution profile

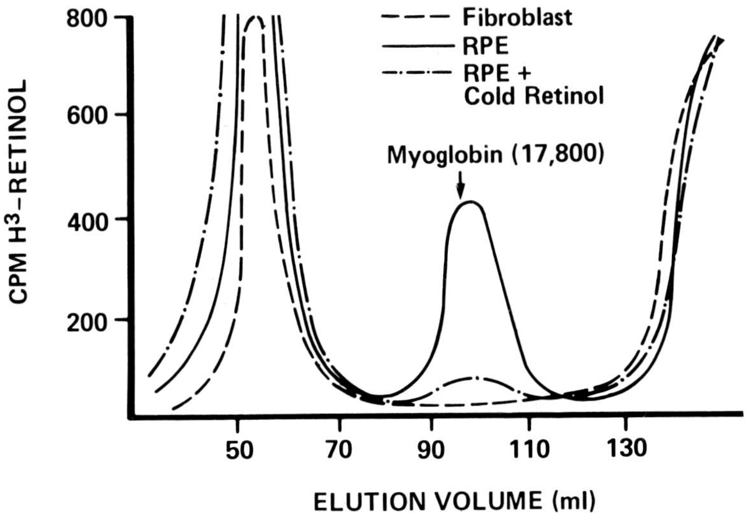

Fig. 6. Sephadex G-75 gel filtration of H^3-retinol incubated with cytosol from cultured human RPE and skin fibroblasts.

obtained from the supernatant of subcultured human RPE cells incubated with H^3-retinol. Three discrete peaks of radioactivity were observed; the first two representing protein bound H^3-retinol and a third free H^3-retinol. The first peak, located in the area of fractions 26-32 (filtration volume 50-62 mls), is a moderately high molecular weight molecule above 75,000 dalton. The second peak, however, which presented in the area corresponding to a filtration volume of 92-102 ml, is probably the specific cytoplasmic retinol binding protein. By comparison with standard proteins of known molecular weights, the estimated molecular weight of the second peak is approximately 17,000 dalton. In addition, this second peak was almost completely eliminated by competitive binding following a chase with cold retinol. These two peaks of bound tritiated retinol were present in subcultured human RPE cells of both the spindle and polygonal morphology. In contrast, the supernatant of human skin fibroblasts showed only two peaks of radioactivity; one bound and of high molecular weight and the other of free H^3-retinol. No binding peak was observed in the 17,000 dalton region.

DISCUSSION

Study of the biochemistry and cell biology of human RPE is only in its infancy. Fortunately, however, with the evolution of tissue culture techniques over the last 20 years, a powerful tool for the study of human RPE has become available. In order to establish the value of cultured human pigment epithelium for the study of human disease, it is necessary to consider two important questions. First, we must determine in what ways in vitro primary and subcultured RPE cells are similar to their in vivo ancestors. That is, which of the important physiological and biochemical RPE functions are retained in culture for possible study. Second, it is important to establish the "normal value" for each parameter from cultured pigment epithelium of normal subjects for later comparison with cultures from patients with various eye disorders.

Studies during the past 20 years have demonstrated that cultured RPE from various experimental animals actively phagocytosed polystyrene latex particles and photoreceptor outer segments (Edwards et al, 1977 ; Essner et al, 1978; Goldman, 1979; Hall, 1978; Hayashi, 1979; Keller, 1977; Tamai, 1979). In this study latex particles were readily phagocytosed by human RPE in tissue culture. Non-specific attachment and ingestion begins almost immediately and can be documented by light and electron microscopy within one half hour. The process of latex engulfment by microvilli, of ingestion of these particles into phagosomes, and of fusion with lysosomes to form secondary lysosomes were all observed with the scanning and transmission electron microscope. Table 1 shows quantitatively the rapid phagocytosis of latex spheres by both morphologocal types of human RPE in culture. Further studies have shown little difference in quantitative phagocytosis between primary cultures and those subcultured up to six times. Human skin fibroblasts showed markedly reduced phagocytic activity in this assay system.

Essner et al (1978) showed that in organ cultures of rabbit and cat RPE, there was a latent period of 12 to 17 hours during which few latex spheres were ingested. Keller and Lauenberger (1977) observed a similar latent period of eight hours in cultured pig RPE. In contrast, studies of rat RPE (Essner et al, 1978) and chick RPE (Hayashi et al, 1979) found no latent period. In the present study, cultured human RPE cells phagocytized latex spheres within one half hour and no latent period was observed.

Recent studies demonstrated the presence of a specific

retinol binding protein in the cytosol of retinal pigment epithelium obtained from several species of animals, both from fresh eyes (chick embryo, rat, guinea pig, and cow) and in tissue culture (chick embryo) (Heller et al, 1978; Israel et al, 1980; Saari et al, 1977; Swanson et al, 1976; Wiggert et al, 1975, 1976). This protein may play an important role in the storage of vitamin A for use by the photoreceptors. There have been no reports, however, concerning the presence of retinol binding protein in cultured human RPE. We therefore studied the uptake and metabolism of H^3-retinol by subcultured human RPE cells. There was a very rapid uptake of the H^3-retinol from the tissue culture medium. As much as 75-80% of added radioactivity was cell bound within two hours. Following gel filtration, two protein bound peaks were observed from cultured human RPE. The first peak, of molecular weight greater than 75,000 dalton, is possibly an aggregate of the lower molecular weight retinol binding protein, or may correspond to the binding by a serum binding protein present in the tissue culture media, or may even represent a separate high molecular weight retinol binding protein as reported by Heller and Bok (1976). The second peak, with estimated molecular weight of approximately 17,000 dalton, corresponds nicely with literature values for cytoplasmic retinol binding protein from animal eyes (Wiggert et al, 1975, 1976). The absence of such a peak from the cytosol of cultured human skin fibroblasts, indicating the lack of specific retinol binding protein, is also consistent with previous literature (Swanson et al, 1976).

The morphology of cultured human pigment epithelial cells has been studied since the early 1970's. Numerous investigators have found a progressive general decrease in the amount of pigment in these cells as tissue culture progresses, probably secondary to the absence of pigment production in culture. Albert et al (1972) were the first to demonstrate changes in the morphologic characteristics of human pigment epithelial cells in culture, some remaining polyhedral and others showing a marked spindle-like growth pattern. In the past in our laboratory, the spindle-shaped cells, which are difficult to distinguish from fibroblasts, were discarded as poorly characterized cells which may be contaminents. In this report, we look more closely at cells of the two major morphologic types, polygonal and spindle. Although there were differences, both cell types retain many epitheloid characteristics, including apical-basal polarity, and microvilli. In addition, we have shown that unlike skin fibroblasts, both morphologic patterns of cultured human RPE continued to demonstrate marked phagocytic activity for latex spheres and contain cytoplasmic retinol binding protein. Certainly, although the capacity for pigment synthesis appears lost in culture, and primary cell morphology becomes more variable, cultured human pigment epithelial cells still possess other characteristic features including phagocytic activity and retinol binding protein.

In conclusion, we have developed a simple assay for the quantitative and qualitative study of phagocytosis in cultured human pigment epithelial cells. This in vitro system, both with latex particles, and later rod outer segments, should be helpful in evaluating the effects of drugs and environmental conditions on the phagocytic activity of human RPE, and should also prove a useful method to explore the role of phagocytosis in various human diseases of the choroid and retina, especially in retinitis pigmentosa. In addition, our studies suggest that human RPE growing in tissue culture continues to produce cytoplasmic retinol binding protein. These in vitro cultures of human RPE should prove useful for the study of vitam A metabolism in normal human retinal pigment epithelium as well as in exploring the role of retinol metabolism in various human retinal disorders.

ACKNOWLEDGMENTS

The authors would like to thank Mrs. Ruth Classon and Mr. Thomas Mitchell for their invaluable assistance in the preparation of this manuscript.

REFERENCES

Albert DM, Tso MOM, Rabson AS (1972). In vitro growth of pure cultures of retinal pigment epithelium. ARch Ophthalmol 88:63-69.

Del Monte MA, Maumenee IH (1980). New techniques for the in vitro sulture of human retinal pigment epithelium. In Danes BS (ed): "In Vitro Epithelia and Birth Defects," New York: Alan R. Liss, p 327-338.

Del Monte MA, Maumenee IH (1981). In vitro culture of human pigment epithelium for biochemical and metabolic study. Vision Research 21:137-142.

Edwards RB, Szamier RB (1977). Defective phagocytosis of isolated rod segments by RCS rat retinal pigment epithelium in culture. Science 197:1001.

Essner E, Roszke JR, Schreiber JH (1978). Phagocytosis and surface morphology in cultured retinal pigment epithelial cell. Invest Ophthalmol 17:1040.

Feeney L, Mixon RN (1976). An in vitro model of phagocytosis in bovine and human retinal pigment epithelium. Exp Eye Res 22:533.

Goldman AI, O'Brien PJ, Masterson E, Ismel P, Teirstein P, Chader G (1979). A quantitative system for studying phagocytosis in pigment epithelium tissue cultures. Exp Eye Res 28:455.

Hall MO (1978). Phagocytosis of light and dark adapted rod outer segments by cultured pigment epithelium. Science 202: 506.

Hayashi M, Matsumoto A, Hamashima Y, Tsukahara I (1979). Phagocytic activity of cultured retinal pigment epithelium: Uptake of polystyrene spheres and staphylococcus aureus. Exp Eye Res 28:427.

Heller J, Bok D (1976). Transport of retinol from the blood to the retina: Involvement of high molecular weight lipoprotein as intracellar carriers. Exp Eye Res 22:403.

Israel P, Masterson E, Goldman AT, Wiggert B, Chader GJ (1980). Retinal pigment epithelial cell differentiation in vitro: Influence of culture medium. Invest Ophthalmol 19:720.

Keller G, Leuenberger PM (1977). Effect of chochicine on phagosome-lysosome interaction in retinal pigment epithelium. II. In vitro observations on histo-organotypical retinal pigment epithelial cells of the pig (a preliminary report). Albrecht v. Graefes Arch Klin Ophthalmol 203:253.

Saari JC, Bunt AH, Futterman S, Berman ER (1977). Localization of cellular retino-binding protein in bovine retina and retinal pigment epithelium, with a consideration of the pigment epithelium isolation technique. Invest Ophthalmol 16:797.

Swanson D, Futterman S, Sarri J (1976). Retinol and retinic acid binding protein: Occurrence in human retina and absence from human cultured fibroblasts. Invest Ophthalmol 15:1017.

Wiggert BO, Chader GJ (1975). A receptor for retinol in the developing retina and pigment epithelium. Exp Eye Res 21: 143.

Wiggert B, Bergsma DR, Chader GJ (1976). Retinol receptors of the retina and pigment epithelium: Further characterization and species variation. Exp Eye Res 22:441.

Wiggert B, Masterson E, Israel P, Chader GJ (1979). Differential retinoid binding in chick pigment epithelium and choroid. Invest Ophthalmol 18:306.

RETINITIS PIGMENTOSA: ELECTRON MICROSCOPY AND CELL CULTURE STUDIES

Merlyn M. Rodrigues, M.D., David Newsome, M.D.
Clinical Branch, National Eye Institute,
National Institutes of Health, Bethesda, MD

Electron microscopic studies of retinitis pigmentosa have been limited to a few reports, generally in advanced cases (Mizuno and Nishida, 1976; Kolb and Gouras, 1974; Szamier and Berson, 1977 and Szamier, Berson, Klein and Myers, 1979). Cell culture studies of this disease have not been previously described.

We report unusual changes in the retinal pigmented epithelium (RPE), predominently of the macula and foveal region, in addition to the more commonly observed degeneration of photoreceptor cells. Scanning electron microscopy of cell cultures of the RPE cells showed a variety of cell types, some compatible with those seen in cultures of normal human RPE (Flood, Gouras and Kjeldbye, 1980) as well as other distinctly abnormal cells.

Case summary: A 51 year old black male had visual deterioration that started at 7 years of age. He had noticed a marked decrease in vision for the past two years and was diagnosed as retinitis pigmentosa. There was no genetic or

Birth Defects: Original Article Series, Volume 18, Number 6, pages 81–94

familial history of retinitis pigmentosa. Both parents had normal vision without eye diseases and two siblings were also normal. The patient did not have children. Systemic examination revealed idiopathic hypertrophic subaortic stenosis with cardiomegaly. Ocular examination revealed light perception vision in both eyes. Intraocular pressures were normal. Both lenses showed moderate anterior and posterior cortical opacifications by slit lamp. Fundoscopy revealed pale discs with markedly attenuated retinal blood vessels, and a prominent bone spicule appearance, 360° in the periphery. There was marked epiretinal membrane change in the maculas. One month after admission the patient expired due to renal failure and congestive cardiac failure.

MATERIALS AND METHODS:

The eyes were obtained approximately 24 hours after autopsy. One eye was fixed in formalin and the other partly frozen and partly used for biochemical estimates of cyclic AMP and cyclic GMP reported elsewhere (Newsome, Fletcher and Chader, 1980). The eyes measured approximately 24 x 24 x 23 mm with 4 mm of optic nerve attached. The iris was brown in color. The lenses were slightly opaque. The retinas showed a marked bone spicule appearance particularly near the periphery and equator. Part of one eye was submitted for cell cultures on which scanning electron microscopy was performed. On the formalin fixed eye, some unstained paraffin sections were examined with ultraviolet light and others were stained with H&E and PAS. A portion of the remaining tissue of this eye was processed for transmission and scanning electron microscopy by standard methods. For transmission electron microscopy the specimens were fixed in glutaraldehyde, postfixed in osmium and embedded in epon. Thin sections were stained with uranyl acetate and lead citrate. For scanning electron microscopy, specimens were postfixed in 1% osmium, dehydrated in graded alcohols, critical point dried and sputter coated with gold.

Cell cultures:

Using sterile procedures, explants of retinal tissue containing pigmented areas were placed in Eagle's Minimal Essential Medium with Earle's salts, 5% fetal calf serum, 100 µg/mL of penicillin and 50 µg/mL of streptomycin. These tissues were placed into polystyrene 60 mm culture dishes, held in position under a glass coverslip, and maintained at 57°C in 95% air and 5% CO_2, 100% humidity atmosphere in a standard water-jacket incubator. Growth medium (3 ml per dish) was changed every three days. Cellular proliferation in the dishes was observed and photographed by a phase contrast inverted microscope equipped with a 35 mm camera. Cellular outgrowths intended for examination by scanning electron microscopy were selected from outgrowths onto the glass coverslips.

RESULTS:

Examination of the routine paraffin sections by light microscopy showed marked absence of the rods throughout the retina with occasional cones present only in the foveal area. Excessive accumulation of lipofuscin pigments was seen on fluorescence microscopy of unstained paraffin sections. The areas of pigment migration in the retina were nonfluorescent with UV light and appeared to consist of melanin.

Transmission electron microscopy of the macular area, particularly of the fovea, showed unusual changes of the retinal pigment epithelium with marked proliferation of endoplasmic reticulum-like profiles, possibly of the smooth surface type (Figs. 1-3); the distance between these profiles was 14 nm. At the apices of these atypical cells, scattered rough endoplasmic reticulum was present. There was a decrease in both melanin and lipofuscin pigment in cells with this unusual alteration (Fig. 4) but in adjacent cells there appeared to be an excessive accumulation of lipofuscin and a decrease of melanin. Some cells displayed a closely packed arrangement of cytoplasmic profiles whereas in others a looser pattern was evident (Fig. 4). The cones showed marked degeneration and attenuation with only occasional remnants of outer and inner segments (Fig. 1). The choriocapillaris and Bruch's membrane appeared normal in the macular area and elsewhere in the retina (Fig. 1). Other areas of retina showed absence of both rod and cone cells. The retinal vessels were surrounded by pigment aggregates, composed mainly of melanin.

The internal limiting membrane was covered by 1-2 layers of pigmented cells (Fig. 5). One focus of pigmented cells extended directly from the retinal pigmented epithelium through the entire thickness of the retina in a mushroom-shaped configuration onto the surface of the internal limiting membrane (Fig. 6). These RPE cells were connected by junctional complexes and contained mostly melanin pigment, mitochondria, and rough and smooth endoplasmic reticulum characteristic of RPE (Fig. 6). In other areas the melanin pigment aggregates appeared to be phagocytosed by glial cells (Fig. 5).

Cells cultured from the primary outgrowth showed prodominantly RPE cells (Fig. 7), occasional macrophages and abnormal cells with filiform cytoplasmic processes and prominent aggregates of melanin granules measuring 1-2 μ in diameter (Fig. 8).

Studies of cyclic nucleotide concentrations showed a five-fold decrease in cyclic GMP (0.5, 0.6 and 2.0 pmol/mg in macula, midzone and periphery respectively) while cyclic AMP levels were essentially normal (Newsome, Fletcher and Chader).

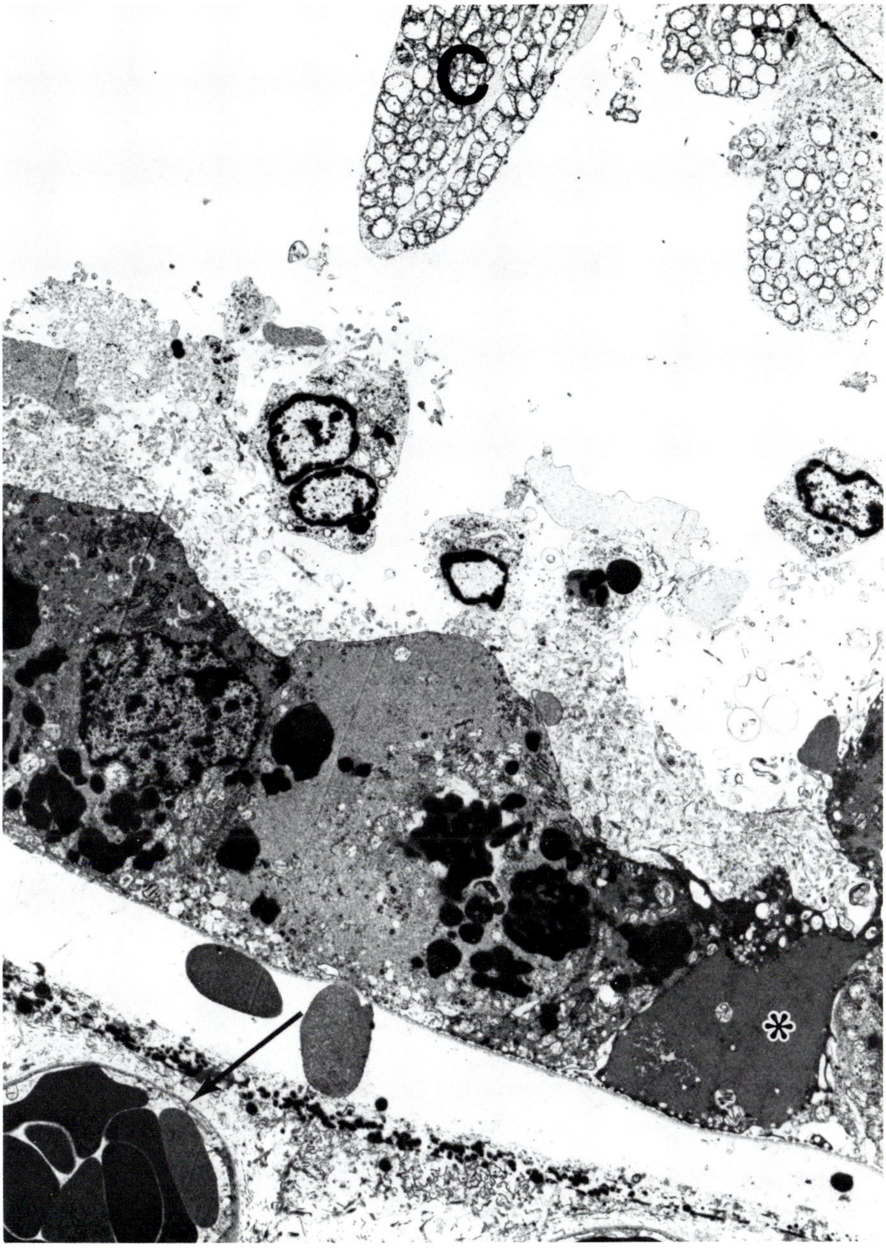

Fig. 1
Foveal region shows scattered atypical RPE cells (*). Cones are indicated (C). The choriocapillaris are normal (arrow) (X3,510).

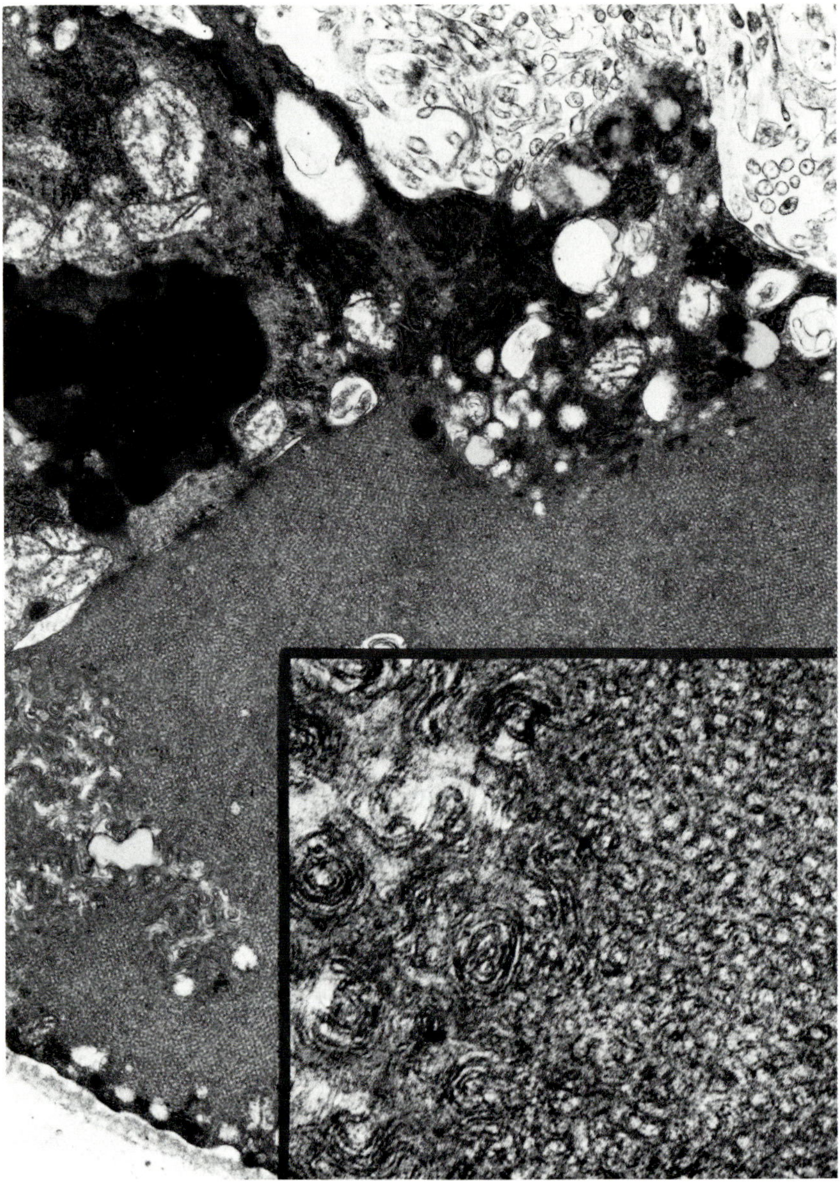

Fig. 2
Higher magnification of unusual RPE cell in Fig. 1. The cytoplasm shows a honeycomb-like packing of profiles (X16,500). Inset shows a higher magnification of the whorl-like and lattice arrangement of these cytoplasmic changes (X27,000).

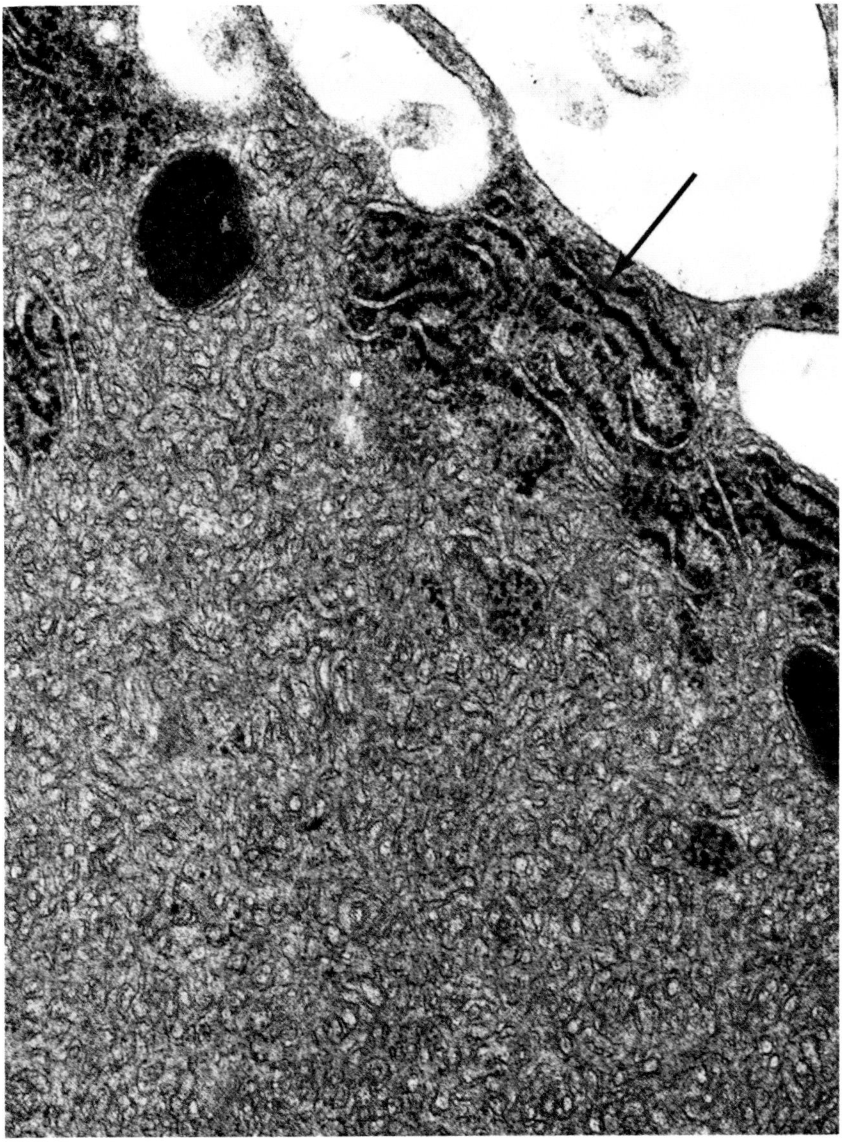

Fig. 3
The foveal RPE shows other cells with similar linear parallel cytoplasmic changes, rough endoplasmic reticulum (arrow) and occasional pigment granules (X58,000).

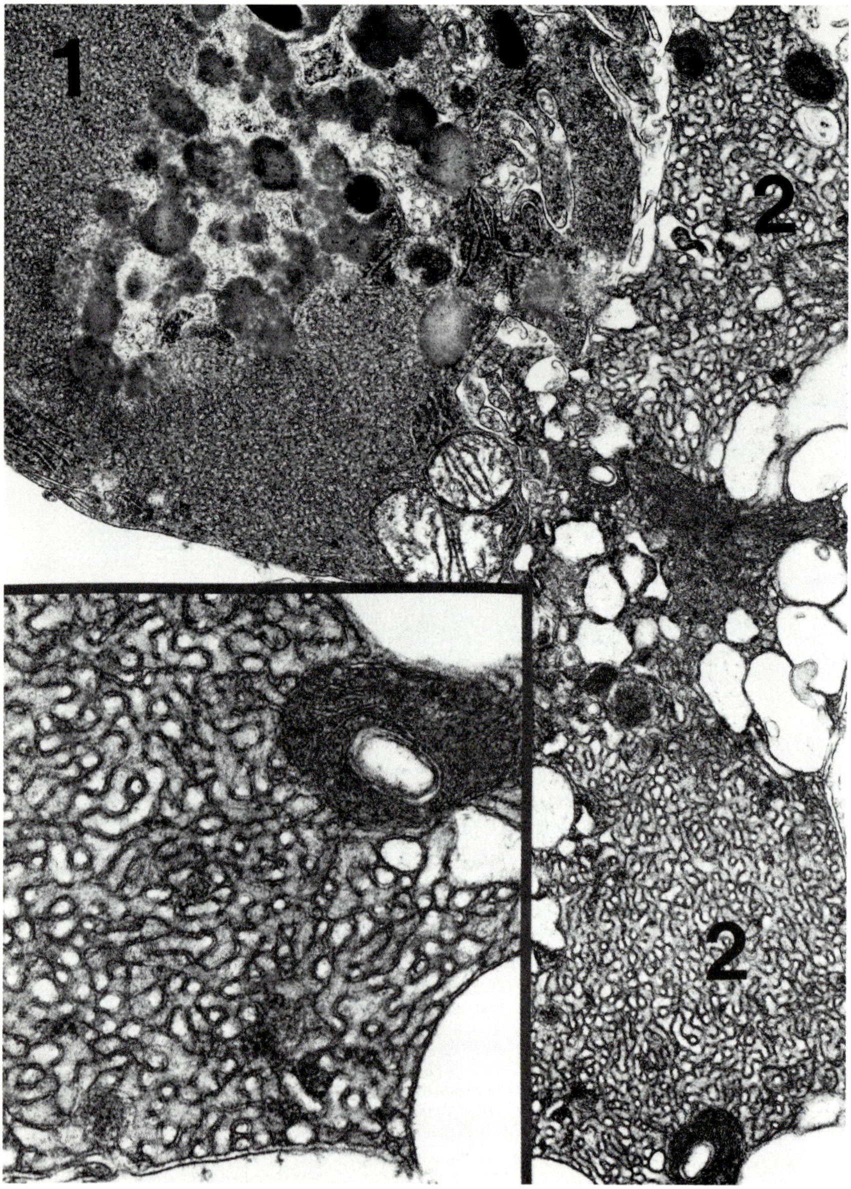

Fig. 4
Foveal RPE cells display two unusual types of cytoplasmic changes: 1 demonstrates an arrangement of closely packed profiles similar to those cells in Figs. 1 and 3. Scattered lipofuscin and melanin pigments are also present. In 2 there is a looser arrangement of cytoplasmic profiles (X21,000). Inset at higher magnification (X35,100).

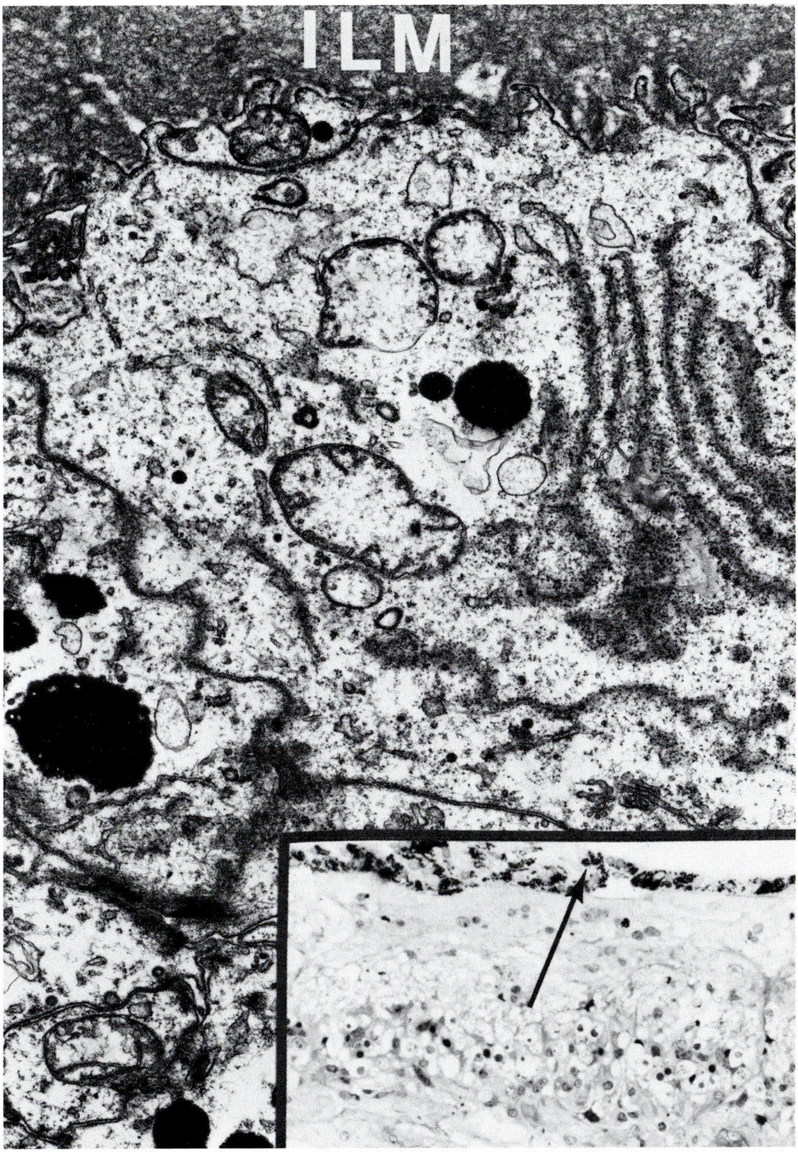

Fig. 5
Inset shows a pigmented cellular layer on the surface of the internal limiting membrane (arrow) (X220). Electron micrograph shows scattered intracellular melanin pigment granules. The internal limiting membrane is indicated (ILM) (X16,500).

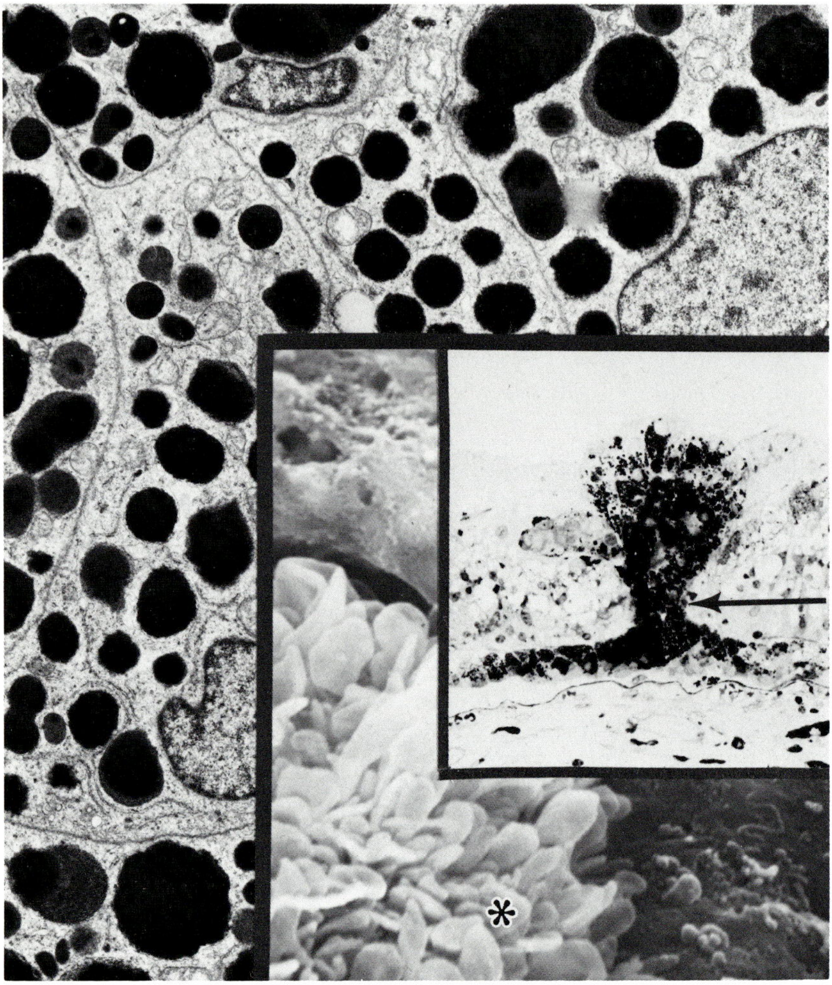

Fig. 6
Inner inset shows a direct extension of RPE cells (arrow) through the full thickness of the retina extending onto the surface of the internal limiting membrane (X200). Scanning electron micrograph in the outer inset shows the mushroom-like extension of RPE cells (*) through the inner retina. Transmission electron micrograph shows intraretinal RPE cells connected by junctional complexes in the mushroom-shaped area in the inner inset (X7,500).

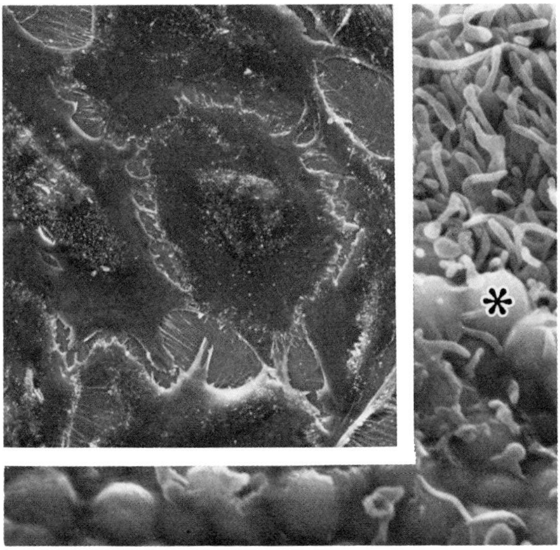

Fig. 7

Inset of a cell culture of pigmented area of the retina shows RPE-like cells (X360). The RPE cells display myriad c cytoplasmic microvillous processes and numerous melanin granules (*) (X660).

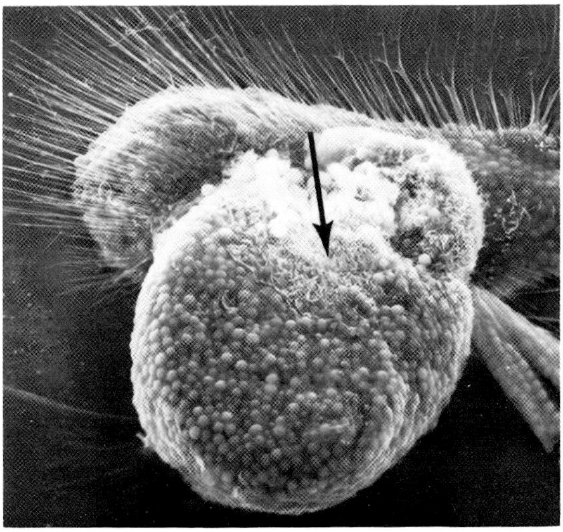

Fig. 8

Cell culture of some atypical RPE cells packed with melanin. Microvillous processes are indicated (arrow). There are numerous filiform cytoplasmic processes (X110).

DISCUSSION:

The inheritance of retinitis pigmentosa usually occurs in three categories: autosomal dominant, autosomal recessive, or sex-linked recessive (Merin and Auerbach, 1976; Bird, 1977). The present case appears to be a sporadic form of retinitis pigmentosa, since there was no evidence of hereditary transmission. There was no history of trauma.

Although there have been extensive clinical and genetic studies of retinitis pigmentosa, only a few cases have been studied by electron microscopy (Mizuno and Nishida, 1967; Kolb and Gouras, 1974; Szamier and Berson, 1977; Szamier, Berson, Klein and Myers, 1979). These reports have generally described extensive degeneration of rod and cone cells. Excessive accumulation of lipofuscin aggregates in the fovea with decreased amounts of melanin was described in one report: the increased lipofuscin was presumably derived from phagocytosis of rod outer segment material (Kolb and Gouras, 1974). Similar changes were observed in our patient. Analysis of the fluorescent spectra of chloroformmethanol extracts of human RPE showed lipofuscin in RPE of individuals over 40 years of age and retinyl ester in RPE of all age groups (Feeney-Burns, Berman and Rothman, 1980). The RPE appears particularly susceptible to the accumulation of lipofuscin because of the daily turnover and renewal process of membranes rich in polyunsaturated fatty acids (Feeney-Burns, Berman and Rothman, 1980; Young, 1977).

In our patient, the nature of the unusual changes of the RPE is uncertain. The origin of the excessive accumulation of tubular profiles could be from smooth endoplasmic reticulum, or less likely, from mitochondria. During hibernation, changes in the smooth endoplasmic reticulum of RPE cells have been described in the ground squirrel (Kuwabara, 1975). The latter changes showed slight similarities to our case, but were not identical. The changes of the RPE in our patient are probably nonspecific and most likely related to the advanced stage of the disease. However, such changes have not to our knowledge been reported in other human retinal diseases or in other cases of retinitis pigmentosa.

An additional feature of interest in our case is the convincing demonstration that the RPE is the source of pigment migration in the inner retinal layers, including those with a perivascular distribution. The glial cells also appear to phagocytose some of the melanin pigment, which in one area extended through the internal limiting membrane.

Human RPE cells in vitro have exhibited epithelioid characteristics with junctional complexes and apical-basal polarity (Flood, Gouras and Kjelbye, 1980). Phagocytosis has also been documented in cultured RPE cells (Essner, Roszka and Schreiber, 1978). In the present report, we noted features of normal RPE cells as well as of abnormal cells of probably RPE origin. In our recent study of cellular constituents in tissues from human massive periretinal proliferation, we observed four distinct types: pigmented epithelioid cells, glial cells, fibroblastic cells and macrophages (Newsome, Rodrigues, Machemer, 1981). We did not observe the unusual configuration of some cells of probable RPE origin noted in the present case (Fig. 8).

The tissue or cellular site of the primary defect in retinitis pigmentosa remains an enigma. Certainly the destruction of visual cells is striking. The extensive migration of RPE we observed and documented both in ocular tissues and in vitro suggests that there may be more than one major pathogenetic component in this disease.

ACKNOWLEDGMENT:

Joseph Hackett and Patricia Donohoo assisted with electron microscopy.

REFERENCES:

Bird AC (1977). Retinitis pigmentosa. A review. Trans Am Ophthalmol Soc NZ 29:51.

Essner E, Roszka JT, Schreiber HJ (1978). Phagocytosis and surface morphology in cultured retinal pigment epithelial cells. Invest Ophthalmol Vis Sci 17:1040.

Feeney-Burns L, Berman ER, Rothman H (1980). Lipofuscin of human retinal pigment epithelium. Am J Ophthalmol 90:783.

Flood MT, Gouras P, Kjeldbye H (1980). Growth characteristics and ultrastructure of human retinal pigment epithelium in vitro. Invest Ophthalmol Vis Sci 19:1309.

Kolb H, Gouras P (1974). Electron microscopic observations of human retinitis pigmentosa, dominantly acquired. Invest Ophthalmol Vis Sci 13:487.

Kuwabara T. (1975) Cytologic changes of the retina and pigment during hibernation. Invest Ophthalmol Vis Sci 14:457.

Merin S, Auerbach I (1976). Retinitis pigmentosa. Surv Ophthalmol. 20:303.

Mizuno K, Nishida S (1967). Electron microscopic studies of human retinitis pigmentosa. Am. J. Ophthalmol 63: 791.

Newsome DA, Fletcher RT, Chader GJ (1980). Cyclic nucleotides vary by area in the retina and pigmented epithelium of the human and monkey. Invest Ophthalmol Vis Sci 19:864.

Newsome DA, Rodrigues MM, Machemer R (1981). Human massive periretinal proliferation. In vitro characteristics of cellular components. Arch Ophthalmol 99:873.

Szamier RB, Berson EL (1977). Retinal ultrastructure in advanced retinitis pigmentosa. Invest Ophthalmol Vis Sci 16:947.

Szamier RB, Berson EL, Klein R, Myers S (1977). Sex-linked retinitis pigmentosa: ultrastructure of photoreceptors and pigment epithelium. Invest Ophthalmol Vis Sci 18:145.

Young RW (1977). Visual cell renewal systems and the problem of retinitis pigmentosa. In Landers MB, Wolbarsht ML, Dowling JE, Laties AM (eds): "Retinitis pigmentosa. Clinical implication of current research," New York and London, p. 93.

GLYCOSAMINOGLYCAN SECRETION BY PRIMARY CULTURES AND SUBCULTURES OF HUMAN RETINAL PIGMENT EPITHELIUM

Ross B. Edwards

Berman-Gund Laboratory for the Study of Retinal Degenerations, Harvard Medical School, Massachusetts Eye and Ear Infirmary
243 Charles Street, Boston, MA 02114, U.S.A.

Some biochemical properties of cultured human retinal pigment epithelial cells (RPE) have been reported to change when the cells are subcultured; for example, retinol content and retinyl palmitate hydrolase activity decrease and actin-like proteins increase (Flood et al, 1981; Haley et al, 1981). The present study was done to determine whether or not cells subcultured from human RPE secrete the same types and proportions of glycosaminoglycans (GAGs) as primary cultures. RPE cells subcultured from a postmortem donor eye of a patient with sex-linked retinitis pigmentosa, primary cultures of normal human choroidal cells, and subcultured normal human skin fibroblasts were also examined.

METHODS

The preparation and maintenance of cultures (human RPE, choroidal cells, and skin fibroblasts), the morphology of the cells, synthesis and secretion of radioactive GAGs from isotopically labeled precursors, isolation of GAGs, analysis of radioactive GAGs by cellulose acetate electrophoresis, and digestion with GAG-degrading enzymes have been described elsewhere (Edwards, in press). Briefly, confluent monolayers of cultured cells were incubated with ^{3}H-glucosamine and $Na_2{}^{35}SO_4$ (30 μCi/ml for each isotope) for 72 hours. Only Falcon Multiwell culture dishes (Oxnard, California) were used for these experiments since initial studies indicated that substantially different GAG profiles were obtained with other brands of culture dishes. The medium was removed and

Birth Defects: Original Article Series, Volume 18, Number 6, pages 95–100

centrifuged to eliminate cellular debris. The radioactive GAGs of the medium were deproteinized by incubating the medium with pronase and purified by precipitation with cetyltrimethylammonium bromide in the presence of added nonradioactive carrier GAGs. Aliquots of the GAG preparations were analyzed by cellulose acetate electrophoresis before or after incubation with enzymes which selectively degrade different classes of GAGs.

RESULTS

The GAGs secreted by primary cultures of RPE into the culture medium during a three-day incubation with ^{3}H-glucosamine and ^{35}S-sulfate could be resolved into three peaks by cellulose acetate electrophoresis (Fig. 1). Peak 1, with the slowest mobility, contained only tritium (^{3}H) and migrated with the hyaluronic acid reference standard. Peak 2 contained tritium and ^{35}S and migrated to a position slightly behind the dermatan sulfate reference standard. Peak 3 contained tritium and ^{35}S and migrated with (Fig. 1) or slightly slower than (Fig. 2) the chondroitin sulfate reference standards. Incubations of GAGs with different enzymes (5 donors) demonstrated that each of the three peaks had different enzyme susceptibilities. Typical results for one donor are shown in Fig. 2. Fungal hyaluronidase, which degrades only hyaluronic acid, removed only peak 1 without significantly altering the other two peaks. Peak 1, therefore, is hyaluronic acid. Chondroitinase AC-II, which degrades hyaluronic acid and chondroitin sulfate, but which does not degrade dermatan sulfate or other GAGs, removed peak 1 and much of peaks 2 and 3; 30 $\pm$ 8% of the radioactive GAGs resisted digestion, and the resistant GAGs migrated with the dermatan sulfate reference standard. Chondroitinase ABC (4.0 units/ml), which degrades hyaluronic acid, chondroitin sulfate and also dermatan sulfate, but no other GAGs, degraded all of the radioactivity. Peaks 2 and 3, therefore, contain chondroitin sulfate and dermatan sulfate. Chondroitinase ABC at 0.2 and 0.02 units/ml degraded only peak 3 without significantly altering the other two peaks. Testicular hyaluronidase had an effect similar to chondroitinase AC-II except that the remaining radioactivity migrated somewhat slower than the dermatan sulfate standard (Fig. 2).

GAGs secreted by cells subcultured for 1, 2, 4, 8, and 11 passages from the RPE of 5 different normal donors were similar, both with respect to proportions and enzyme suscep-

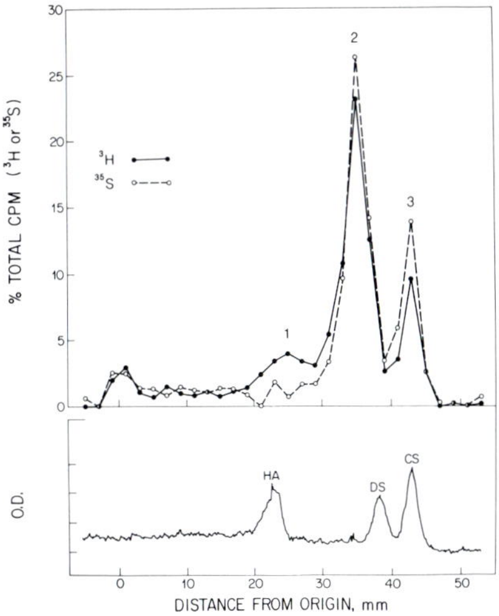

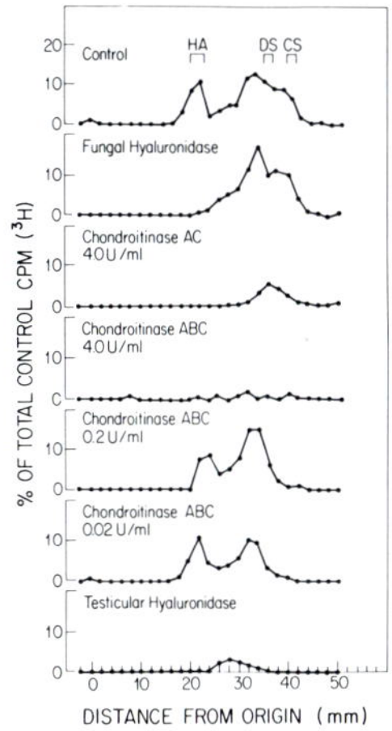

Figure 1 (left): Cellulose acetate electrophoresis of GAGs synthesized and secreted into the medium by a primary RPE culture prepared from the postmortem eyes of a normal donor aged 69 years. The cells were incubated for 72 hours with medium containing ^{3}H-glucosamine and ^{35}S-sulfate. The upper graph illustrates the distribution of radioactivity. The total radioactivity of the electropherogram was 923 counts/min ^{3}H and 168 counts/min ^{35}S and was 8.5% of the total radioactive GAGs secreted by this culture in 72 hours. The lower graph is an optical scan showing the distribution of reference standards: HA, hyaluronic acid; DS, dermatan sulfate; CS, a mixture of chondroitin-4-sulfate and chondroitin-6-sulfate.

Figure 2 (right): Enzyme digestion analysis of GAGs secreted by a primary culture of RPE prepared from postmortem eyes of a normal donor aged 29 years. Each aliquot contained 780 counts/min ^{3}H before enzyme digestion, which was 4.4% of the total radioactive GAG secreted by this culture in 72 hours. Brackets indicate the positions of reference GAGs abbreviated as in Fig. 1.

tibilities, to GAGs secreted by primary cultures of RPE (Fig. 3). The GAGs secreted by cells subcultured for 7 and

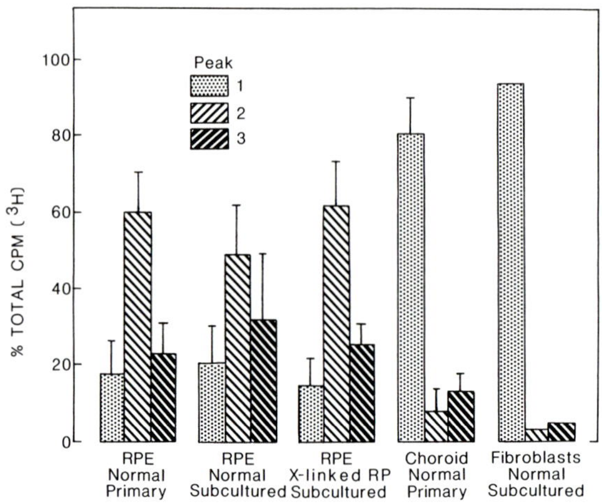

Figure 3: Distribution on ^3H among the three peaks of radioactive GAGs secreted in 72 hours and analyzed by cellulose acetate electrophoresis. Peak numbers are as in Fig. 1. Each bar represents the mean percent of ^3H in the indicated peak; the vertical lines equal one standard deviation. Each set of bars represents analysis of the following number of donors: RPE normal primary, 8; RPE normal subcultured, 5; RPE X-linked RP, 3 cultures at 7th passage and one culture at 18th passage from the donor aged 24 years with sex-linked retinitis pigmentosa; choroidal cells, 3; skin fibroblasts, one (2 electropherograms).

18 passages from the RPE of a patient aged 24 years with sex-linked retinitis pigmentosa (Figs. 3 and 4) were also similar in proportions and enzyme susceptibilities to the GAGs secreted by normal primary RPE cultures.

In contrast, primary cultures of normal human choroidal cells secreted GAGs with a higher proportion of peak 1 and a lower proportion of peak 2 than the GAGs secreted by RPE cells. For both peaks 1 and 2, the difference between cultured choroidal cells and cultured RPE cells was statistically significant (P less than 0.001). Likewise, the distribution of GAGs secreted by normal human skin fibroblasts in seventh passage differed markedly from that of cultured RPE (Fig. 3).

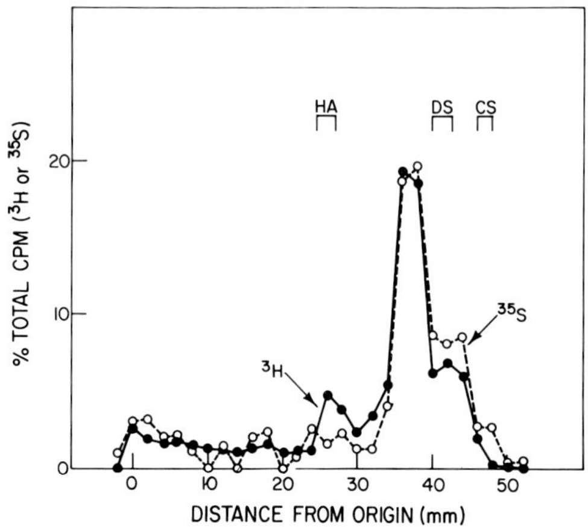

Figure 4: Cellulose acetate electrophoresis of GAGs secreted by subcultured RPE at 7th passage from the donor with sex-linked retinitis pigmentosa. Details are as in Fig. 1. The total radioactivity of the electropherogram was 1434 counts/min ^{3}H and 110 counts/min ^{35}S and was 4.5% of the total radioactive GAGs secreted by this culture in 72 hours.

Enzyme digestion of GAGs secreted by primary choroidal cells and subcultured skin fibroblasts gave results similar to the effects of enzymes on GAGs secreted by cultured RPE.

DISCUSSION

These results show that the profile of radioactive GAGs secreted by cultured human RPE is stable after extensive cell division in vitro. Cells have been subcultured from human RPE for up to 18 passages with no significant alteration of the GAG profile. This profile is not a general characteristic of cells in culture; primary cultures of human choroidal cells and subcultured human skin fibroblasts maintained under the same conditions as RPE cells secreted GAGs with a distinctly different profile compared to RPE. Thus, the GAG secretion profile is a stable biochemical characteristic of cultured human RPE and should prove to be useful in helping to distinguish cell strains subcultured from the RPE from other possible contaminating cells.

ACKNOWLEDGMENTS

The author thanks Junelle Taylor Brandt, Anthony Maranto, and Judith Boruchoff for technical assistance and Jean Mannagh for helpful discussions on culture methodology. The author also thanks the New England Eye Bank for providing normal postmortem donor eyes and the University of Wisconsin Eye Bank for their cooperation in helping to obtain the postmortem donor eyes of the patient with retinitis pigmentosa. This work was supported in part by National Eye Institute Specialized Research Center Grant EY02014 and in part by the National Retinitis Pigmentosa Foundation, Baltimore, Maryland, and the George Gund Foundation, Cleveland, Ohio.

REFERENCES

Edwards RB (in press). Glycosaminoglycan synthesis by cultured human retinal pigment epithelium from normal postmortem donors and a postmortem donor with retinitis pigmentosa. Invest Ophthalmol Vis Sci.

Flood MT, Blaner WS, Smith JE, Haley JE, Gouras P (1981). Biochemical studies on human retinal pigment epithelium in vitro. Invest Ophthalmol Vis Sci 20(ARVO Suppl.):165.

Haley JE, Flood MT, Gouras P (1981). Changes of protein patterns in human retinal pigment epithelial cells in vitro. Invest Ophthalmol Vis Sci 20(ARVO Suppl.):165.

HUMAN RETINAL PIGMENT EPITHELIAL CELLS IN TISSUE CULTURE: A MEANS OF STUDYING INHERITED RETINAL DISEASES.

M.E.Boulton, J.Marshall* and J.Mellerio

Polytechnic of Central London
Institute of Ophthalmology*

INTRODUCTION

The laboratory investigations of inherited retinal disease in man are significantly impeded by the lack of suitable tissues. This situation arises due to a variety of reasons; socioreligous, ethical and medical. The major problems are (1) that biopsy of retinal tissue for experimental investigation is not considered ethical by many centres, (2) that such diseases are not life threatening and therefore postmortem tissue generally becomes available many years after the manifestation of initial clinical symptoms and (3) that most patients die remote from eye hospitals so even this grossly diseased material is lost for laboratory analysis.

The establishment of patient groups in a number of countries, and their interaction with research workers, has recently enabled a significant restructuring of research into the retinal dystrophies. These groups are actively involved on a volunteer basis in investigations aimed at subclassifying the R.P. syndrome in investigations using a variety of techniques (e.g. genetic, psychophysical and electrophysiological). These groups are also participating in direct laboratory studies in which tissue or biopsies are obtained, for example blood and samples of nasal cilia (Airaksinen et.al.,1979; Arden and Fox, 1979).

Birth Defects: Original Article Series, Volume 18, Number 6, pages 101–118

These studies are far more than the normal doctor-patient relationship of clinical investigation and are an active collaboration of the informed volunteer in research projects.

This association of sufferers and scientists has resulted in the emergence of eye donor schemes in the U.K., the U.S.A. and Canada. The mechanics of such schemes vary but in the U.K. volunteer R.P.sufferers carry plastic cards which confirm the patients' willingness for their eyes to be used for research purposes in event of their death. Eyes of young sufferers with early disease-induced changes most commonly become available as the result of a fatal accident. Even with donor schemes and the prior consent of the patient, legal proceedings often delay laboratory access to tissue so that its subsequent uses are limited. A more promising source of material exhibiting mild or early disease is female carriers of X-linked disease who, in many cases, retain useful vision into the 6th or 7th decade of life.

In reality however, the majority of eyes obtained by donor schemes will be in an advanced state of the disease with few, if any photoreceptor cells. But in contrast, all cases will have retinal pigment epithelium. In these situations with limited amounts of tissue and delayed access to organs, tissue culture techniques, although confined to a single cell type, seem to offer one of the few means of dynamic investigations of genetic defects.

Our research therefore has three primary aims:-

(1) To culture human retinal pigment epithelial cells and to characterise such cultures.

(2) To compare the cultured cells with those *in vivo*.

(3) To compare and contrast human pigment epithelial cells from normal and diseased individuals to assess any genetically induced defect.

ISOLATION

In our study control eyes with no known ophthalmic disease are collected from hospital mortuaries and diseased tissue obtained via the British Retinitis Pigmentosa Eye Donor Scheme.

Human retinal pigment epithelial cells are isolated using a modification of the technique described by Ross Edwards (1981). In this the eye cup, devoid of vitreous and neural retina, is filled with 0.25% trypsin and incubated at 37°C for 1-2 hours followed by gentle aspiration to remove retinal pigment epithelial cells. Our method involves the above trypsinisation procedure but on discrete areas of pigment epithelium contained within stainless steel cylinders whose external boundaries are sealed in place with vaseline (Fig.1). The size of the cylinders may

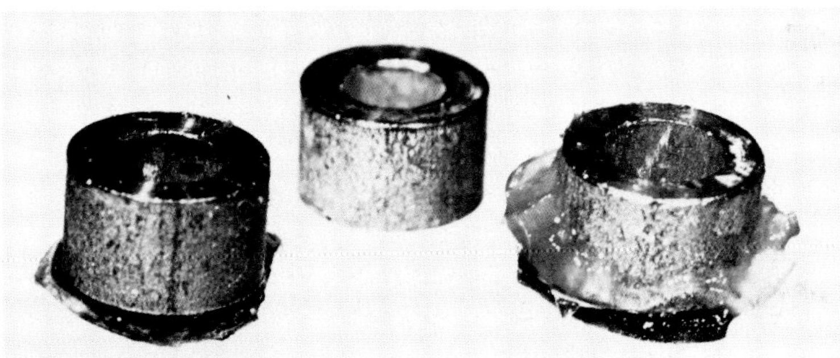

Fig.1. The cylinders used for isolating human retinal pigment epithelial cells.

be made larger or smaller depending on the size of tissue available. Our modification facilitates: (1) the isolation of cells from different foci within the retina, (2) the use of small pieces of tissue when individual eyes need to be shared between laboratories and (3) may allow the utilisation of retinal biopsy material from either conventional surgical or vitrectomy procedures.

GROWTH CHARACTERISTICS

Isolated cells are placed in plastic culture vessels containing Ham's F10 medium supplemented with 20% foetal calf serum, 0.4% glucose and antibiotics (penicillin, streptomycin and kannamycin). Cells are usually plated out in concentrations of 5 - 10 x 10^4 cells/17mm diameter multiwells. Within 9 days 10-35% of cells become attached to the culture vessel. Plating efficiency can be increased by 10-18% if the plastic substrate is precoated with rat tail collagen (Paul, 1975). Cell attachment appears to be dependent on both donor age and postmortem time (i.e. time between death and enucleation) of the eye (Fig.2). Following adherence individual cells flatten dorso-ventrally, their diameter increase by 3-8 times that of their dormant <u>in vitro</u> size. At the same time cytoplasmic processes appear randomly distributed around each cell. Usually during the second and third weeks in culture a fraction of the cells begin to divide and from this stage onwards three distinct cell types are observed:-

(1) Giant multinucleate cells which are heavily pigmented containing up to seven nuclei and do not divide.

(2) Stationary cells which are heavily pigmented and remain at the outgrowth stage (Fig.3).

(3) Actively dividing cells (Fig.3) which are smaller and are formed from the division of cells at the outgrowth stage. These cells progressively depigment as a result of sharing the initial complement of pigment granules amongst an increasing number of daughter cells.

The ratio of stationary to dividing cells is related to donor age (Fig.4). Also, both the initial lag phase (the time between isolation and cell division) and the rate of proliferation show an age dependence with eyes from young donors exhibiting a shorter lag phase and increased division rate when compared with eyes from older donors (Fig.5). These results support those previously published (Flood and Gouras, 1981). The

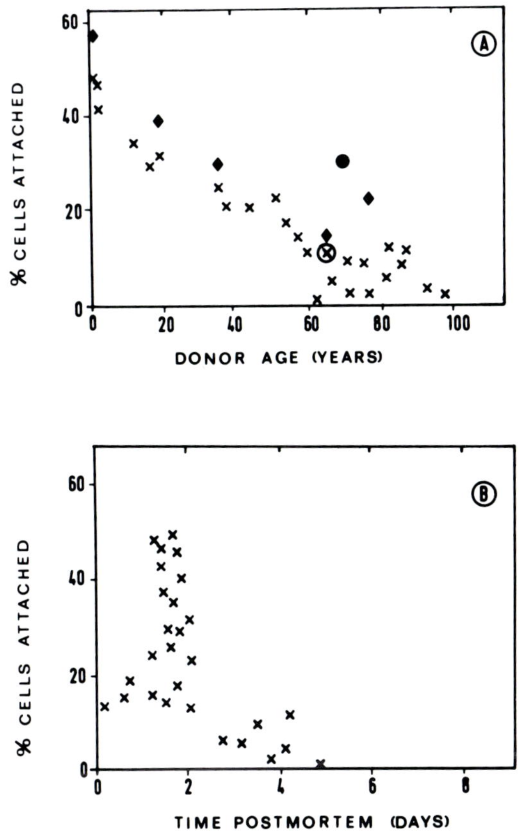

Fig.2. The effect of donor age and time post-mortem on the attachment of human retinal pigment epithelial cells. (A) × = control cells on a plastic substrate; ⊗ = RP cells on plastic substrate; ● = abnormal control cells (71yr) on plastic substrate; ◆ = control cells on rat tail collagen substrate. (B) Results are derived from control cells from donors less than 45 years old. All data points are from a minimum of two cultures from the same donor.

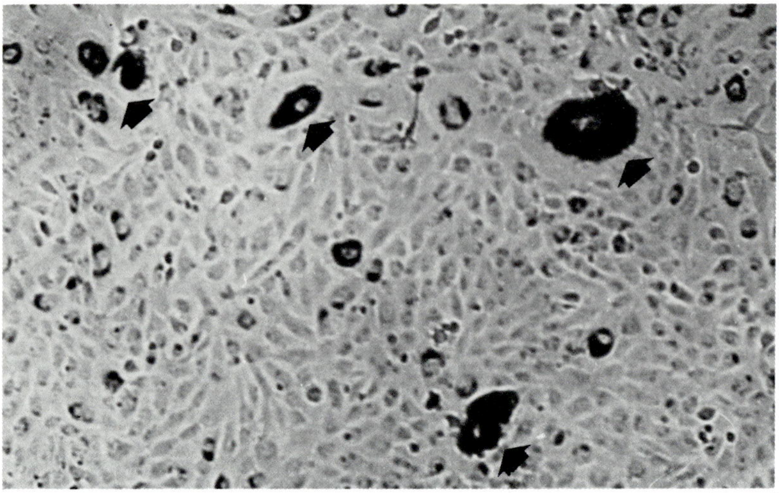

Fig.3. Photomicrograph of cultured human retinal pigment epithelial cells 27 days after isolation from a 48 year old donor. Large heavily pigmented cells (arrowed) are interspersed with smaller less-pigmented actively dividing cells. x 220.

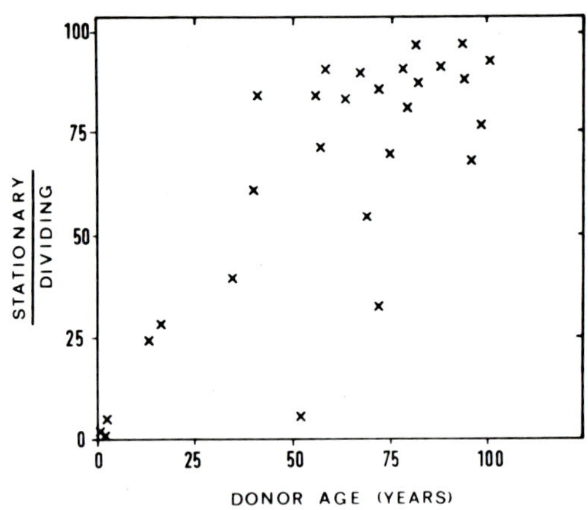

Fig.4. A graph of the ratio of stationery to actively dividing human retinal pigment epithelial cells in primary culture isolated from donors of varying ages. Each point represents data from a minimum of two cultures from the same donor.

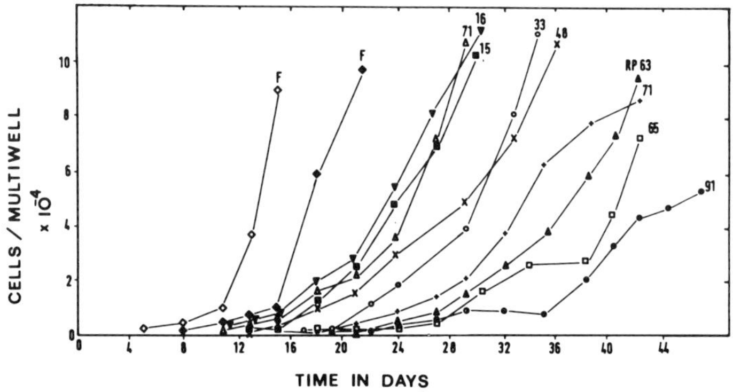

Fig. 5. A graph showing growth curves of human retinal pigment epithelial cells isolated from donors of different ages. Cells were grown in 17mm diameter wells, and cell numbers obtained by counting different areas within each well and calculating the total number per well. Donor ages are given at the top of each curve. F = foetal donors, RP = autosomal recessive Retinitis Pigmentosa eye mentioned in the text.All data are from a minimum of two cultures from the same donor.

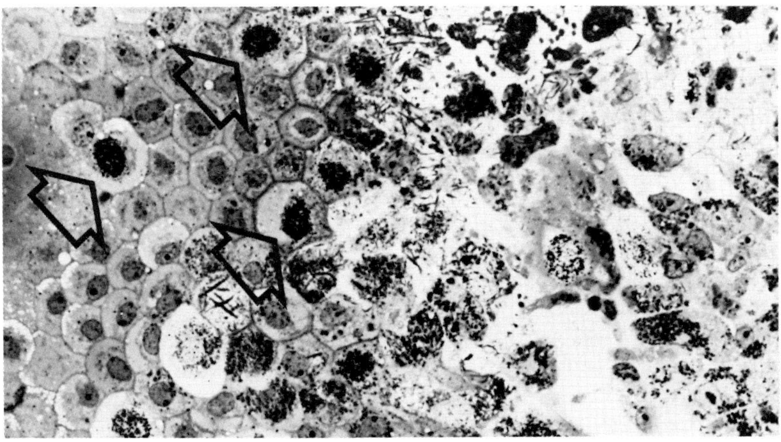

Fig.6. Light microscopic autoradiograph of adult pig pigment epithelium four days after exposure to argon laser radiation, showing incorporation of ^{3}H-thymidine into the nucleus of dividing cells. x 822.

growth curve for retinal pigment epithelial cells isolated from a 63 year donor suffering from an autosomal recessive R.P. show a normal fit. We have cells from a 71 year control eye with no observed ophthalmic disease which demonstrate atypical characteristics for such an age.

It should be mentioned at this stage that retinal pigment epithelial cells in vivo only divide under conditions of severe stress e.g. photocoagulation (Fig.6). We must therefore assume that dividing cells in vitro are a result of a stressful experience.

Actively dividing cells continue undergoing division until a confluent monolayer of non-pigmented hexanocuboidal cells is formed (Fig.7).

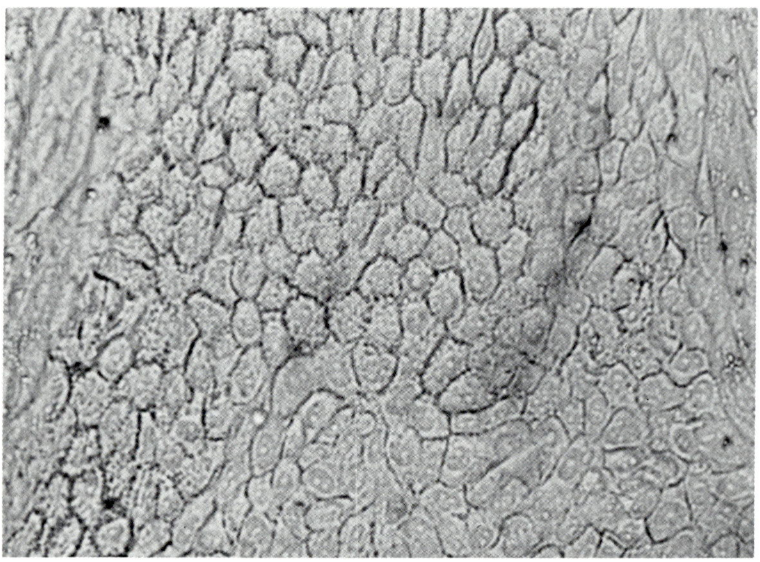

Fig.7. Light micrograph of a confluent culture of human retinal pigment epithelial cells established from a 33 year old donor. x 580

These cells can be repeatedly subcultured; however, in all cultures there are a maximum number of subcultures, which varies between donors, before a crisis period occurs and the cells no longer exhibit cell division. Cells may be stored at any stage during their growth phase using standard liquid nitrogen freezing techniques (May, 1972). Freezing enables storage of cells until new specialised techniques become available and allow cultures to be sent to other laboratories.

MORPHOLOGY

Confluent cultures are examined by both scanning and transmission electron microscopy and component cells are seen to retain many of their *in vivo* characteristics.

Cells re-establish polarity under culture conditions and exhibit similar morphology to the *in vivo* situation. The apical surface is covered with microvilli (Fig.8), which are shorter and thicker than those seen *in vivo*. This is perhaps not surprising considering the growth conditions and lack of rod outer segment pigment epithelium contact. In contrast, the complex basal invaginations seen *in vivo* are either greatly reduced or lost altogether in cells grown on a plastic substrate. However, the cells are capable of producing a collagenous basement membrane.

In confluent cultures cell-to-cell contact is associated with the development of gap junctions, but, as yet, tight junctions are not observed. The cells retain a large basal nucleus but the numbers of cytoplasmic organelles (i.e. golgi bodies, mitochondria, and endoplasmic reticulum) are depleted (Fig.9) compared with *in vivo* cells (Hogan et al., 1971). No pigment granules are observed in subcultured cells and only reduced numbers are identified in primary cultures. *In vivo*, pigment is produced during a limited induction period in embryogenesis and is only seen to be made in later life during pathology such as melanoma. It has been reported (Eguchi, 1979) that

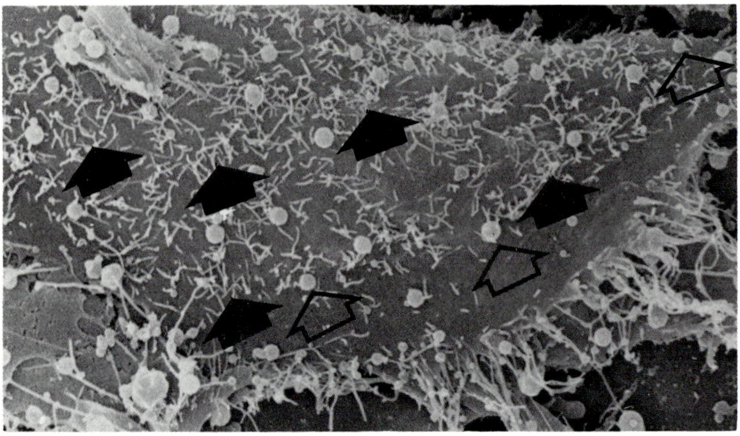

Fig.8. Scanning electron micrograph of a human retinal pigment epithelial cell in vitro, isolated from a 33 year old donor. The apical surface is covered with short microvilli (fine arrows) and as the cell had previously been challenged with latex microspheres (open arrows) these are visible on the surface. x 3,700.

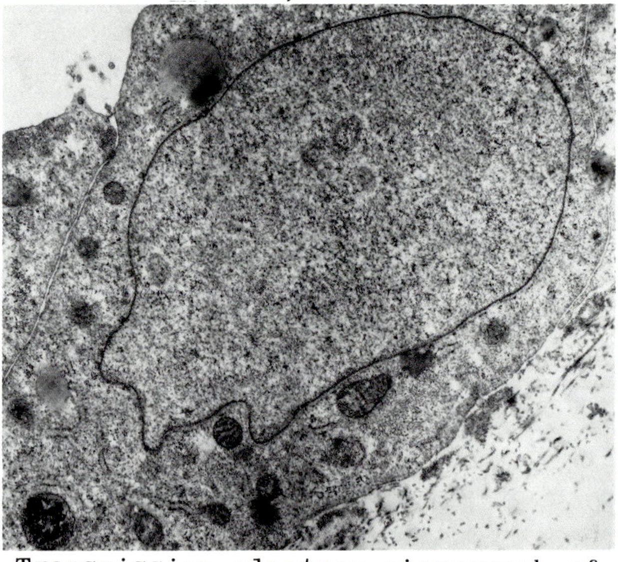

Fig.9. Transmission electron micrograph of a cultured human retinal pigment epithelial cell. x 10,000. (Courtesy of Dr.B.P.Hayes).

foetal chick and human retinal pigment epithelial cells in culture do repigment indicating that melanogensis is occurring, but cells isolated from more mature donors, despite the stress of *in vitro* techniques, do not repigment in culture. This absence of pigmentation in cultured retinal pigment epithelial cells may result in alteration of cellular characteristics, which *in vivo* are interrelated with the presence of pigment (i.e. enzyme action, transport and binding properties and electrophysiological responses).

TRANSEPITHELIAL TRANSPORT

A major difficulty in studying transport systems in retinal pigment epithelium cells *in vitro* is that cells are normally cultured on an impermeable plastic substrate and thus it is impossible to challenge the choroid side of the cells (i.e. the side through which the metabolites normally enter). We have overcome this problem by growing cells to confluence on a commercially available polycarbonate membrane precoated with rat tail collagen (Fig.10a). This membrane plus cell layer may then be placed in a specially constructed chamber (Fig.10b) where the composition of the fluid on either side may be varied at will. The biochemistry of membrane receptor sites, transepithelial transport, and if barrier functions are present, the electro-potential of cell monolayers may thus be studied. The obvious experiment to start with is to study retinol binding protein receptor sites and retinol transport since *in vivo* characteristics are well documented (Bok and Heller, 1976; Saari et al., 1977; Bok and Heller, 1980).

PHAGOCYTOSIS

Since it has been shown in the RCS rat that the defective gene is expressed solely in the retinal pigment epithelium and renders these cells incapable of ingesting rod outer segments (Mullen, 1976), we consider it worthwhile to

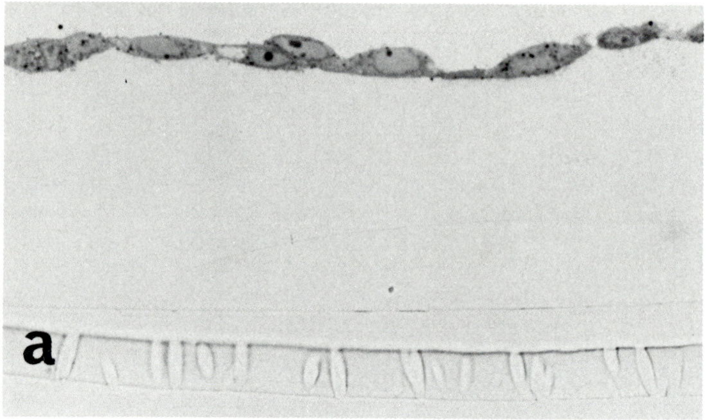

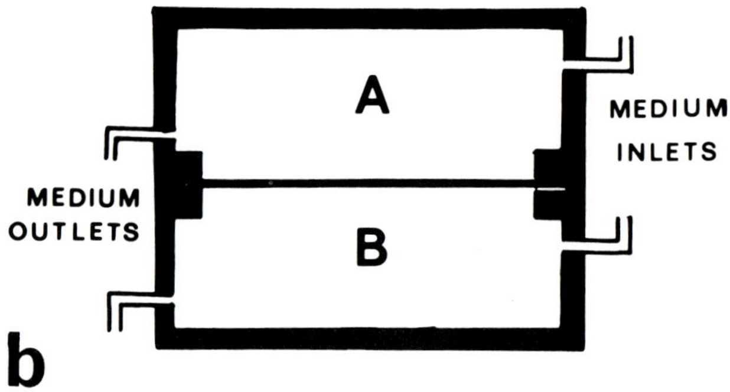

Fig.10. (a) Photomicrograph of human retinal pigment epithelial cells cultured on a polycarbonate membrane pre-coated with rat tail collagen. x 600. The cell monolayer has detached from the membrane during preparation. (b) Diagrammatic representation of the chamber we intend to use for transport studies.

examine the phagocytic capability of cultured human retinal pigment epithelial cells.

In an initial series of experiments human retinal pigment epithelial cells in culture were challenged with latex microspheres. Electron microscopy shows ingestion of such abiotic particles occur (Fig.11a) after an initial lag phase of 2-4 hours. Obviously, it would be preferable to challenge the cells with rod outer segments but the supply of fresh human rod outer segments is limited. Experiments using these outer segments cannot exploit labelling techniques other than those involving surface sugars. Clearly, the phagocytosis of discs in isolated rod outer segments may demonstrate selectivity with a preference for older discs near the rod tip. This has to be investigated and can only be demonstrated using animal rod outer segments. Electron microscopy shows that our cells will phagocytise human, bovine, rat and mouse rod outer segments (Fig.11b) prepared by the technique of O'Brien and Muellenberg (1974).

Quantitation of phagocytosis is easily obtained using scintillation counting techniques and we have examined the uptake of rod outer segments prelabelled with tritiated choline. Retinae are isolated and then incubated in culture medium supplemented with H^3-choline for 1 hour (Goldmann et al., 1979). Rod outer segments are subsequently prepared as previously described. Confluent monolayers of retinal pigment epithelial cells are challenged with these rod outer segment preparations for different time periods. The uptake of radioactivity within the pigment epithelial cells is measured with a scintillation counter. Figure 12 shows that in both human and C57 mouse retinal pigment epithelial cells, bovine rod outer segments are progressively ingested over an initial 2 hour period. This is followed by a plateau phase when little or no further uptake occurs. A second burst of ingestion follows after 8-10 hours. This plateau or rest period may result from the lack of suitable apical membrane due to its initial loss in phagocytosis. That is to say phagocytosis

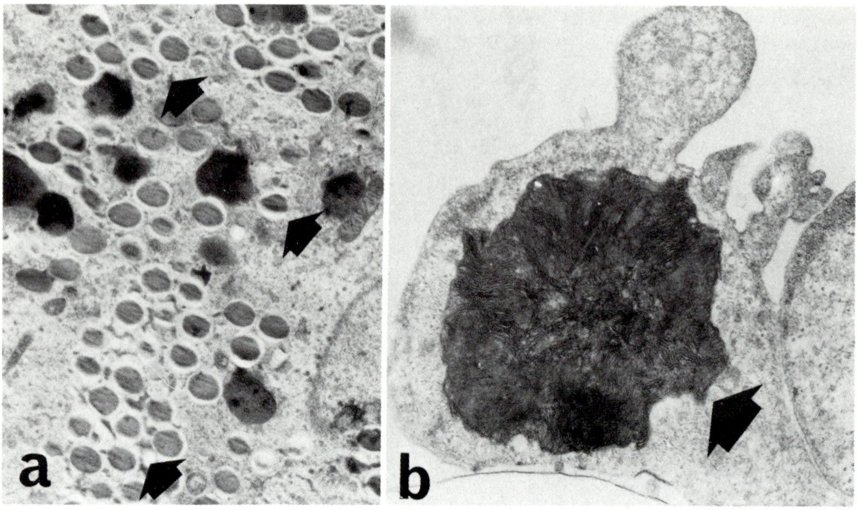

Fig.11. Transmission electron micrograph of human retinal pigment epithelial cells in culture showing engulfment of (a) latex microspheres (arrowed) x 5,000 and (b) bovine rod outer segments (arrowed) x 10,000.

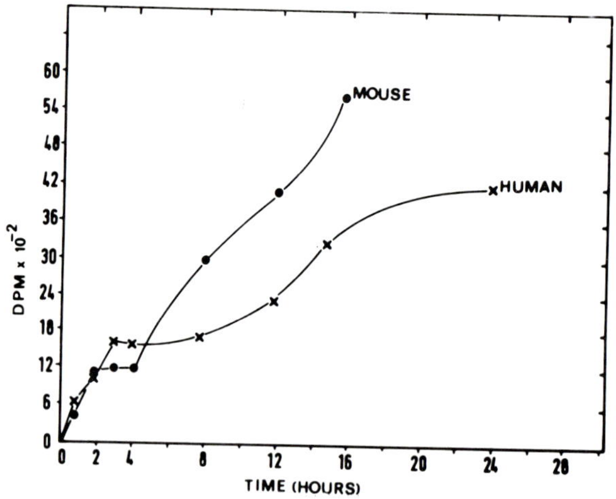

Fig.12. Graph of the uptake of bovine rod outer segments pre-labelled with H^3-choline.

consists of a particle being wrapped in cell membrane before both particle and membrane components are taken into the cell. Thus each phagosome involves a significant loss of retinal pigment epithelium apical cell membrane and at some point insufficient new membrane is available on the cell's production line to support further engulfment.

Since, in practice, each individual retinal pigment epithelial cell culture will be challenged with different rod outer segment preparations, it is imperative that some attempt be made to standardise before comparison of phagocytic capability can be made in different cultures or cells from different origins (e.g. control v dystrophic). This may be overcome by storing all cell lines in liquid nitrogen and at a suitable date challenging these cultures with the same rod outer segment preparation. Since the latter is not always expedient an attempt is being made to obtain standardisation by measuring the variable factors involved; (1) the amount of label incorporated by rod outer segment preparations on any given exposure, (2) the surface area of pigment epithelial cells exposed to labelled outer segments and the number of cells/unit area, (3) the relative numbers of rod outer segments engulfed per individual cell in any given time, and (4) the rate at which label is lost from the retinal pigment epithelium. Values for each of these factors should hopefully provide an index for the phagocytic capability of different cell cultures.

In vivo, engulfed phagosomes pass through a degredation sequence and the resulting products may be; (1) re-incorporated into the cell metabolism, (2) voided into the choriocapillaries and (3) retained within the cell as residual bodies (i.e. lipofuschin). The rate of decay of phagosomes is related to age, being more rapid in young individuals than in the old. In the aged both the reduction in rate and the capacity of the degredation process lead to build up of waste products both within and beneath the retinal pigment epithelium, e.g. drusen. If the rate of loss of labelled material from cultured cells is monitored a ratio of voiding of lytic products to re-incorporated label in relation to age of donor may be tabulated. Such data will thus enable comparison of rod outer segment degredation between normal and dystrophic eyes.

CONCLUSIONS

Using human material we have:-

(1) Developed an isolation technique suitable for topographic sampling of eyes and biopsy material.

((2) Established cell lines for a range of normal and one pair of dystrophic eyes.

(3) Accumulated data on growth and morphology characteristics in relation to age.

(4) Developed an artificial membrane system in order to study transport and barrier problems.

(5) Begun to assess phagocytosis with regard to donor age, time in culture and disease.

ACKNOWLEDGEMENTS

We are grateful to the British Retinitis Pigmentosa Society, the Wellcome Trust and the Smith Kline and French Foundation for financial support. We thank Doctors G. Clover and C.F.J. Grindle and colleagues for enabling us to obtain human eyes and Mr.P.West for assistance in the scanning electron microscopy results.

REFERENCES

Airaksinen EM, Airaksinen MM, Shivola P, Shivola M, Tuovinen E (1979). Uptake of taurine by platelets in Retinitis Pigmentosa. Lancet Mar.3rd: p474.

Arden GB, Fox B (1979). Increased incidence of abnormal nasal cilia in patients with Retinitis Pigmentosa. Nature 279:p534.

Bok D, Heller J (1976). Transport of blood to the retina: An autoradiographic study of the pigment epithelial cell surface receptor for plasma retinol-binding protein. Exp Eye Res 22: 395.

Bok D, Heller J (1980). Autoradiographic localisation of serum retinol-binding protein receptors on the pigment epithelium of dystrophic rat retinas. Invest Ophthalmol Visual Sci 19: 1405.

Edwards RB,(1981). Culture of mammalian retinal pigment epithelium and neural retina. In Packer L (ed): "Visual pigments and purple membranes," A volume of Methods of Enzymology: New York: Academic Press (In Press).

Eguchi G (1979). "Transdifferentiation" in pigmented epithelial cells of vertebrate eyes in vitro. In Ebert and Okada (eds): "Mechanisms of cell change," Wiley, 273.

Flood MT, Gouras P (1981). The organisation of human retinal pigment epithelium in vitro. Vision Res 21: 119.

Goldmann AI, O'Brien PJ, Masterson E, Israel P, Tierstein P, Chader G (1978). A quantitative system for studying phagocytosis in pigment epithelium tissue culture. Exp Eye Res 28: 455.

Hogan MJ, Alvarado JA, Weddell JE (1971). "Histology of the Human Eye" Philadelphia: Saunders, p 405.

May J (1972). Sub-zero cell storage. In Wasley G (ed): "Animal Tissue Culture: Advances in Technique," Butterworths, p139.

Mullen R, LaVail M (1976). Inherited retinal dystrophy: A primary defect in pigment epithelium determined with experimental rat chimeras. Science 192: 799.

O'Brien PJ, Mullenberg CG (1974). The biosynthesis of rhodopsin in vitro. Exp Eye Res 18: 241.

Paul J (1975). "Cell and Tissue Culture." Edinburgh London and New York: Churchill Livingstone,p77.

Saari JC, Bunt AH, Futterman S, Berman E (1977). Localization of cellular retinol-binding protein in bovine retina and retinal pigment epithelium, with a consideration of the pigment epithelium isolation technique. Invest Ophthalmol Visual Sci 16: 797.

HEREDITARY RETINAL DEGENERATIONS IN THE DOG: SPECIFICITY OF ABNORMAL CYCLIC NUCLEOTIDE METABOLISM TO DISEASES OF ARRESTED PHOTORECEPTOR DEVELOPMENT.

Gustavo Aguirre,[1] Gregory Acland,[2] Gerald Chader,[3] University of Pennsylvania Schools of Veterinary Medicine (1) and Medicine (1, 2) and Laboratory of Vision Research, National Eye Institute (3).

University of Pennsylvania, 3800 Spruce Street
Philadelphia, Penna. 19104

The cyclic nucleotides, cyclic 3':5'-adenosine or guanosine monophosphate (cAMP or cGMP, respectively) are found in high concentration in the vertebrate retina. The role of cGMP in normal rod photoreceptor maintenance and function is suggested by the high intracellular concentration, nucleotide compartmentalization and modulation of levels in a light-dependent manner (Miki et al., 1973; Chader et al., 1974; Fletcher and Chader, 1976; Orr et al., 1976; Woodruff et al., 1977). A similar role has been proposed more recently for cAMP function in cone photoreceptors (Farber, 1981).

Cyclic nucleotide concentration is regulated by the enzymes responsible for synthesis (nucleotide cyclase) and hydrolysis (nucleotide phosphodiesterase (PDE)). The phosphodiesterase is the only enzyme capable of metabolizing the cyclic nucleotides and is, therefore, crucial in controlling the concentration of these intracellular messengers (Chader et al., in press).

Visual cell viability depends on the maintenance of normal intracellular cyclic nucleotide levels by the carefully balanced processes of cyclic nucleotide synthesis and hydrolysis. <u>In vitro</u> studies with differentiating amphibian (Lolley, et al., 1977) or adult human (Ulshafer and Hollyfield, 1981) retinas have shown that arrested photoreceptor differentiation and/or degeneration occurs when PDE activity is inhibited. These <u>in vitro</u> studies followed earlier reports demonstrating the association between abnormal cyclic nucleotide function and hereditary photoreceptor degeneration (Farber and Lolley, 1974; 1976).

In C3H mice with recessively inherited retinal degenera-

Birth Defects: Original Article Series, Volume 18, Number 6, pages 119–133

tion (rd), photoreceptor development is normal during the early postnatal period. Then, just as inner segments are elongating and outer segments start to form, differentiation arrests; visual cells fail to develop further and subsequently degenerate. The entire process of arrested photoreceptor differentiation, degeneration and loss of visual cells and nuclei from the retina takes place between 10 and 20 days of age (Farber and Lolley, 1974, 1976; Lolley and Farber, 1976).

An abnormality in retinal cGMP metabolism occurs before the visual cells of rd mice begin to degenerate. Microdissection of normal mouse retinas shows that 2 kinetic classes of cGMP-PDE are present: a high and a low Km enzyme localized, respectively, in the photoreceptor and inner retinal layers. In rd mice, a deficient activity of the photoreceptor specific (high Km) cGMP-PDE results in the marked elevation of retinal cGMP levels; this appears to cause the subsequent photoreceptor degeneration. The elevation of cGMP levels precedes morphologic evidence of visual cell disease. Levels rise rapidly to peak at the stage of maximal visual cell degeneration and fall after visual cells and their nuclei disappear from the photoreceptor layer (20 days of age) (Farber and Lolley, 1974, 1976; Lolley and Farber, 1976).

These elegant studies emphasize the importance of proper regulation of cyclic nucleotide levels in maintaining photoreceptor viability. We were prompted to ask if similar abnormalities in retinal cyclic nucleotide metabolism might exist in other inherited retinal degenerations. If so, then photoreceptor diseases in different species could have similar pathogenetic mechanisms. This could then be extrapolated to selected retinal degenerative diseases that affect man, thus providing guidance for studies of the very limited supplies of human retinal tissues.

To address this question we have examined inherited retinal degenerative diseases in different breeds of dogs (Table 1). These diseases, known collectively as progressive retinal atrophy (PRA), are characterized by: 1) night blindness followed by day blindness; 2) histologically confirmed outer retinal degeneration; 3) ophthalmoscopically visible retinal thinning, vascular attenuation and loss (Aguirre, 1976). They are analogous to retinitis pigmentosa (RP) in man (Cogan and Kuwabara, 1965). PRA is recessively inherited in all breeds so far examined; however, the diseases are genetically distinct at least in three different affected breeds (Table 1) (Acland, et al., 1980; Aguirre, 1976). The diseases present in these 3 breeds of dogs are examples, respectively, of arrested differentiation, abnormal development, and degeneration of photoreceptors. These are discussed individually.

Table 1: Characteristics of Retinal Diseases in Three Canine Breeds

	IRISH SETTER	NORWEGIAN ELKHOUND	MINIATURE POODLE
Disease	Rod-cone dysplasia	Rod dysplasia	Progressive rod-cone degeneration
Age of Ophthalmoscopic Diagnosis	12-16 weeks	1-2 years	2½-4 years
Age of Blindness	6m-1 year	1-3 years	3-5 years
Electro-retinography	Absent rod mediated responses; cone mediated responses lower in amplitude, prolonged in latency.	Absent rod mediated responses.	Rod and cone mediated responses develop normally; with degeneration reponse amplitude decreases.
Pathology	Arrested differentiation of rods and cones. Rod damage more extensive than cone damage.	Abnormal development of rod photoreceptors.	Normal photoreceptor development; slow degeneration of outer segments.
References	Aguirre, 1976 Aguirre and Rubin, 1975 Aguirre et al., 1978; 1981 (in press) Buyukmihci et al., 1980 Chader et al., 1981, (in press) Liu et al., 1979	Acland, et al., 1980 Aguirre, 1978	Aguirre, 1976 Aguirre and Rubin, 1973 Aguirre et al., 1981 (in press)

ARRESTED PHOTORECEPTOR DIFFERENTIATION (Rod-Cone Dysplasia in Irish Setters)

The canine retina is undeveloped at birth. Between 5-7 days of age, photoreceptor inner segments begin to elongate through the external limiting membrane and contact the pigment epithelium. Waves of maturation, beginning at the posterior pole and progressing to the periphery, gradually result in the formation of the outer segment; the outer and inner segments continue to elongate, and the retina matures by 6 weeks of age (Fig. 1).

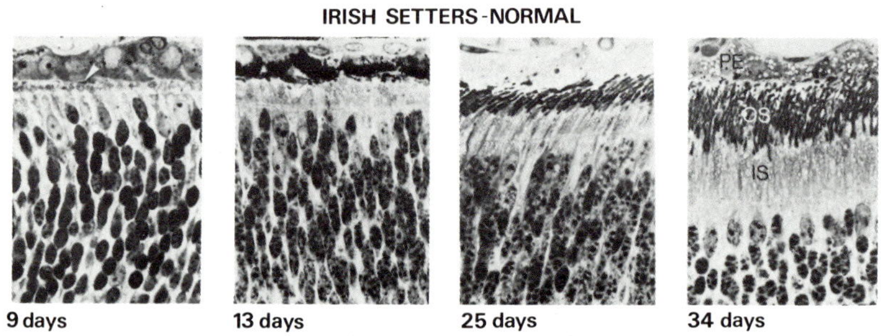

Figure 1: Developing retina of normal Irish setters. At 9 days or age, outer segment material (white arrowhead) is limited in the yet undeveloped photoreceptor layer. By 34 days of age, inner and outer segments (IS: OS) have developed. PE=pigment epithelium. (x440).

In Irish setters homozygous recessive for the rod-cone dysplasia gene, the retina is indistinguishable from normal between 5 and 13 days of age; this is the stage of photoreceptor inner segment elongation and initial formation of the outer segment. After 16 days of age, however, photoreceptor development fails to progress. This arrested development is most prominent in rods which remain diminutive without a well-formed outer segment (Figure 2).

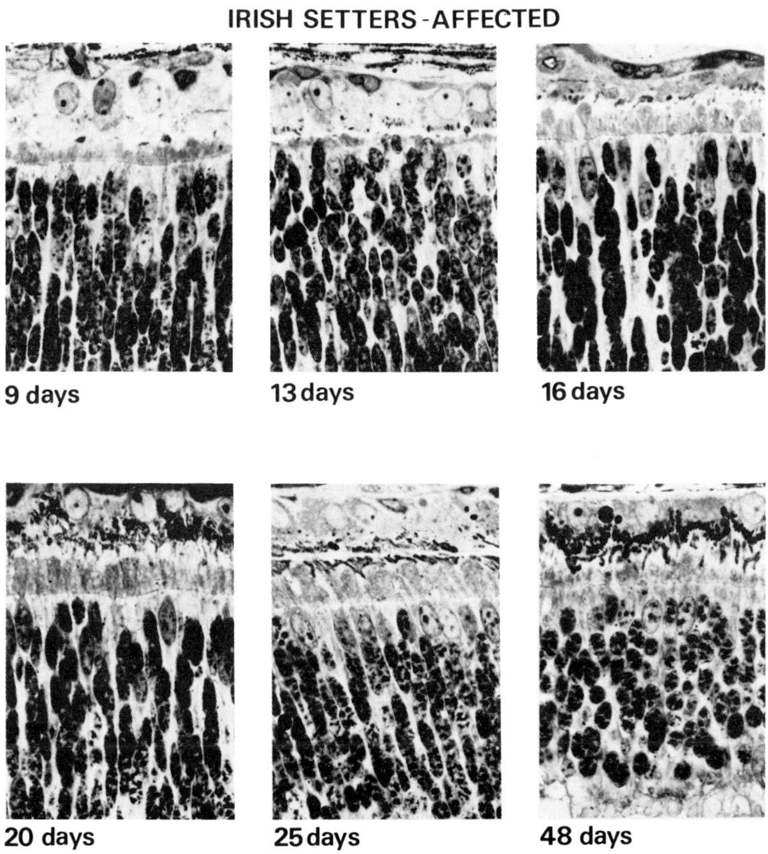

Figure 2: Developing retina of affected Irish setters. Retina is normal at 9 and 13 days. By 16 days, photoreceptors fail to develop as in normals; rod inner segments remain small and outer segments (note 20 and 25 days) fail to elongate as in normals. Visual cell degeneration reduces width of outer nuclear layer by 48 days. (x625).

Degeneration of visual cells begins at this time and gradually results in a decrease in the thickness of the outer nuclear layer (Figure 2). The initial, rapid photoreceptor degeneration is limited to rods, and broad prominent cones remain in the photoreceptor layer (Fig. 3).

With time, continual loss of photoreceptors and their nuclei progresses (Fig. 4). By approximately one year of age, the inner nuclear layer is adjacent to the pigment epithelium (Aguirre, 1976; Aguirre et al., in press; Aguirre and Rubin, 1975; Buyukmihci et al., 1980).

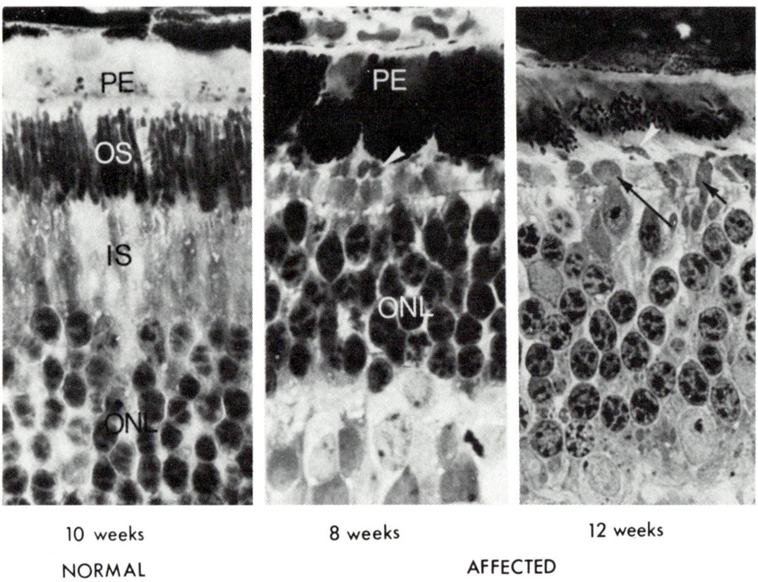

Figure 3: Photoreceptor layer from normal and rod-cone dysplasia affected Irish setters. In affected dogs, the photoreceptor layer is reduced in width, and there is minimal outer segment (OS) material (arrowheads). Loss of rods results in increased prominence of cones (black arrows) and a decreased outer nuclear layer (ONL) width. (PE=pigment epithelium; IS=inner segment) (x965). From Aguirre et al., 1978.

Even though rod-cone dysplasia in Irish setters differs temporally from rd in mice, the diseases are similar in the evolution of the photoreceptor abnormalities. By both light and electron microscopy, the photoreceptors in both species are normal in the initial stages of postnatal differentiation. Similarly in both, the disease becomes evident when photoreceptor outer segments begin to form. Afterwards, arrested visual cell differentiation and the degeneration occurs.

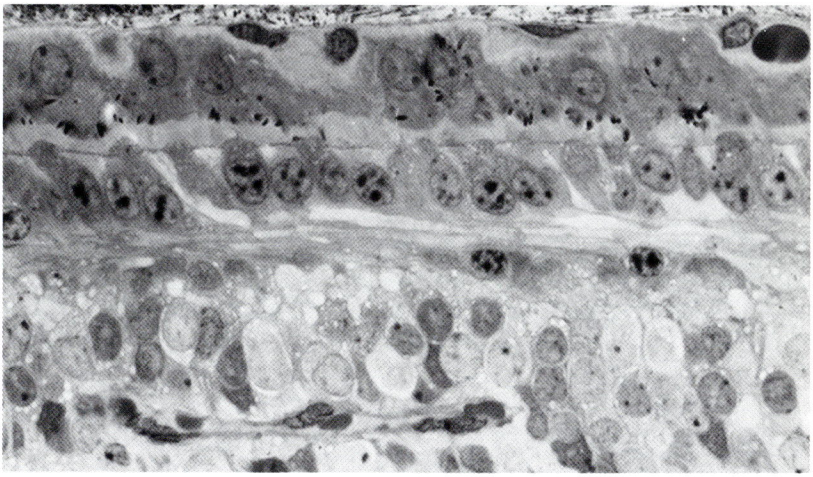

Figure 4: Retina from the posterior pole of an 8½-month old rod-cone dysplasia affected Irish setter. There is loss of photoreceptors and their nuclei. The single cell wide outer nuclear layer consists primarily of cone nuclei. Inner retinal layers are normal. (x1000).

As in rd mice, a defect in retinal cGMP metabolism is also present in affected Irish setters. In dogs whose retinas show advanced retinal degeneration, i.e. 8-12 weeks of age (Fig. 3), there is approximately a 10-fold elevation in retinal cGMP compared to control (Table 2). This abnormality is restricted to cGMP in the retina since other tissues, including the pigment epithelium-choroid complex, show no abnormalities. Cyclic AMP levels are normal (Aguirre et al., 1978; Chader et al., in press).

In retinal homogenates of control-dog retina, two kinetic types (low and high Km) of PDE activity are observed. In the affected retinas, however, only the low Km type is found (Table 2) (Aguirre et al., 1978). The abnormally high concentration of cGMP appears to result from the deficient activity of the high Km enzyme. By analogy to the situation that exists in the rd mouse, the high Km, photoreceptor specific, cGMP-PDE is absent in both rd in mice and rod-cone dysplasia affected Irish setters.

Table 2: Rod-Cone Dysplasia (Irish Setters); Retinal Cyclic Nucleotide Concentrations

Group	Neural Retina*			
	cGMP-PDE		Cyclic Nucleotides (pmol/mg protein)	
	High Km	Low Km	cAMP	cGMP
Control	1.2×10^{-4}M	2.0×10^{-5}M	12	12±0.7
Affected	0	1.8×10^{-5}M	12	102±8.6

*Neural retinas obtained from 8- and 12-week old affected (n=10 eyes) and 10-week old control (n=8 eyes) animals.

(Table modified from Aguirre, et al., 1978.)

Table 3: Correlation of Retinal cGMP Levels and Morphology During Postnatal Retinal Development

Postnatal Age (Days)	Control* RETINA		Affected RETINA	
	cGMP**	Morphology***	cGMP**	Morphology***
5	2	Normal	-	Normal
6	(2)	Normal	.1	Normal
7	1	Normal	-	-
9	1	Normal	3	Normal
10	(1), 2	Normal	9	Normal
11	-	-	3	Normal
12	-	-	3	Normal
13	-	-	23	Normal
14	(2), 4	Normal	-	-
16	-	-	36	Affected

*Control animals consist of homozygous normal and (heterozygotes).

**Retinal cGMP concentration (pmol/mg protein).

***Retinal morphology - masked light and electron microscopic examination to determine status.

(Table modified from Aguirre et al., in press.)

These studies do not establish a causal relation between the cGMP metabolic defect and visual cell degeneration in the dog. Since the retinal degeneration was at an advanced stage at the time the cGMP levels were elevated, it is possible that the observed changes were secondary to the photoreceptor abnormality rather than being primary.

We now know, however, that the elevation in cyclic nucleotide levels precedes morphologic evidence of degeneration (Table 3). Although levels are higher than control values at 10 and 13 days of age, it is not until 16 days of age that morphologic abnormalities are evident (Aguirre et al., in press).

ABNORMAL PHOTORECEPTOR DEVELOPMENT (Rod Dysplasia in Norwegian Elkhounds)

Not all the retinal diseases that occur during postnatal development result in the marked arrest in photoreceptor differentiation evident in Irish setters with rod-cone dysplasia. At least one disease (rod dysplasia) results in a structurally more developed albeit abnormal visual cell (Aguirre, 1978).

In rod dysplasia, rod differentiation is abnormal. At the time when the normal dog retina has matured, the rod dysplastic retina has well-developed structurally normal cones but diseased rods (Fig. 5). Unlike rod-cone dysplasia where the diminutive rod inner segments fail to form a distinct and broad outer segment layer, the rods in rod dysplasia form more developed but structurally abnormal rod outer segments. Lamellar disorientation and disorganization are characteristic of these diseased rods.

Because of the limited number of affected dogs available for study, the sequence of aberrant rod photoreceptor morphogenesis is unknown at this time. However, the more advanced state of development of the rods in this disease suggests that the lesion occurs at a later time in development or is, alternatively, less severe.

Retinal cyclic nucleotide content of affected elkhounds at the peak of the developmental defect (prior to the onset of photoreceptor degeneration (Fig. 5)) does not differ from that of littermate controls (Table 4). In contrast to rod-cone dysplasia, rod dysplasia in the Norwegian elkhound does not appear to represent a defect in cyclic nucleotide metabolism.

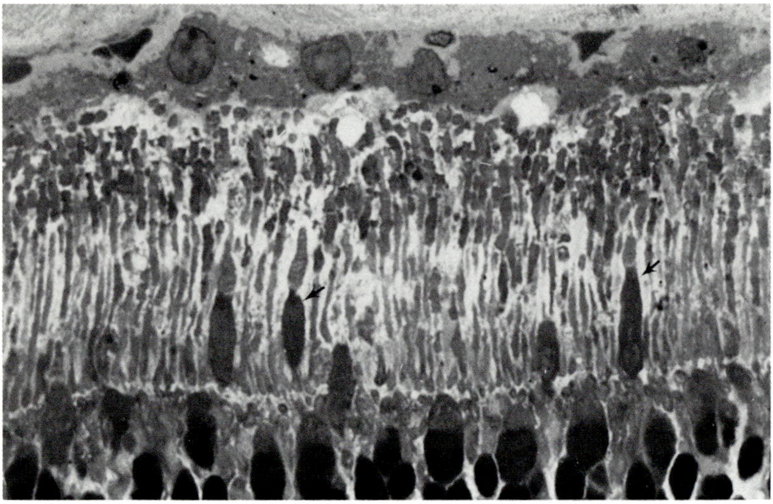

Figure 5: Photoreceptor layer from 6-week old rod-dysplasia affected Norwegian elkhound. Cones (small arrow) are normal. Outer segment layer contains disorganized and disoriented rod outer segment material. (x1150).

Table 4: Rod Dysplasia (Norwegian Elkhounds): Cyclic GMP Concentration in Ocular Tissues

	cGMP Concentration (pmol/mg protein)	
Group	Neural Retina	Pigment Epithelium-Choroid
Control (6-8 wks.)	9.5±2.7	1.7±.8
Affected (6-6½ wks.)	9.5±.5	1.9±.3

PHOTORECEPTOR DEGENERATION (Progressive Rod-Cone Degeneration in Miniature Poodles)

Progressive rod-cone degeneration (PRCD) in miniature poodles is a late-onset slowly progressive disease of both rod and cone photoreceptors. Unlike rod-cone dysplasia and rod dysplasia, photoreceptor development is normal as measured by electrophysiology and ultrastructure (Aguirre, 1976; Aguirre et al., in press; Aguirre and Rubin, 1972).

Early in the disease, however, photoreceptor outer segments show disorientation of the lamellar discs and apparent ruptures or excrescences from the cell membrane of the outer segment (Aguirre, 1976; Aguirre et al., in press). These ultrastructural abnormalities occur by 6-9 weeks of age in the distal half of the outer segment of visual cells located in the posterior pole. Although subject to temporal variation, the proximal half of the outer segment is similarly involved in most dogs by 25-35 weeks of age (Fig. 6).

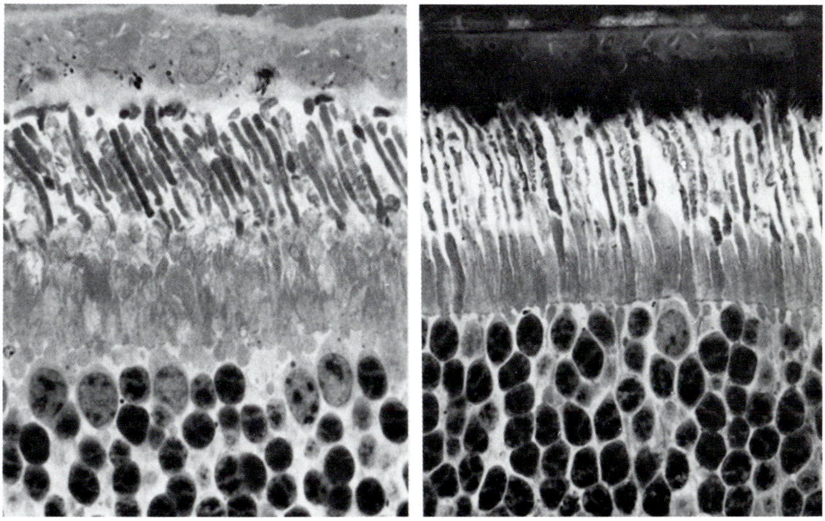

Figure 6: Photoreceptor layer from 14.5- (left) and 30-week old (right) PRCD-affected miniature poodles. By 30 weeks of age, the disease affects the entire length of the rod outer segment; there is loss of lamellar orientation and sides appear indented and irregular. Variation in pigment epithelial pigmentation is normal. (x1000)

The sequence of visual cell degeneration also has a spatial component; in animals younger than one year of age, the disease is more advanced in the posterior pole and equatorially than in the periphery. In older animals, however, progressive outer retinal atrophic changes begin in the periphery and advance centrally. The posterior pole is the best preserved region in these older retinas (Fig. 7).

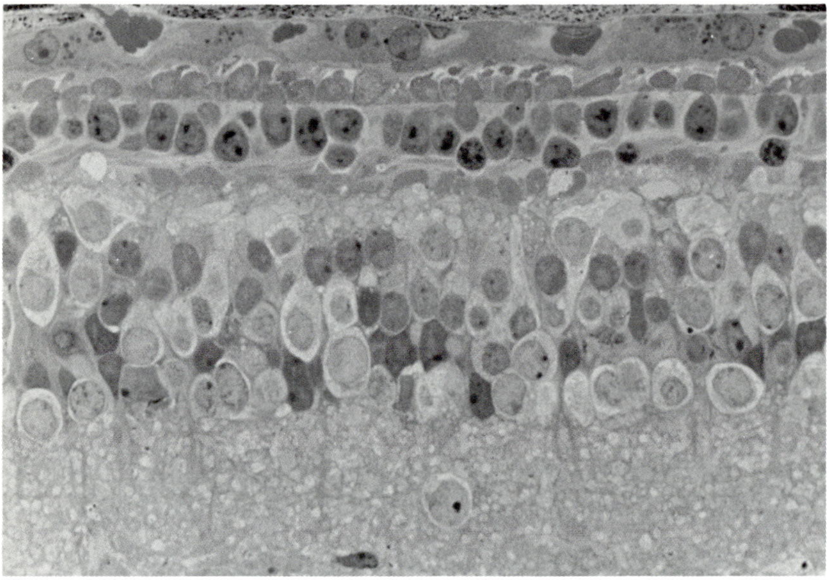

Figure 7: Parapapillary retina of a 3½-year old PRCD affected miniature poodle. The photoreceptor layer is narrowed and the remaining cell type is the cone. The outer nuclear layer is reduced to 1-2 nuclei in width. Inner retinal layers and pigment epithelium are normal. (x800).

Retinal cGMP concentration from affected animals at different ages and disease stages are similar to control values (Table 5). When the outer segment lamellar disc changes are only apparent ultrastructurally (14.5 weeks of age) or when more extensive (23 weeks of age), cGMP levels are normal. Similarly, retinal cGMP levels are normal during the course of the degeneration and loss of the visual cells.

Table 5: Progressive Rod-Cone Degeneration (Miniature Poodles): Retinal cGMP Concentration

Group	cGMP Concentration (pmol/mg protein)
Control*	8.7±3.3
Affected:	
14.5 weeks	8.6
23 weeks	7.9
1.5 years	4.1
2.5 years	6.4
3.5 years	3.4
5-8 years	5.9±1.4

*Control category consists of phenotypically normal animals (n=17) older than 7 weeks of age of the following breeds: miniature poodle, Irish setter, Norwegian elkhound, Irish setter x Norwegian elkhound and beagle.

At two time points (23 weeks and 2½ years) in the course of the disease, retinal cGMP levels were determined for selected 4 mm trephined areas from the posterior pole, equatorial and peripheral retinal zones. These values were also similar to the normal controls.

CONCLUSION

A similar biochemical defect is present in different animal species with early onset retinal degeneration (rd in mice and rod-cone dysplasia in Irish setters). The biochemical abnormality is expressed early during the development of visual cells and arrests photoreceptor differentiation. These cells develop improperly and subsequently degenerate. The causal relationship between the biochemical defect and cell degeneration is inferred since the accumulation of cGMP precedes visual cell degeneration.

Thus, abnormal cGMP metabolism is a feature of early onset rapidly progressing retinal disease. As has been demonstrated by *in vitro* studies (Lolley et al., 1977; Ulshafer and Hollyfield, 1981), the elevated cGMP levels are not compatible with normal visual cell differentiation and maintenance.

In retinal diseases characterized either by qualitatively abnormal rather than arrested development (rod dysplasia) or by degeneration (progressive rod-cone degeneration), retinal cyclic nucleotide levels are normal. However, we cannot rule out the presence of a more limited defect in cyclic nucleotide metabolism. If present, such a defect could affect photoreceptor viability without appreciably raising nucleotide levels in whole retinal homogenates.

Nevertheless, we conclude that elevated retinal cGMP levels do not represent a nonspecific response of a degenerating retina. Cyclic GMP is elevated only in those diseases with a specific cyclic nucleotide metabolic abnormality and remains elevated during visual cell degeneration.

It is not yet possible to determine the relevance of our findings to the retinal degenerations of man. The normal human retina is more developed at birth than that of the dog or the mouse. Those retinal diseases in man characterized by blindness shortly after birth may result from abnormal cyclic nucleotide metabolism.

REFERENCES

Acland G, Aguirre G, Chader G, Fletcher R, Farber D (1980). Canine early onset hereditary retinal degeneration: genetic and biochemical distinction of three diseases. Suppl Inv Ophth Vis Sci 19:250.

Aguirre G (1976). Inherited retinal degenerations in the dog. Trans Am Acad Ophth Otol 81:667.

Aguirre G (1978). Retinal degenerations in the dog: I rod dysplasia. Exp Eye Res 26:233.

Aguirre G, Farber D, Lolley R, Fletcher RT, Chader GJ (1978). Rod-cone dysplasia in Irish setters: a defect in cyclic GMP metabolism in visual cells. Science 201:1133.

Aguirre G, Farber D, Lolley R, O'Brien P, Alligood J, Fletcher RT, Chader G (in press). Retinal degenerations in the dog: III abnormal cyclic nucleotide metabolism in rod-cone dysplasia. Exp Eye Res.

Aguirre G, O'Brien P, Alligood J, Buyukmihci N (in press). Pathogenesis of progressive rod-cone degeneration in the miniature poodle. Inv Ophth Vis Sci.

Aguirre G, Rubin L (1972). Progressive retinal atrophy in the miniature poodle: an electrophysiologic study. J Am Vet Med Assoc 160:191.

Aguirre G, Rubin L (1975). Rod-cone dysplasia (PRA) in Irish setters. J Am Vet Med Assoc 166:157.

Buyumihci N, Aguirre G, Marshall J (1980). Retinal degenerations in the dog: II development of the retina in rod-cone dysplasia. Exp Eye Res 30:575.

Chader G, Herz L, Fletcher R (1974). Light activation of phosphodiesterase activity in retinal rod outer segments. Biochim Biophys Acta 347:491.

Chader GJ, Liu YP, Fletcher RT, Aguirre G, Santos-Anderson R, T'so M (in press). Cyclic GMP phosphodiesterase in early onset inherited retinal degenerations.

Cogan D, Kuwabara T (1965). Photoreceptive abiotrophy of the retina in the elkhound. Path Vet 2:101.

Farber D, Lolley R (1974). Cyclic guanosine monophosphate: elevation in degenerating photoreceptor cells of the C3H mouse retina. Science 186:449.

Farber D, Lolley R (1976). Enzymic basis for cGMP accumulation in degenerative photoreceptor cells of mouse retina. J Cyclic Nucleot Res 2:139.

Farber DB, Souza DW, Chase DG, Lolley RN (1981). Cyclic nucleotides in cone dominant retinas: reduction of cyclic AMP levels by light and by cone degeneration. Inv Ophth Vis Sci 20:24.

Fletcher R, Chader G (1976). Cyclic GMP: control of concentration by light in retinal photoreceptors. Biochem Biophys Res Comm 70:1297.

Liu YP, Krishna G, Aguirre G, Chader GJ (1979). Involvement of cyclic GMP phosphodiesterase activator in an hereditary retinal degeneration. Nature 280:62.

Lolley RN, Farber DB (1976). Abnormal guanosine 3', 5' monophosphate during photoreceptor degeneration in inherited retinal disorders of C3H/HeJ Mice. Ann Ophth 8:469.

Lolley R, Farber D, Rayborn M, Hollyfield J (1977). Cyclic GMP accumulation causes degeneration of photoreceptor cells: simulation of an inherited disease. Science 196:664.

Miki N, Keirns J, Marcus F, Freeman J. Bitensky M (1973). Regulation of cyclic nucleotide concentrations in photoreceptors: an ATP-dependent stimulation of cyclic nucleotide phosphodiesterase by light. Proc Natl Acad Sci USA 76:3820.

Orr H, Lowry O, Cohen A, Ferrendelli J (1976). Distribution of 3':5'-cyclic AMP and 3':5'-cyclic GMP in rabbit retina in vivo: selective effects of dark and light adaptation and ischemia. Proc Natl Acad Sci USA 73:4442.

Ulshafer R, Hollyfield J (1981). The effects of PDE inhibitors and ouabain on cultured human retina. Suppl Invest Ophth Vis Sci 20:40.

Woodruff M, Bownds, D, Green S, Morrisey J, Shedlovsky A (1977). Guanosine 3', 5'-cyclic monophosphate and the in vitro physiology of frog photoreceptor membranes. J Gen Physiol 69:667.

APPROACHES TO HUMAN RETINITIS PIGMENTOSA THROUGH STUDIES OF VITAMIN A METABOLISM IN THE RCS (DYSTROPHIC) RAT

E.R. Berman, S. Merin, N. Segal and S. Photiou
Department of Ophthalmology, Hadassah University Hospital
Jerusalem, Israel

INTRODUCTION

Considerable progress has been made in recent years in delineating the enzymatic or biochemical bases of heredity diseases in which retinal pigmentary degeneration forms part of a generalized syndrome (e.g. abetalipoproteinemia, mucopolysaccharidoses II and III, gyrate atrophy of the choroid and retina and Refsum's syndrome). Because the genetic defects in these X-linked or autosomal recessive disorders are expressed systemically, it has been possible to identify aberrant enzymes in extraocular tissues or in circulating fluids. This is not the case however for retinitis pigmentosa (RP), the generic term applied to the heterogeneous group of inherited disorders localized to the retina, and characterized by night blindness, photoreceptor degeneration and pigment migration. There is at present no clue as to the nature of the enzyme defect(s) in any of the forms of this disorder, but one could postulate that a variety of different biochemical insults could produce what the clinician recognizes as RP in any particular patient. An inherited disease localized to the eye is not easily amenable to direct biochemical approach because even if post-mortem material were available, the deterioration of the tissue would probably be so advanced as to preclude reliable enzymatic measurements. Moreover the problem of time elapsed until autopsy material reaches the laboratory adds another uncertainty to this approach.

Many investigators have turned to animal models which, in spite of their limitations, offer many advantages. Rodents

Birth Defects: Original Article Series, Volume 18, Number 6, pages 135–148

and other small animals reaching inbred status, usually after about 20 generations (LaVail, 1979), provide a convenient source of material not only for studying the pathogenesis of the disease but also for manipulating environmental factors such as light or diet in order to examine possible influences on the progress of the retinal dystrophy. Caution must however be exerted since although some animal dystrophies share many features in common with human RP, it has yet to be established that we are in fact dealing with identical disease processes. The best that could be expected is that an animal model may resemble one of the many forms of human RP, but it is highly unlikely that it could serve as a general model for all of the forms. The most widely used used rodent models include several strains of rd mice, and the RCS and Wag/Rij rats. Among canine models the Irish setter with a rod-cone dysplasia resembling some human forms has aroused considerable interest. The biochemical defects in the rd mice and the Irish setter dog involve specific aspects of cyclic nucleotide metabolism (Farber and Lolley, 1974; Aguirre et al, 1978) while in the RCS rat, the inherited defect appears to be a deficiency of retinol esterifying enzyme in the pigment epithelium (Berman et al, 1981a). The relevance of any of these findings to human RP remains to be established. The present communication summarizes our recent observations on vitamin A metabolism in general and in the RCS rat in particular, and in addition describes some preliminary results on the uptake and esterification of retinol by cultured skin fibroblasts from RP patients.

VITAMIN A AND THE PIGMENT EPITHELIUM

The retinal pigment epithelium (RPE) plays a vital role in the visual cycle through storage and release of vitamin A produced during light- and dark-adaptation (Dowling, 1960a). Apart from the rat, whose stores are minimal in the dark-adapted state, in most animal species, the pigment epithelium represents a major storage site for vitamin A. It is found almost exclusively in the endoplasmic reticulum in the form of the ester in the cattle eye (Berman et al, 1979). In rodents, lipid droplets can only be demonstrated after systemic administration of vitamin A (Hirosowa and Yamada, 1976; Robison and Kuwabara, 1977). Although the visual cycle is probably the major source of retinol in the pigment epithelium, the vitamin also reaches these cells from phagocytized rod outer segment disks (Young and Bok, 1969) and from the circulation.

Storage and mobilization of vitamin A in the pigment epithelium

Metabolic transformations of vitamin A in mammalian pigment epithelium, regardless of its source, have received relatively little attention. Krinsky (1958) found remarkably high retinol esterifying activity in cattle RPE, and recent quantitation of the assay for this enzyme using labeled retinol has shown that as much as 80% of the substrate can be esterified by as little as 30-40 µg of microsomal protein in 15 min at 30° (Berman et al, 1980a). By contrast, the mobilization of retinol through hydrolysis of retinyl ester proceeds at only about 1/100 of this rate. The cytosol of the pigment epithelium from a variety of species is a rich source of retinol binding protein (Wiggert and Chader, 1975; Saari et al, 1977), which forms a 1:1 complex with retinol; it is only in this form that vitamin A alcohol (retinol) is

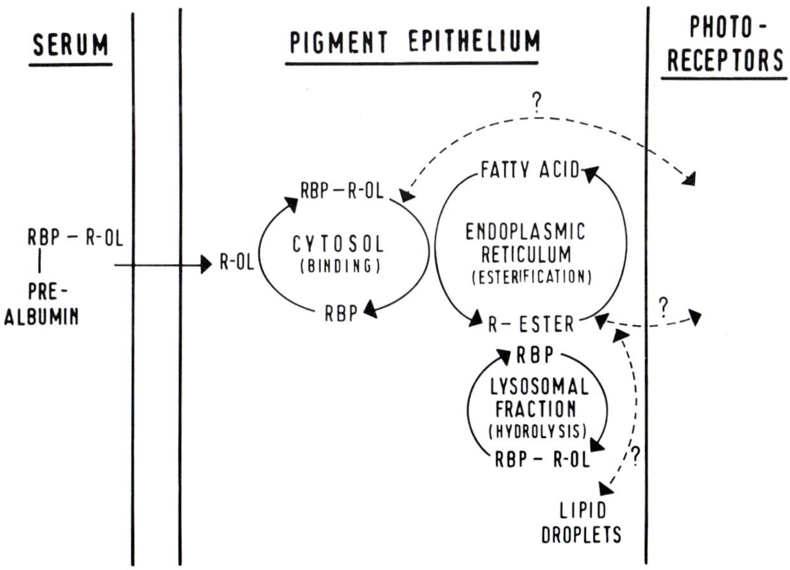

Figure 1. Metabolic interconversions of vitamin A in the pigment epithelium of cattle eye (From Berman et al, 1980b)

present in the pigment epithelium (Berman et al, 1979). Free retinol is a highly membranolytic substance (Lucy et al, 1963) and would cause considerable cell damage if allowed to accumulate intracelularly. Thus there may be control mechanisms in the RPE for regulating the various metabolic transformations of vitamin A. This may take the form of a cycle (Fig. 1) through which vitamin A entering the cell from various sources is channeled into a form (either the ester or a complex with retinol binding protein) that maintains a proper physiological balance (Berman et al, 1980b). We now know that both a deficiency (Dowling, 1960b; Delmelle et al, 1975; Berman et al, 1982) and an excess (Berman et al, 1981a) of vitamin A, either induced through dietary manipulations, or acquired as a result of hereditary disease, are associated with specific forms of retinal degeneration in experimental animals. Efforts to extrapolate some of these findings to humans will be discussed below.

Although the classic work on translocation of vitamin A between the photoreceptors and the pigment epithelium during light and dark adaptation was carried out on the rat eye (Dowling, 1960a), its small size and the limited amount of material have necessitated development of new techniques for studying the pigment epithelium. These cells have been successfully cultured in many laboratories (Flood et al, 1980) but because they may dedifferentiate under certain conditions (Masterson et al, 1978), we prefer using cell homogenates, which can be prepared in good yield from the optic cup after removal of the neural retina (Berman et al, 1981a). The retinol esterifying activity in these preparations (Fig. 2) is similar to that found in cattle eyes.

The findings in vitro on the remarkably high retinol esterifying activity in cattle and rat have been corroborated by in vivo studies on rabbits in our laboratory. Labeled retinol perfused through the vortex vein is converted to retinyl ester within 10 min, and continues to be esterified for as long as 40 min, the maximum length of time studied (Zauberman et al, 1981). It is reasonable to suppose that, regardless of its source in the pigment epithelium (whether from the visual cycle or the circulation) retinol is rapidly esterified, stored and then further metabolized. These may be transformations of major importance for normal development and function of the retina.

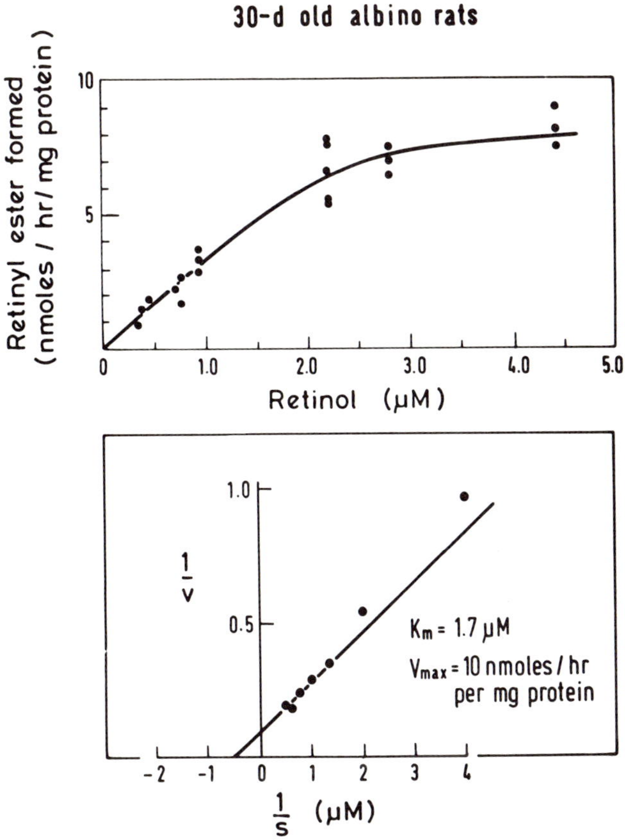

Figure 2. Retinol esterifying activity in homogenates of albino retinal pigment epithelium. The upper panel shows velocity as a function of substrate concentration; the lower panel is a double reciprocal plot from which apparent Km and Vmax values can be calculated

VITAMIN A METABOLISM IN THE RCS RAT

This model of retinal degeneration has been extensively studied in many laboratories for nearly two decades. First discovered in the animal colony of the Royal College of

Surgeons (Bourne et al, 1938), the morphological hallmark of the dystrophy is the accumulation of lamellar photoreceptor debris, probably the consequence of faulty phagocytosis by the pigment epithelium (Dowling and Sidman, 1962; Herron et al, 1969; Bok and Hall, 1971). Studies with chimeric rats have established that the site of the inherited disorder is the RPE, not the neural retina (Mullen and LaVail, 1975) and the defect may involve faulty receptors in the plasma membrane of the RPE cells which cannot recognize and phagocytize rod outer segment disks in a normal way. A specific enzymatic defect in the pigment epithelium has not been demonstrated until recently when it was shown that there is a pronounced deficiency of retinol esterifying enzyme in this cell layer of the RCS rat (Berman et al, 1981a and 1981b). The defect is demonstrable as early as the 10th postnatal day and until about the 55th day. Afterward the pigment epithelium itself begins to degenerate (Battelle and LaVail, 1975), hence measurements of enzyme activity would likely give rise to artifactuous results. Our studies showed that, on the average, the pigment epithelium of RCS rats contained only about 25% of the retinol esterifying activity found in aged-matched controls, the defect being particularly striking at high substrate concentrations. A more precise understanding of the abnormality can be obtained by drawing double-reciprocal plots of enzyme activity as a function of substrate concentration (Fig. 3). Calculations of the intercepts show that the apparent Km for both RCS and control animals is in the range of 0.5 to 1.5 x 10^{-6} M, i.e., there is very little difference between the mutant animals and controls. In contrast to this, the apparent Vmax values for esterification in control rats at maturity (beyond the 20th day) are about 5 times higher than those of the RCS rats. It is tempting to speculate that the inability of the pigment epithelium to esterify retinol through its normal pathway may be the primary inherited defect in the RCS rat.

How then can we explain the pathogenesis of lamellar debris accumulation and faulty phagocytosis in terms of a deficiency in retinol esterification in the pigment epithelium? It is possible that the common denominator in these two seemingly unrelated phenomena may be faulty synthesis of membrane glycoconjugates through the retinylmannosyl phosphate pathway (De Luca, 1977). The failure of the pigment epithelium to esterify retinol could in some way affect the synthesis of surface glycoprotein receptors required for recognition and phagocytosis of rod outer segment disks.

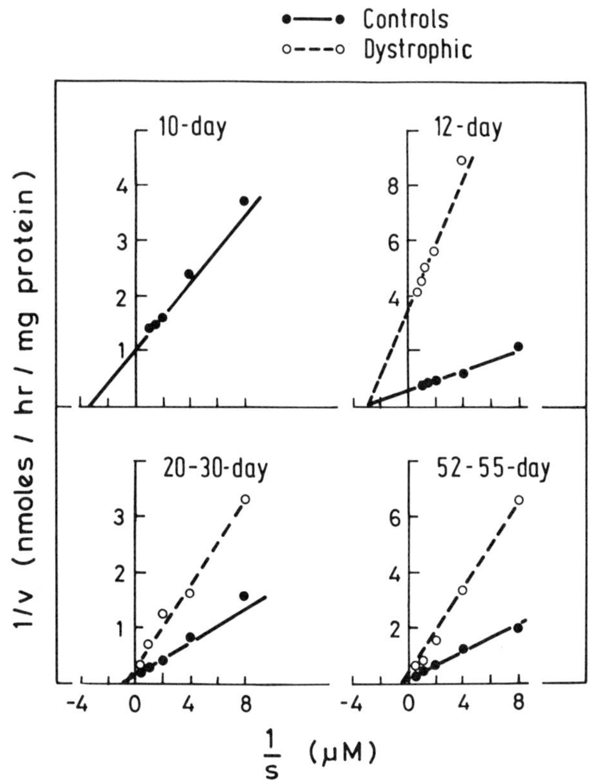

Figure 3. Double reciprocal plots of velocity data for esterification of retinol in pigment epithelial homogenates from RCS (dystrophic) and RCS-rdy$^+$ (congenic) rats. The apparent Km and Vmax values calculated from these plots are given in the text

As interesting as this working hypothesis may be, recent investigations suggest that, in addition to the specific retinol esterifying defect, the RCS strains also carry a generalized abnormality in retinoid metabolism (Kaitz, 1982; Berman et al, 1982). We have found that both the RCS (dystrophic) and the RCS-rdy$^+$ (congenic) strains do not utilize retinoic acid as a substitute for vitamin A for growth and differentiation of epithelia to the same extent as albino rats. Future investigations in these strains of rats could shed important light on the pathogenesis of retinal degenerations in this species, and perhaps in humans, in terms of abnormalities in retinoid metabolism.

VITAMIN A AND HUMAN RETINITIS PIGMENTOSA

The possibility that RP may represent a special form of localized vitamin A deficiency (Cogan, 1950) was at one time considered an attractive hypothesis. However the observation that serum vitamin A levels tended to be lower in RP patients than in controls (Campbell et al, 1964) could not be confirmed by other investigators, and it is now firmly established that there are no abnormalities in either vitamin A (Mehra and Khare, 1965; Krachmer et al, 1966) or retinol binding protein (Gouras and Chader, 1974; Maraini, 1974; Futterman et al, 1974) in the blood of RP patients. Added to this, the negative results of clinical trials with vitamin A for RP patients (Bergsma and Wolf, 1977) strengthens the view that vitamin A is not directly involved in the etiology of RP, at least as far as this is detectable in circulating levels of either the vitamin or its binding protein, or by dietary manipulations. The possibility still exists however that, as in the RCS rat, there may be an intracellular defect in retinol - or retinoid - metabolism in the neural retina or pigment epithelium in one (or more?) of the forms of human RP. However the unavailability of ocular tissue from RP patients except under rare circumstances precludes direct testing for this hypothetical enzymatic defect, and necessitates examination of extra-ocular tissues in the expectation that they may express the metabolic abnormality. Cultured skin fibroblasts are widely used as the most convenient source of tissue for studying enzymatic or biochemical defects in a variety of genetic disorders. For our purposes, skin biopsies were taken from a series of RP patients and controls (individuals with no obvious signs of retinal disease). The cells were grown in either Eagle's MEM or Ham's F-10 medium supplemented with 10% fetal calf serum in an atmosphere of 95% air - 5% CO_2. Confluent monolayers of skin fibroblasts obtained after 5-10 passages were used for all studies. The cells were trypsinized and homogenates made by brief sonification. Preliminary studies carried out to establish optimum conditions for assaying the enzyme from this source showed that it is present in measurable amounts (Fig. 4). The average Vmax for eight out of the ten controls was about 5 pmoles of ester formed

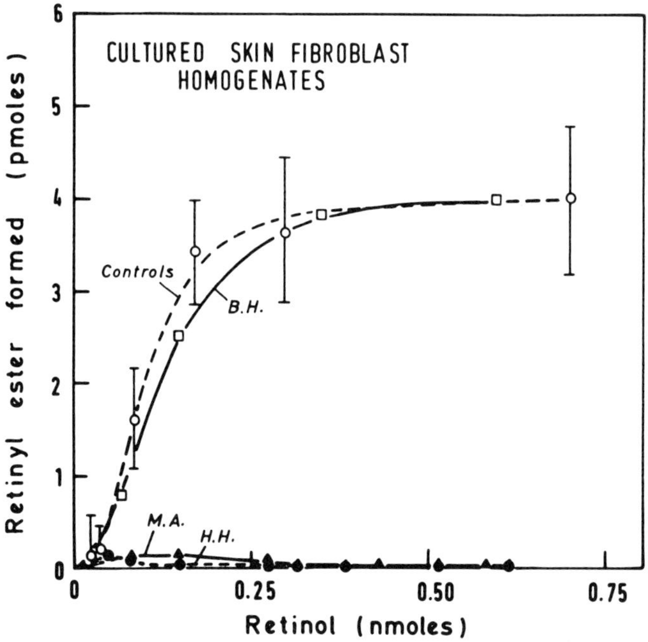

Figure 4. Esterification of ^{3}H-retinol by cell-free extracts of cultured skin fibroblasts. The dotted line (○--○) represents the means ± S.E.M. of 8 controls, and the other lines (□,▲,●) the values measured in three patients with retinitis pigmentosa. The incubation mixtures of 0.4 ml contained 400-600 μg of protein in 0.1 M phosphate buffer, pH 7.4 and varying concentrations of ^{3}H-retinol. All incubations were at 30° for one-half hour

under the conditions used. It should however be pointed out that 2 of the controls had almost undetectable activity. All RP patients were established as autosomal recessive forms on the basis of either parental consanguinity or sibships with two or more affected individuals. As shown in Fig. 4, two of the three RP patients had no detectable retinol esterifying activity while the third one fell within the range of normal controls. These results are still inconclusive and more work is required to improve the assay. For example we do not know why there are such large variations in activity among the controls, nor do we know why two out of ten controls were inactive.

Further experiments were carried out using intact cultured cells. Unlike cell-free extracts which showed relatively low activity, cultured skin fibroblasts are able to esterify up to 70% of exogenous retinol over a period of 24 hr (Fig. 5). When fibroblasts from two RP patients were compared to those of controls, they were found to have similar activity.

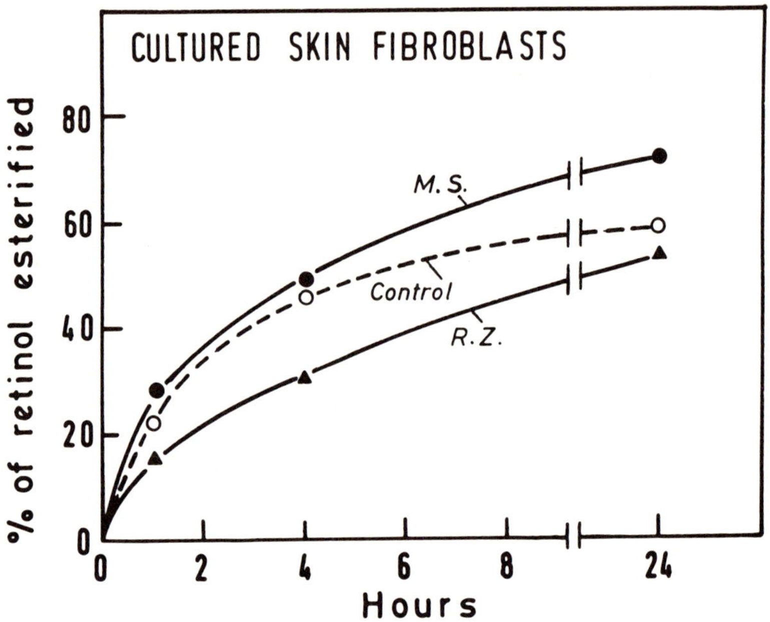

Figure 5. Esterification of ^{3}H-retinol by cultured skin fibroblasts from controls (o--o) and from two patients with retinitis pigmentosa (●,▲). The ^{3}H-retinol was added to the culture media of a series of flasks, which were then removed and analyzed at intervals of 4, 8, 12 and 24 hr.

These experiments suggest that there may be a defect in retinol esterifying enzyme in cultured fibroblasts of certain

RP patients. However, large numbers of additional patients must be examined before we can assess the potential usefulness of this enzyme assay as a tool in the diagnosis of any of the forms of human RP.

SUMMARY AND CONCLUSIONS

The RCS (Royal College of Surgeons) rat has been used as a model of retinal dystrophy for many decades. The retinal degeneration is characterized by an accumulation of photoreceptor debris which is believed to be the consequence of impaired phagocytic capabilities in the pigment epithelium. It has been established by studies on chimeric rats that the pigment epithelium is the site of the inherited defect (Mullen and LaVail, 1975) and recent biochemical studies have shown a marked deficiency of retinol esterifying enzyme in this cell layer (Berman et al, 1981a and 1981b). Since post-mortem material is not generally available from RP patients, we have examined extra-ocular tissue sources, e.g. cultured skin fibroblasts, as a tissue source in which the inherited defect could possibly be expressed. Studies on retinol esterifying enzyme showed a striking deficiency in two RP patients and normal values for another one, using cell-free homogenates. When intact cultured cells were examined for enzyme activity, two RP patients were found to have normal values. Further work with a larger number of patients is required before any relationship can be established between RP and intracellular defects in vitamin A metabolism.

ACKNOWLEDGMENTS

We wish to thank Hoffmann-LaRoche, Basle for providing some of the labeled and unlabeled retinoids used in these studies. This work was supported in part by the Chief Scientist's Office, Ministry of Health, Israel and the U.S.-Israel Binational Science Foundation

REFERENCES

Aguirre G, Farber D, Lolley R, Fletcher RT and Chader GJ (1978). Rod cone dysplasia in Irish setters: a defect in cyclic GMP metabolism in visual cells. Science 201:1133

Bergsma DR and Wolf ML (1977). A therapeutic trial of vitamin A in patients with pigmentary retinal degenerations: A negative study. In: "Retinitis Pigmentosa. Clinical Implications of Current Research", Ed. by M.B. Landers, III, M.L. Wolbarsht, J.E. Dowling and A.M. Laties, Plenum Press, New York/London, p. 197

Berman ER, Segal N and Feeney L (1979). Subcellular distribution of free and esterified forms of vitamin A in the pigment epithelium of the retina and in liver. Biochim Biophys Acta 572:167

Berman ER, Horowitz J, Segal N, Fisher S and Feeney-Burns L (1980a). Enzymatic esterification of vitamin A in the pigment epithelium of bovine retina. Biochim Biophys Acta 630:36

Berman ER, Segal N, Schneider A and Feeney L (1980b). An hypothesis for a vitamin A cycle in the pigment epithelium of bovine retina. Neurochemistry 1:113

Berman ER, Segal N, Photiou S, Rothman H and Feeney-Burns L (1981a). Inherited retinal dystrophy in RCS rats: a deficiency in vitamin A esterification in pigment epithelium. Nature 293:217

Berman ER, Segal N, Photiou S and Rothman H (1981b). Esterification of vitamin A in mammalian retina: Impaired activity in the RCS rat. In: "New Directions in Ophthalmic Research", Ed. by M.L. Sears, Yale University Press, New Haven/London, p. 223

Berman ER, Kaitz M and Segal N (1982). Effects of vitamin A deprivation on RCS (dystrophic) and RCS-rdy$^+$ (congenic) rats. In: "Proceedings of the International Workshop on Problems of Normal and Genetically Abnormal Retinas, Ed. by R. Clayton et al, Academic Press, New York/London, in press

Bok D and Hall MO (1971). The role of the pigment epithelium in the etiology of inherited retinal dystrophy in the rat. J Cell Biol 49:664

Bourne MC, Campbell DA and Tansley K (1938). Hereditary degeneration of the rat retina. Brit J Ophthalmol 22:613

Campbell DA, Harrison R and Tonks EL (1964). Retinitis pigmentosa. Vitamin A serum levels in relation to clinical findings. Exp Eye Res 3:412

Cogan DG (1949). Symposium: Primary chorioretinal aberrations with night blindness. Pathology. Trans Amer Acad Ophthal and Laryng 44:629

Delmelle M, Noell WK and Organisciak DT (1975). Hereditary retinal dystrophy in the rat: rhodopsin, retinol, vitamin A deficiency. Exp Eye Res 21:369

De Luca LM (1977). The direct involvement of vitamin A in glycosyl transfer reactions of mammalian membranes. Vitam Horm 35:1
Dowling JE (1960a). Chemistry of visual adaptation in the rat. Nature 188:114
Dowling JE (1960b). Night blindness, dark adaptation, and the electroretinogram. Amer J Ophthal 50:875
Dowling JE and Sidman RL (1962). Inherited retinal dystrophy in the rat. J Cell Biol 14:73
Farber DB and Lolley RN (1974). Cyclic guanosine monophosphate: elevation in degenerating photoreceptor cells of the C3H mouse retina. Science 186:449
Flood MT, Gouras P and Kjeldbye H (1980). Growth characteristics and ultrastructure of human retinal pigment epithelium in vitro. Invest Ophthalmol Vis Sci 19:1309
Futterman S, Swanson D and Kalina RE (1974). Retinol in retinitis pigmentosa: evidence that retinol is in normal concentration in serum and the retinol-binding protein complex displays unaltered fluorescence properties. Invest Ophthalmol 13:798
Gouras P and Chader G (1974). Retinitis pigmentosa and retinol-binding protein. Invest Ophthalmol 13:239
Herron WL, Riegel BW, Myers OE and Rubin ML (1969). Retinal dystrophy in the rat - A pigment epithelial disease. Invest Ophthalmol 8:595
Hirosawa K and Yamada E (1976). Localization of vitamin A in the mouse retina as revealed by radioautography. In: "Structure of the Eye III", Ed. by E. Yamada and S. Mishima, Jap J Ophthalmol, p. 165
Kaitz M (1982). Acceleration of retinal degeneration in RCS (dystrophic) rats by vitamin A deficiency. Submitted
Krachmer JH, Smith JL and Tocci PM (1966). Laboratory studies in retinitis pigmentosa. Arch Ophthalmol 75:661
Krinsky NI (1958). The enzymatic esterification of vitamin A. J Biol Chem 232:881
LaVail MM (1979). The retinal pigment epithelium in mice and rats with inherited retinal degeneration. In: "The Retinal Pigment Epithelium", Ed. by K.M. Zinn and M.F. Marmor, Harvard University Press, Cambridge/London, p. 357
Lucy JA, Luscombe M and Dingle JT (1963). Biochem J 89:419
Maraini G (1974). The vitamin A transporting protein complex in human hereditary pigmentous retinal dystrophy. Invest Ophthalmol 13:288
Masterson E, Israel P and Chader GJ (1978). Pentose shunt activity in developing chick retina and pigment epithelium:

A switch in biochemical expression in cultured pigment epithelial cells. Exp Eye Res 27:409

Mehra KS and Khare BA (1965). Vitamin A in retinitis pigmentosa. Oriental Arch Ophthalmol 3:80

Mullen RJ and LaVail MM (1976). Inherited retinal dystrophy: primary defect in pigment epithelium determined with experimental rat chimeras. Science 192:799

Robison WG Jr and Kuwabara T (1977). Vitamin A storage and peroxisomes in retinal pigment epithelium and liver. Invest Ophthalmol Vis Sci 16:1110

Saari JC, Bunt AH, Futterman S and Berman ER (1977). Localization of retinol-binding protein in bovine retina and retinal pigment epithelium. Invest Ophthalmol Vis Sci 16:797

Wiggert BO and Chader GJ (1975). A receptor for retinol in the developing retina and pigment epithelium. Exp Eye Res 21:143

Young RW and Bok D (1969). Participation of the retinal pigment epithelium in the rod outer segment renewal process. J Cell Biol 42:392

Zauberman H, Segal N, Photiou S and Berman ER (1981). Perfusion of the choriocapillaris through the vortex vein. In: "Proceedings of the Conference on Subretinal Space", Ed. by H. Zauberman, Dr. W. Junk bv Publishers, The Hague-Boston-London, p. 93

Retinitis Pigmentosa: Genetic Types, Epidemiology, and Clinical and Laboratory Studies

GENETIC ANALYSIS OF HETEROGENEITY AND VARIATION IN RETINITIS PIGMENTOSA

Joann A. Boughman, Ph.D.

Department of Human Genetics
Medical College of Virginia, Box 33
Richmond, Virginia 23298 U.S.A.

INTRODUCTION

The study of retinitis pigmentosa (RP) poses several interesting clinical genetic problems that can best be solved by careful and deliberate integration of multiple methodologies. Ophthalmologic observations can provide information regarding clinical variation among cases and describe the many and sometimes subtle clinical differences among types of RP. Genetic analysis, on the other hand, can provide methods to analyze pedigree and population data to clarify the inheritance of this heterogeneous group of disorders. While the ultimate answers will surely come through molecular biological studies, our immediate problems include the definition of the phenotypes of retinitis pigmentosa and careful delineation of the clinical population to permit appropriate patient care and counseling.

There are several reasons why RP represents an important clinical genetic problem. First, it is a relatively common group of disorders, with an estimated frequency in Europe of 1 in 7000 (Ammann et al, 1965); 1 in 2000 to 3000 in the U.S. for recessive forms (Boughman et al, 1980); and 1 in 2000 in Israel (Merin and Auerbach, 1976). Second, the psychological, social, and economic impact of RP can be devastating to the individual, the family, and the community at large. Third, because RP is genetically heterogeneous, there remain many unanswered questions regarding diagnosis and prognosis. Retinitis pigmentosa can pose difficult genetic counseling problems because of our inability to assign many persons unambiguously to a partic-

Birth Defects: Original Article Series, Volume 18, Number 6, pages 151–160

ular genetic category. And finally, there are still many challenging areas for genetic research. These include improved discrimination of genetic entities from possible non-genetic causes, development of reliable carrier detection and antenatal testing procedures, and application of modern techniques of recombinant DNA technology as an approach to isolation of the genetic determinants of RP and discovery of their physiologic function.

Although RP is known to represent a genetically heterogeneous group of disorders, the number and relative frequency of the separate genetic entities is still unresolved. Genotypes of cases and relatives cannot be identified, except in a few situations, and the assignment of isolated cases to genetic categories, especially when family size is small, is frequently impossible. It is important to understand, however, that methods of analysis can be utilized to clarify such issues as the importance of non-mendelian factors in the determination of the RP phenotype and degree of clinical variability expressed within specific RP genotypes. Systematically coded data on probands and relatives are required for such analyses.

In 1975, a National Survey Data Base was established in conjunction with the National Retinitis Pigmentosa Foundation. It consists of systematic information obtained from 1,004 probands and includes some data on a total of 18,886 family members. The 10-page survey questionnaire consisted of four parts. Systematic medical history data were gathered on the presence and severity of 14 ocular and 26 extraocular symptoms and ratings obtained on the progression of the disorder and age of onset. Pedigree information includes names, demographic variables, and information on ocular and general health status of relatives. The probands were not systematically examined, although nearly all had been diagnosed by ophthalmologists and >40% had diagnostic electroretinography. Because probands were ascertained from the general RP population, we believe that the sample may realistically approximate the population of RP patients seen in genetic counseling clinics. Rather than being a weakness in the data base, the heterogeneous nature of the population provides us with the opportunity to compare results with those obtained from clinical centers such as the study by Massof et al (this volume).

Analysis of pedigree data will help us understand

variation among genetic types by the comparison of cases that follow specific inheritance patterns. However, a large proportion of RP cases are simplex--only one affected in the family. These cases present special problems for diagnosticians and counselors. Every effort should be made to gain understanding about the possible etiology and associated familial risks in these cases, because this subset of patients may be further confounding the issue of genetic heterogeneity.

The separation of families into high- and low-risk groups and the estimation of associated recurrence risks can be accomplished by performing segregation analysis as developed by Morton (1959). This approach permits the evaluation of large numbers of nuclear families and maximum likelihood estimation of the following parameters:

$\underline{\pi}$ = ascertainment probability
$\underline{p}$ = segregation ratio
$\underline{x}$ = proportion of low-risk (sporadic) cases

The first parameter to be estimated in segregation analysis is $\underline{\pi}$, the probability of a person being independently ascertained (i.e., a proband). If every affected individual is ascertained independently, as in complete or truncate selection, then $\underline{\pi} = 1$. If ascertainment is such that no family is ascertained more than once, as in single selection, then $\underline{\pi}$ approaches zero. Usually, a sample is ascertained under what is termed "multiple selection," where the value of $\underline{\pi}$ falls between 0 and 1 and must be estimated from the data. In the National Survey, $\underline{\pi}$ was estimated to be 0.086, indicating that nearly every family had only one proband. It is important to recognize that any method of ascertainment is acceptable; as long as $\underline{\pi}$ is known, an appropriate adjustment for the bias can be made.

The segregation ratio, $\underline{p}$, is the frequency of affecteds for various mating types and has expected values of 0.50 for dominant disorders, and 0.25 for recessives. In segregation analysis, the basic hypothesis that the distribution of affected individuals in a sample can be explained by a mendelian segregation ratio is tested and maximum likelihood estimate of the value of $\underline{p}$ obtained. The proportion of low-risk or sporadic cases, $\underline{x}$, can also be estimated from the excess of families in which only the proband is affected. In many families at-risk for mendelian disorders, only one child by chance is affected, thus giving rise to an isolated case. This is especially true in populations consisting of small families. Segregation analysis evaluates, over all sibships, the expected proportion of these high-risk, but chance-isolated, cases. If an excess number of isolated cases is found, they are assumed to represent "low-risk" or "sporadic" cases for which the recurrence risk is negligible.

Sporadic cases may be present in a patient population for many reasons. Some may be environmentally determined phenocopies of the mendelian disorders. Cases carrying new mutations would also represent "low-risk" cases for their parents, although the affected child could transmit the genes to future generations. In addition, cases caused by multifactorial or polygenic inheritance would be categorized as "sporadic" in this type of analysis because they would be associated with low recurrence risk in the nuclear families of unaffected parents.

RESULTS AND DISCUSSION

TABLE 1 shows the results of the segregation analysis of 624 informative sibships from the National Survey. Each family has parents of known phenotype and at least two offspring. The families are then divided by mating type, affected by normal or normal by normal, and the associated mendelian hypotheses tested.

Of the informative matings, 103 had one parent reported to be affected. Because ascertainment was through an affected child and one parent was also affected, these cases are hypothesized to be dominant ($\underline{p}$ = 0.5) and we assume that no cases are sporadic ($\underline{x}$ = 0.0). This hypothesis was rejected (χ^2 = 28.02), and subsequent calculation of $\hat{\underline{p}}$ yielded a maximum likelihood estimate of $\hat{p}$ = 0.309. Because there should be no low-risk cases in these families, this reduced value for $\hat{\underline{p}}$ indicates a reduction in the segregation ratio of the RP phenotypes in these families. From this estimate, penetrance for the dominant phenotype is calculated to be: 0.31/0.5 = 0.62. This estimate is based on the assumption that there is no primary disturbance in the segregation of the RP gene. This value for reduced penetrance quite likely reflects variation in age of onset as well as incomplete penetrance,

Table 1: Segregation Analysis of 624 Sibships ($\Pi = 0.86$)

Mating type and hypothesis tested	χ^2_p	χ^2_x	No. of sibships	No. of sibs Aff.	No. of sibs Nl.
AFFECTED X NORMAL					
H_o: p=0.5, x=0.0	28.02	--	103	202	201
NORMAL X NORMAL					
H_o: p=0.25, x-0.0	48.12	62.01	521	756	1183
H_1: p=0.25, $x=\hat{x}=0.323$	3.41	--	521	756	1183
H_o: p=0.25, x=0.0 multiplex sibships	4.77	--	146	396	345

since some at-risk family members had not yet passed through age of risk for developing symptoms.

In the 521 normal by normal matings, the hypothesis that all cases are segregating as high-risk cases ($\underline{p}$ = 0.25; $\underline{x}$ = 0.0) was also rejected as indicated by the high χ^2 values for $\underline{p}$ and $\underline{x}$. Simultaneous iteration yielded maximum likelihood estimates of $\hat{\underline{p}}$ = 0.27 and $\hat{\underline{x}}$ = 0.32, suggesting the presence of a large proportion of low-risk or sporadic cases in this sample. From this analysis alone it is not immediately obvious whether a reduced segregation ratio, as in the dominants, could also be contributing to this high proportion of simplex cases.

However, in the analysis of multiplex sibships the hypothesis of $\underline{p}$ = 0.25 and $\underline{x}$ = 0 could not be rejected. It appears that among the offspring of normal by normal matings known to be at high-risk, the segregation ratio is not reduced by the same magnitude as in the dominant families, suggesting that the presence of sporadic cases, rather than reduced penetrance, is the more likely explanation for the failure of the original model.

The interpretation of the parameter $\underline{x}$ must be made carefully. Segregation analysis does not reveal which of the simplex cases are sporadic and does not imply specific etiology for these cases. The results clearly show, however, that the traditional definition of retinitis pigmentosa as consisting of a group of simple mendelian traits cannot account for the observed distribution of affected individuals in these families. By looking at families showing reduced penetrance for the dominant phenotype of RP, and by examining the large proportion of simplex cases, we can conclude that genetic-environmental interactions, environmental factors, or possibly polygenic background variation are of importance either in the etiology or the clinical expression of the RP phenotype.

These results suggest that appropriate analysis and comparisons of the simplex and multiplex cases may yield invaluable information regarding the diagnosis and nosology of the disease and insight may be gained regarding etiological factors by examination of multiple parameters of interest. To illustrate the genetic and clinical approaches that should be included in sibship analysis, age of onset has been analyzed for the National Survey population.

All probands were asked to report the age of onset of the first symptom. The most common initial symptom was night blindness which was reported as present in 97% of the probands. Previous studies have variously shown differences in age of onset among genetic types. Krill (1972) suggested that age of onset is earlier in recessive and X-linked cases than in dominant, Tanino et al (1976), showed a significantly earlier onset in recessives than dominants, while Berson et al (1980) found earlier onset of night blindness in X-linked and dominant cases than in other groups.

TABLE 2: Reported Age of Onset for Different Genetic Types

	Recessive	Dominant	X-linked
No. of probands	188	62	19
Mean, in years	16.2±0.96	18.7±2.0	9.1±1.2
Range, in years	0-54	0-57	3-18
95% symptomatic by	40 yrs.	50 yrs.	18 yrs.

TABLE 2 summarizes the age of onset for probands meeting probabilistic criteria for specific modes of inheritance described elsewhere (Boughman et al, 1980). The mean age of onset for X-linked cases in the National Survey was 9.1, and differed significantly from the means of the autosomal recessive and dominant groups. The X-linked cases also showed a more restricted range in age of onset of the first symptom, with all probands reported to be symptomatic prior to child-bearing years.

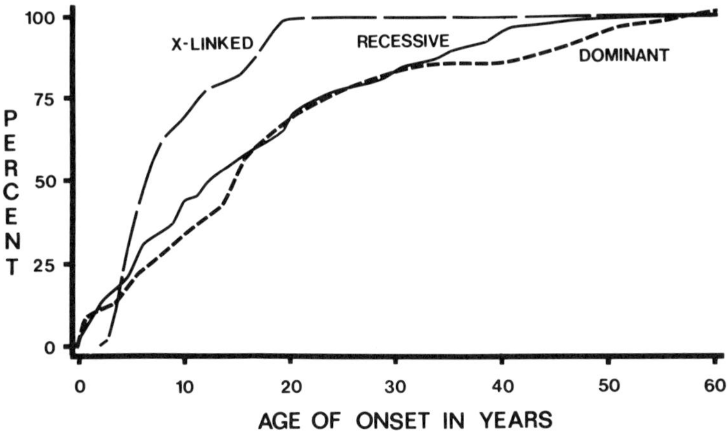

Figure 1: Cumulative age-of-onset distribution

A comparison of cumulative age-of-onset distributions is shown in FIGURE 1. These distributions graphically illustrate the difference in age of onset between the X-linked and autosomal forms of retinitis pigmentosa. The extended range in age of onset for the autosomal forms, occurring well into adult life in many cases, is easily apparent by the shapes of the distributions.

Extending the reasoning from contrasting well defined genetic types, we performed an analysis to compare probands from multiplex sibships, presumed to be genetic, and simplex cases which would include both high-risk (genetic) and low-risk (sporadic) cases. In TABLE 3, results are shown for each sex as well as pooled data.

Comparison of the means for simplex and multiplex male probands showed significant differences ($t = 2.26$; $p = 0.02$).

Table 3: Age of Onset of First Symptom

Simplex Probands	Males	Females	Total
Mean	17.2	21.8	19.5
SE	1.0	1.1	0.7
range	0-60	0-71	0-71
N	203	202	405
Multiplex Probands			
Mean	14.4	17.9	16.2
SE	0.8	9.9	0.6
range	0-66	0-67	0-67
N	249	254	503
t	2.26	2.76	3.50
p	0.02	<0.01	<0.001

Differences between females and for the pooled sexes were highly significant (p = <0.01), with the simplex cases having later onset in each group. These results suggest that low-risk cases may be contributing to variation between groups by having a later onset than high-risk genetic cases, a plausible hypothesis since age of onset has been shown to differ among genetic groups.

In the analysis of a clinical variable measured in any heterogeneous genetic disorder, the demonstration of group differences does not, in itself, provide sufficient information to be used in any predictive way. The variation within a genetic type must be measured. Only if the within-family variation is small, in comparison to the differences between groups, will the variable in question be useful as a discriminator between genetic types.

In FIGURE 2, the range in age of onset within sibships is illustrated. Age of onset of the first symptom showed wide ranges between sibs, with the proband usually, but not consistently, having earlier age of onset than affected siblings. Only siblings have been used in this analysis to avoid reporting differences across generations. The top histogram shows sibships considered dominant, since a parent was also affected. The mean difference in age of onset in these sibships was 11.5 years; the median, 7 years; and the range more than 40 years in some families. For multiplex sibships with normal parents, the range was more restricted. In sibships in which only males were affected (including recessive and X-linked cases), the median difference was 3 years. For male-female and female only sibships, the median was 4 years. The results of within-sibship differences indicate that variation is sufficiently large within sibships for us to question whether group differences in age of onset can be utilized as a reliable discriminating variable.

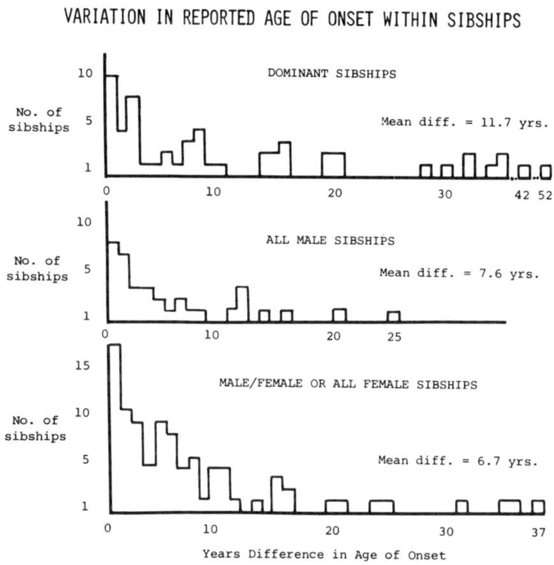

Figure 2

CONCLUSION

These results on reported age of onset illustrate some of the approaches that should be utilized in the analysis of any clinical variable to be utilized as a potential discriminator between types of retinitis pigmentosa. It is intuitively obvious that the combination of many different parameters may be useful to discriminate between genetic types, and possibly to eventually show diagnostic significance for high- versus low-risk cases. Many clinicians are presently studying clinical variables that should be analyzed in the context of family structure. Parameters that are obtained on nearly every patient at clinical centers and should be available for analysis include progression of the disease, including field loss and change in visual acuity; cataract development; electroretinographic changes; and correlation with other ocular and extraocular symptoms such as hearing loss. Conclusions based on careful within- and among-family comparisons and population genetic analyses will provide valuable clinical and genetic information for patients and their families.

ACKNOWLEDGEMENT

This is paper #142 from the Department of Human Genetics of the Medical College of Virginia, and was supported by a grant from the Retinitis Pigmentosa Foundation (5-31369). The assistance of A. Walton and T. Mayo in the preparation of the manuscript, is gratefully acknowledged.

REFERENCES

Ammann F, Klein D, Franceschetti A (1965). Genetic and epidemiological investigation of pigmentary degeneration of the retina and allied disorders in Switzerland. J Neurol Sci 2:183-196.

Berson EL, Rosner B, Simonoff E (1980). Risk factors for genetic typing and detection in retinitis pigmentosa. Am J Ophthalmol 89:763-775.

Boughman JA, Conneally PM, Nance WE (1980). Population Genetic studies of retinitis pigmentosa. Am J Hum Genet 32: 223-235.

Krill AE (1972). Retinitis pigmentosa: a review. Sight Sav Rev 42:21-28.

Merin S, Auerbach E (1976). Retinitis pigmentosa. Surv Ophthalmol 20:303-346.

Morton NE (1959). Genetic tests under incomplete ascertainment. Am J Hum Genet 11:1-16.

Tanino T, Ohba N (1976). Studies on pigmentary retinal dystrophy. I. Age of onset of subjective symptom and the mode of inheritance. Jap J Ophthalmol 20:474-481.

GENETIC ANALYSIS OF SUBGROUPS WITHIN SIMPLEX AND MULTIPLEX RETINITIS PIGMENTOSA

Robert W. Massof, Ph.D. and Daniel Finkelstein, M.D., Wilmer Institute, The Johns Hopkins University School of Medicine, Baltimore, MD, 21205 U.S.A.

Joann A. Boughman, Ph.D., Dept. of Human Genetics, Medical College of Virginia, Virginia Commonwealth University, Richmond, VA, 23298 U.S.A.

Typical retinitis pigmentosa (RP) is a clinical syndrome defined as: 1) nightblindness, 2) loss of vision in the midperipheral and peripheral visual field, 3) retention of good central vision until relatively late in the natural course of disease progression, 4) ophthalmoscopically visible, midperipheral, black, intra-retinal, bone-spicule-like pigmentation, 5) retinal arterioles of abnormally small caliber, and 6) no known systemic metabolic, inflammatory, toxic, traumatic, or dietary cause of the retinal disorder. Although in practice the term RP is often applied to a wide variety of retinal dystrophies and degenerations, the term "typical" RP is reserved for those patients who meet, or those who are expected to meet the above defining criteria.

Genetic Hypothesis

It is widely believed that all typical RP is heritable. Although autosomal dominant with full penetrance, autosomal dominant with incomplete penetrance, autosomal recessive, and X-linked recessive inheritance patterns have been described, and are well- accepted subdivisions of RP, the assumption of a genetic basis for all RP is unwarranted; the majority (60% to 70%) of RP cases are simplex (no family history) or are multiplex (affected siblings). Thus, as opposed to inheriting the disease, it is equally likely that this majority of typical RP patients has acquired the disease; especially considering that the first five defining

Birth Defects: Original Article Series, Volume 18, Number 6, pages 161–166

signs and symptoms are met by a variety of known acquired disorders (e.g. quinine retinopathy). Indeed, this important fact is explicitly recognized in the practice of referring to such acquired retinal degenerations as "pseudo-RP"; "pseudo", because they fail to meet the sixth criterion, idiopathy.

A compromise hypothesis, that the present study examines, is that simplex/multiplex RP, as a group, represents a mix of genetic and nongenetic cases. Krill (1972), Maumenee, et al (1975), and Palmer et al (1980) have concurred that there is large variability in the age of symptom onset among autosomal recessive (sic) RP patients. The observed variability led these authors to speculate that their respective patient subgroup was inhomogeneous with respect to retinal disease.

Figure 1 illustrates a histogram of reported age of nightblindness onset for our cohort of 200 simplex/multiplex RP patients. The distribution is bimodal with the first mode occurring in the first quinquenniad and the second mode occurring in adulthood (greater-than or equal-to age 21). This bimodality suggests that there may be at least two different population distributions represented in our sample.

Subclassifications of Simplex/Multiplex RP

In earlier studies, we presented evidence that simplex/multiplex RP patients can be subdivided according to the pattern of visual function loss (Massof and Finkelstein, 1979; Massof and Finkelstein, 1981). One group of patients, who we refer to as "type 1" simplex/multiplex RP, have the following characteristics: 1) rod function is not measurable throughout the visual field, regardless of field size, 2) the rod function loss occurs at an early age, and 3) cone function is progressively and diffusely lost, more in the periphery than in the center. Another group of patients, who we refer to as "type 2" simplex/multiplex RP, have the following characteristics: 1) an early combined loss of rod and cone sensitivity in the midperiphery, 2) normal or near normal rod sensitivity in the central and far peripheral field during early stages, and 3) progression by deepening of the sensitivity loss and widening of the affected zone in the midperipheral ring.

From those simplex/multiplex RP patients who have

enough remaining visual function to permit classification, we find that type 1 simplex/multiplex RP patients account for the first mode in the age of nightblindness onset distribution and that type 2 simplex/multiplex RP patients account for the second mode (figure 2). This result suggests that we may be converging on the identification of two separate disease entities, both of which are labeled typical RP.

Taken alone, the above-described functional subclassifications of simplex/multiplex RP do not bear upon the genetic question. For example, we may have separated two different autosomal recessive diseases, or we may have separated two different acquired diseases. Furthermore, the possibility exists that type 1 and/or type 2 may represent a mix of genetic and nongenetic cases.

Segregation Analysis

In order to test the genetic hypothesis for simplex/multiplex RP, we have employed a statistical tool called segregation analysis (Morton, 1959; Boughman, this volume). This analysis tests the hypothesis that for all cases in the sample, the relevant trait is recessively inherited. Two parameters are returned by the analysis; p, which corresponds to the proportion affected, and x, which corresponds to the excess of simplex cases. The predicted values from the recessive hypothesis are $p = 0.25$ and $x = 0.0$. To find the maximum likelihood values for p and x, $\hat{p}$ and $\hat{x}$ respectively, a simultaneous convergence technique can be employed, or alternatively, either $\hat{p}$ and $\hat{x}$ can be constrained to the predicted value while the maximum liklihood value is computed for the unconstrained parameter. the success of the simultaneous convergence technique depends, among other things, on sample size.

We performed the segregation analysis on 95 sibships of simplex/ multiplex RP. The hypothesis that all cases in the sample are recessive was rejected on the basis of the simultaneous interation results ($\hat{p} = .27$; $\hat{x} = .31$; $X^2 = 34.76$). These results mean that simplex/multiplex RP, taken as a group, most likely is a mix of genetic and nongenetic diseases (cf. Boughman, this volume).

When those simplex/multiplex RP patients who could be classified as type 1 or type 2 were examined separately, we found that the number of sibships was too small to perform a successful simultaneous iteration (n = 23 for type 1 and n = 29 for type 2). Nevertheless, by constraining $\hat{p}$ and $\hat{x}$ to 0.25 and 0.0 respectively, we obtained values of $\hat{p}$ = .22 and $\hat{x}$ = .12 for the type 1 subgroup and $\hat{p}$ = .14 and $\hat{x}$ = .39 for the type 2 subgroup (to be compared to $\hat{p}$ = .16 and $\hat{x}$ = .27 when the same analysis is performed on all simplex/multiplex RP patients as a group). Thus, type 1 simplex/multiplex RP appears to be consistent with the recessive hypothesis; whereas, for type 2 simplex/multiplex RP, the hypothesis that all cases are segregating as recessive is rejected.

Conclusions

The results presented here must be considered preliminary. The segregation analyses will be performed again after we have increased our sample sizes of type 1 and type 2 simplex/multiplex RP. Nevertheless, the results do strongly imply that the type 1 simplex/multiplex RP patients may have a recessive disorder and that the type 2 simplex/multiplex RP patients include a large proportion of cases who have an acquired or sporadic retinal disease. Thus, from these preliminary results it appears that the functional RP subclassifications that we have proposed, may have potential for discriminating genetic from nongenetic forms of RP.

References

Boughman JA (1982). "Genetic Analysis of Heterogenity and Variation in Retinitis Pigmentosa." (In this volume.)

Krill AE (1972). Retinitis Pigmentosa: A Review. Sight-sav Rev 42:21.

Massof RW, Finkelstein D (1979). Rod Sensitivity Reltive To Cone Sensitivity in Retinitis Pigmentosa. Invest Ophth Vis Sci 18:263.

Massof RW, Finkelstein D (1981). Subclassifications of Retinitis Pigmentosa From Two-Color Scotopic Static Perimetry. Docum Ophthal Proc Ser 26:219.

Maumenee IH, Pierce ER, Bias WB, Schleutermann DA (1975). Linkage Studies of Typical Retinitis Pigmentosa and Common Markers. Amer J Human Genet 27:505.

Morton NE (1959). Genetic Tests Under Incomplete Ascertainment. Am J Hum Genet 11:1.

Palmer RW, Massof RW, Finkelstein D (1980). Heterogeneity Within Subgroups of Retinitis Pigmentosa. Invest Ophthal Vis Sci Suppl p 78.

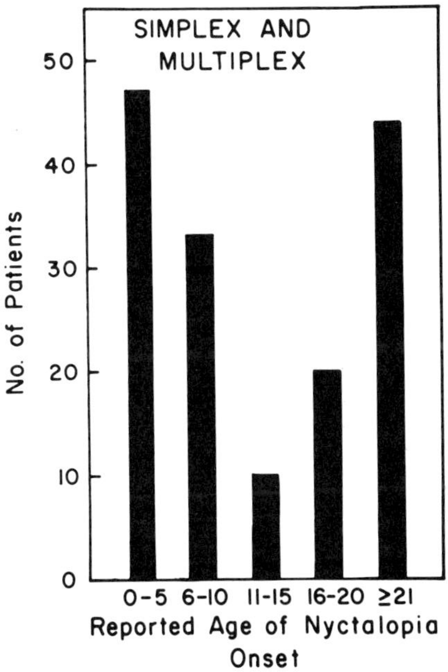

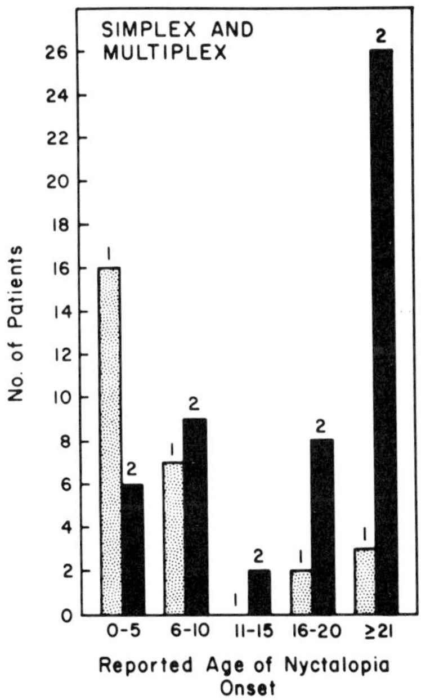

Fig. 1 Histograms of age of nightblindness onset as reported by simplex and multiplex retinitis pigmentosa patients.

Fig. 2 Nightblindness onset age histograms for type 1 simplex/multiplex RP (stippled bars) and type 2 simplex/multiplex RP (solid bars).

FIGURES AND FANTASIES: THE FREQUENCIES OF THE DIFFERENT GENETIC FORMS OF RETINITIS PIGMENTOSA.

Marcelle Jay, PhD

Moorfields Eye Hospital, London, England

The relative frequencies of the various genetic forms of retinitis pigmentosa have been a topic in several studies performed on large series of patients all over the world (Ammann et al, 1965; Boughman, 1978; Faber, 1970; Francois and Verriest, 1962; Imaizumi, 1971; Jay, 1972, 1974, 1978; Panteleeva, 1969). The proportions vary from one series to another, and they reflect to some extent the ethnic and other socio-economical factors which influence the prevalence of any genetically determined disease in a given population. It has often been assumed that all sporadic cases are autosomal recessive, and it is only occasionally that their true genetic status has been questioned.

The results from our previous publications (Jay, 1972, 1974, 1978) have been based on a series of consecutive patients seen in the Genetic Clinic at Moorfields Eye Hospital, and in view of the bias inherent in any series, it is pertinent to question to what degree these results are representative of the population of Moorfields, and of the population in the British Isles.

The Genetic Clinic at Moorfields Eye Hospital is a specialised department of an eye hospital which sees almost ¼ million out-patients a year. 70% of these out-patients are drawn from London and the surrounding counties, and the remainder live all over the British Isles. Patients are referred to the Genetic Clinic for assessment of their disease, for advice on management and for genetic counselling, and their referral from the general clinics of the hospital is likely to be influenced by the known

Birth Defects: Original Article Series, Volume 18, Number 6, pages 167-173

research interests of the clinicians.

These factors are apparent when considering the 453 families seen at the Genetic Clinic up to July 1979 (Table 1). Since the criteria used for the definition of autosomal recessive transmission differ in some respects from those currently used, it is relevant to define their use in this context. The term "autosomal recessive" is applied to all cases with evidence of parental consanguinity in a sibship with one or more affected sibs, or to affected individuals with parents who were believed to be homozygous or heterozygous for autosomal recessive retinitis pigmentosa on the basis of their family history. The term multiplex is used when two or more sibs are affected in a family with unaffected and unrelated parents, male multiplex being used where only males are affected, and mixed multiplex for all other cases. Similarly, simplex cases are those where only one member of the sibship is affected. These subdivisions of possibly autosomal recessive cases identify those groups where the true genetic status may be in doubt: for example, some of the male multiplex sibships may be calculated to be X-linked.

TABLE 1

GENETIC CLINIC SERIES - NUMBER OF FAMILIES

Autosomal Dominant	104
X-linked	67
Autosomal Recessive	29
Male Multiplex	19
Mixed Multiplex	28
Simplex	175
Usher Syndrome	27
Adopted	4
TOTAL	453

There are 247 families (54% of the total) with a positive family history, either of another affected member, or with parental consanguinity and one or more affected members in the same generation. The frequency of X-linked families is 15% when identified by their pedigree and by the clinical diagnosis of affected males and obligate heterozygotes.

It is interesting to note that almost 10% of all probands are unaffected, although in the X-linked group 18 of the 19 unaffected females were shown on examination to be obligate heterozygotes. There is a remarkable excess of female probands in the autosomal dominant families (Table 2) which can only be interpreted as reflecting the greater concern of affected females for the genetic consequences of this form of retinitis pigmentosa and for its high genetic risk.

TABLE 2

GENETIC CLINIC SERIES

	Families	Probands	
		Male	Female
Autosomal Dominant	104	33	71
X-linked	67	48	19
Autosomal Recessive	29	18	12
Male Multiplex	19	18	2
Mixed Multiplex	28	6	26
Simplex	175	103	72
Usher Syndrome	27	13	14
Adopted	4	2	2
TOTAL	453	241	218

The bias of ascertainment can be demonstrated by considering the frequency of the different genetic forms observed among all affected individuals in each pedigree (Table 3). The total number of affected individuals in each group is based on those born after 1910, and the information is collated from probands and their relatives who were subsequently seen in the Genetic Clinic, although not every individual has been examined.

The frequency of genetic forms among probands and among all affected individuals can be compared. The frequency of autosomal dominant transmission among all affected individuals is high (44%). The proportion of X-linked cases is identified as 19%; the obligate heterozygotes are not included in the total. The true proportion of X-linked cases is higher than 19%, since 16 of the 103 simplex cases have been calculated as being X-linked. These calculations are made on the basis of those applied to male sibships, and cannot be adjusted for individual cases among male sibships. The true proportion of X-linked cases is therefore at least 21% in this series.

TABLE 3

GENETIC CLINIC SERIES

	Families	Affected	
		Male	Female
Autosomal Dominant	104	211	228
X-linked	67	189	(187)
Autosomal Recessive	29	25	22
Male Multiplex	19	44	
Mixed Multiplex	28	27	42
Simplex	175	103	72
Usher Syndrome	27	18	16
TOTAL	449	617	380

These figures are all based on patients seen in the Genetic Clinic and are not representative of the Moorfields Eye Hospital population as a whole. A number of patients with retinitis pigmentosa is seen in the Electrodiagnostic Department either for diagnostic or for research purposes. A search of their records has yielded a further 309 probands who were not previously ascertained in the Genetic Clinic. No fewer than 203 (66%) are simplex cases and any divisions according to genetic form have to be based on probands only because reliable family details are incomplete in the Electrodiagnostic series. It is nonetheless interesting to consider the two hospital series together as they probably account for 95% of all patients with retinitis pigmentosa seen at Moorfields Eye Hospital.

The combined series is therefore based on probands and, if all simplex and multiplex cases are grouped together, it would appear that the autosomal recessive form predominates (Table 4). It cannot be assumed, however, that these are all autosomal recessive. An X-linked pedigree can simulate an autosomal recessive pedigree if obligate heterozygotes are considered as unaffected. Obligate heterozygotes are not always available for examination, the mother may be dead, and either the affected males only have sons, or their daughters are too young for tests to be conclusive. It has been estimated, from calculations performed on the Genetic Clinic series, that the true proportion of X-linked in this combined series is at least 14%, and this increase is at the expense of some male multiplex and simplex cases.

TABLE 4

COMBINED MOORFIELDS SERIES

	Families	%
Autosomal Dominant	147	19.3
X-linked	78	10.2
Autosomal Recessive	33	4.3
Male Multiplex	31	4.1
Mixed Multiplex	41	5.4
Simplex	378	49.6
Usher Syndrome	47	6.2
Adopted	7	0.9
TOTAL	762	

It is also likely that the true proportion of autosomal dominant families is slightly higher, and that of mixed multiplex and simplex slightly lower, than indicated due to the problems in obtaining reliable details of older members of a family.

A third source of patients with retinitis pigmentosa became available from the replies to a very simple questionnaire sent to members of the British Retinitis Pigmentosa Society. The membership is drawn from local groups throughout the country, and the geographical distribution is quite different to that of the hospital series, although the ethnic distribution is the same. The lack of clinical information makes any comparisons invidious, particularly as some cases ascertained by this means were subsequently ascertained at Moorfields and were found to have a variety of retinal dystrophies. The genetic status has been altered from autosomal dominant to X-linked in a number of these cases.

The replies to the questionnaire show that the number of affected females exceeds that of affected males which is contrary to the findings in both hospital series (Table 5). The true proportion of X-linked retinitis pigmentosa is likely to be much higher than the 4.7% indicated, in this case at the expense of the mixed multiplex group where the so-called affected females are actually obligate heterozygotes. This whole series is to be regarded with great caution since it is even more biased than others. There is no clinical information which is essential in the accurate diagnosis of retinitis pigmentosa in general, and the recognition of the X-linked form in particular. When other factors are taken into consideration, such as the age distribution of the membership which is heavily weighted in favour of middle-aged and elderly females, it cannot be considered as representative of retinitis pigmentosa in the British Isles.

TABLE 5

BRITISH RETINITIS PIGMENTOSA SOCIETY SERIES

	Families	Probands	
		Male	Female
Autosomal Dominant	130	55	102
X-linked	27	25	4
Autosomal Recessive	5	3	2
Male Multiplex	24	27	
Mixed Multiplex	76	28	64
Simplex	292	129	163
Usher Syndrome	16	9	7
Adopted	1		1
TOTAL	571	276	343

It is far more pertinent to regard the combined Moorfields Eye Hospital series as showing a genetic distribution which is probably similar to that found in Britain. The salient features are a proportion of 50% of families with only one member affected and no evidence of parental consanguinity, and an X-linked proportion of at least 14% of families. While 70% of the X-linked families may live at present in or around London, they originate from all over the British Isles and some even from Europe, but that is the subject of a different study which has yet to be completed.

REFERENCES

Ammann F, Klein D, Franceschetti A (1965). Genetic and epidemiological investigations on pigmentary degeneration of the retina and allied disorders in Switzerland. J Neurol Sci 2:183.

Boughman JA (1978). "Population Genetic Studies of Retinitis Pigmentosa". PhD Thesis, Indiana University.

Faber F (1970). "Retinitis Pigmentosa in Israel. Statistical-Clinical Survey". MD Thesis, Hebrew University, Jerusalem.

François J, Verriest G (1962). Etude Biométrique de la retinopathie pigmentaire. Ann Oculist 195:937.

Imaizumi K (1971). Stastical investigation on retinitis pigmentosa. Jap J Clin Ophthalmol 25:293.

Jay B (1972). Hereditary aspects of pigmentary retinopathy. Trans Ophthalmol Soc UK 92:173.

Jay B (1974). Recent advances in ophthalmic genetics: genetic counselling. Brit J Ophthalmol 58:427.

Jay B (1978). Retinitis pigmentosa in childhood - diagnosis, counseling and prevention. Metab Ophthalmol 2:221.

Panteleeva OA (1969). On the hereditary tapeto-retinal degenerations. Vestn Oftalmol 1:53.

RETINITIS PIGMENTOSA IN ONTARIO - A SURVEY

WILLIAM G. MACRAE, M.D., F.R.C.S.(C)

DEPARTMENT OF OPHTHALMOLOGY, University of
Toronto and Hospital for Sick Children
Toronto and 555 University Avenue, Toronto Canada

This report is the result of a study on the genetics of Retinitis Pigmentosa as found in the province of Ontario, (Canada). The study was undertaken with a three-fold purpose:

1. To ascertain the genetic distribution of RP in Ontario (both proven mendelian and indeterminate simplex).

2. To explore particular aspects of the natural progression of the disorder.

3. To utilize the information on the genetics and natural history of RP to aid in genetic counselling.

METHODS.

Cases for this study were ascertained in two ways. First, ophthalmologists throughout the province submitted names of patients with "typical RP". The patients were then requested to complete an extensive questionnaire including pedigree. Those completed questionnaires with sufficient data were then used in the study. Second, a smaller number were referred to our Eye Genetic Clinic at the Hospital for Sick Children for examination. The criteria used for assignment of genetic modes were based on Fishman's study in 1978.[1] Autosomal dominant required direct vertical transmission in at least three generations with other criteria of autosomal dominant traits. Autosomal dominant (probable) required direct vertical transmission in two generations with other criteria of an autosomal dominant trait. X-linked recessive inheritance required that

Birth Defects: Original Article Series, Volume 18, Number 6, pages 175–185

in a particular pedigree, males were almost exclusively involved with no male to male transmission and was assigned to those simplex male families whose carrier mothers had typical changes described by Bird.[2] Autosomal recessive inheritance required that more than one member of a sibship was affected and no other member from a previous generation. In addition other criteria of autosomal recessive inheritance had to be present. Autosomal recessive (probable) was assigned to those simplex cases with parental consanguinity and included simplex cases whose mothers had no symptoms or signs of X-linked RP. The simplex cases were those in whom only one affected member was present without a history of parental consanguinity. The term "simplex" is preferable to that of "sporadic" or "isolated" as genetic descriptions. Sporadic indicates non-genetic, and isolated is often confused with uncomplicated which means no other systemic anomaly. For example, Usher's Syndrome is a form of complicated Retinitis Pigmentosa. "Simplex" is not a restrictive term denoting genetic or non-genetic but rather refers to the only known affected family member.

GENETIC TYPES OF RP.

In Ontario through questionnaire and referral we identified 874 cases in 431 families with possible RP. Out of this total 2/3 had isolated RP (no other systemic anomaly) and the remaining 1/3 were as follows. Six percent had various manifestations of the Lawrence-Moon-Bardet-Biedle syndrome. Two percent had Leber's congenital amaurosis, 12% had RP associated with hearing loss in various forms, and 17% had insufficient information for proper categorization. Isolated RP was identified in 698 cases in 274 families, and of this total we examined personally 130 from 110 families. By questionnaire and by examination we estimated the following genetic percentages in families with Retinitis Pigmentosa: autosomal dominant 16%, autosomal recessive 28%, X-linked recessive 8%, and simplex 48%. Of the families that we examined personally we determined that 19% were autosomal dominant, 26% autosomal recessive, 9% X-linked recessive and 46% simplex. Thus, all modes of inheritance were well represented but in almost one half of the cases an identifiable genetic mode could not be established. There was no appreciable difference between the combined group (questionnaire and referral) and the examined group alone. When our data was compared to previously published studies (Table 1) interesting similarities and differences could be noted.

TABLE 1: PERCENT OF GENETIC TYPES IN FAMILIES WITH RP

Genetic Category	JAY[4]	PANTELEEVA[3]	FISHMAN[1]	MACRAE	AMMANN[5*]
Autosomal Dominant	39	12.7	19	16	9
Autosomal Recessive	15	27.9	19	28	90
X-linked Recessive	25	1.1	8	8	1
Undetermined Genetic Type	-	-	2	-	-
Simplex	21	58.3	52	48	0

*based on patients not families

ANALYSIS.

Our study closely parallels that of Fishman with the only major difference being the larger number of autosomal recessive cases in our study. Of interest however is that similarly to Fishman we found that almost one half of our cases could not be identified genetically. Other studies have shown a different genetic distribution perhaps reflecting different geographical influences as well as the vigor with which simplex families were investigated.

NATURAL HISTORY OF RETINITIS PIGMENTOSA.

The second aim of the project was to explore particular aspects of the progression of the disorder. In this instance cases were studied individually according to known genetic type where possible, and the data utilized was from personal examination only. Our sample was biased somewhat because the majority of our patients were young, often with severe disease, and frequently in the child-bearing years and interested in genetic counselling. We also utilized only those with isolated RP in the typical form. For the purpose of this study we defined "typical" Retinitis Pigmentosa as those found in patients with a history of night blindness and tunnel vision before central involvement and we excluded those cases with Leber's congenital amaurosis. We expected a typical ring scotoma but in most cases the field had been reduced to only a central island. In addition we expected to find waxy pallor of the optic disc, attenuated blood vessels, bone spicule pigmentation and, where necessary, typical electroretinographic changes.

We found that night blindness and eventual severity of RP were not closely correlated. We found many with night blindness since infancy with severe early central vision loss and others who had useful central vision for decades. We also noted late onset of night blindness associated with mild disease and others with a rapid visual decline. The onset of night blindness and development of tunnel vision correlated closely as expected and for this reason field determination was not used for assessment of progression. Anticipation played a significant role in many dominant families particularly with reference to the onset of symptoms. To assess severity we elected to compare central vision with age. For various reasons there was a large discrepancy in many cases between the vision in each eye and we elected to correlate age with the optimum corrected vision in the better eye.

RESULTS.

In the autosomal dominant families (Table 2) it was evident that most had excellent vision until after child-bearing years when vision slowly deteriorated. In the autosomal recessive group (Table 3) a large number maintained reasonable vision until the thirties although not as good as the dominant group and a few had significant early central loss. In a small group of X-linked recessive patients (Table 4) good vision was maintained for only a short period of time before a more rapid visual decline. Many of the simplex patients (Table 5) had good vision past child-bearing years although variability characterized this group.

OBSERVATIONS.

Our data was biased in favour of younger people. The young were examined often because they were more severely involved or were interested in genetic counselling. The older

TABLE 2 - AUTOSOMAL DOMINANT

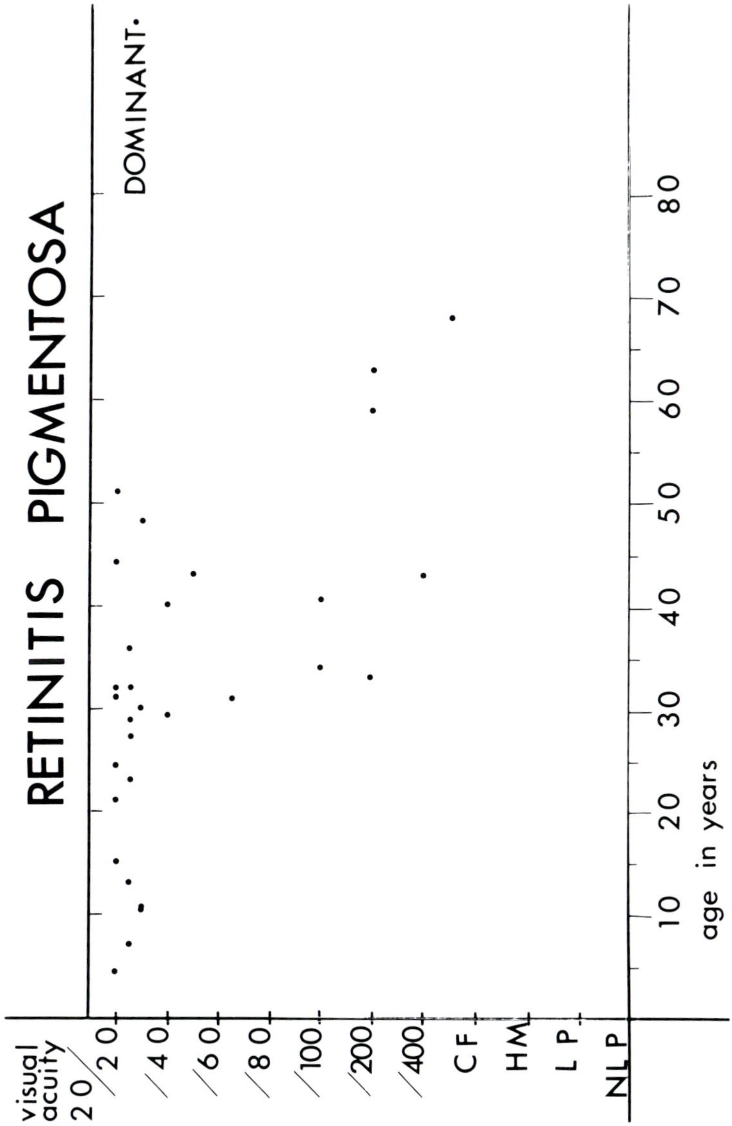

TABLE 3 - AUTOSOMAL RECESSIVE

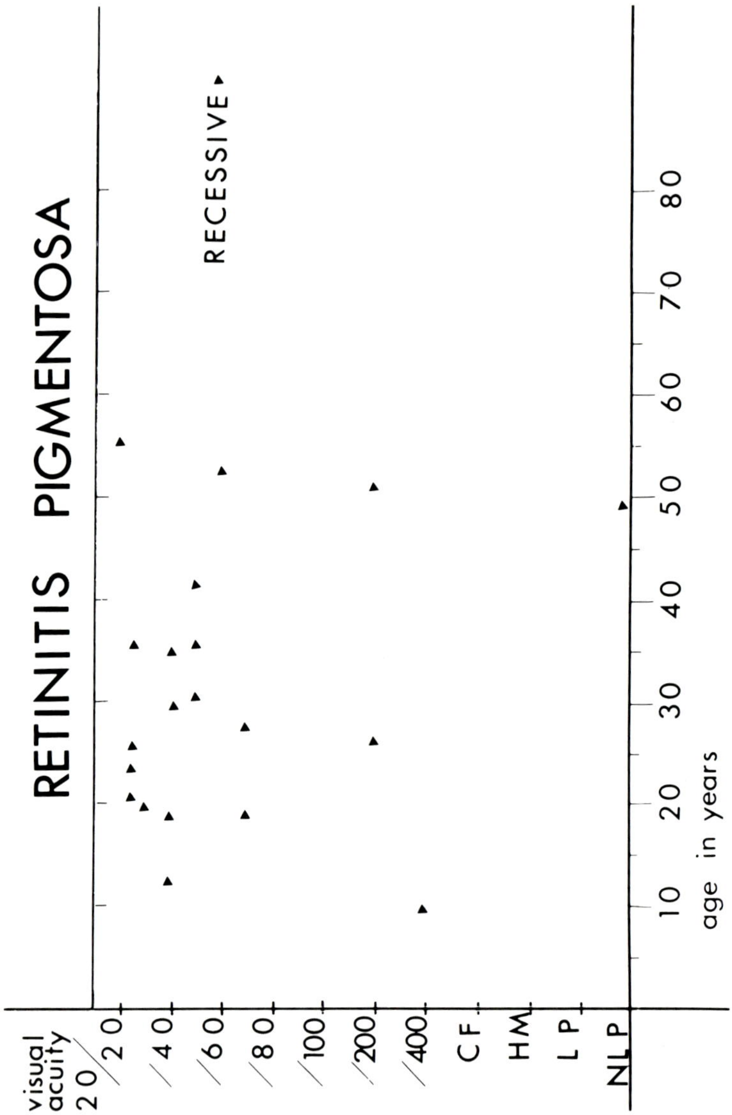

TABLE 4 - X-LINKED RECESSIVE

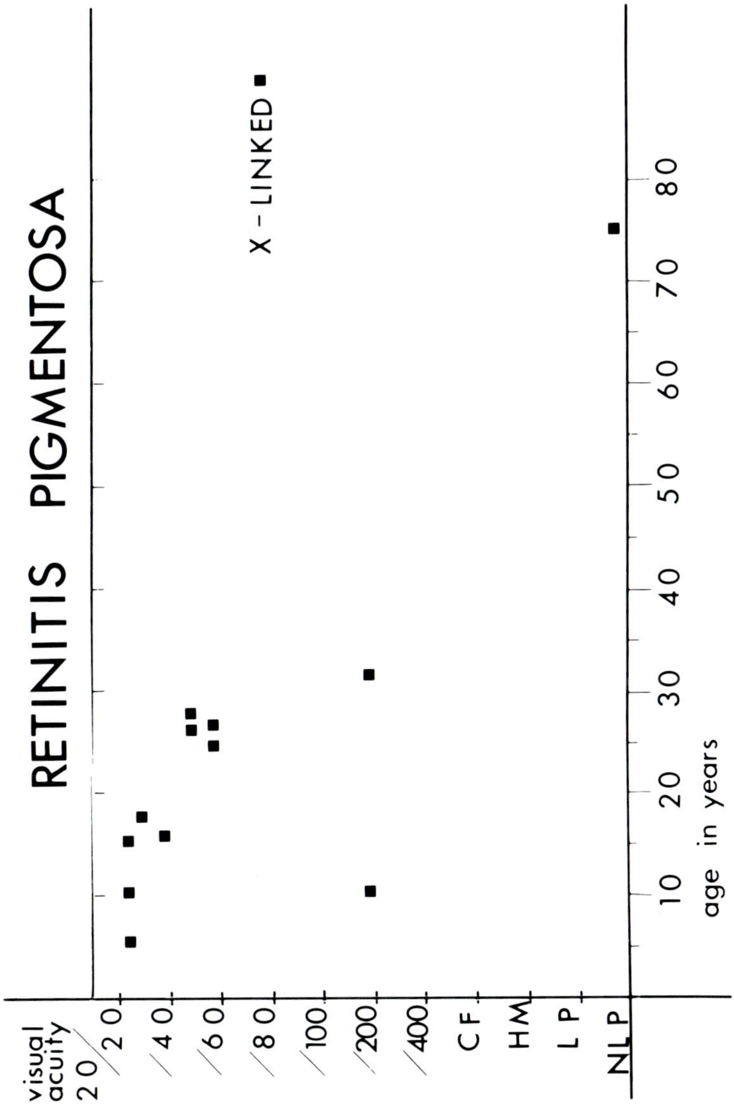

TABLE 5 - SIMPLEX

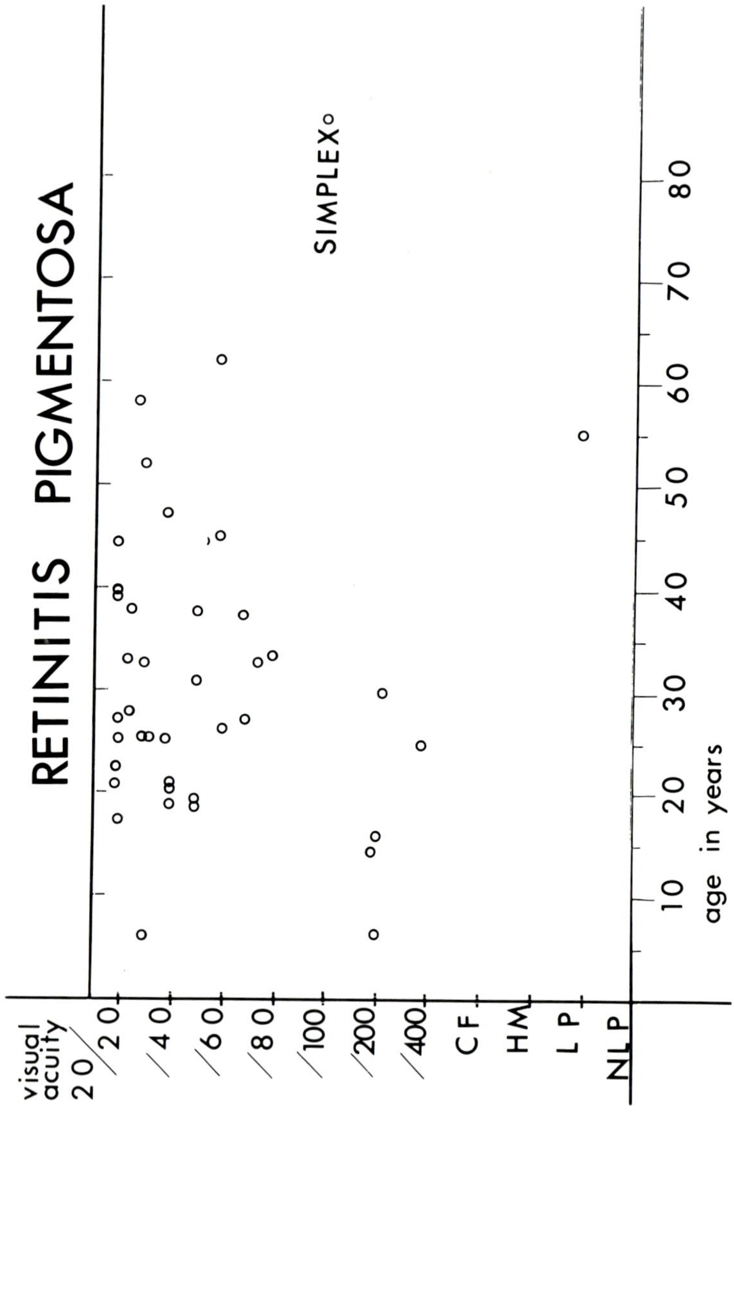

affected were often severely involved but had no interest in coming in for an examination. The dominant and simplex in most cases tended to have a milder course compared to the autosomal recessive and X-linked recessive. The etiology of the simplex cases is of course complex. Undoubtedly many reflect mendelian disease isolated by chance although it cannot be ruled out that some cases are purely non-genetic. Undoubtedly the marked clinical variability of the simplex group suggested several etiologic possibilities. Genetic heterogeneity was consistent with our data particularly in the autosomal recessive mode as it appeared to be two distinct form of the disease, a mild and severe.

GENETIC COUNSELLING IN RP.

The third aspect of the study was to see how the information accumulated on the genetics and natural history of the disease could be utilized to assist us in genetic counselling.

Examination.

1. We saw many patients diagnosed as having RP and referred to our clinic for genetic counselling, who after examination had a genocopy or more rarely a phenocopy of true RP. The main genocopies encountered in order of importance was the cone-rod dystrophies, paravenous retinal atrophy, undiagnosed cases of the Lawrence-Moon-Bardet-Biedle syndrome, choroideremia, diffuse choroidal atrophy, and stationary night blindness, with and without high myopia. The uncommonly encountered phenocopies were rubella and toxoplasmosis.

Our attempt at diagnostic specificity had three purposes. Firstly we wished to determine an accurate diagnosis as accurate genetic counselling depends upon a specific diagnosis. For example choroideremia, an X-linked recessive trait, has many clinical similarities to an autosomal recessive RP but their recurrence risks are different. Secondly, we wished to determine whether the RP was "isolated" or "complicated". We examined many patients who had prelingual speech who were either unaware of their hearing deficit or not aware of its genetic importance. Each of our 50 families with RP and hearing loss had a mode of inheritance consistent with autosomal recessive disease. Thirdly, we wished to have an exact diagnosis even when the mode of inheritance was known because far more often than not patients were concerned more with their visual than with their genetic prognosis.

2. Visual prognosis. From our data it is evident that it was difficult to predict the visual outlook for an individual patient, particularly when seen at a young age without a family history. It was only slightly more accurate when the mode of inheritance could be established. However, total blindness in our study was rare. Of the 130 patients examined only 7 had a visual acuity of 20/400 or worse. Of these, 3 had early visual loss and the remainder were after age 50.

3.Genetic Prognosis. Accurate genetic counselling depends upon establishing a correct diagnosis along with a mode of inheritance in a particular family. Examination of supposed normal relatives was often helpful in establishing a positive family history in otherwise simplex cases. However, in one half of our families a specific mode could not be established. Thus without a family history recurrence risks in RP have to be given cautiously.

4.Disability. On a more positive note our analysis of the questionnaires and the interviews with patients suggests that the disability caused by the disease does not correlate closely with its severity. Our experience indicates that RP is a predominantly chronic ocular disease of very slow progression and as Jean Real Brunette[6] has pointed out, people become aware of their disease well before it becomes a handicap. Most people we see are not blind and a large number in all likelihood will maintain some vision throughout life. For most, the reading vision is maintained through the high school years and beyond. Apart from the small number with hearing loss and the other rare syndromes of RP, there is no loss of intellectual or physical functioning. In all likelihood even after symptoms present, useful vision will be maintained for years if not decades thus enabling resourceful people to modify their life and adapt.

This study was supported by the National Retinitis Pigmentosa Foundation of Canada.

The assistance of my genetic associate, Mrs. Debbie MacIntosh, is gratefully acknowledged.

REFERENCES:

1. Fishman, G.A.: Retinitis Pigmentosa: Genetic Percentages Arch Ophthalmol - Vol 96, 822 , May 1978

2. Bird, A.C.: X-linked retinitis Pigmentosa Br J.Ophthalmol 59:177-197, 1975

3. Panteleeva, O.A.: On hereditary tapetoretinal degeneration (Russia) Vesta Oftalmol 82:53-56, 1969

4. Jay, B.: Hereditary aspects of pigmentary retinopathy. Trans Ophthalmol Soc UK 92:173-178, 1972

5. Ammann, F. Klein D. Franceschetti A: Genetic and epidemiological investigations on pigmentary degeneration of the retina and allied disorders in Switzerland. J. Neurol Sci 2:183-196, 1965

6. Brunette, J.R.: Personal Communication

CATARACT FORMATION IN RETINITIS PIGMENTOSA

Saul Merin, M.D.

Department of Ophthalmology

Hadassah University Hospital, Jerusalem, Israel

INTRODUCTION

Patients suffering from retinitis pigmentosa have also an increased incidence of cataract. Such patients may be seen to have cataracts relatively early in their life. This cataract may cause visual disturbance, in addition to and beyond the visual impairment caused by the retinal degenerative process.

The purpose of the present study was to find out the incidence of cataract in patients with retinitis pigmentosa, the age at which it appears, and the relation of cataract formation and vitreous changes.

MATERIALS AND METHODS

Patients suffering from retinitis pigmentosa and attending the retinitis pigmentosa clinic of the Hadassah Hospital department of ophthalmology were included in the study. Ninety-two consecutive patients were examined for the study. All had complete ophthalmological examination, including slit-lamp biomicroscopy, ophthalmoscopy, refraction, visual acuity and visual fields tests, color vision tests, electroretinography and visual evoked responses. Most had also electrooculographic tests. The diagnosis of retinitis pigmentosa was confirmed in all patients. The lens and vitreous were examined by biomicroscopy and the findings were recorded accordingly.

Birth Defects: Original Article Series, Volume 18, Number 6, pages 187–191

RESULTS

The typical cataract found in patients with retinitis pigmentosa was a posterior subcapsular cataract.

Sixty-one percent had clear lenses and 39% had cataracts. Of these about half had mild changes, disturbing the vision only a little while the other half had severe disturbance of vision from the lens changes.

The youngest patient with cataract was 17 years old. No patient in the first decade of life had cataracts. In the second decade of life 15% had cataracts, in the third - 40%, in the fourth - 60%, while 74% above age 40 had cataracts. (Table 1).

TABLE 1: PSC CATARACT AND AGE OF R.P. PATIENTS

Age group	Number of eyes		% with cat.
	total	with cat.	
< 10	14	0	0
11 - 20	60	9	15
21 - 30	42	17	40
31 - 40	30	18	60
> 41	38	28	74

Two types of changes were found in the vitreous, and were classified as outlined in Table 2.

TABLE 2: VITREOUS CHANGES IN R.P.

I. "Cells": fine, semitranslucent particles of one size

Grades:
- 0 - none
- +1 - several
- +2 - multiple
- +3 - heavy

II. Breakdown of vitreous structure

Grades:
- 0 - none
- +1 - posterior detachment and increase in fluidity
- +2 - floating fibers
- +3 - multiple floating fibers and large particles

Table 3 compares the state of the lens with the two types of vitreous changes as graded in Table 2. All patients with zero grade of "V-cells" had clear lenses. With increase in grade of "V-cells", the incidence and severity of lens changes increased. This relation was also present for "V-breakdown" but to a lesser degree.

TABLE 3: 146 EYES WITH R.P.: COMPARISON OF VITREOUS AND LENS CHANGES

Lens	"V-cells"				"V-breakdown"			
	0	1	2	3	0	1	2	3
Clear	53	36	12	0	35	35	26	5
PSC incip.	0	16	9	2	1	8	14	4
PSC progr.	0	0	9	9	0	2	8	0

Twenty of 146 eyes had a different grading of "V-cells" and "V-breakdown". In all of these the grading of "cells" fitted more than "breakdown" with the lens appearance. Six patients had in one eye a clear lens or an incipient cataract and a progressent cataract in the other. In all these, the vitreous of the more affected eye had more "cells" than the less affected eye.

DISCUSSION

This study confirms the clinical impression that in patients with retinitis pigmentosa a cataract tends to form early in life, that it is age related and that, in some patients, it affects vision, in addition to the basic disease process.

What causes the cataract in retinitis pigmentosa?

Theoretically, the lens changes could be caused by genetic factors acting directly on the lens, or be secondary to some other local ocular changes induced by the retinal degenerative process. The evidence for a genetic factor would be that some types of retinal dystrophy cause cataracts and others do not. Dystrophic rats develop cataracts, while some dystrophic mice do not (Merin and Auerbach, 1976). Sorsby (1970) claimed that some genetic types in human R.P.

develop cataracts, while others do not. On the other hand, there is evidence that ocular diseases affecting the vitreous may cause secondary lens opacification. This includes such diseases like persistent hyperplastic primary vitreous, retrolental fibroplasia, uveitis, vitreous hemorrhage or metallosis. Actually, the cataract which is frequently found in "pars planitis" or vitreous hemorrhage is of the same type of posterior subcapsular as found by us in retinitis pigmentosa.

Our study indicates that the cataract formation in retinitis pigmentosa is related to the vitreous changes. Pruett (1975) showed several years ago that such vitreous changes are very common in retinitis pigmentosa. These vitreous changes could, possibly, be secondary to the retinal degeneration or be a result of some other unknown factor. Of the two vitreal abnormalities, it is the inflammatory or pseudo-inflammatory appearance of vitreal cells which is related to the lens changes, rather than the structural breakdown.

SUMMARY

We studied the lens and the vitreous in 92 patients with tapetoretinal degenerations. Sixty-one percent of the eyes had a clear lens and the rest had a cataract or were aphakic. The typical cataract was posterior subcapsular, often with a nuclear cataract or with stellate projections. The vitreous showed frequently two types of abnormal changes: a pseudo-inflammatory reaction in the form of multiple "cells" and/or breakdown of the normal vitreous structure in the form of separation of the gel into fibers of collagen and fluid.

We found a definite correlation between the appearance of the cataract and the number of the "cells" and concluded that the pseudo-inflammatory vitreous response found in retinitis pigmentosa may be the cause of the cataract frequently found in this disease.

REFERENCES

Merin S and Auerbach E (1976). Retinitis pigmentosa. Surv Ophthalmol 20:303.
Pruett RC (1975). Retinitis pigmentosa, a biomicroscopical study of vitreous abnormalities. Arch Ophthalmol 93:603.
Sorsby A (1970). "Ophthalmic Genetics". 2nd edition, London: Butterworths, p. 136.

PRESERVED PARA-ARTERIOLE RETINAL PIGMENT EPITHELIUM (PPRPE) IN RETINITIS PIGMENTOSA

John R. Heckenlively, M.D.

Jules Stein Eye Institute and The Department of Ophthalmology, UCLA School of Medicine, Los Angeles, CA 90024 USA

Distinctive fundus patterns have been used to name many retinal dystrophies. In general the patterns have been the result of loss or degeneration of the retina or adjacent tissues. One example is pigmented paravenous retinochoroidal atrophy in which a pigment degenerative pattern next to retinal veins has been associated with typical retinitis pigmentosa (RP), cone-rod degeneration, sarcoidosis, and Stickler syndrome. Retinitis punctata albescens and sector RP are further examples of morphological fundus patterns that have been used to describe retinal disease states, but in which the etiology is unknown.

Retinitis pigmentosa is the generic name given to a group of retinal disease characterized by a slowly progressive panretinal degeneration that typically starts in the equator region, resulting in a ring scotoma earlier in the disease. Later, many patients have severely contracted visual fields but maintain central vision, as the macula, for unknown reasons, usually is more resistant to these disease processes.

Why the retina is preserved or degeneration is retarded in certain areas despite the panretinal nature of the process is an important question, as the answer to this question has the potential for aiding in the development of treatment for these conditions. A group of RP patients have been evaluated at the Jules Stein Eye Institute with a different form of retinal preservation which is adjacent to retinal arterioles.

Five unrelated individuals with RP, three with an inheritance pattern consistent with autosomal recessive disease and two with sporadic occurrence, have been identified with

Birth Defects: Original Article Series, Volume 18, Number 6, pages 193–196

a unique pattern of preservation of retinal pigment epithelium (RPE) under retinal arterioles (Heckenlively, 1982). The RPE preservation is relative with most of the patients demonstrating the pattern in isolated areas in the equator or anterior retina (Figure 1). One patient has had documented loss of the PPRPE pattern over one year. The clinical findings for these patients are presented in Table I.

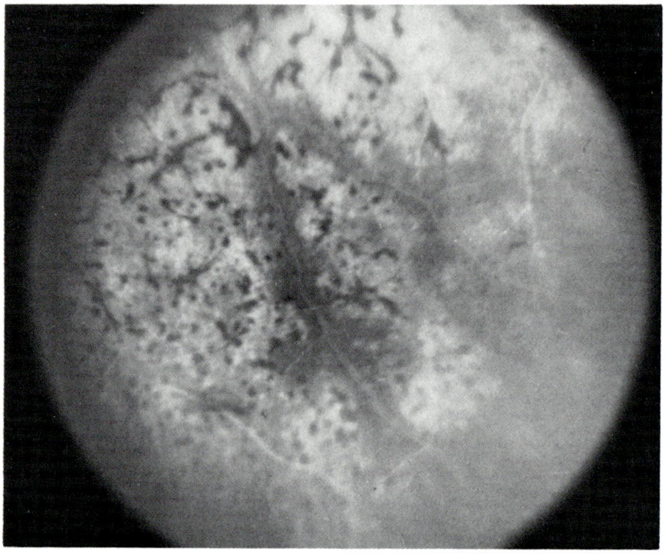

Fig. 1 Fluorescein angiogram of PPRPE pattern in a 33-year-old Iranian woman with advanced autosomal recessive RP. Retinal pigment epithelium under retinal arteriole blocks the transmission of the dye, giving hypofluorescent pattern.

All patients are significantly hypermetropic (group average absolute refractive error is +3.77) while RP patients tend to be myopic as a group (Sieving and Fishman, 1978). All patients with the PPRPE pattern had advanced disease, with severe night blindness, contracted fields, and abnormal electroretinogram.

These patients appear to have a specific type of RP in which the retinal arteriole plays a role in retarding the RP process. There are many hypotheses for explaining this phenomenon. One possible explanation is that a permeable factor is being released by the retinal arteriole that

Table 1 Summary of clinical findings in 5 patients with PPRPE

Case	Age	Age of Onset	Inheritance Pattern	Eye	Visual Acuity	Refraction
1	9	6	Sporadic	OD	20/30	+6.00+1.00 x 75
				OS	20/40	+6.00+1.00 x 105
2	33	5	Parents	OD	CF	+3.00+.75 x 120
			1st cousins	OS	4/200	+2.50
3	18	8	Mat. Aunt	OD	20/60	+2.00+2.25 x 90
			Blind	OS	20/50	+1.50+2.75 x 95
4	65	35	Sister, Mat.	OD	20/200	+3.75
			GGM had RP	OS	20/400	+2.75
5	15	3	Sporadic	OD	20/300	+3.00+.75 x 90
				OS	20/400	+2.50+.75 x 90

temporarily retards the degeneration locally in the areas of the retinal arteriole. Proving the existence of such a factor may be difficult, since the etiology of the disease process is not known.

Table 2 Summary of electrophysiological/psycholphysical data in 5 patients with PPRPE

Case	Dark Adaptation rod threshold	ERG findings	Goldmann visual fields (IV-4 isopter)		
1	4.6 log units	rod-cone	OD	30°	
		degeneration	OS	15°	
2	4.2 log units	nonrecordable	OD	-	peripheral
			OS	3°	islands OU
3	3.2 log units	nonrecordable	OD	3°	
			OS	3°	
4	5.0 log units	nonrecordable	OD	5°	
			OS	4°	
5	3.2 log units	nonrecordable	OD	7°	peripheral
			OS	7°	islands OU

The PPRPE pattern is not common; the frequency in our RP population is less than 1%. This pattern is seen best with indirect ophthalmoscopy and should be sought especially in hypermetropic RP patients. It is hoped that identifying subtypes of RP will allow research efforts to be focused more effectively, and will aid practitioners to diagnose more precisely the various types of RP.

Another interesting clinically identified sub-group is Usher's syndrome, in which retinitis pigmentosa is associated with profound hearing loss from an early age. This well known observation led us to routine audiologic testing of all our RP patients; we found additional RP patients who show a subclinical hearing loss for high frequencies, and this occurred in up to 10-15% of patients with retinitis pigmentosa who did not know previously of this hearing loss (and who had no other otologic disease or acoustic trauma that could explain the deficit at high frequency).

This relationship of hearing deficit to retinal degeneration may be of more than passing interest. Recognizing that retinal receptors are modified cilia and the hearing defect of Usher's syndrome could be based on a ciliary defect as well, the suggestion arose that retinitis pigmentosa might be associated with a more generalized ciliary abnormality in other parts of the body. To test this hypothesis, recently, Arden and Fox (1979) analyzed the ultrastructure of nasal cilia obtained by nasal biopsy from patients with retinitis pigmentosa. Their study was motivated as an etiological investigation with an awareness of the possible role of cilia in disease. Arden and Fox reported a statistically significant abnormality of nasal cilia ultrastructure in 14 patients with retinitis pigmentosa as compared to normal controls.

We have examined cilia from 13 patients with retinitis pigmentosa and compared them with nasal cilia from six healthy controls, performing an ultrastructure analysis similar to that of Arden and Fox. We confirm the study of Arden and Fox in demonstrating a significant abnormality in the ultrastructure of patients with retinitis pigmentosa.

Cilia are finger-like protrusions of the cell surface with a well defined internal structure (Fawcett and Porter, 1954). When motile, they fulfill important transport functions in the respiratory (Mossberg et al., 1978) and in the reproductive (Afzelius, 1979) systems. They are also a constant feature in many sensory receptors, although their exact role in these functions has not been determined (Barber, 1974). It is not surprising, then, that ciliary abnormalities may be manifest as wide-spread systemic disease, including infertility and respiratory infections (Afzelius, 1979).

The internal structure of cilia (Warner, 1974) is characterized by nine peripheral microtubular doublets surrounding a central a central microtubular pair (Fig. 1). In motile cilia, each peripheral microtubular doublet exhibits two protrusions: these constitute the dynein arms. In addition, there are periodic transversal links, called radial spokes, between the central sheath and each of the peripheral doublets; less prominent periodic linkages called nexin links occur between adjacent peripheral doublets. The dynein arms have ATPase activity which appears to provide the energy for ciliary motility. It is generally accepted that in motile cilia, microtubule sliding occurs to produce ciliary bending and it has been supposed that the radial spokes and nexin bridges, along with the central microtubules and central sheath, may act as mechanical supports during bending (Satir, 1974).

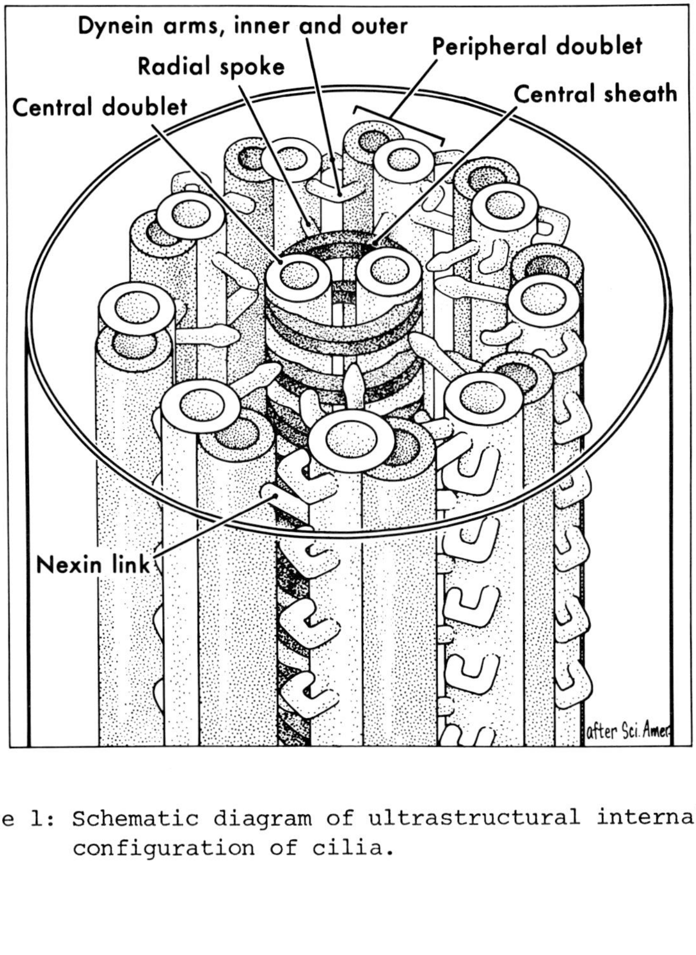

Figure 1: Schematic diagram of ultrastructural internal configuration of cilia.

METHODS

We examined cilia from 13 patients with retinitis pigmentosa and compared them with nasal cilia from six healthy controls. Table 1 summarizes the clinical features. The tissue samples were obtained from the nasal epithelium. Dr. Haskins Kashima, an otolaryngologist skilled in this technique, obtained these specimens by curette without premedication or topical anesthesia. Samples ranging in size from one to two millimeters square were obtained without discomfort. At the same time, a clinical ENT examination and relevant history were obtained from patients and controls. The samples were fixed in 2% gluteraldehyde in 0.1 molar cacodylate buffer, pH 7.2, and processed for transmission electron microscopy. The sections were mounted on single hole grids to visualize as many cilia as possible. All fields which showed perpendicular cilia, that is where the microtubular pattern was clearly discernable, were photographed for counting and analysis of possible abnormalities. The cilia included in the count had to meet two essential conditions: the cilium should not be counted twice at two different levels and sections of cilia that could be close to the tapering tip where some of the microtubules may have already ended, particularly in the bent position, were excluded from the count. This analysis was performed independently by Dr. Reissig and by Dr. Finkelstein. From 70 to 444 cilia were examined from each subject. Analysis was with respect to the 9+2 arrangement of microtubules only. Other ultrastructural features of the cilia were not examined, such as the presence of dynein arms.

RESULTS

In RP patients, the abnormal cilia ranged from 1.9% to 15%, with a median of 4.0%. In the normal control group, the abnormal cilia ranged from 0.0% to 3.0%, with a median of 1.2%. Even though there is some overlap in the percentage of abnormal cells between RP patients and normal controls, the rates in the RP group are significantly higher than in the controls ($P < 0.01$ by Wilcoxon's non-parametric test for ranked data) (Snedecor and Cochran, 1967).

Figure 2 demonstrates two types of ciliary abnormalities that were frequently observed.

SEX	AGE	RACE	TYPE	HEREDITY	ACUITY OD; OS	FIELD LOSS	PERCENT ABNORMAL CILIA	NUMBER CILIA COUNTED
F	33	W	Class II*	Dominant	20/20; 20/25	Mild-moderate O.U.	15.0%	293
F	34	B	Class I	Simplex	20/150; 20/40	Mild O.U.	7.4%	418
F	44	W	Usher's	Simplex	20/40; 20/40	Severe O.U.	5.3%	113
F	63	W	Class II	Recessive vs Dominant with incomplete penetrance	20/60; 20/60	Moderate O.U.	1.9%	267
F	32	W	Usher's	Simplex	20/25; 20/20	Severe O.U.	7.6%	70
M	38	W	Usher's	Recessive	20/50; 20/50	Severe O.U.	4.0%	173
M	53	W	X-linked	X-linked	20/50; 20/60	Severe O.U.	2.0%	199
M	53	W	X-linked	X-linked	20/200; 20/80	Severe O.U.	2.0%	264
F	38	W	Usher's	Recessive	HM; HM	Severe O.U.	2.0%	441
M	60	W	Usher's	Simplex	20/60; 20/50	Severe O.U.	2.2%	316
F	53	W	Class I	Simplex	20/25; 20/25	Severe O.U.	3.0%	342
F	29	W	Class I	Recessive	20/40; 20/50	Severe O.U.	6.8%	444
F	25	W	Class I	Dominant with incomplete penetrance	20/50; 20/160	Mild O.U.	6.3%	144
M	22	W	Normal				2.0%	183
M	40	W	Normal				3.0%	437
M	32	W	Normal				0.0%	252
M	29	W	Normal				1.4%	354
F	38	W	Normal				0.0%	339
F	27	B	Normal				0.9%	112

*Class I & II, see Reference 12

Table 1: Summary of clinical features of RP patients and controls.

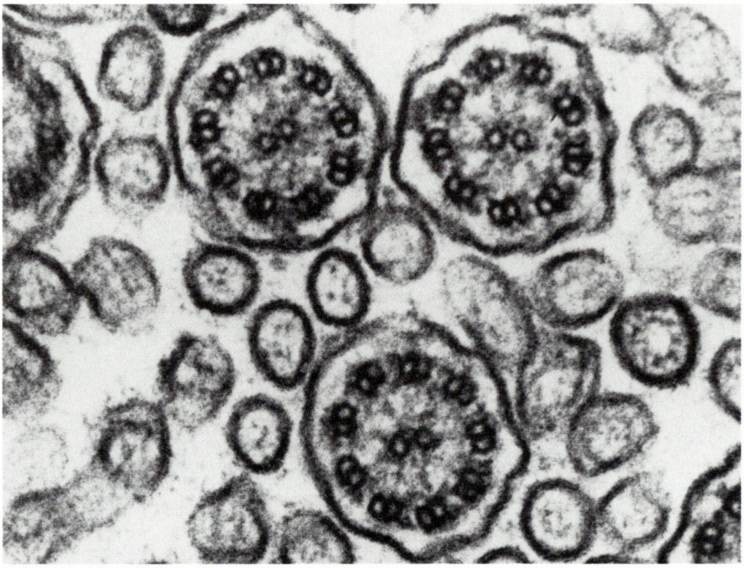

Figure 2a: EM cross section of three cilia demonstrating normal 9+2 arrangement of microtubules.

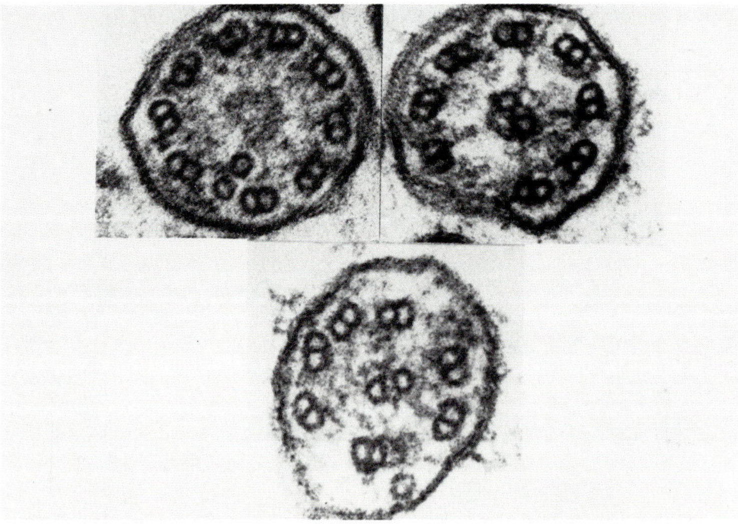

Figure 2b: EM cross section of three cilia demonstrating, in each, an abnormality of the 9+2 arrangement.

DISCUSSION

The importance of this statistically significant abnormality is unknown. Our data, and that recorded by Arden and Fox (1980), suggest that there might be a more generalized cilia abnormality in some patients with retinitis pigmentosa. In reviewing our data, we have not identified any sub-group of RP (i.e., Usher's syndrome, genetic type, psychophysical type) that appears to be more highly associated with the cilia abnormality. We want to caution that nasal cilia ultrastructure is technically difficult to evaluate. Electron microscopic sperm tail ultrastructure provides better definition of ultrastructural features (Afzelius, 1981), but that has not yet been evaluated in males with retinitis pigmentosa. However, it is relevant that several investigators have established that cilia ultrastructure abnormalities can be associated with a clinical disease entity termed the immotile-cilia syndrome. In 1933, Kartagener (1933) described a triad of bronchiectasis, chronic sinusitis, and situs inversus. Some males with Kartagener's syndrome had infertility as well, with living, but immotile sperm. In 1975, Afzelius et al. evaluated the immotile sperm and noted that they lack dynein arms, an ultrastructural component of cilia important to ciliary motility. This observation led to the discovery that cilia from nasal biopsy as well similarly lacked dynein arms (Eliasson et al, 1977; Pedersen and Mygind, 1976), explaining the decreased muco-ciliary transport and clinical respiratory disease in Kartagener's syndrome. Further clinical investigations have shown that immotile sperm and nasal cilia are associated with a somewhat broader clinical disease entity that is now termed the immotile-cilia syndrome, clinically characterized (Afzelius and Mossberg, 1980) as:

A. Cases with complete Kartagener's syndrome (triad of chronic sinusitis, bronchiectasis, and situs inversus)

B. Men without situs inversus but with a typical clinical history (chronic bronchitis and rhinitis since early childhood) and with living, but immotile spermatozoa

C. Women or children without situs inversus but with typical clinical signs and a sibling with complete Kartagener's syndrome

D. Individuals without situs inversus but with clinical signs, if biopsy shows characteristic ultrastructural defects in cilia

An excellent review of clinical considerations, ciliary studies and speculations is presented by Afzelius (1979).

Our RP patients were not analyzed for abnormalities of nasal cilia dynein arms because of the much greater technical difficulties with that analysis beyond that associated with analysis of the 9+2 microtubular arrangement; our analysis of the 9+2 arrangement alone developed from our interest in the data of Arden and Fox (1979) who have previously suggested the more easily analysed 9+2 arrangement may be abnormal. Interestingly, in this rapidly advancing new field of cilia ultrastructure abnormalities in relation to clinical disease, several reports have shown that the absence of dynein arms is not the only abnormality. Sturgess et al (1979) in studying three siblings with chronic respiratory disease, showed an absence of the radial spokes in nasal cilia but the dynein arms were present. This absence of radial spokes was associated with decreased muco-ciliary clearance and, in the male sibling, with sperm immotility. Sturgess et al. proposed that absence of the radial spokes is another cause of the immotile-cilia syndrome.

Afzelius and Eliasson (1979) have described five types of ultrastructural abnormalities from patients with living but immotile sperm:

1. Absence of both dynein arms
2. Absence of inner dynein arms
3. Absence of outer dynein arms
4. Probable absence of part of the radial spoke
5. Absence of one or both central microtubules and lacking the central sheath

Interestingly, the fifth category of patients did not have the other clinical aspects of the immotile-cilia syndrome. This heterogeneity of ultrastructure and clinical presentation suggests that other ciliary abnormalities may exist that affect function of only some ciliated organs, and not others, supporting a rationale for continued research in the relation of cilia abnormalities to various disease entities, including that of the eye. Svedbergh et al (1981) have performed ophthalmic and visual function evaluation of 10 patients with the immotile-cilia syndrome. No retinal abnormalities could be appreciated.

Schneeberger et al (1980) demonstrated heterogeneity in respiratory cilia of three male patients with the immotile-cilia syndrome. One patient had an absence of inner dynein arms, unusually prominent outer dynein arms, a spoke defect in 46% of cilia, and no detectable nexin links. A second patient had absence of both dynein arms. A third patient had absence of both dynein arms and almost 40% had one to nine extra microtubules peripheral to the nine outer doublets. These case reports by Schneeberger et al. were of particular interest in relation to our case reports in demonstrating an abnormality of the 9+2 arrangement and in demonstrating that a given ultrastructural abnormality may be present in some, but not all, biopsied cilia.

These studies of the heterogeneity of ciliary disease demonstrate the rationale for continued cilia ultrastructural studies in patients with retinitis pigmentosa.

REFERENCES

Afzelius B (1979). The immotile-cilia syndrome and other ciliary diseases. Int Rev Exp Path 19:1-43

Afzelius B (1981). Personal communication.

Afzelius B and Eliasson R (1979). Flagellar mutants in man: on the heterogeneity of the immotile-cilia syndrome. J Ultrastructure Res 69:43-52

Afzelius B, Eliasson R and Johnson O (1975). Lack of dynein arms in immotile human spermatozoa. J Cell Biol 66:225-232

Afzelius B and Mossberg B (1980). Editorial. Thorax 35: 401-404

Arden GB and Fox B (1979). Increased incidence of abnormal nasal cilia in patients with RP. Nature 279:534-536

Barber V (1974). Cilia in sense organs. In: "Cilia and Flagella", Ed. by M. Sleigh, Academic Press, New York, p. 403

Eliasson R, Mossberg,B, Camner P and Afzelius B (1977). The immotile-cilia syndrome. New Engl J Med 297:1-6

Fawcett DW and Porter KR (1954). A study of the fine structure of human nasal cilia including abnormalities found in retinitis pigmentosa.

Fox B, Bull TB and Arden GB (1980). Variations in the ultrastructure of human nasal cilia including abnormalities found in retinitis pigmentosa. J Clin Pathol 33:327-335

Kartagener M (1933). Zur pathogenese der bronchiektasien. I. Bronchiektasien bei situs viscerum inversus. Beitr Klin Tuberk 83:489-501

Massof R and Finkelstein D (1979). Rod sensitivity relative to cone sensitivity in RP. Invest Ophthalmol Vis Sci 18:263

Mossberg B, Afzelius B, Eliasson R and Camner P (1978). On the pathogenesis of obstructuve lung disease. Scan J Resp Dis 59:55-65

Pedersen H and Mygind N (1976). Absence of axonemal arms in nasal mucosa cilia in Kartagener's syndrome. Nature 262:494-495

Satir P (1974). The present status of the sliding microtubule model of ciliary motion. In: "Cilia and Flagella", Ed. by M. Sleigh, Academic Press, New York, p. 131

Schneeberger EE, Mc Cormack J, Issenberg HJ, Schuster SR and Gerald PS (1980). Heterogeneity of ciliary morphology in the immotile-cilia syndrome in man. J Ultrastructural Res 73:34-43

Snedecor SW and Cochran WG (1967). "Statistical Methods", Ames, Iowa: The Iowa State University Press, p. 130

Sturgess JM, Chao J, Wong J, Aspin N and Turner JAP (1979). Cilia with defective radial spokes. New Engl J Med 300:53-56

Svedbergh B, Josson V and Afzelius B (1981). Immotile-cilia syndrome and the cilia of the eye. Graefes Arch Ophthalmol 215:265-272

Warner F (1974). The fine structure of the ciliary and flagellar axoneme. In: "Cilia and Flagella", Ed. by M. Sleigh, Academic Press, New York, p. 11

Therapy of Gyrate Atrophy of Retina and Choroid

A TWO YEAR TRIAL OF LOW PROTEIN, LOW ARGININE DIETS OR VITAMIN B_6 FOR PATIENTS WITH GYRATE ATROPHY

Eliot L. Berson, Arthur H. Hanson, III, Bernard Rosner, and Vivian E. Shih

Berman-Gund Laboratory for the Study of Retinal Degenerations, Harvard Medical School, Massachusetts Eye and Ear Infirmary
243 Charles Street, Boston, MA 02114, U.S.A.

INTRODUCTION

Patients with gyrate atrophy of the choroid and retina have 10-20 fold elevations in plasma ornithine (Simell and Takki, 1973; Takki and Simell, 1974; Takki, 1974) in association with a deficiency of ornithine ketoacid transaminase (OKT) activity (Trijbels et al, 1977; Valle et al, 1977; Kennaway et al, 1977; Shih et al, 1978; O'Donnell et al, 1978; Berson et al, 1978). The concentrations of ornithine in the plasma can be lowered toward normal with low protein, low arginine diets in all cases so far studied (Stoppolini et al, 1978; Valle et al, 1980; McInnes et al, 1981; Shih et al, 1981; Berson et al, 1981), and with vitamin B_6 (pyridoxine hydrochloride) in some cases (Berson et al, 1978; Weleber et al, 1978; Kaiser-Kupfer et al, 1980; Kennaway et al, 1980; Berson et al, 1981; Weleber et al, 1981; Shih et al, 1981). However, it is not known whether any decline in the hyperornithinemia will modify the course of the ocular disease over the long term. We have been following five patients with gyrate atrophy whose plasma ornithine levels have been lowered toward normal for about two years. This report summarizes our observations on the ocular findings in these patients.

MATERIALS AND METHODS

Five patients, ranging in age from 12-30 years, with gyrate atrophy of the choroid and retina were admitted to the

Birth Defects: Original Article Series, Volume 18, Number 6, pages 209-218

Mallinckrodt General Clinical Research Center at the Massachusetts General Hospital in early 1979 for a five-week period during which time their food protein was gradually lowered to 10-15 grams per day (about 0.25-0.5 grams of arginine per day). A mixture of essential amino acids (EAA) (Shih et al, 1981), based on nutritional requirements of normal human adults (Meister, 1965; Kopple and Swendseid, 1975), was given in capsules each day so that the total of food protein and amino acid supplement together was maintained at 35 grams per day. This low arginine diet was supplemented with multiple vitamins and minerals including calcium, phosphorus, zinc, and iron to ensure that Recommended Daily Allowances (Food and Nutrition Board, National Council, National Academy of Science, 1974) were met. All five patients were given 300 mgm of vitamin B_6 orally per day. During the hospital admission patients were taught to keep daily food records which were reviewed by a nutritionist; this procedure was continued after discharge. Plasma amino acids were measured at each level of protein intake during hospital admission and monthly after discharge to help assure compliance with the prescribed diet. Over the five-week in-hospital period, all showed substantial declines in plasma ornithine levels (Table 1). No harmful systemic side effects were observed, in particular, no hyperammonemia (Shih et al, 1981).

Table 1

PLASMA ORNITHINE LEVELS IN PATIENTS ON LOW-PROTEIN, LOW-ARGININE DIETS OR VITAMIN B_6

Patient	Age§	Baseline* (Pre-Diet)	In Hospital (5 Weeks)	Lowest Ornithine	Average† (4 Mo-2 Yrs)
1	30	706	280	153	315
2	21	1,185	630	390	680
3	12	1,000	600	400	713
4	13	975	500	390	658
5	16	800 (434‡)	177	177	402‡

§Age at onset of trial.

*Normal range for plasma ornithine 50-102 nmol/ml.

†Average based on monthly determinations of plasma ornithine.

‡On vitamin B_6 300 mgm/day alone.

Following discharge, patient 1 achieved her lowest plasma ornithine concentration of 153 nmol/ml on an intake of 15 grams per day at week 13; at her request, dietary protein intake was then increased to 20 grams per day and EAA were decreased to 15 grams per day at home and her plasma ornithine concentration rose to an average level of about 315 nmol/ml. Patient 2 could not continue a 15 gram per day protein diet beyond week 14 but with a 25 to 35 gram diet, his plasma ornithine concentration gradually rose and stabilized around 680 nmol/ml. Patient 3 achieved a plasma ornithine level of 400 nmol/ml five to seven weeks after starting the diet; then, on modified protein restriction (20-25 grams), her level rose to an average of 713 nmol/ml. Patient 4, a sibling of patient 3, also achieved her lowest plasma ornithine level of 390 nmol/ml shortly after discharge from the hospital; then, on a modified food protein restriction (20-25 grams), her ornithine level rose to around 658 nmol/ml. Withdrawal of vitamin B_6 tablets after year 1 had no effect on plasma ornithine levels of patients 1-4. Patient 5, the only vitamin B_6 responsive patient, showed an additive effect of the diet compared with vitamin B_6 alone. After five weeks of protein restriction (15 grams per day), his plasma ornithine level decreased from 434 nmol/ml to 177 nmol/ml. After returning home, he discontinued all dietary restrictions and vitamin B_6 due to personal considerations. His plasma ornithine increased to 870 nmol/ml. Reinstitution of vitamin B_6 (300 mg per day) alone again lowered his plasma ornithine to the 400 nmol/ml range, and he has been followed at this level for about two years.

Ocular examinations were performed prior to institution of this diet, at four weeks after onset of the diet, and then at one- to six-month intervals. Each examination included measurements of best corrected Snellen visual acuity, slit-lamp examination, kinetic visual fields on the Goldmann perimeter, dark adaptation testing on the Goldmann-Weekers dark adaptometer, full-field electroretinograms (ERGs), and fundus photographs. Dark adaptation thresholds were measured with an 11° white test light centrally fixated after 45 minutes of dark adaptation. A given threshold measurement was based on the average of at least two determinations per eye during each test period. Full-field ERGs were monitored with a bipolar Burian-Allen contact lens electrode placed on the topically anesthetized cornea after dilation of the pupils with 10% phenylephrine hydrochloride and 1% cyclopentolate hydrochloride. Responses were elicited with single flashes of white light presented at 0.5 Hz and at 30 Hz; for both test conditions, stimulus flash duration was 10 μsec and stimulus flash intensity was 16 x 10^3 ft-Lamberts. Responses were computer averaged (n = 64), displayed on an oscilloscope, and photographed. Two to three consecutive runs were averaged for each test condition. Responses under 2 μV could not be reliably quantitated with this technique.

For visual acuity, Goldmann visual fields, dark adaptation thresholds, and ERG amplitudes, the intra- and inter-visit patient variability was monitored and the amount of change required between two visits to indicate a statistically significant ($p < 0.05$) change was determined for an average patient with gyrate atrophy. For each parameter, results from both eyes at a given visit were averaged. In the case of visual acuity, the natural log of the Snellen fraction was used to better normalize the distribution of acuities. Based on an assessment of the median between-visit and within-visit variability (Snedecor and Cochran, 1967), it was determined for our patients that a change in average visual acuity of one or more lines (i.e., change in minus the natural log of Snellen fraction $\geq$ 0.241), or a change in the area of the average visual field over both eyes with a V-4 white test light of $\geq$ 41%, or a change of $\geq$ 0.3 log units in final dark-adapted thresholds averaged over both eyes, or a change of > 25% in ERG amplitude for single flashes of white light dark-adapted or > 50% for 30 Hz white flicker in both eyes would be required to show a statistically significant ($p < 0.05$) difference between the mean of two to three measurements at one visit with the mean of two to three measurements at a follow-up visit. Linear regression analyses were also used to assess trends over time for individual patients for each of the above parameters. Fundus photographs were considered significantly changed if two observers could independently observe enlarged areas of chorioretinal atrophy or new foci of atrophy.

RESULTS

Although all patients showed substantial declines in plasma ornithine levels on low protein, low arginine diets or vitamin B_6 (Table 1), findings on ocular examinations over about two years showed no significant improvement compared with baseline measurements (Table 2). Taking into account intra- and inter-visit variability, no patient showed a one line or greater improvement in visual acuity averaged over both eyes (i.e., change in minus the natural log of Snellen

Table 2

OCULAR FINDINGS IN PATIENTS WITH GYRATE ATROPHY OF THE CHOROID AND RETINA ON LOW-PROTEIN, LOW-ARGININE DIETS OR ON PYRIDOXINE

Pt.	Weeks on Diet	Visual Acuity OD	Visual Acuity OS	Natural Log of Snellen Fraction*	Change†	Visual Field‡ OD	Visual Field‡ OS	Change†	Dark Adaptation OU	Dark Adaptation Change†	Electroretinograms OU (μV) 0.5 Hz	Change	30 Hz	Change
1	0	20/60	20/50	1.008		25°‡	25°		0.9§		4.2‖		ND‖	
	4	20/60	20/50	1.008		25°	25°		0.9		5.2		ND	
	16	20/60	20/60	1.099		25°	25°		0.9		NA		ND	
	46	20/60	20/60	1.099		29°	28°		0.9		3.8		ND	
	76	20/70	20/60	1.173		28°	28°		0.8		4.1		ND	
	103	20/70	20/60	1.173	0.165	27°	28°	17%	0.9	0.0	3.3	21%	ND	--
2	0	20/70	20/100	1.431		23°	25°		0.9		ND		ND	
	4	20/70	20/100	1.431		25°	24°		1.0		ND		ND	
	8	20/70	20/100	1.431		NA	NA		NA		ND		ND	
	20	20/70	20/100	1.431		23°	27°		1.1		ND		ND	
	52	20/60	20/100	1.354		26°	21°		1.0		ND		ND	
	86	20/60	20/100	1.354		NA	NA		0.6		ND		ND	
	99	20/60	20/100	1.354		15°	20°		0.6		ND		ND	
	115	20/60	20/100	1.354	0.077	17°	20°	41%	0.9	0.0	ND	--	ND	--
3	0	20/50	20/60	1.008		~40°**	~40°		0.2		74.2		14.5	
	4	20/50	20/70	1.085		~40°	~40°		0.2		67.5		14.0	
	8	20/50	20/50	0.916		NA	NA		0.2		71.0		12.0	
	24	20/50	20/50	0.916		~40°	~40°		0.3		59.5		10.5	
	59	20/50	20/70	1.085		~40°	~40°		0.2		68.0		5.7	
	82	20/50	20/50	0.916		~40°	~40°		0.6		63.4		6.3	
	95	20/50	20/50	0.916		~40°	~40°		0.1		38.5		2.9	
	113	20/50	20/50	0.916	0.092	~40°	~40°	0%	0.0	0.2	54.6	26%	5.4	62%
4	0	20/40	20/40	0.693		full**	full		1.3		ND		ND	
	4	20/40	20/40	0.693		full	full		1.2		ND		ND	
	8	20/40	20/40	0.693		NA	NA		NA		ND		ND	
	24	20/40	20/40	0.693		full	full		1.2		ND		ND	
	56	20/40	20/50	0.805		full	full		1.2		ND		ND	
	82	20/50	20/30	0.629		full	full		1.5		ND		ND	
	95	20/30	20/30	0.406		full	full		1.0		ND		ND	
	113	20/40	20/30	0.539	0.154	full	full	0%	1.2	0.1	ND	--	ND	--
5	0	20/25	20/25	0.223		full**	full		2.6		4.3		ND	
	4	20/25	20/25	0.223		full	full		2.4		3.9		ND	
	20***	20/25	20/20	0.112		full	full		2.4		3.9		ND	
	67***	20/25	20/25	0.223		full	full		2.5		5.0		ND	
	97***	20/25	20/30	0.310		full	full		2.1		3.6		ND	
	124***	20/25	20/25	0.223	0.0	full	full	0%	2.4	0.2	4.3	0%****	ND	--

*Results from both eyes were averaged for each visit. Numbers represent minus the natural log of the Snellen fraction.

†Average change over both eyes compared with average from both eyes at time zero.

‡Goldmann perimeter, isopter designated for V-4 white test light (i.e., 25° is field constricted to 25° in all quadrants with V-4 white test light).

§Goldmann-Weekers dark adaptometer (11° white test light centrally fixated); dark adaptation thresholds expressed as log units above normal.

‖Normal range for amplitudes: white (0.5 Hz dark adapted) 350-700 μV; white flicker (30 Hz) 50-125 μV; NA, Not available; ND, non-detectable ERG as tested (< 2 μV).

**Visual fields to a V-4 white light in patient 3 extended to the 35° isopter nasally, 30° superiorily, 50° isopter temporally, and 35° isopter inferiorly in each eye. Patients 4 and 5 had full fields with a V-4 white test light but fields OU constricted to about the 8-10° (patient 4) and 5-6° (patient 5) isopters with a I-4 white test light.

***On pyridoxine hydrochloride 300 mg/day alone.

****Measurements from right eye only.

fraction $\geq$ 0.241). None showed an enlargement in the area of visual field averaged over both eyes of $\geq$ 41%, or an improvement of final dark-adapted threshold of $\geq$ 0.3 log units averaged over both eyes. No increases in ERG amplitudes of > 25% to single flashes (0.5 Hz) of white light or > 50% to white 30 Hz flicker could be detected. Furthermore, none of these patients reported any subjective improvement in visual function. Slit-lamp examination revealed moderate posterior subcapsular cataracts in patient 1 and slight posterior subcapsular cataracts in patients 2 and 3 that remained unchanged.

Based on an assessment of both baseline to last visit comparisons and linear regression analyses, patients 1, 4, and 5 showed no significant change ($p > 0.05$) for any of the parameters of visual function tested. Patient 2 had a significant loss of visual field and patient 3 showed a significant decline in her full-field ERGs. Comparison of fundus photographs of all patients taken prior to onset of the diet and at 1-1/2 to 2 years after onset of the diet or vitamin B_6 showed enlargement and posterior extension of areas of chorioretinal atrophy in both eyes. Representative fundus photographs to illustrate these changes are shown for patients 1 and 5 in Figure 1.

DISCUSSION

Other laboratories have reported improvements in visual acuity (Kaiser-Kupfer et al, 1980; McInnes et al, 1981), visual fields (McInnes et al, 1981), dark adaptation thresholds (Kaiser-Kupfer et al, 1980; Kaiser-Kupfer et al, 1981), and/or ERGs (Weleber et al, 1978; Kaiser-Kupfer et al, 1980; Weleber and Kennaway, 1981; Kaiser-Kupfer et al, 1981) in some patients with gyrate atrophy after onset of a low protein, low arginine diet or vitamin B_6, but these reports are difficult to evaluate without more information about the amount of intra- and inter-visit variability for these parameters in their patients. Taking into account the intra- and inter-visit variability in our patients with respect to measurements of Snellen visual acuity, area of visual fields, final dark-adapted thresholds, and full-field ERG amplitudes, we could not document any significant improvement over the first two years despite substantial declines in plasma ornithine levels. Moreover, serial fundus photographs revealed progression in all five of our patients including two who have maintained plasma ornithine levels at 50-60% (i.e., 300-400 nmol/ml) of

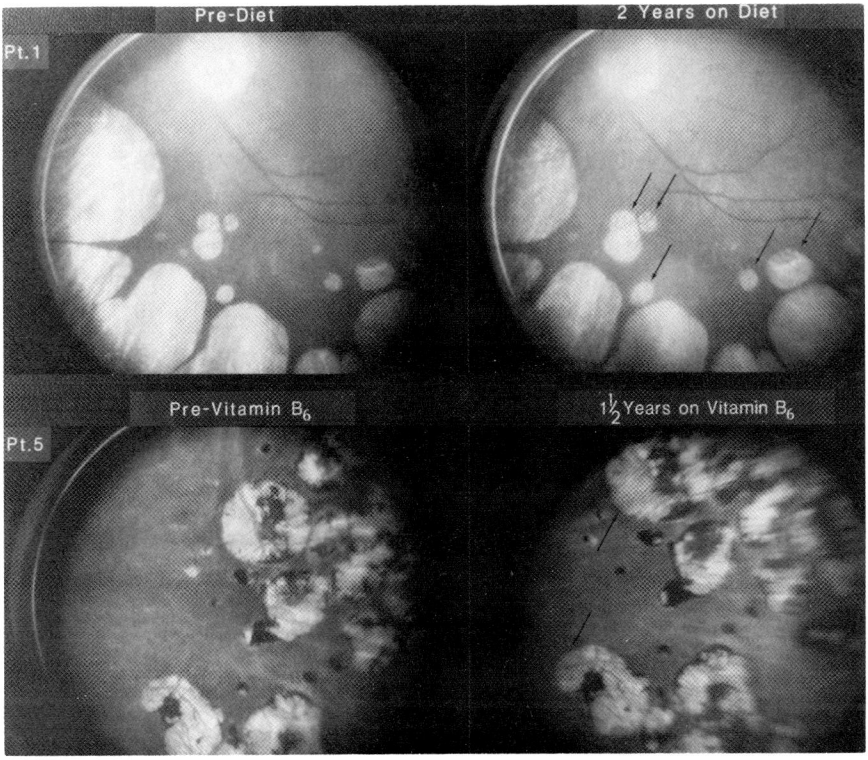

Figure 1: Fundus photographs from patient 1 (inferonasal fundus, left eye) taken prior to onset (left photo) and two years after onset of a low protein, low arginine diet and from patient 5 (far temporal fundus, left eye) taken prior (i.e., week 20, see Table 1) to onset (left photo) and 1-1/2 years after onset of vitamin B_6 (300 mgm/day). Both patients show enlarged areas of chorioretinal atrophy (see arrows) compared to pre-trial photos.

pretrial levels.

Although enlargement of areas of chorioretinal atrophy was observed in all five patients within two years, only two have shown significant declines in retinal function over this period. This discrepancy between visible fundus changes and lack of functional changes in some patients could reflect the fact that the functional tests used in this study are not sensitive enough to monitor slight losses of photoreceptor function in association with slight increases in the areas of midperipheral chorioretinal atrophy. Another possibility is that the areas of functioning retina have remained virtually unchanged in three of these five patients after two years because of the declines in plasma ornithine levels. These patients continue to be followed in this trial of diet or vitamin B_6 to determine whether declines in plasma ornithine concentrations will result in stabilized retinal function.

SUMMARY

Four patients with gyrate atrophy on low protein (20-35 g/day), low arginine diets and one on vitamin B_6 (300 mgm/day) have maintained their plasma ornithine concentrations in the range of 30-60% of pre-therapeutic trial levels for about two years. After two years, three of the five patients have shown no significant change in Snellen visual acuity, visual fields, final dark-adapted thresholds or full-field electroretinograms. All five patients have shown slight enlargement of areas of chorioretinal atrophy in the midperiphery. These patients continue on low protein, low arginine diets or on vitamin B_6 to determine whether any reduction in the hyperornithinemia will result in stabilization of retinal function.

ACKNOWLEDGMENTS

This work was supported in part by National Eye Institute Specialized Research Center Grant EY02014 (Dr. Berson), by USPHS Grant NS 05096 (Dr. Shih), by the National Retinitis Pigmentosa Foundation, Baltimore Maryland, and the George Gund Foundation, Cleveland, Ohio (Dr. Berson), and by USPHS Grant RR 1066 to the Mallinckrodt General Clinical Research Center, Massachusetts General Hospital.

REFERENCES

Berson EL, Schmidt SY, Shih VE (1978). Ocular and biochemical abnormalities in gyrate atrophy of the choroid and retina. Ophthalmology 85:1018-1027.

Berson EL, Shih VE, Sullivan PL (1981). Ocular findings in patients with gyrate atrophy on pyridoxine and low-protein, low-arginine diets. Ophthalmology 80:311-315.

Kaiser-Kupfer MI, de Monasterio FM, Valle D, Walser M, Brusilow S (1980). Gyrate atrophy of the choroid and retina: improved visual function following reduction of plasma ornithine by diet. Science 210:1128-1131.

Kaiser-Kupfer MI, de Monasterio FM, Valle D, Walser M, Brusilow S (1981). Visual results of a long-term trial of a low-arginine diet in gyrate atrophy of choroid and retina. Ophthalmology 88:307-310.

Kaiser-Kupfer MI, Valle D, Bron AJ (1980). Clinical and biochemical heterogeneity in gyrate atrophy. Am J Ophthalmol 89:219-222.

Kennaway NG, Weleber RG, Buist NRM (1977). Gyrate atrophy of choroid and retina: deficient activity of ornithine ketoacid aminotransferase in cultured skin fibroblasts. N Engl J Med 297:1180.

Kennaway NG, Weleber RG, Buist NRM (1980). Gyrate atrophy of the choroid and retina with hyperornithinemia: biochemical and histologic studies and response to vitamin B_6. Am J Hum Genet 32:529-541.

Kopple JD, Swendseid ME (1975). Evidence that histidine is an essential amino acid in normal and chronically uremic man. J Clin Invest 55:881-891.

McInnes RR, Arshinoff FA, Bell L, Marliss EB, McCulloch JC (1981). Hyperornithinemia and gyrate atrophy of the retina: improvement of vision during treatment with a low-arginine diet. Lancet 1:513-517.

Meister A (1965). The role of amino acids in nutrition. In Biochemistry of the Amino Acids, Vol 1 2nd Edn, pp 201-230, Academic Press, New York.

O'Donnell JJ, Sandman RP, Martin SR (1978). Gyrate atrophy of the retina: inborn error of L-ornithine: 2-oxoacid aminotransferase. Science 200:200-201.

Recommended Dietary Allowances, 8th Edn (1974). Food and Nutrition Board, National Council, National Academy of Sciences, Washington D C.

Shih VE, Berson EL, Gargiulo M (1981). Reduction of hyperornithinemia with a low protein, low arginine diet and pyridoxine in patients with a deficiency of ornithine-ketoacid transaminase (OKT) activity and gyrate atrophy of the choroid and retina. Clin Chim Acta 113:243-251.

Shih VE, Berson EL, Mandell R, Schmidt SY (1978). Ornithine ketoacid transaminase deficiency in gyrate atrophy of the choroid and retina. Am J Hum Genet 30:174-179.

Simell O, Takki K (1973). Raised plasma ornithine and gyrate atrophy of the choroid and retina. Lancet 1:1030-1033.

Snedecor GW, Cochran WG (1967). Statistical Methods, 6th Edn, Ames, IA: Iowa State University Press, pp 289.

Stoppolini G, Prisco F, Santinelli R, Tolone C (1978). Hyperornithinemia and gyrate atrophy of choroid and retina. Helv Paediatr Acta 33:429-433.

Takki K (1974). Gyrate atrophy of the choroid and retina associated with hyperornithinaemia. Br J Ophthalmol 58:3-23.

Takki K, Simell O (1974). Genetic aspects in gyrate atrophy of the choroid and retina with hyperornithinaemia. Br J Ophthalmol 58:907-916.

Trijbels JMF, Sengers RCA, Bakkeren JAJM, DeKort AFM, Deutman AF (1977). L-Ornithine-ketoacid-transaminase deficiency in cultured fibroblasts of a patient with hyperornithinemia and gyrate atrophy of the choroid and retina. Clin Chim Acta 79:371-377.

Valle DA, Kaiser-Kupfer M, Del Valle LA (1977). Gyrate atrophy of the choroid and retina: deficiency of ornithine aminotransferase in transformed lymphocytes. Proc Natl Acad Sci USA 74:5159-5161.

Valle D, Walser M, Brusilow SW, Kaiser-Kupfer MI (1980). Gyrate atrophy of the choroid and retina. Amino acid metabolism and correction of hyperornithinemia with an arginine-deficient diet. J Clin Invest 65:371-378.

Weleber RG, Kennaway NG (1981). Clinical trial of vitamin B_6 for gyrate atrophy of the choroid and retina. Ophthalmology 88:316-324.

Weleber RG, Kennaway NG, Buist NRM (1978). Vitamin B_6 in management of gyrate atrophy of choroid and retina. Lancet 2:1213.

GYRATE ATROPHY OF THE CHOROID AND RETINA: CLINICAL AND BIOCHEMICAL HETEROGENEITY AND RESPONSE TO VITAMIN B_6

Richard G. Weleber, M.D., Mary K. Wirtz, B.S.,
Nancy G. Kennaway, D. Phil.
Oregon Health Sciences University

3181 SW Sam Jackson Park Road
Portland, Oregon 97201

INTRODUCTION

Gyrate atrophy of the choroid and retina is an autosomal recessive genetic dystrophy which begins within the first decade of life as gradually enlarging areas of atrophy of peripheral choroid and retina (1-5). Marked constriction of peripheral visual field occurs within the next several decades, cataracts may further reduce central acuity, and most patients become legally, if not functionally, blind by 40 to 50 years of age (5). These patients may have relatively normal dark adaptation thresholds in early adulthood but eventually develop severe defects of dark adaptation. Most, if not all patients have been myopic, with spherical correction ranging from -4 to -20 diopters. Abnormalities of muscle occur, with atrophy of type II muscle fiber associated with subsarcolemmal inclusions which on EM appear as tubular aggregates (6-9). Other systemic manifestations may include seizure (4,8), abnormalities on electroencephalography (4,6,9-11), or electrocardiography (7), and abnormalities of hair on microscopy (9).

In 1973 Simell and Takki (13) reported that gyrate atrophy is associated with 10-20 fold elevation of plasma ornithine. Deficient activity of ornithine aminotransferase (OAT) (L-ornithine:2-oxoacid

Birth Defects: Original Article Series, Volume 18, Number 6, pages 219–230

TABLE 1

CLINICAL FEATURES OF B_6 RESPONSIVE PATIENTS WITH GYRATE ATROPHY

PATIENT	1	2	3	6
Age 1)	31	34	41	90
Sex	F	F	F	F
Visual Acuity				
OD	20/30	20/20-2	10/400	20/50+2
OS	20/30	20/20	20/20-1	LP (no projection)
Refraction				
OD	-16.00+0.50x150°	-4.75+0.25x35°	-3.00+2.25x70°	+10.50+2.50x168°
OS	-16.00 sphere	-4.50 sphere	-3.25+2.25x90°	--
Horizontal Visual Field 2)				
OD	70° [77°]	130° [130°]	63° [63°]	29°
OS	78° [85°]	115° [124°]	71° [75°]	--
Lens and Anterior Segment				
OD	early coronary lens opacities	normal	dense PSC	aphakic
OS	early coronary lens opacities	normal	minimal PSC	dense cataract
Dark Adaptometry 3)				
OD 3.1[2.3] 6)	3.0[3.3-4.3]	2.2[2.1-2.7]	3.4[3.1-3.6]	NT
OS 3.0[2.3]	2.9[3.4-4.4]	2.2[2.2-2.6]	2.1[2.0-2.1]	NT
ERG 4)				
OD	82[146-187]	[86-97]	20[30] 7)	NT
OS	76[143-185]	[100-113]	99[109]	NT
EOG 5)				
OD	1.14[1.74]	[1.38-1.43]	1.00[1.27] 7)	NT
OS	1.00[1.56]	[1.34-1.41]	1.18[1.55]	NT

NT = not tested; LP = light perception; PSC = posterior subcapsular cataract.
Values within brackets were after patient was given supplemental oral pyridoxine HCl, in most cases most recent evaluation.

1) At most recent evaluation.
2) Maximal horizontal diameter of Goldmann perimetric visual field using IV-4e test object.
3) Final 30 minute Goldmann Weekers dark adaptometry threshold in log micro micro Lamberts.
4) Maximal scotopic corneal positive peak amplitude (μV) after at least 30 minutes dark adaptation.
5) Electro-oculogram (EOG) light-to-dark ratio. Normal is over 1.85.
6) Tests performed at another institution.
7) After 3 years of stable ERG's and EOG's, over the last 1 year the maximal scotopic ERG amplitude has fallen to <10 μV OD and 82-85 μV OS and the EOG ratios have fallen to 1.00 OD and to 1.23-1.38 OS. This variance makes uncertain the significance of the initial improvement.

TABLE 2

CLINICAL FEATURES OF VITAMIN B_6 NONRESPONSIVE PATIENTS WITH GYRATE ATROPHY

PATIENT	4	5	7
Age[1)]	43	64	28
Sex	M	F	F
Visual Acuity			
OD	20/60	NLP	20/200
OS	5/400	20/200+	20/200
Refraction			
OD	-6.25+2.50x96°	--	-2.75+1.00x115°
OS	-7.00+3.00x82°	+6.00+1.25x180°	-3.25+0.75x90°
Horizontal Visual Field[2)]			
OD	74[65°]	--	57°
OS	67[53°]	3-5°	59°
Lens and Anterior Segment			
OD	early PSC	corneal leukoma, glaucoma	early PSC
OS	dense PSC	aphakic	moderate PSC
Dark Adaptometry[3)]			
OD	3.3[3.1-4.0]	NT	4.7-5.2
OS	4.3[4.2-5.0]	NT	4.7-5.2
ERG[4)]			
OD	30[29-44][6)]	NR	NR
OS	15[18-29]	NR	NR
EOG[5)]			
OD	1.00[1.00]	NT	1.00
OS	1.00[1.00]	NT	1.00

NT = not tested; NR = non-recordable; NLP = no light perception; PSC = posterior subcapsular cataract.

Values within brackets were after patient was given supplemental oral pyridoxine HCl, in most cases most recent evaluation.

1) - 5) See footnote to Table 1.

6) When first studied prior to B_6 supplementation (without computer averaging) an ERG was barely discernible over background noise. Following B_6 supplementation this small ERG response varied in its ability to be detected by single flash technique. Computer averaging was done once at 15 months following vitamin B_6 supplementation. No significant improvement or worsening of ERG responses was seen over 19 months of observation.

TABLE 3

FASTING SERUM ORNITHINE LEVELS AND INCORPORATION OF RADIOACTIVITY FROM ^{3}H-ORNITHINE INTO PROTEIN IN CULTURED SKIN FIBROBLASTS *IN SITU*

Patient	Pyridoxine HCl mg/day	Serum Ornithine µmol/ml*	^{3}H incorporation dpm/µg protein*
Responders			
1	0	0.64 ± 0.17	233 ± 62
	750	0.34 ± 0.10	
2	0	0.57 ± 0.02	268 ± 34
	600-750	0.25 ± 0.01	
3	0	0.77 ± 0.08	237 ± 33
	600-750	0.34 ± 0.07	
6**	uncertain	0.52 ± 0.08	482 ± 91
Non-responders			
4	0	0.68 ; 0.69	66 ± 17
	600-750	0.71 ± 0.07	
5	0	0.83 ; 1.00	58 ± 28
	50 ; 250	0.87 ; 0.88	
7	0	1.05 ± 0.10	66 ± 32
	750	0.97 ± 0.17	
Controls	0	0.083 ± 0.030	859 ± 129

* Mean ± std. dev.

** Patient 6 is included as a responder on the basis of her milder disease and fasting serum ornithine levels.

patients 1 and 2 (8). Obviously, constancy among siblings in the capacity to respond to vitamin B_6 suggests that this capacity is genetically controlled.

Most patients, including all those of Finnish extraction are non-responders; of the 6 reported responsive patients, three (patients 1-3) have been followed by us over a period of several years and one of our other patients (patient 6) probably also belongs in this category. Our remaining three patients are non-responders. Thus, we have had the opportunity to study the clinical and biochemical heterogeneity between these two groups of patients.

Our B_6 responsive patients (Table 1) with gyrate atrophy have milder disease compared to our nonresponsive patients (Table 2) and especially when compared to the natural history originally described by Takki (4) and elaborated by Takki and Milton (5). The detailed case histories of our patients will be the subject of another paper; however, our B_6 responsive patients (patients 1-3), in general, have greater retention of visual field, better dark adaptometry, and retained ERG and EOG responses compared to our non-responders. Additionally, they lack the early peripapillary and perimacular chorioretinal atrophy reported with some B_6 non-responsive patients (4,5,12). Adequate evaluation for *in vivo* biochemical vitamin B_6 responsiveness has not been possible for patient 6. However, she probably is a responder, based on her mild clinical findings, her lower fasting serum ornithine levels and results in her cultured fibroblasts (Table 3). Clinical heterogeneity in gyrate atrophy has also been suggested by Kaiser-Kupfer *et al* (10) on the basis of two women who had milder clinical features and symptoms and somewhat lower blood ornithine levels than most reported patients. One of these patients also demonstrated a 27% reduction of plasma ornithine with vitamin B_6 supplementation. The milder symptoms and clinical findings may result from chronically lower blood and hence tissue levels of ornithine in B_6 responders rather than differences in pathogenetic mechanisms in comparison to non-responders. Even small doses of dietary or supplemental B_6 can reduce ornithine levels (8,23) and thereby may slow down the progression of the disease.

All patients with gyrate atrophy with hyperornithinemia have deficient activity of OAT. This is usually measured in tissue homogenates by generation of Δ^1-pyrroline-5-carboxylate, which reacts with o-aminobenzaldehyde to form a yellow condensation product which is measured colorimetrically, radiochemically or by high pressure liquid chromatography. The level of residual enzyme activity does not appear to correlate with the ability to respond to vitamin B_6 *in vivo* (10,18,21). Similar lack of correlation between level of residual enzyme activity and *in vivo* responsiveness has also been reported in a few patients with homocystinuria, another B_6-responsive condition (26,27), although in the majority of patients with that disease, there is such correlation (28). It should be noted that accurate determination of very low enzyme levels is both difficult and sometimes of questionable validity. Furthermore, levels of residual enzyme activity vary with the conditions of assay, in particular the concentration of pyridoxal phosphate, so that comparison of values obtained in different laboratories must be viewed with caution. Additionally as discussed earlier, the measurement of OAT activity at increasing levels of pyridoxal phosphate in the assay medium has not proved a reliable indicator of B_6 response _in vivo_, possibly because of the difficulty of obtaining accurate values for very low activities, but more likely because the concentrations of pyridoxal phosphate that are used in these studies are artificially high and do not reflect the intracellular concentrations attained _in vivo_ during pyridoxine supplementation. Evidence for this has recently been obtained in homocystinuria where it was shown that if cells were first depleted of pyridoxal by growth in low-pyridoxine medium, then the response of these cells to pyridoxine, as measured by the Km for pyridoxal phosphate, was indeed distinct in B_6-responders, non-responders, and controls (29).

An alternative, and perhaps more reliable, indicator of residual OAT activity is the measurement of the incorporation of radioactivity from ^{3}H-ornithine into protein, presumably in the form of proline or glutamate, in cultured skin fibroblasts _in situ_. As shown in Table 3, this activity is greatly reduced in all patients with gyrate atrophy. Moreover, this activity is clearly greater in our B_6-responsive patients than in the non-responders, suggesting that this technique may prove to be a reliable indicator of B_6 response _in vivo_.

Genetic heterogeneity in gyrate atrophy could reflect mutations at two separate loci, perhaps each coding for a separate subunit of the enzyme, or perhaps reflecting both structural and regulatory defects. There is no evidence to suggest the existence of more than one subunit of OAT, and the question of a regulatory defect in certain patients has not been examined. Presumably at least the patients in whom abnormal pyridoxal phosphate (8,18,22) or ornithine (30) kinetics were reported, all represent structural gene mutations. It seems more likely that genetic heterogeneity in gyrate atrophy reflects the occurrence of at least two mutant alleles at the locus for OAT. Our inability to demonstrate complementation in heterokaryons derived from B_6 responsive and non-responsive patients lends support to this conclusion (31).

ACKNOWLEDGMENT

This work was supported by National Eye Institute grant EY-02527 and National Foundation - March of Dimes grant 1-621. Travel Funds for Richard G. Weleber, M.D. were supplied in part by the National Foundation - March of Dimes and the National Retinitis Pigmentosa Foundation. Dr. Robert Kalina and Dr. Frederick Miller kindly provided clinical data on patient 5.

REFERENCES

1. Jacobsohn E (1888). Ein fall von retinitis pigmentosa atypica. Klin Mbl Augenheilk 26:202-206.
2. Cutler CW (1895). Drei Ungewöhnliche Fälle von Retino-Chorioideal-Degeneration. Arch Augenheilk 30:117-122.
3. Fuchs E (1895). Ueber zwei der Retinitis pigmentosa verwandte Krankheiten (Retinitis punctata albescens und Atrophia gyrata chorioideae et retinae). Arch Augenheilk 32:111-116.
4. Takki K (1974). Gyrate atrophy of the choroid and retina associated with hyperornithinaemia. Br J Ophthalmol 58:3-23.
5. Takki KK, Milton RC (1981). The natural history of gyrate atrophy of the choroid and retina. Ophthalmol 88:292-301.
6. McCullough C, Marliss EB (1975). Gyrate atrophy of the choroid and retina with hyperornithinemia. Am J Ophthalmol 80:1047-1057.

7. Sipilä I, Simell O, Rapola J, Sainio K, Tuuteri L (1979). Gyrate atrophy of the choroid and retina with hyperornithinemia: tubular aggregates and type 2 fiber atrophy in muscle. Neurol 29:996-1005.
8. Kennaway NG, Weleber RG, Buist NRM (1980). Gyrate atrophy of the choroid and retina with hyperornithinemia: biochemical and histologic studies and response to vitamin B_6. Am J Hum Genet 32:529-541.
9. Kaiser-Kupfer MI, Kuwabara T, Askanas V, Brody L, Takki K, Dvoretzky I, Engel WK (1981). Systemic manifestions of gyrate atrophy of the choroid and retina. Ophthalmol 88:302-306.
10. Kaiser-Kupfer MI, Valle D, Bron AJ (1980). Clinical and biochemical heterogeneity in gyrate atrophy. Amer J. Ophthalmol 89:219-222.
11. Valle D, Walser M, Brusilow SW, Kaiser-Kupfer M (1980). Gyrate atrophy of the choroid and retina: amino acid metabolism and correction of hyperornithinemia with an arginine-deficient diet. J Clin Invest 65:371-378.
12. Kaiser-Kupfer MI, Valle D, Del Valle LA (1978). A specific enzyme defect in gyrate atrophy. Am J Ophthalmol 85:200-204.
13. Simell O, Takki K (1973). Raised plasma ornithine and gyrate atrophy of the choroid and retina. Lancet 1:1031-1033.
14. Sengers RCA, Trijbels JMF, Brussaart JH, Deutman AF (1976). Gyrate atrophy of the choroid and retina and ornithine-ketoacid aminotransferase deficiency (abstr). Pediatr Res 10:894.
15. Kennaway NG, Weleber RG, Buist NRM (1977). Gyrate atrophy of the choroid and retina: deficient activity of ornithine ketoacid aminotransferase in cultured skin fibroblasts. N Engl J Med 297:1180.
16. O'Donnell JJ, Sandman RP, Martin SR (1977). Deficient L-ornithine:2-oxoacid aminotransferase activity in cultured fibroblasts from a patient with gyrate atrophy of the retina. Biochem Biophys Res Commun 79:396-399.

17. Trijbels JMF, Sengers RCA, Bakkeren JAJM, DeKort AFM, Deutman AF (1977). L-Ornithine-ketoacid-transaminase deficiency in cultured fibroblasts of a patient with hyperornithinaemia and gyrate atrophy of the choroid and retina. Clin Chim Acta 79:371-377.
18. Shih VE, Berson EL, Mandell R, Schmidt SY (1978). Ornithine ketoacid transaminase deficiency in gyrate atrophy of the choroid and retina. Am J Hum Genet 30:174-179.
19. O'Donnell JJ, Sandman RP, Martin SR (1978). Gyrate atrophy of the retina: inborn error of L-ornithine:2-oxoacid aminotransferase. Science 200:200-201.
20. Valle D, Kaiser-Kupfer MI, Del Valle LA (1977). Gyrate atrophy of the choroid and retina: Deficiency of ornithine aminotransferase in transformed lymphocytes. Proc Natl Acad Sci USA 74:5159-5161.
21. Berson EL, Schmidt SY, Shih VE (1978). Ocular and biochemical abnormalities in gyrate atrophy of the choroid and retina. Ophthalmol 85:1018-1027.
22. Tada K, Saito T, Omura K, Hayasaka S, Mizuno K (1981). Hyperornithinaemia associated with gyrate atrophy of the choroid and retina: in vivo and in vitro response to Vitamin B_6. J Inher Metab Dis 4:61-62.
23. Weleber RG, Kennaway NG, Buist NRM (1978). Vitamin B_6 in management of gyrate atrophy of choroid and retina. Lancet 2:1213.
24. Weleber RG, Kennaway NG (1981). Clinical trial of vitamin B_6 for gyrate atrophy of the choroid and retina. Ophthalmol 88:316-324.
25. Lowry OH, Rosebrough NJ, Farr AL, Randall RJ (1951). Protein measurement with the Folin phenol reagent. J Biol Chem 193:265-275.
26. Uhlendorf BW, Conerly EB, Mudd, SH (1973). Homocystinuria: studies in tissue culture. Pediat Res 7:645-658, 1973.
27. Fowler B, Kraus J, Packman S, Rosenberg LE (1978). Homocystinuria: evidence for three distinct classes of cystathionine β-synthase mutants in cultured fibroblasts. J Clin Invest 61:645-653.

BATTEN DISEASE: NEW RESEARCH FINDINGS ON THE BIOCHEMICAL DEFECT

Leonhard S. Wolfe, Ph.D., M.D. and N. M. K. Ng Ying Kin, Ph.D
Montreal Neurological Institute and Hospital
3801 University Street
Montréal, Québec, Canada H3A 2B4

The term Batten disease covers the late infantile and juvenile forms of familial (autosomal recessive inheritance) cerebromacular degenerations also classified as the neuronal ceroid lipofuscinoses (NCL) by Zeman (Zeman, Donahue, Dyken et al, 1970). The first clinical descriptions date back over 100 years but despite much effort by pediatric neurologists, ophthalmologists, neuropathologists and neurochemists the basic biochemical defect in these fatal, not uncommon neurogenetic diseases remains elusive. On clinical and pathological grounds, four genetically distinct phenotypes are recognized which historically have been associated with a complex of eponyms.

(1) Infantile NCL or Santavuori-Haltia-Hagberg type usually onsets in the second year of life with ataxia, seizures, myoclonic jerks, rapid deterioration of movement, vision and mental status progressing to a vegetative state and death usually between 5 and 9 years of age. At death the cerebral cortex contains virtually no neurones and astrocytes are loaded with autofluorescent storage material with a finely granular ultrastructure.

(2) Late infantile NCL, late infantile Batten disease or Jansky-Bielschowsky type onsets around three to four years with ataxia, seizures often intractable to antiepileptic medication, deterioration of vision to blindness and motor and mental deterioration with death between eight to twelve years. Retinal pigmentary changes may be present, retinal vessels are attenuated and optic atrophy is present. Neurones contain membrane bound accumulation of autofluorescent material that usually has aggregates with curvilinear profiles by electronmicroscopy.

Birth Defects: Original Article Series, Volume 18, Number 6, pages 233–239

(3) Juvenile NCL, Batten-Mayou, Spielmeyer-Vogt-Sjögren or Stengel-Spielmeyer-Vogt-Stock type presents between 5 and 10 years with blindness followed by seizures or seizures followed by blindness with motor and intellectual deterioration over a longer period and death may occur as late as the early twenties dependant upon the quality of nursing care. The autofluorescent cytosomes in this type of NCL most often have a fingerprint type or granular pattern.

(4) The rarer adult NCL or Kufs disease onsets in early adulthood often with extrapyramidal symptoms, dysarthria and myoclonus epilepsy, but amaurosis and visual impairment are either absent or milder and the disease progresses more slowly than the other forms. Storage of autofluorescent ceroid-lipofuscin in the retina and central nervous system is present in the form of fingerprint, granular or curvilinear ultrastructures.

It is important to appreciate that in all forms of NCL the autofluorescent accumulations are not restricted to the retina and neurones but are in most extra-neural tissues. Thus the disease is generalized in nature with the central nervous system and the retina being the main target of the dysfunction. Skin biopsy including the sweat glands is the mainstay of pathological diagnosis at present. Electrophysiological findings are summarized in Table 1. The progresssive loss of the electroretinogram response is due to the degeneration and loss of rods and cones from the photoreceptor cells.

Table 1.
Electrophysiological Studies in Batten Disease

	Late Infantile (Jansky-Bielschowsky)	Juvenile (Spielmeyer-Vogt)
EEG	Irregular slow wave activity with rhythmic spike and wave complexes	
ERG	Small to absent b wave	
VER	Very enlarged major positive wave	Small and delayed or absent major positive wave

The hypothesis that the autofluorescent accumulations result from a peroxidation of polyunsaturated fatty acids with coupling of released malondialdehyde to amines and proteins has little support at present. Previous reports of a paraphenylene diamine leukocyte peroxidase deficiency have not been substantiated by many laboratories in North America and Europe and the analysis has no practical clinical value (Wolfe, Ng Ying Kin, Baker, 1981). During the period of this controversy our group succeeded in isolating pure fractions of the ceroid-lipofuscin storage material (Wolfe, Ng Ying Kin, Baker, Carpenter, Andermann, 1977) with the expectation that further knowledge of its chemical nature might lead to the enzymatic defect as was the case in the sphingolipidoses. We obtained suggestive evidence that the autofluorescent highly solvent-insoluble residue obtained after extensive chloroform-methanol extraction contained retinoid-like structures complexed to protein or peptides. Because of the inherent instability of retinoid polyenes to acid and base treatments required to solubilize the residues progress on the precise chemical nature of these components has been slow. Recently, however, we have concentrated on analysis of the chloroform-methanol extracts of the storage material. Although unesterified cholesterol and phospholipids constitute the major lipid types, in agreement with the histochemical staining properties, we discovered the presence of highly significant amounts of a class of polyisoprenols termed dolichols and were able to analyse these long chain dolichols by high performance liquid chromatography (HPLC). I wish to briefly summarize our progress in this area.

Analyses of the total brain dolichol content of late infantile and juvenile Batten disease cases compared with age matched control subjects has revealed highly significant increases in these compounds in NCL patients (Table 2). Figure 1 illustrates the type of HPLC profiles obtained.

A very important and interesting point which showed up in these studies was that in the non-Batten 'disease' controls there was a marked increase in brain dolichol content with age and this is more clearly illustrated in Figure 2. We were fortunate in being able to obtain small cerebral cortex tissue samples from patients undergoing neurosurgery for the treatment of temporal lobe epilepsy and also tissue from Huntington's disease patients from Dr. E. G. Bird of the Brain Tissue Bank, McLean Hospital, Harvard Medical School. We have found that this age related increase in brain dolichols also occurs in rats (Wolfe, Ng Ying Kin, unpublished observations). Whether this is related to the known increase in lipofuscin accumulation in brain with age is worthy of further investigation.

Since electron microscopy of the urinary sediment in NCL patients shows the presence of curvilinear and fingerprint bodies derived from the renal tubular epithelium (DeBaecque, 1975; DeBaecque, Pollack and Suzuki, 1976) we decided to look at the dolichol content of the urinary sediment from a series of patients with appropriate controls. The results are shown in Table 3.

Table 2. DOLICHOL CONTENT OF HUMAN CEREBRAL CORTEX

Diagnosis	Age	Dolichols C90-C105 μg/g Tissue	
Late infantile Batten	9-11	460.3 ± 146.3	(3)*
Juvenile Batten	16-20	149.5 ± 29.2	(5)*
Tay Sachs	5-8	29.5 ± 4.5	(3)
Seizure patients, biopsy	4-10	41.6 ± 21.5	(7)
Juvenile Huntington	9-12	65.1 ± 16.5	(5)
Seizure patients, biopsy	11-20	89.9 ± 25.9	(11)
Seizure patients, biopsy	21-30	132.3 ± 42.0	(7)
Seizure patients, biopsy	31-50	183.2 ± 53.1	(7)
Various diseases, biopsy and post-mortem	51-81	207.4 ± 44.8	(16)

*$p<0.01$ for disease controls in 4-20 age bracket. Total dolichols obtained by saponification and extraction from 300-500 mg of cerebral cortex tissue. HPLC analysis was on a 10 μm C_{18} Bondapak column eluted with methanol-isopropanol mixtures at a flow rate of 2 ml/min.

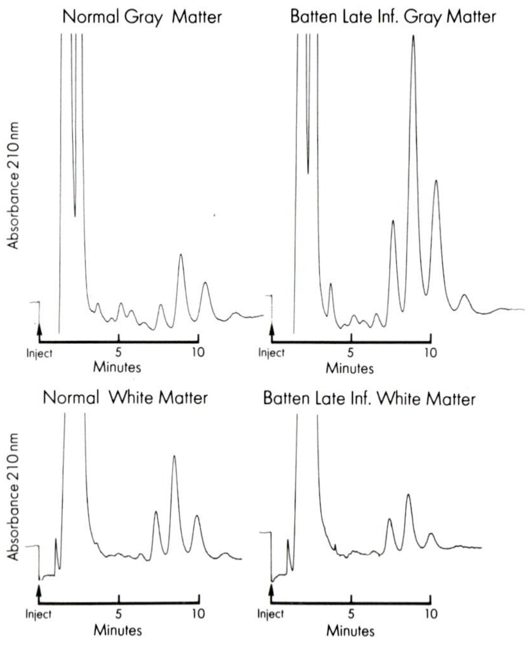

Figure 1. HPLC profiles of brain dolichols of carbon chain lengths of C90-C105 in normal compared to a Batten disease patient.

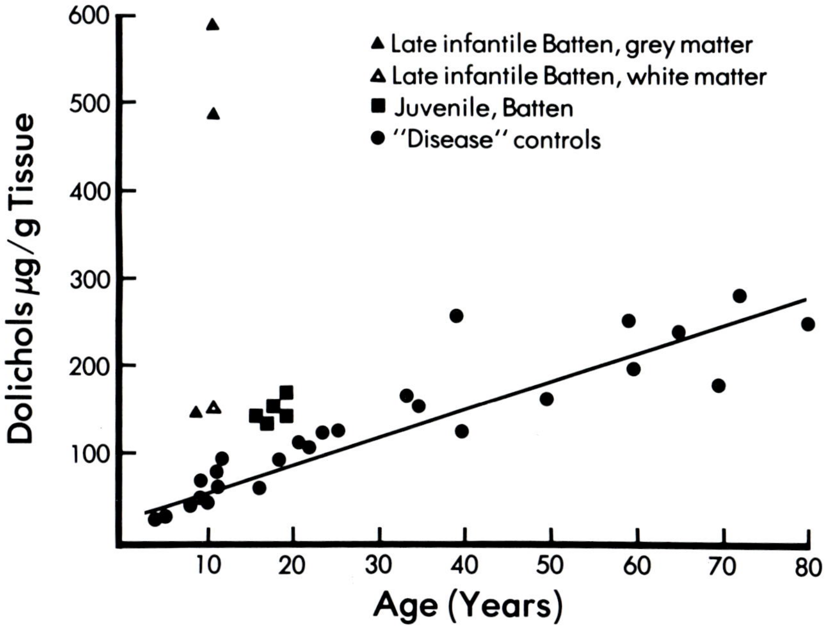

Figure 2. Brain Dolichol Content in Batten Disease Related to Disease Controls at Different Ages.

Table 3. Dolichols in Urinary Sediment from Batten Disease and Other Subjects

Diagnosis	µg Dolichols/mg Total Lipid
Infantile NCL	6.25 ± 1.71 (3)
Late infantile Batten	5.68 ± 2.52 (4)
Juvenile Batten	4.78 ± 1.33 (4)
Neurological disease, various	0.16 ± 0.15 (11)
Normal, age 10-20	0.09 ± 0.12 (9)

Analysis by HPLC as described in Table 2.

Highly significant increases in dolichols in the urinary sediment of NCL patients were found. Although this work is still in an early stage, we believe that forthe first time this biochemical test can be useful in the diagnosis of NCL patients when taken together with the clinical picture and the results of skin biopsy.

The structure of dolichols is illustrated below.

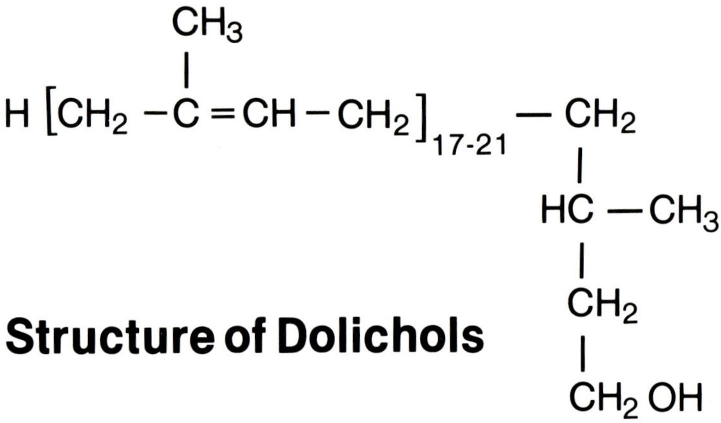

Structure of Dolichols

These lipids are key intermediates as their phosphate and pyrophosphate derivatives in the transfer of oligosaccharides to N-glycosidically linked glycoproteins. The enzymatic mechanisms controlling the utilization of dolichols is little understood but our studies suggest that the basic biochemical defect in NCL lies on path-ways involving polyisoprenol or isoprenoid metabolism (dolichols and retinoids).

Conclusions

1. Polyisoprenols are significantly increased in brain and urinary sediment in NCL patients.
2. Brain dolichol content increases with age.
3. HPLC analysis of urinary sediment is of value in supporting the diagnosis of NCL.
4. The genetic defect is associated with an abnormality in dolichol and retinoid metabolism.

Acknowledgements

This research was supported by a grent MT-1345 from the Medical Research Council of Canada. We thank Dr. J. Palo and Dr. M. Haltia of the Department of Neurology, University of Helsinki for the infantile NCL urine samples and a grant NIH-ROI MH/NS-31862 to the Brain Tissue Bank, Harvard Medical School for frozen samples of human brain.

References

De Baecque C (1975). Diagnosis of neuronal ceroid lipofuscinosis by electron microscopy of urinary sediment. New Engl J Med 292:1408.

De Baecque C, Pollack AM, Suzuki K (1976). Systemic pathology in, late infantile neuronal storage disease with curvilinear bodies. Arch Pathol Lab Med 100:139.

Wolfe LS, Ng Ying Kin NMK, Baker RR, Carpenter S, Andermann F (1977). Identification of retinoyl complexes as the autofluorescent component of the neuronal storage material in Batten disease. Science 195:1360.

Wolfe LS, Ng Ying Kin NMK, Baker RR (1981). Batten disease and related disorders. In Callahan JW, Lowden JA (eds): "Lysosomes and Lysosomal Storage Diseases," New York: Raven Press, p 315.

Zeman W, Donahue S, Dyken P, et al (1970). The neuronal ceroid lipofuscinoses. In Vinken PJ, Bruyn GW (eds): "Handbook of Clinical Neurology Vol 10," Amsterdam: Elsevier, p 588.

ULTRASTRUCTURAL STUDIES ON THE RETINA IN HUMAN AND CANINE NEURONAL CEROID-LIPOFUSCINOSES AND OTHER LYSOSOMAL DISORDERS

Hans H. Goebel[1], Bernd Köhnecke[1], and Nils Koppang[2]
[1]Department of Neuropathology, University of Göttingen, D-3400 Göttingen, Fed. Rep. Germany
[2]National Veterinary Institute, Oslo, Norway

Long before the concept of lysosomal disorders had been elaborated almost 20 years ago by Hers (1963), certain lysosomal entities were already well known to the clinician though not as such, owing e.g. to the work of Tay, Batten and Vogt. These and other clinicians had observed the cherry-red spot due to extensive storage of lipid material in macular ganglion cells and retinal degeneration similar to retinopathia pigmentosa, culminating in the now obsolete term "amaurotic idiocy". These two funduscopic lesions indicate two different morphological processes, accumulation of non-catabolized lipid compounds within the intracellular lysosomal compartment typical of neuronal storage disorders, such as gangliosidoses and Niemann-Pick disease, and degeneration of photoreceptors with subsequent retinal atrophy encountered in the neuronal ceroid-lipofuscinoses (NCL) and certain mucopolysaccharidoses. In these two latter groups of lysosomal disorders, retinal pigmentary degeneration develops in addition to and probably independent of the intralysosomal storage of disease-specific compounds.

The cherry-red spot - or black-cherry spot in a patient with a heavily pigmented fundus (Burck et al. 1980) - only illustrates the ophthalmological "tip" of the accretion of lysosomal material within nerve cells, actually one of the few sites where "storage" in lysosomal disorders is apparent in the living patient without biopsy.

As histopathology may reveal enlargement of retinal neuronal perikarya due to intracellular storage, electron microscopy may be a more subtle technique to document such intralysosomal accumulation. In this respect, membranous cyto-

Birth Defects: Original Article Series, Volume 18, Number 6, pages 241-253

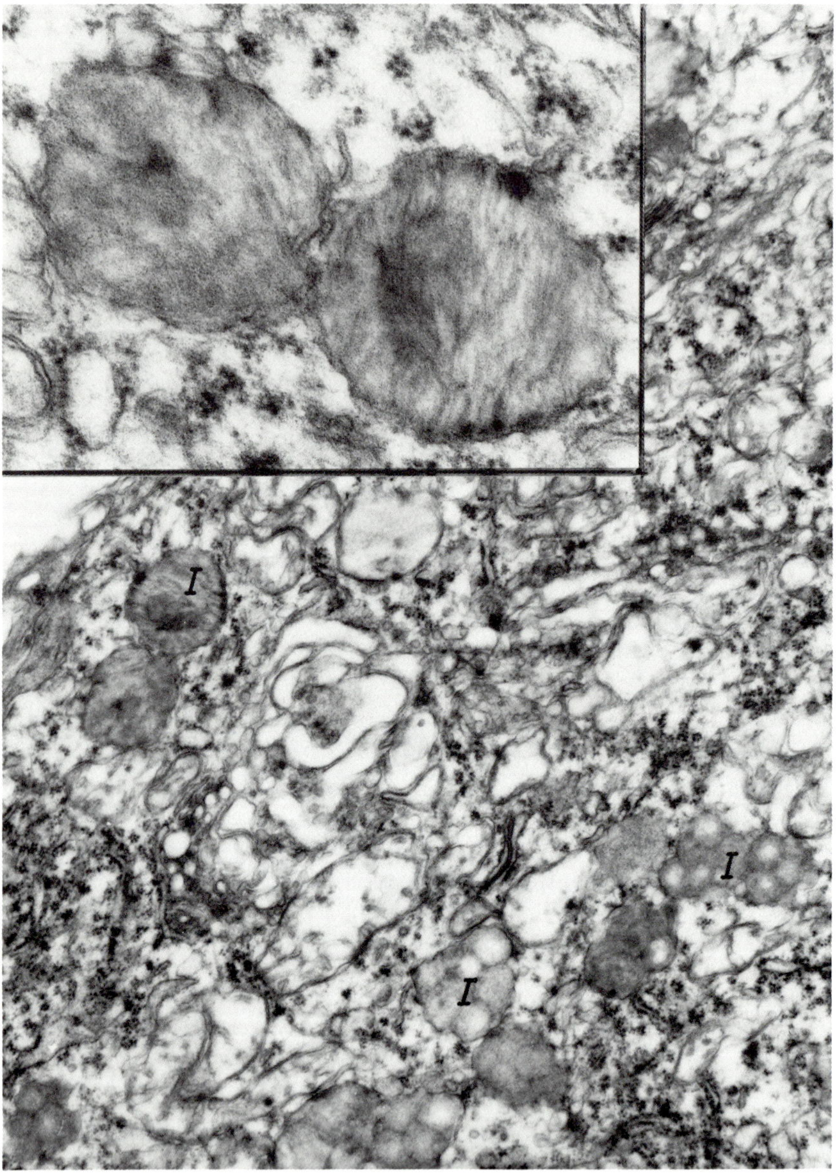

Fig. 1. A retinal cell contains numerous membrane-bound inclusions (I). Adult metachromatic leukodystrophy; X 22,400. Inset: Membranes in finely granular material fill these membrane-bound inclusions. X 63,800.

plasmic bodies, typical of the accumulation of gangliosides in nerve cells, are present in retinal ganglion cells in GM_1-gangliosidosis, even when funduscopic findings are negative. Ganglion cells seem to be affected first by neuronal storage, but with increasing severity of the gangliosidosis, other retinal cells may be also affected as gangliosides accrete in other retinal cells in the GM_2-gangliosidoses.

The accumulation of intralysosomal lipids depends on the role of these lipids in cell metabolism. As sulfatides are predominantly involved in the metabolism of the myelin sheath, a lysosomal block in the catabolism of sulfatides in metachromatic leukodystrophy (MLD) results in accumulation of sulfatides in oligodendroglial cells, in Schwann cells of the peripheral nervous system, but also in astrocytes, possibly due to phagocytosis of sulfatides from decaying oligodendrocytes. However, sulfatides also play a minor role in the metabolism of nerve cells and, therefore, in MLD, membrane-bound sulfatides accrete in retinal nerve cells. In adult MLD, ganglion cells exclusively harbour membrane-bound sulfatides (Fig. 1). These intraganglionic sulfatides are not derived from myelin breakdown as the human retina does not contain myelinated axons which acquire their myelin sheaths at the optic nerve level.

As glycogen is metabolized in almost every cell type, in type II glycogenosis intralysosomal glycogen will accrue in almost every cell type as well. This is reflected in the retina in that membrane-bound sacs of glycogen (Fig. 2) are present in each cell type. Impaired function due to this intracellular storage, though, is not apparent morphologically - different from the striking lesions in striated muscle fibers -, and retinal atrophy or degeneration cannot be demonstrated. As the course of type II glycogenosis progresses too rapidly to death, refined electrophysiological and ophthalmological assessment of retinal cell function has not been reported.

Similarly, the intracellular accumulation of lipopigments is widespread in canine neuronal ceroid-lipofuscinosis (NCL) of English setters (Fig. 3) without obvious morphological damage to the affected cells (Goebel et al. 1979; Neville et al. 1980). The various cell types of the retina encompass the entire ultrastructural spectrum of lipopigments in canine NCL (Fig. 4), similar to those seen in non-retinal cells and in human NCL. Whether these diversely structured lipopigments are also chemically different is so far unknown.

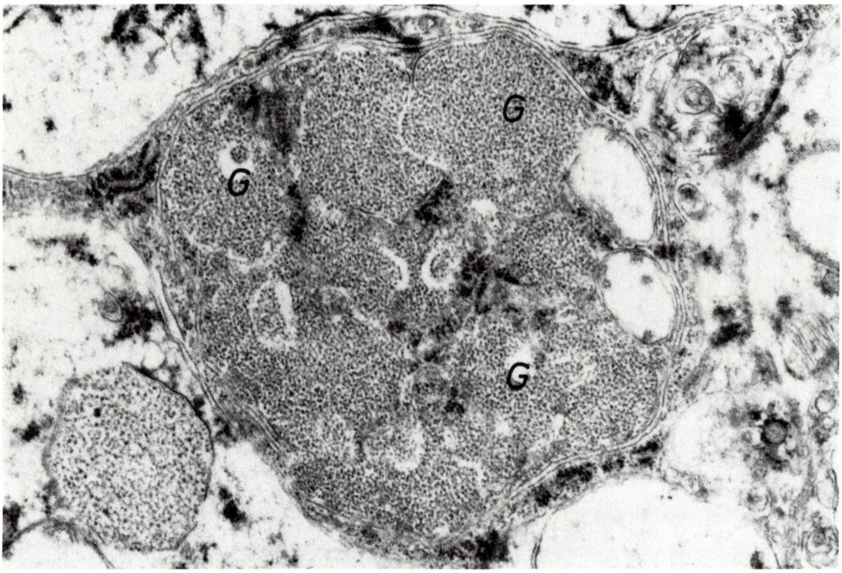

Fig. 2. A retinal cell process contains membrane-bound sacs of glycogen (G). Type II glycogenosis; X 24,000.

But such an ultrastructural diversity of lipopigments certainly presents a challenge to the biochemist to bear such morphological differences in mind when analysing NCL-lipopigments biochemically. The photoreceptors are also heavily endowed with lipopigments (Fig. 3), but morphological damage of either the perikarya or the photoreceptor inner or outer segments is not obvious. This is in striking contrast to the damage and later to the loss of photoreceptors in human NCL (Goebel et al. 1974, 1977).

The retinal pigment epithelium (RPE) in canine NCL shows peculiar circular, semicircular and straight stacks of lamellae (Fig. 5). Such layered membranes have consistently been seen in the RPE of homozygously NCL-affected English setters, overlying both the tapetal (Fig. 5a) and non-tapetal (Fig. 5b) areas, but not in non-affected English setters (Fig. 6). These stacks of lamellae may not always be surrounded by a limiting membrane (Fig. 7a), and they may be found incorporated within other cytosomes of the RPE (Fig. 7b), and also within lipofuscin (Fig. 7c). Morphology alone cannot establish whether these peculiar layered membranes actually manifest an impaired phagocytotic process of photoreceptor outer segments

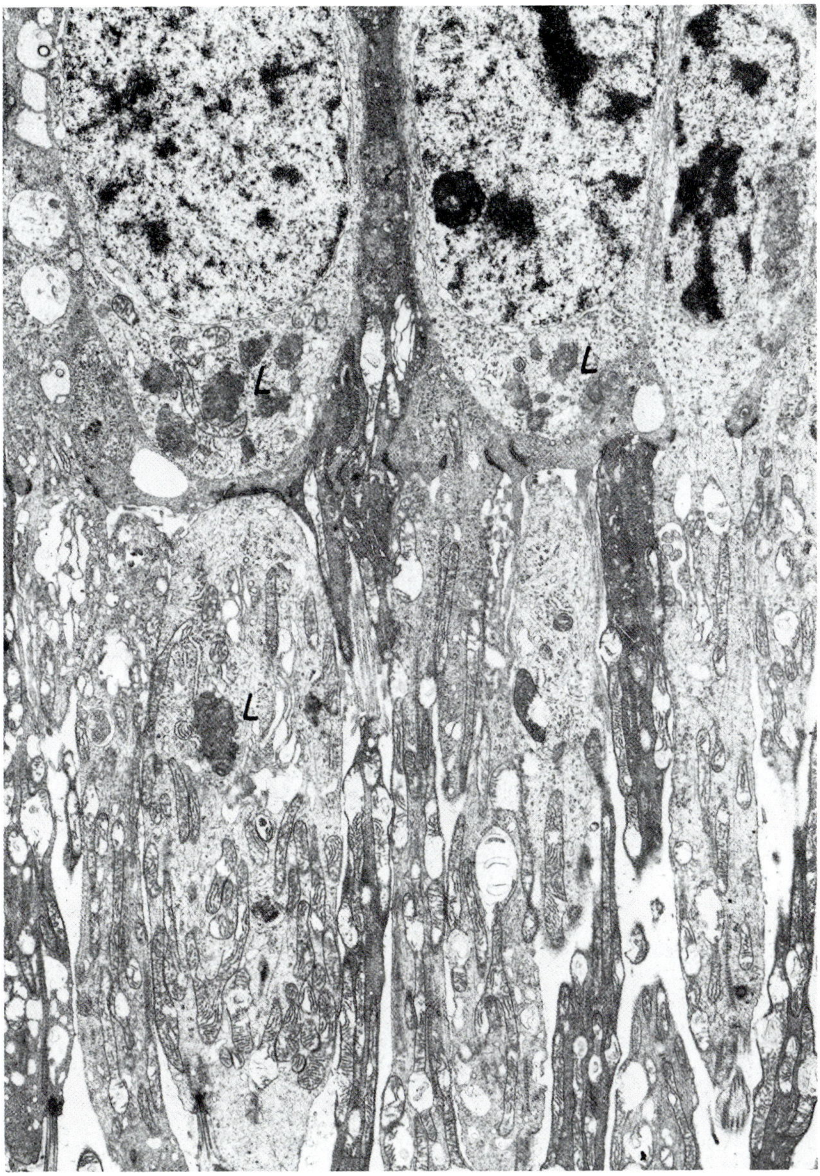

Fig. 3. The perikarya and inner segments of photoreceptors contain NCL-specific lipopigments (L). NCL-affected English setter; X 6,720.

Fig. 4. Retinal lipopigments in canine NCL

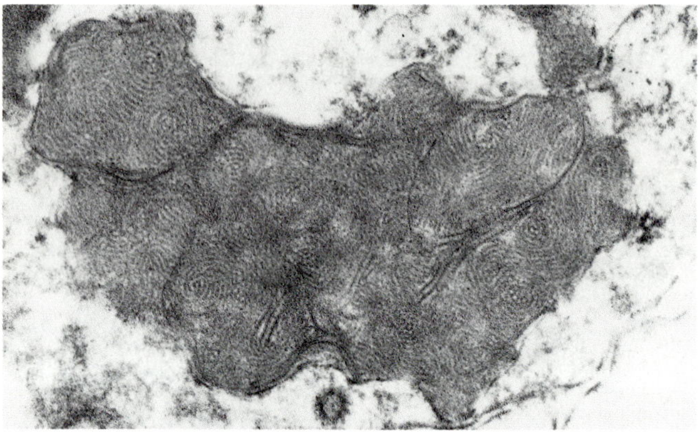

a. Fingerprint type; X 49,400

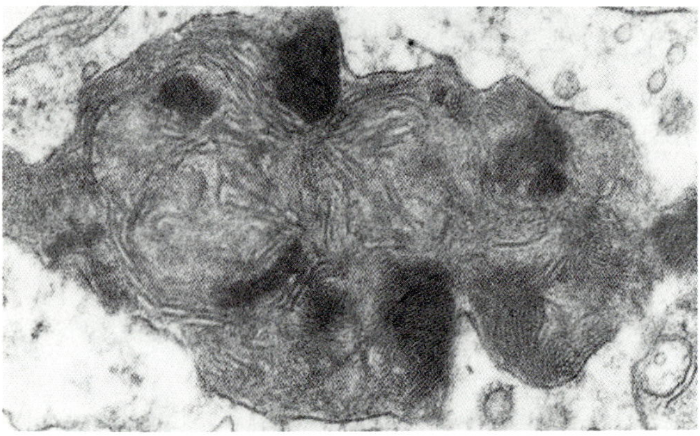

b. Composite membranous type; X 49,400

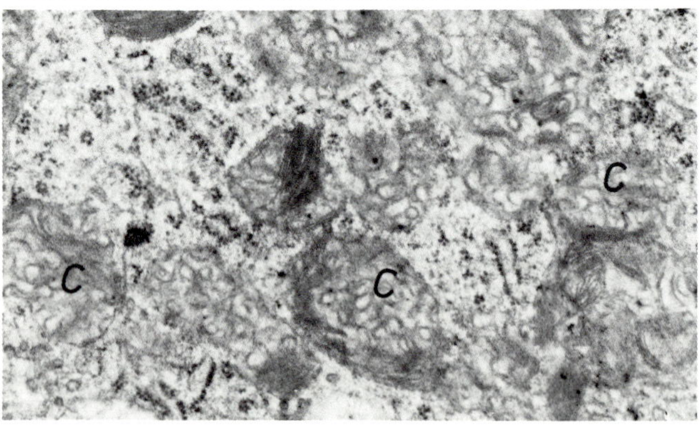

c. Curvilinear (C) type; X 19,200.

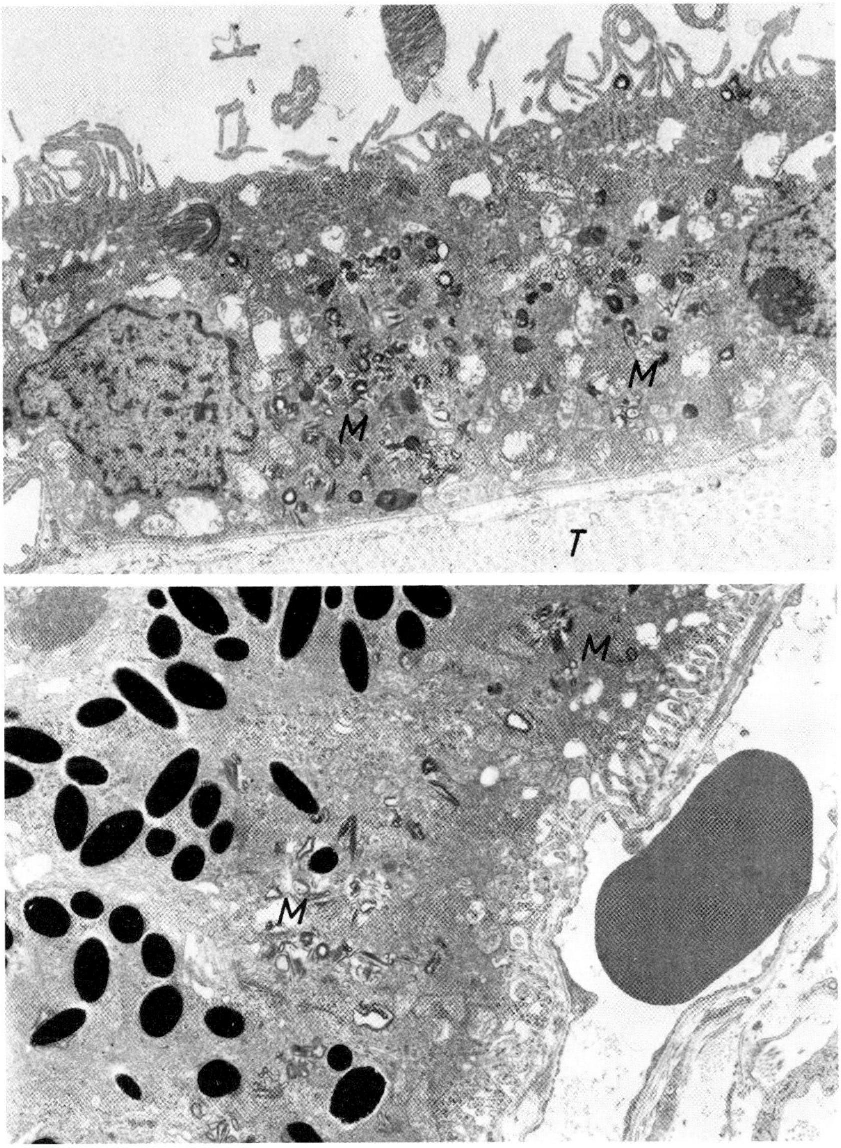

Fig. 5. Peculiar circular and semicircular layered membranes (M) in RPE cells, overlying the tapetum (T), X 5,700 (a), and the non-tapetal area, X 7,770 (b).

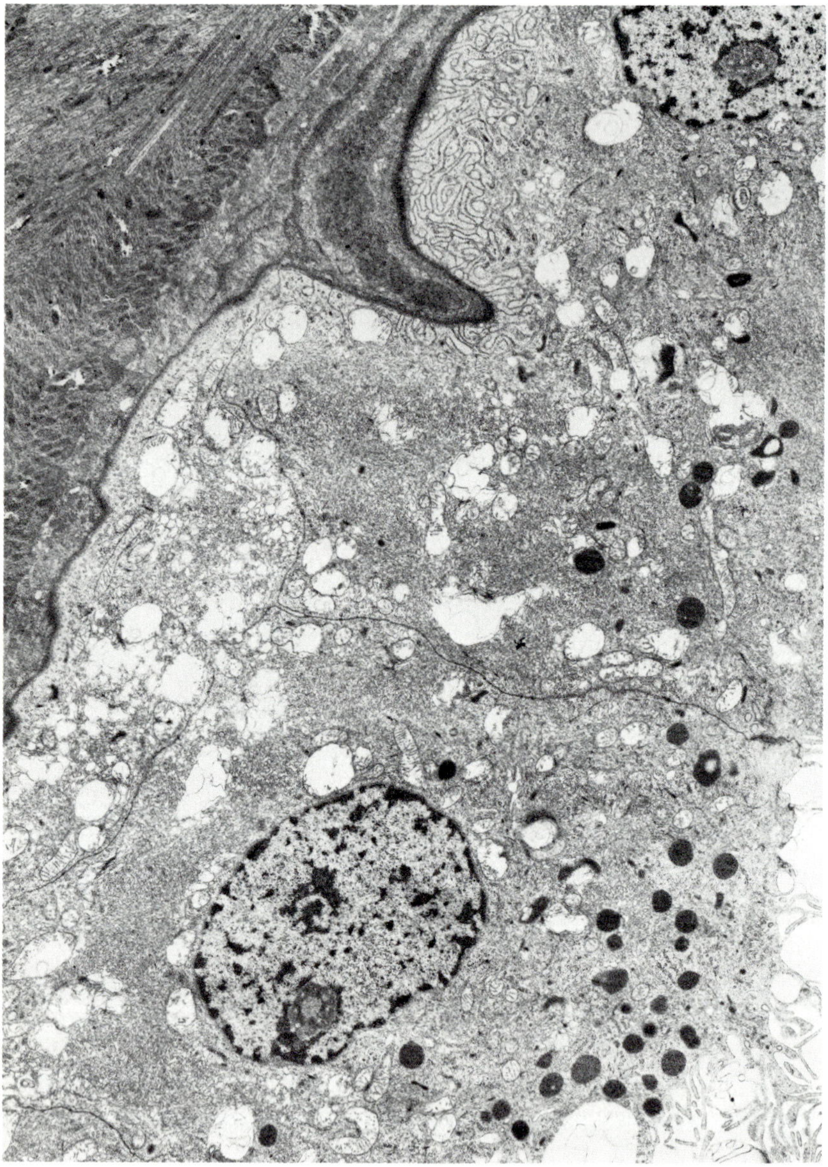

Fig. 6. RPE of a normal English setter, overlying the tapetum, contains numerous lipopigment granules, but no circular or semicircular layered lamellae. X 6,650.

Fig. 7. Layered membranes in RPE in canine NCL,

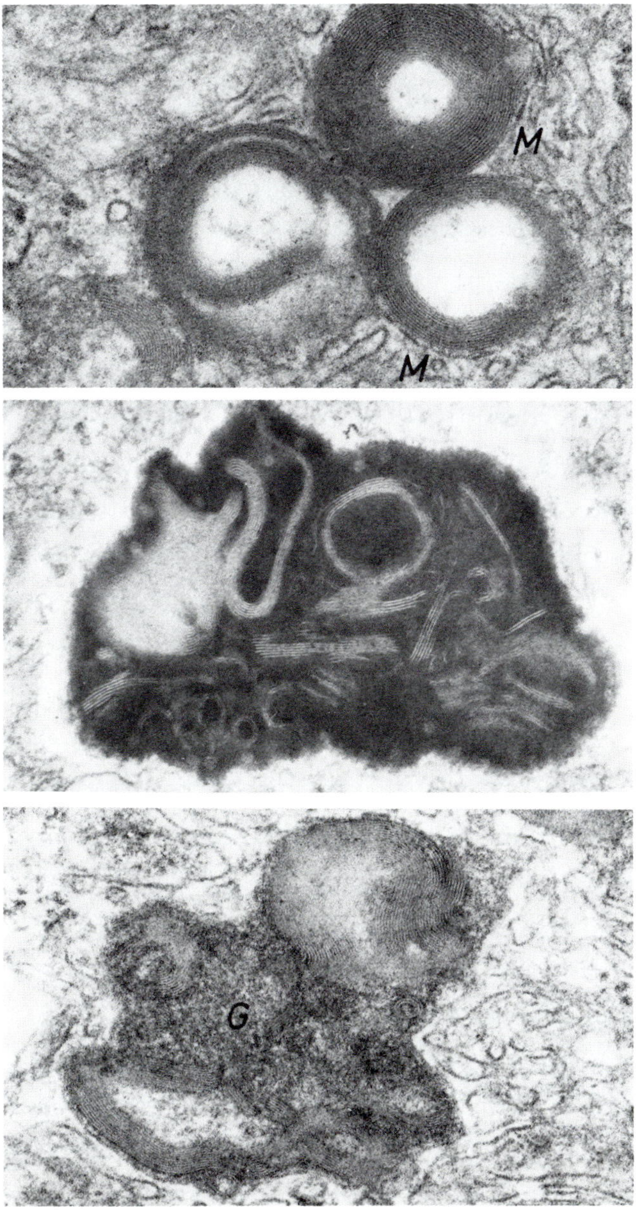

a.
partly surrounded by a membrane (M); X 78,300,

b.
incorporated into a dense cytosome; X 58,000,

c.
enclosed in a membrane-bound granular (G) matrix; X 78,300.

or whether they merely represent an unrelated, but NCL-specific phenomenon, although occasional close spatial proximity of these membranous stacks to phagocytosed photoreceptor outer segments morphologically suggests such a pathogenetic relation (Fig. 8).

Ultrastructural studies of the retina in human NCL have hitherto illustrated the endstages (Goebel et al. 1974, 1977) of the disease. They are identical in infantile (Tarkkanen et al. 1972), late infantile (Goebel et al. 1977), juvenile (Fig. 9) (Goebel et al. 1974) and possibly adult (Dom et al. 1979) forms of NCL. Retinopathy in NCL does not significantly differ form the endstage ultramorphology of non-NCL retinopathia pigmentosa, apart from the composition of the lipopigments and melanolysosomes.

As so often during the long-lasting process of elucidating a genetically determined disease in man, morphological studies may provide the basis for further biochemical and physiological questions as the former are frequently merely descriptive. Electron microscopy may not only disclose early lesions and their distribution, not obvious to the histopathologist, but may propose additional research for the physiologist and biochemist. The exclusive intralysosomal accumulation of sulfatides in ganglion cells in MLD certainly challenges the biochemist to investigate the sulfatide catabolism of individual cell types rather than of a tissue or organ homogenate. The peculiar membrane complexes encountered in RPE in canine NCL also should attract investigators to study the function of RPE cells in normal and NCL-diseased English setters. The common accumulation of NCL-specific lipopigments within photoreceptors in canine and human NCL, but the preservation of these cells in canine NCL and the degeneration of these cells in human NCL illustrate the question whether accumulation of lipopigments damages the cell or whether primary damage of the cell may result in intracellular lipopigment accumulation.

ACKNOWLEGEMENTS

The presentation of these studies has been supported by the "Deutsche Forschungsgemeinschaft" (Go 185/4 and 477/877/80).

We are grateful to Ms. Rose Kosswig for her excellent technical and photographic aid.

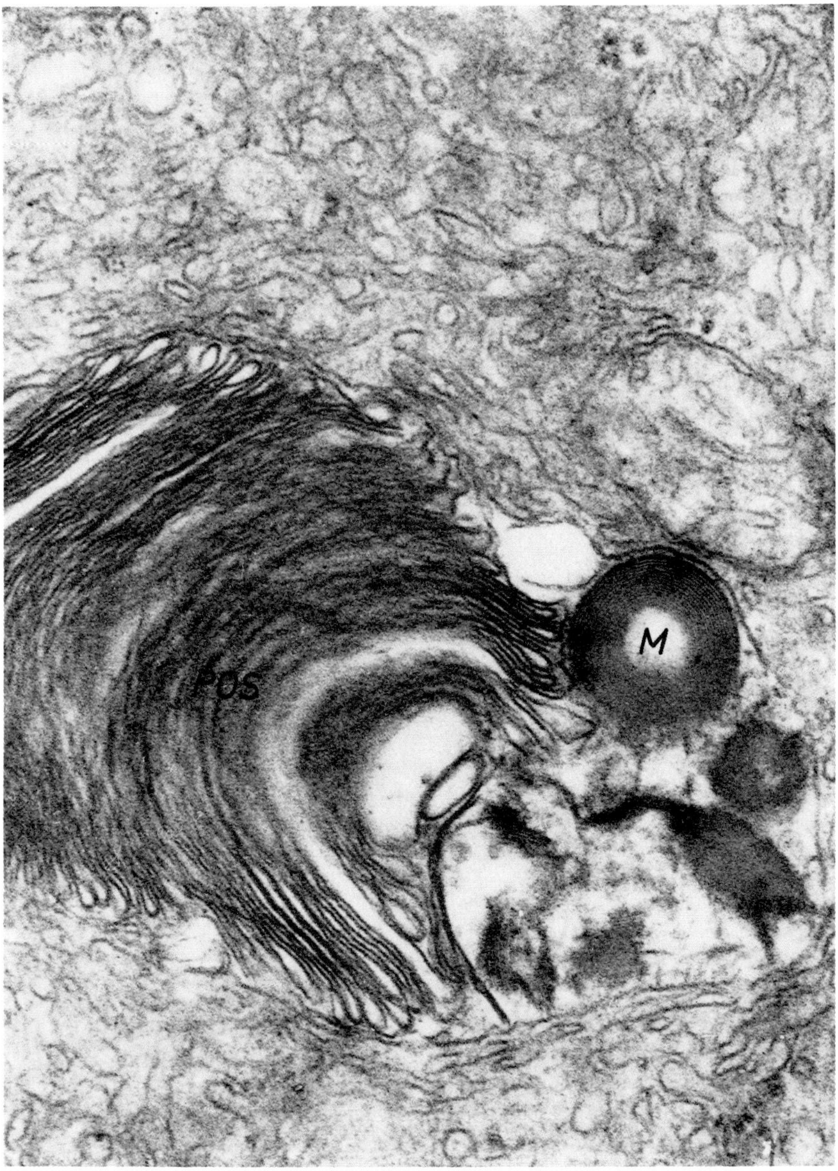

Fig. 8. Layered circular membranes (M) are in close spatial proximity to phagocytosed photoreceptor outer segment (POS). RPE, NCL-affected English setter; X 81,200.

ELECTRORETINOGRAPHY (ERG) AND HEREDITARY TRANSMISSION IN SOME NEUROLOGIC HEREDO-DEGENERATIVE DISEASES.

Bianca Stanescu*, Jean Michiels* , Gilles Lyon**

*Service d'Ophtalmologie, **Service de Neurologie Pédiatrique, Université de Louvain, Bruxelles (Belgium)

Retinitis pigmentosa (RP) is not a homogeneous disorder, but a group of diseases with variable phenotypic expression.

Classically the ERG was considered to be extinguished in RP. However modern recording techniques, by averaging ERG, reveal recognisable signals.

More recent studies using the "Ganzfeld" (full field), have demonstrated that in patients with early or mild forms of RP and with minimal or no ophthalmoscopic changes, the ERG was subnormal but large enough to permit separation into cone and rod components (Berson, 1968, Berson et al., 1968, 1969, 1970; Weinstein, 1977).

Some patients with RP can be genetically typed, by family history, into autosomal dominant, autosomal recessive and X-linked recessive forms (Berson et al., 1968, 1969, 1970, 1976, 1980), François et al., (1974), Berson et al., 1968, 1969, 1970, 1974, 1979, 1980). François et al.(1974) found some correlations between ERG abnormalities and the type of hereditary transmission in RP. Marmor (1979) however did not find appreciable differences in ERG characteristics in recessive, dominant and X-linked cases of RP.

Retinitis pigmentosa is a constant or frequent manifestation in several heredo-degenerative diseases of the nervous system (NHDD).

In the past decade several studies have supported the view that there are constant ERG alterations in lipofuscinosis (Pinkers, 1974; Stanescu et al., 1974, 1975),

Birth Defects: Original Article Series, Volume 18, Number 6, pages 255–262

Steinert's dystrophia myotonica (Burian & Burns, 1966; Stanescu et al., 1970, 1975), Laurence-Moon-Bardet-Biedl syndrome (L.M.B.B.) (Stiggelbaut, 1969; Michiels et al., 1973; Stanescu et al., 1974), spino-cerebellar degenerations (SCD) (Björk et al., 1951; François, 1974; Stanescu et al., 1972, 1979, 1980).

In the present study, based on ERG investigations of patients with different NHDD, we attempted to investigate a possible relation between the type of genetic transmission and the pattern of ERG abnormality.

MATERIAL AND METHOD

32 patients with different types of NHDD where investigated (table 1) : 11 patients had Steinert's dystrophia myotonica, 6 had different clinical forms of SCD, 5 patients had L.M.B.B. syndrome and 10 had a lipofuscinosis.

Initially, the group of NHDD was larger, but patients with uncertain diagnosis or with unclear hereditary transmission were discarded.

The ERG was recorded on a cathode ray storage oscilloscope connected to an electroretinograph and its photostimulator (Van Gogh and Tektronix). The recording was done in "Ganzfeld" with a single low intensity flash stimulation and neutral filters that attenuated the stimulus 200 times (2,3 u log).

TABLE 1

ERG VALUES IN HEALTHY AND PATIENTS WITH N.H.D.D

Diagnosis	Nb of cases		Mean age	b wave amplitude, μv		b wave, I.T, msec	
				photo	scoto	photo	scoto
Healthy	30		34,2	85 ± 45	148 ± 30	41,4 ±5.7	60 ± 7.2
Steinert's Myotonia	11		44,01	58.2± 17.3	61.8± 14	41.3 ±5	83.6± 6
S.C.D.	6		27,2	41,7± 16	80,8± 27,3	53 ±2.4	79 ± 10
L.M.B.B.	5	3	20	extinguished			
		2		30 ± 16.2	59 ± 25	50 ± 6	80 ± 10.3
Lipofuscinosis	10		13	extinguished			

The tests for implicit time (IT) were done in complete darkness after twenty minutes of dark adaptation, for scotopic conditions, and after three minutes adaptation to a light of 750 Lux, for photopic conditions. The b wave "Implicit time" was measured as the time interval between the onset of the stimulus and the major cornea positive peak for the rod and cone responses. The control group comprised 30 healthy subjects ranging age between 6-55 years.

RESULTS

In the group with Steinert's dystrophia myotonica, all patients had ERG alterations consistent with the "rod dysfunction syndrome", with low amplitude and delayed IT of the b wave in scotopic conditions, and in photopic conditions (table 1).

In a second group of 6 patients with SCD, including 1 Friedreich disease and 5 sporadic cases of uncertain classification, ERG recordings revealed a "cone- rod dysfunction syndrome", with diminished amplitude and delayed implicit time respectively in photopic and scotopic conditions (table 1).

Five patients had Laurence-Moon-Bardet-Biedl syndrome; three of them had extinguished ERG records, while 2 patients presented a "cone rod dysfunction" syndrome (table 1).

In the last group of 10 patients with lipofuscinosis, the ERG was extinguished in all (table 1).

Previous investigations indicated a possible connection between ERG alterations and the type of hereditary transmission of RP (table 2) (Berson, 1968, 1976, 1979; Berson et al., 1968, 1969, 1970, 1975, 1980; François et al., 1974).

François et al. (1974) summarizing partially Berson's results described mainly 3 types of ERG dysfunction syndromes (table 3) :

- The "rod dysfunction syndrome" or "progressive rod degeneration" characterised by a low amplitude and delayed IT of the b wave in scotopic conditions and of normal amplitude and IT in photopic conditions. This type of ERG abnormality was observed in families with dominant forms of RP.
- The "cone rod dysfunction syndrome" or"progressive cone-rod degeneration" with a predominant loss of cone function. The ERG is extinguished or very low and delayed in photopic conditions, in the presence of low rod amplitu-

TABLE 2

ERG IN WIDESPREAD , PROGRESSIVE RETINITIS PIGMENTOSA (R.P)

TYPE OF DEGENERATION	CASES	CONE ERG (b-wave) Amplitude	CONE ERG (b-wave) Implicit Time	ROD ERG (b-wave) Amplitude	ROD ERG (b-wave) Implicit Time
Dominant RP with complete penetrance	11	Normal or reduced	Normal	Reduced	Delayed
Dominant RP with reduced penetrance	8	Normal or reduced	Delayed	Reduced	Delayed
Autosomal recessive RP	75	Reduced	Delayed	Reduced	Normal or reduced
Sex-Linked reccessive RP	7	Reduced	Delayed	Reduced	Delayed

Ganzfeld , clear media, dilated pupil,large enough responses to separate into cone, and rod components
D'après Berson 1976

TABLE 3

ERG Syndromes in different hereditary types of R.P.

ERG Syndrome	Type of hereditary transmission
Rod dysfunction	autosomal dominant
Rod cone dysfunction	(X linked ?)
Cone Rod dysfunction	autosomal recessif

Data from François and all.(1974)

de, and normal latency in scotopic conditions. This type of ERG abnormality was noted in families with recessive forms of retinitis pigmentosa.

- The "rod-cone dysfunction syndrome" or "progressive rod-cone degeneration" with extinguished ERG and, when registrable, with loss of rod and cone functions : low amplitude and delayed implicit time in scotopic and photopic conditions. It is a combined degeneration of both receptors systems. This type of ERG abnormality has been seen by Berson (1976) in families with sex linked forms of RP.

Marmor (1979) did not find the same link between patterns of ERG and the genetic type of transmission in patients with RP.

He explains the discrepancy between Berson's and his results by the limited number of patients studied. Indeed the dominant RP is not very frequent in the U.S.A. and the number of cases studied by both Marmor and Berson, including dominant and X-linked transmission, is to small to permit definite conclusions. Moreover, pedigree informations are frequently incomplete so that some patients are arbitrarly considered to have either a recessive or a dominant inheritance with reduced penetrance.

We suggest that the study of the ERG in NHDD, could contribute to shed some light on this problem. Indeed, the genetic transmission in several of these diseases is well established and one has not to rely on sometimes vague family data.

The hereditary transmission is dominant in dystrophia myotonica Steinert's, recessive in lipofuscinosis, L.M.B.B. syndrome, Friedreich disease, etc.

Our study shows that the ERG alteration in Steinert's disease, which is a dominant disease, is of the "rod dysfunction" type, an ERG pattern previously found by Berson et al., 1968, 1969, 1975, 1976, 1980 and François et al., 1974), in the dominant forms of RP (table 4).

ERG recordings in lipofuscinosis and L.M.B.B., which have a recessive hereditary transmission, were either extinguished or showed a "cone rod dysfunction" syndrome, as respectively, in the advanced forms and early forms of RP with a recessive transmission (Berson, 1968, 1976; Berson

TABLE 4

NEUROLOGIC DIAGNOSIS	NOMBRE OF CASES (32 PATIENTS)	ERG SYNDROM	TYPE OF HEREDITARY TRANSMISSION
Dystrophia myotonica Steinert	11	Rod-dysfunction	dominant
Spino cerebellar degeneration of atypical pattern	5	Cone-rod dysfunction	recessive
Friedreich disease	1	Cone-rod dysfunction	recessive
Laurence-Moon-Bardet-Biedl-syndrome	5	3 cases : abolished 2 cases : rod-cone dysfunction	recessive
Lipofuscinosis	10	abolished	recessive

et al., 1970, 1975; François et al., 1974) (table 4). In SCD the hereditary transmission, is variable : it is autosomal recessive in Friedreich's disease, in olivo-pontocerebellar degeneration, cerebello-olivar atrophy or Hunt's dysgenesia cerebello-myoclinica.

In the patients we studied 5 had sporadic SCD with high probability of autosomal recessive transmission, another patient had a Friedreich's disease, which is always inherited as an autosomal recessive tract. ERG records showed in all of them a "cone-rod dysfunction syndrome" that was previously reported to occur in families with recessive RP.

Our results suggests the possibility of a link between the ERG pattern and the type of genetic transmission in some NHDD. The number of patients studied by us in some diseases is however to small to draw definite conclusions. More data are needed to support our findings.

REFERENCES

Berson E (1968). Progressive cone rod degeneration. Arch Ophthalmol 80:68.

Berson E, Gouras P, Gunkel R (1968). Rod response in retinitis pigmentosa dominantly inherited. Arch Ophthalmol 80:58.

Berson E, Gouras P, Gunkel R, Myriantopoulos M (1969).

Dominant retinitis pigmentosa with reduced penetrance. Arch Ophthalmol 81:215.
Berson E, Kanters L (1970). Cone and rod responses in family with recessively inherited retinitis pigmentosa. Arch Ophthalmol 89:288.
Berson E (1975). Retinitis pigmentosa, the electroretinogram and Mendel's laws. Communication : The annual meeting of the Pensylvania Academy of Ophtalmology and Otolaryngology.
Berson E (1976). Hereditary retinal disease : classification with full-field electroretinogram. Doc Ophthalmol 13:149.
Berson E (1979). Dominant retinitis pigmentosa with reduced penetrance. Arch Ophthalmol 97:1286.
Berson E, Rosner B, Simonoff E (1980). Genetic typing and retinitis pigmentosa. Arch Ophthalmol 89:763.
Bjork A, Lindblom H, Waldenstein L (1951). Retinal degeneration in hereditary ataxia. J Neurol Surg Psych 19:186.
Burian H, Burns C (1966). Electroretinography and dark adaptation in patients with myotonic dystrophy. Amer J Ophthalmol 61:1044.
François J, De Rouck A, Cambie E, Zanen A (1974). L'électrodiagnostic des affections rétiniennes. Bull Soc Belge Ophtalmol 166:257.
François J (1974). Tapeto-retinal degenerations in spino cerebellar degenerations (heredoataxia). Acta Genet Med Gemell 23:3.
Marmor MF (1979). The electroretinogram in retinitis pigmentosa. Arch Ophthalmol 97:1300.
Michiels J, Stanescu B (1973). La rétinopathie du syndrome de Laurence-Moon-Bardet-Biedl. Bull Soc Belge Ophtal 163:103.
Pinckers A, Bremer S (1974). Neuronal ceroid-lipofuscinosis (ERG and EOG). Ann Oculist 207:529.
Stanescu B, Wawernia E (1970). Electroretinographic and electro-encephalographic changes in dystrophia myotonica Steinert. Ophthalmol 160:157.
Stanescu B, Wawernia E (1970). Electroretinogram and electro-encephalogram in Laurence-Moon-Bardet Biedl syndrome. Confin Neurol 32:423.
Stanescu B, David M, Wawernia E (1972). L'importance de l'électrorétinographie dans les atrophies optiques héréditaires. Arch Ophthalmol 32:203.
Stanescu B, Spiritus M, Michiels J (1974). L'importance de l'électrophysiologie rétinienne dans la maladie de Batten-Mayou-Spielmeyer-Vogt. Acta Genet Med Gemell 23:367.
Stanescu B, Michiels J (1975). Temporal aspecta of electro-

retinography in patients with myotonic dystrophy. Amer J Ophthalmol 80:2.

Stanescu B, Michiels J (1979). Heredoataxia (spino-cerebellar degeneration) ERG alterations, temporal aspects. Ophthalmol 178:267.

Stanescu B, Evrard Ph, Michiels J, Lyon G (1980). Electroretinographic changes in a case of spino-cerebellar degeneration (SCD). Metab Pediat Ophthal 4:221.

Stiggelbaut W (1969). The Laurence-Moon-Bardet-Biedl syndrome. Van Gorcum. Assen.

Weinstein G (1977). The natural history of retinitis pigmentosa. In Landers M, Wolbarsht M, Dowling J, Laties A (eds) : "Retinitis pigmentosa, clinical implications of current research", Plenum Press, New York, p 3.

Zeman W., Dycken P (1969). Neuronal ceroid-lipofuscinosis (Batten's disease). Relationship to amaurotic idiocy. Pediatrics 44:570.

KEARNS-SAYRE SYNDROME

PINHAS NEMET MD, VICTOR GODEL MD PhD,
MOSHE LAZAR MD
Department of Ophthalmology, Ichilov
Hospital, Tel Aviv University Medical
School, Israel.

Since Kearns and Sayre (1958) described the syndrome bearing their names, several cases have been recorded and abundant evidence has been forthcoming to convey a relationship between external ophthalmoplegia, retinal degeneration and cardiac disturbances.

Such cases appear usually as sporadic occurrences in their families, however some instances of hereditary transmission, operating through autosomal dominant genes, have been reported (Leveille & Newell 1980).

This paper describes the familial occurrence of chronic progressive external ophthalmoplegia, retinal degeneration and cardiac anomalies associated with arachnodactily, pectus excavatum, highly arched palate, and severe myopia. The distribution of this syndrome in this kindred is compatible with autosomal recessive inheritance.

CASE REPORTS

This Jewish-Iranian family (Fig 1) was ascertained through a 30 year-old female (II-3) with progressive external ophthalmoplegia. Physical examination revealed some limb weakness, arachnodactily, pectus excavatum, a highly arched palate and high myopia. The ophthalmoscopic

Birth Defects: Original Article Series, Volume 18, Number 6, pages 263–268

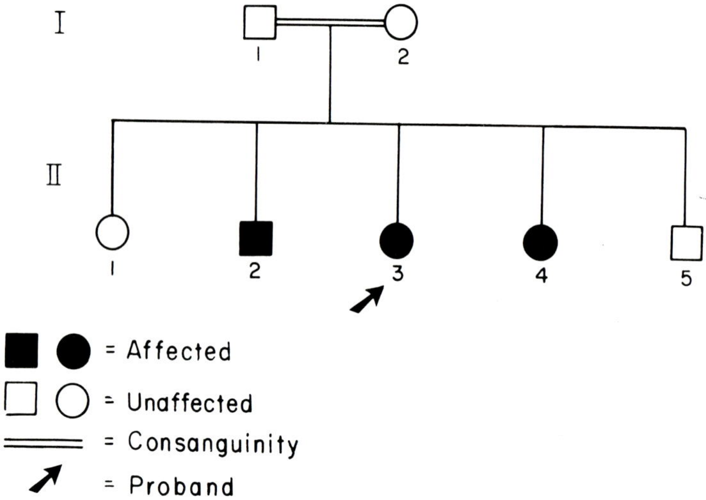

Fig 1. Family pedigree

examination revealed an atypical pigmentary distrophy of the retina and the electroretinographic results confirmed the diagnosis. Cardiologic investigations showed a prolapse of the aortic valve. Electromyographic recordings from the extraocular muscles showed potentials of low amplitude. In order to improve her eye motility status a squint operation was performed but the improvement was only minimal. An extraocular muscle biopsy showed a high degree of destruction of the muscle fiber and characteristic mitochondrial abnormalities. Further laboratory examinations showed a high protein content in the cerebrospinal fluid. Later she underwent an extracapsular cataract extraction.

The 32 year-old brother of the proband(II-5) was also high myopic. He presented arachnodactily, pectus excavatum and highly arched palate. He presented minimal ocular movements and suffered from retinal pigmentary degeneration confirmed by electroretinography. Electromyography of the extraocular muscles showed potentials of reduced duration and low amplitude. Following squint surgery his esotropia was successfully corrected. Cardiologic investigation showed a clear degree of right axis deviation and a significant delay in intraventricular conduction.

Another 28 year-old sister of the proband (II-4) was operated on both eyes because cataract. Her physical examination revealed arachnodactily and pectus excavatum. Ophthalmoscopy showed atypical retinal pigmentary dystrophy with very low amplitudes of the electroretinograms. Some restrictions of her eye movements were disclosed and the electromyography showed potentials of normal duration but slightly attenuated amplitudes. Electrocardiographic investigations revealed synus arrhytmia with premature contractions.

The parents of these cases were second cousins and all the family members were originating from the same small Iranian village. From their history it appeared that intrafamilial marriages were a frequent phenomenon between their ancestors. Two other children in this family were normal as concerns the ocular and neurologic examination.

DISCUSSION

The different symptoms accompanying the chronic progressive external ophthalmoplegia in our family members were interesting and difficult to classify (Table 1). The ophthalmoplegia associated with the retinal degeneration and cardiac disturbances justified in our opinion the inclusion of these cases in the Kearns Sayre syndrome. The elevated concentration of cerebrospinal fluid protein in one case and the histopathologic findings confirming mitochondrial alterations were strongly supporting such a diagnosis.

Table 1. Clinical findings of the affected family members.

Anomaly	II-2	II-3	II-4
Ocular			
High myopia	+	+	+
Ophthalmoplegia	+	+	−
Cataract	−	+	+
Retinal dystrophy	+	+	+
Abnormal ERG	+	+	+
Abnormal EMG	+	+	+
Skeleto-muscular			
High palate	+	+	−
Arachnodactily	+	+	+
Limb weakness	−	+	−
Pectus excavatum	+	+	−
Mitochondrial defect	?	+	?
Cardiac	+	+	+
CSF hyperproteinemia	?	+	?

Although the arachnodactily, highly arched palate, pectus excavatum and high myopia were suggestive of Marfan's syndrome, the lack of other characteristic findings for this disorder made such a diagnosis unlikely.

The nature of the basic defect in this complex disorder is not properly understood. Some morphological and biochemical observations have been brought to indicate that the primary disturbance of the metabolic process is at the level of the mitochondria (Karpati et al 1973). As the mitochondrial development can fail in various systems and organs, the disease may appear with different symptomatology. Such a concept of primary mitochondrial disorder at various targets account for the spectrum of the clinical expression and the multitude of its clinical variants. Given the complexity of such mitochondrial responses, pathogenetic heterogeneity should be a likely rather than a surprising event. It is in this context that the extreme variability found in this disorder must be viewed and names like oculo-cranio-somatic neuromuscular disease interpreted (Olson et al 1972).

There is some unequivocal evidence for the familial occurrence of Kearns Sayre syndrome. The disease is felt to be inherited by an autosomal dominant mechanism with variable expressivity, explaining pseudo-sporadicity, pseudo-recessivity and pleiotropy (Bastiaensen 1978). However, no simple hypothesis can be put forward for the genetic factors involved in the vast majority of cases.

In our family, the consanguinity between the parents, their freedom from any discernible abnormalities, the occurrence of the trait in both sexes and the res emblance of the phenotypic expression constitues convinving evidence of autosomal recessive inheritance. As this family derived from the same place in one of the most inbred areas of Iran, it is possible that more consanguineous marriages took place in their ancestors.

Increasing knowledge of the pathology of Kearns Sayre syndrome doubtless will stem from more accurate diagnosis through awareness of the condition and more widespread appreciation of its clinical features.

SUMMARY

A family with Kearns Sayre syndrome, characterized by a distinctive type of progressive external ophthalmoplegia,retinal pigmentary dystrophy and cardiac disturbances is described. Additional malformations as arachnodactily, sternal deformity, high arched palate and severe myopia are reported. The spectrum of the variable phenotypic expression is delineated. The occurrence of the disease in these patients, offspring of a consanguineous mating, reinforce the assumption that hereditary transmission may play a role in the pathogenesis of at least some cases. The pedigree analysis suggest autosomal recessive inheritance.

REFERENCES

Bastiaensen LAK (1978). Chronic Progressive External Ophthalmoplegia. Winchester Mass. Sijthoff-Noordhoff Int Publ.

Karpati G, Carpenter S, Larbrisseau A, LaFontaine R (1973). The Kearns-Shy syndrome. A multisystem disease with mitochondrial abnormality, demonstrated in skeletal muscle and skin. J Neur Sci 19:133.

Kerns TP, Sayre GP (1958). Retinitis pigmentosa, external ophthalmoplegia and complete heart block. Arch Ophth 60:280.

Leveille AS, Newell FN (1980). Autosomal dominant Kearns Sayre syndrome. Ophthal 87:99.

Olson W, Engel WK, Walsh GO, Einaugler R(1972). Oculocraniosomatic neuromuscular disease with "ragged-red" fibers. Histochemical and ultrastructural changes in limb muscles of a group of patients with idiopathic progressive external ophthalmoplegia. Arch Neurol 26:193.

Reprint requests: Pinhas Nemet MD, Department of Ophthalmology, Ichilov Hospital, Tel Aviv 64239, Israel.

INCOMPLETE ACHROMATOPSIA: DIAGNOSIS IN INFANCY

C. G. Keith,

Royal Children's Hospital, Melbourne.

Flemington Road, Parkville, Victoria.

Congenital cone dysfunction can manifest itself as complete achromatopsia (rod monochromatism) and the incomplete or atypical achromatopsias. The latter terms are often inappropriate because the subject can frequently detect different colours, even when the visual acuity is poor. The features of fifteen children with cone dysfunction are discussed, including four who had a recordable photopic ERG. It is suggested that these represent incomplete cone dysfunction (incomplete achromatopsia). Two of these children were siblings, and other members of their kindred are also affected to a varying degree; this family is discussed briefly.

MATERIAL AND METHODS.

Over the past four and a half years at the Royal Children's Hospital in Melbourne, infants and children with persistently poor vision and/or nystagmus have had a full ocular examination under general anaesthesia. This includes slit-lamp examination, retinoscopy, ophthalmoscopy with scleral indentation, fundus photography, fluorescein angiography, electroretinography and recording of the visually evoked potentials. Most of these children have had a generic diagnosis of Leber's disease applied. Electroretinography was performed using the Medical Workshop electroretinography lens of Echte and Papst. The stimuli were provided by bright flash photostimulators with appropriate filters, and the responses were recorded on a Medelec MS6 apparatus. Subjects were tested under photopic

Birth Defects: Original Article Series, Volume 18, Number 6, pages 269–280

TABLE 1. DETAILS OF CONE DYSFUNCTION CASES WITH NO RECORDABLE PHOTOPIC ERG.

CASE/SEX	NYSTAGMUS	PHOTOPHOBIA	V.A.	REFRACTION	COLOUR VISION	ERG POTENTIALS SCOTOPIC a.	b.
1. M.M. M.				+1.00/+2.00 x 90°		50	240
	Yes	Yes	6/60		Some		
18.11.68				0/+2.00 x 90°		25	140
2. E.C. F.*				+6.00/+2.00 x 90°		160	340
	Yes	Yes	5/60		None		
12.6.75				+6.00/+2.00 x 90°		160	420
3. A.C. F.*				+2.00/+2.50 x 90°		140	360
	Yes	Yes	-		-		
26.7.78				+0.50/+0.50 x 90°		140	420
4. T.H. M.				-1.25/-1.25 x 160°		60	280
	Yes	Yes	6/30		Red/Blue		
21.1.73				-1.50/-1.00 x 10°		80	320
5. D.R. F.				0/+1.50 x 90°		20	75
	Yes	No	< 6/60		-		
26.4.78				0/+2.00 x 90°		18	70

* Sisters

TABLE 1 cont.,

CASE/SEX	NYSTAGMUS	PHOTOPHOBIA	V. A.	REFRACTION	COLOUR VISION	ERG POTENTIALS SCOTOPIC a	b
6. J. S. M.	Yes	Yes	6/120	$-3.00/-0.50 \times 180^0$	-	25	100
25. 9. 78				$-3.00/-0.50 \times 180^0$		10	145
7. D. T. M.	Yes	No	6/36	+2.00	Blue, Yellow	10	70
7. 3. 77				+2.00		10	65
8. M. P. M.	Yes	-	6/120	-11.00	Blue, Yellow Green	25	75
6. 5. 70			6/120	-12.00		15	60
9. G. T M.	Yes	Yes	6/36	$-3.00/-1.50 \times 180^0$	No.	50	55
5. 12. 77				$-3.50/-3.50 \times 180^0$		45	50
10. E. O. F. *	Yes	Yes	6/36	$-3.00/-4.00 \times 180^0$	Yellow	55	155
27. 8. 71				$-3.50/-3.50 \times 180^0$		40	110
11. P. T. F. *	Yes	Yes	6/72	$+5.00/+1.00 \times 90^0$	-	40	115
6. 4. 77				$+3.00/+1.00 \times 90^0$		25	110

* Cousins

TABLE 2. **DETAILS OF CONE DYSFUNCTION CASES WHO HAD A RECORDABLE PHOTOPIC ERG.**

CASE/SEX/D.O.B.	NYSTAGMUS	PHOTOPHOBIA	V.A.	REFRACTION	COLOUR VISION	ERG POTENTIALS PHOTOPIC a.	PHOTOPIC b.	SCOTOPIC a.	SCOTOPIC b.
12. H.C. M.	Yes	No	?>6/60	-9.00	Red, Yellow, Blue	20	25	60	50
2.12.77				-9.00		21	25	50	38
13. T.T. M.	Yes	No	6/36	0	-	15	30	40	70
18.4.71			6/36	0/-1.50 x 180°		20	35	60	70
14. N.R. M.	Ceased	No	6/18	-2.00/-2.00 x 180°	-	12	32	14	37
27.7.78			6/18	-0.05/-2.00 x 180°		8	15	6	18
15. D.R. M.	Yes	No	6/60	0	Red, Green	7.5	25	55	70
3.8.76				0		-	15	20	40

illumination (1080 lux), scotopic illumination and after fifteen minutes dark adaptation. Colour vision was tested with primary projected colours, and when appropriate, with Ishihara plates (1978), Farnsworth D. 15 test, and the Farnsworth Munsell 100-Hue test in daylight.

RESULTS.

Fifteen children were detected with features suggestive of achromatopsia, in four of these a photopic ERG (Fig 1.) was recordable, while in the remaining eleven only a scotopic ERG was found (Fig 2.).

The other details of the subjects are shown in Tables 1. and 2., and it can be seen that visual acuities tended to be worse in those patients with no recordable photopic ERG (Group 1.), and these are summarized below (one patient was too young for V.A. assessment).

<6/60	6/60	6/36	6/30
5	1	3	1

while those with a recordable photopic ERG (Group 2.) tended to be slightly better.

<6/60	6/60	6/36	6/18
1	1	1	1

All eleven cases in Group 1. had nystagmus, while eight had photophobia, one had no photophobia, and in one the datum is lacking. Another child had difficulty only with a change in illumination. Of the four cases in Group 2., none had photophobia, three had persistant nystagmus, and in the fourth child it was only present for a few months, and then ceased. The refractive disorders were varied, but astigmatism was common, and high myopia was found in two of the children. The colour vision was very difficult to assess accurately in most cases, but some were obviously completely colour blind, while others seemed to distinguish primary colours, and two of the children in Group 2. could definitely distinguish primary colours.

The fundus appearances were within normal limits in most

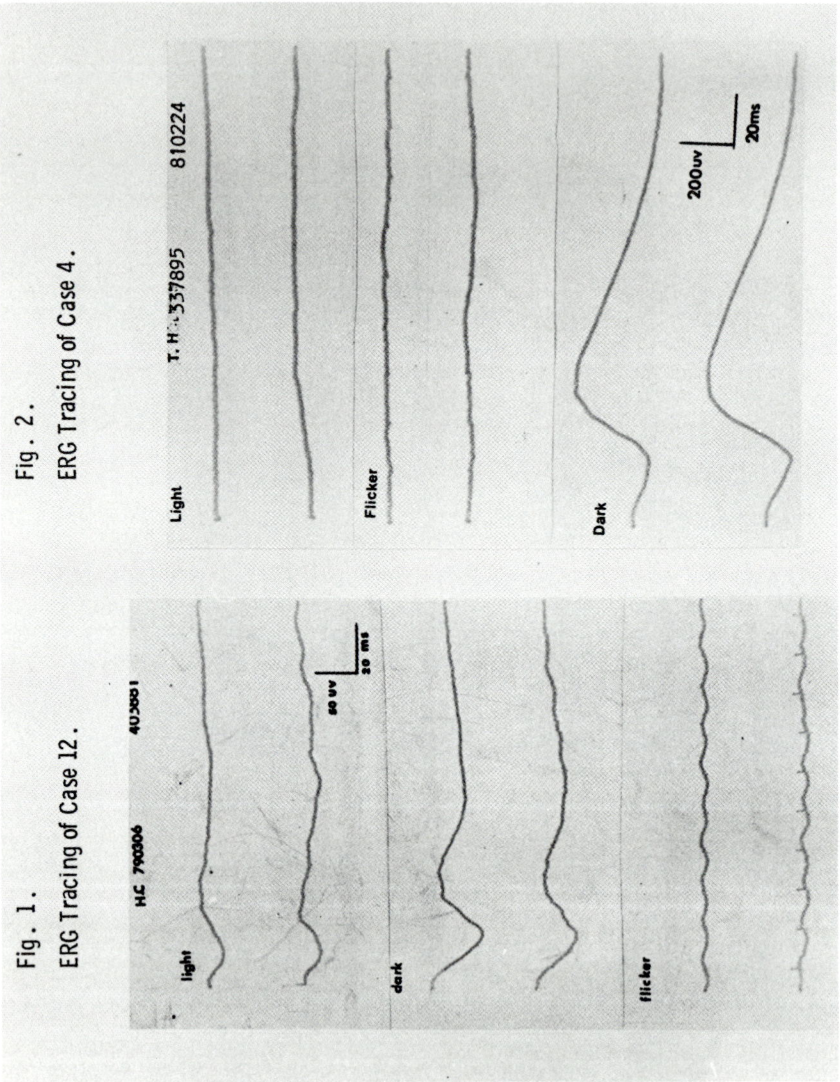

Fig. 1.
ERG Tracing of Case 12.

Fig. 2.
ERG Tracing of Case 4.

cases, and in none was there any evidence of macular hypoplasia or abnormal pigmentation. A few cases had been suspected of albinism before the ERG was performed. In three cases a diagnosis of optic nerve hypoplasia had been made, and certainly the optic nerve head appeared smaller than usual in these children, and might represent a reduction in nerve fibres from the retina, but again the ERG results demonstrated a cone dysfunction.

In the four children who showed a photopic response, the potentials obtained were all very low, and far below the normal parameters, but the peak implicit times were normal. In no case was a flicker ERG obtainable. The potentials in the dark adapted states were also abnormally low in many cases, but the implicit times were all normal. There did not seem to be any correlation between ERG potentials and the level of visual acuity or the degree of colour vision. No children had difficulty with night vision, and none of the children have shown any progression suggestive of cone dystrophy.

A family history was found in several instances. Cases two and three were sisters, and cases ten and eleven were cousins (case thirteen had a brother who we did not examine, but is reported to have nystagmus with a visual acuity of 6/9 in each eye). Case fourteen (IV. 1.) and case fifteen (IV. 2.) were brothers, and the family tree is shown in Fig.3. Five other members of their kindred have been examined, and all had abnormal ocular features, which are summarized in Table 3. The mode of inheritance seems to be autosomal dominant, with great variation in expressivity of the gene.

DISCUSSION

The features of incomplete cone dysfunction have been described by many authors, inter alia, François and Verriest (1959, 1960), Waardenburg (1963), Krill (1977). In a recent paper Smith, Pokorny and Newell (1979) stressed that the visual acuity is usually better in incomplete (6/60 - 6/18) than in the complete cone dysfunctions (<6/60). This was also found in our series. However it is not invariable, as eleven out of 25 of the complete cone dysfunction cases reported by Goodman, Ripps and Siegel (1963) had a visual acuity of better than 6/60, and two of their incomplete cases had visual acuity worse than 6/60. Light aversion

Fig. 3: FAMILY TREE OF CASES 14 AND 15.

FAMILY D. R. 368605

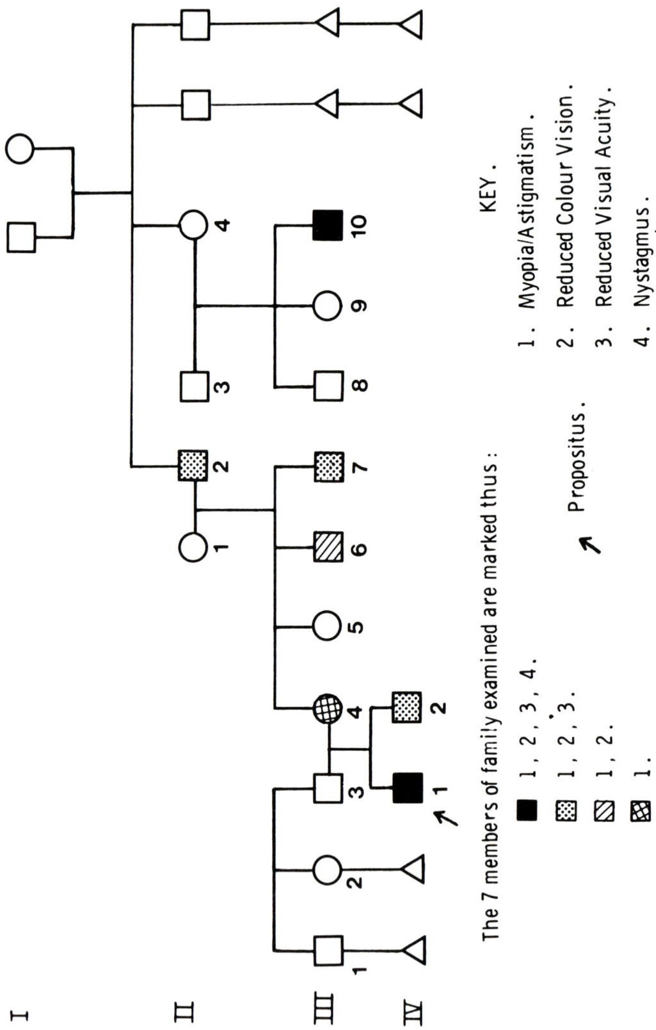

TABLE 3. OCULAR FEATURES FOUND IN FAMILY D. R. 368605.

SUBJECT	II 2	III 4*	III 6	III 7	III 10	IV 1	IV 2
REDUCED COLOUR VISION	+		+	+	+	+	+
REDUCED VISUAL ACUITY	+			+	+	+	+
MYOPIA/ ASTIGMATISM	+	+	+	+	+	+	+
NYSTAGMUS					+	+	

* Female.

and nystagmus are common features, and some colour discrimination is usually present. Both deutan defects (Smith et al, 1979) and protan defects (Smith et al, 1978) have been described, and also the X-linked recessive blue monocone-monochromacy has been reported by several authors (Blackwell and Blackwell (1961), Spivey et al (1964), Spivey (1965), Alpern et al (1965). The photopic ERG has been reported as being absent in incomplete cone dysfunction (Krill, 1977), however Waardenburg (1963), cites several cases of so-called achromatopsia with a reduced but present photopic ERG, and suggested that these represent an incomplete form of achromatopsia. Smith et al (1978) also found a photopic ERG in four cases of atypical cone dysfunction with a deutan defect. Since two of the cases were female siblings the inheritance was presumed to be autosomal recessive. The two male siblings that we report with a photopic ERG both belong to a kindred in which the inheritance appears to be autosomal dominant, but further studies are in progress to evaluate the family more fully.

Children with incomplete cone dysfunction are more likely to have reasonable vision and some colour discrimination than the complete rod-monochromat, and from the cases reported here, it seems that detection of a photopic ERG, however small, is a significant sign that the dysfunction is incomplete, and a slightly more optimistic prognosis can be given to the parents when counselling. In our study of infants and children with poor vision, most of whom had been diagnosed as Leber's disease, it was found that congenital cone dysfunction was by far the commonest cause of poor vision, and true cases of Leber's disease were extremely rare.

SUMMARY.

Infants and children with persistant poor vision and/or nystagmus had a full ocular examination under general anaesthesia. This included corneal electroretinography and fluorescein angiography. Eleven children were found with features of complete, and four with incomplete, cone dysfunction. The four incomplete cases had a small but recordable photopic ERG, but no flicker response. None had photophobia, while three had nystagmus. The visual acuity was 6/60 or less in two, 6/36 in one, and 6/18 in the other. They all seemed to have some degree of colour vision discrimination. The children with no recordable photopic ERG were considered to be complete cone dysfunctions, and in these the V.A. was worse (6/60 or less in six, 6/36 in three, and 6/30 in one), few seemed to have any colour discrimination. Two of the incomplete cone dysfunction cases were siblings, and other members of their family showed reduced visual acuity, colour vision defects, nystagmus, and myopia/astigmatism. The pedigree strongly suggests autosomal dominant inheritance, with a variable degree of expressivity.

In our study of infants and children with poor vision, most of whom had been diagnosed as Leber's disease, it was found that congenital cone dysfunction was by far the commonest cause of poor vision, and true cases of Leber's disease were extremely rare.

REFERENCES

Alpern M, Lee G, Arbor A (1965). Π_1 Cone monochromatism. Arch Ophthal 74: 334.

Blackwell HR, Blackwell OM (1961). Rod and cone receptor mechanisms in typical and atypical congenital achromatopsia. Vision 1: 62.

Francois J, Verriest G (1959). Contribution a l'etude des dyschromatopsies congenitales a symptomes intermediaires entre ceux des systemes dichromatiques classiques et ceux de l'achromatopsie typique: observation personnelle et revue de la litterature. Ann Oculist 192: 81.

Francois J, Verriest G (1960). Trois nouvelles observations d'achromatopsie congenitale atypique. Ann Oculist 193: 123.

Goodman G, Ripps H, Siegel I (1963). Cone dysfunction syndromes. Arch Ophthal 70: 214.

Krill AE (1977). Congenital color vision defects. In Archer DB (ed): 'Krill's Hereditary Retinal and Choroidal Diseases'. Vol 2. Clinical Characteristics, Hegerstown, Harper and Tow, Inc. p. 355.

Smith V, Pokorny J, Newell F (1978). Autosomal recessive incomplete achromatopsia with protan luminosity function. Ophthalmologica, Basel 177: 197.

Smith V, Pokorny J, Newell F (1979). Autosomal recessive incomplete achromatopsia with deutan luminosity. Am J Ophthal 87: 393.

Spivey B (1965). The X-linked recessive inheritance of

atypical monochromatism, Arch Ophthal 74: 327.
Spivey B, Pearlman J, Burian H (1964). Electroretinographic findings (including flicker) in carriers of congenital X-linked achromatopsia. Docum Ophthal XVIII: 367.
Waardenburg PJ (1963). Achromatopsia congenital. In Waardenburg PJ, Franseschetti A, Klein D (eds). Genetics and Ophthalmology vol 2. Assen, Netherland, Royal van Gorkum, p 1695.

AN INHERITED CENTRAL RETINAL PIGMENT EPITHELIAL DYSTROPHY

Ronald Klein, M.D. MPH, George Bresnick, M.D.

University of Wisconsin, Department of Ophthalmology

Madison, Wisconsin 53792

INTRODUCTION

Hereditary macular dystrophies are generally classified by fundus appearance, fluorescein angiographic findings, retinal function studies, and mode of inheritance. The more common of these relatively rare conditions, such as Best's vitelliform dystrophy, fundus flavimaculatus-Stargardt's disease, and cone dystrophies have been classified in this manner as specific nosologic entities. Occasionally, families present with macular degenerations which do not fit the more common diagnostic entities. The following report describes one such family which shares many clinical features of two very rare disorders, central areolar pigment epithelial dystrophy (Fetkenhour et al. 1976) and dominant progressive foveal dystrophy (Frank et al. 1974).

The etiologies of the hereditary macular dystrophies are poorly understood. Recent laboratory studies in animal models of vitamin E deficiency suggest that there may be an association of retinal pigment epithelial degeneration with low levels of this vitamin (Hayes 1974). This association may be due to abnormalities in lipid peroxidation of photoreceptor membranes in vitamin deficient animals (Feeney-Burns, Berman, Rothman 1980). We investigated vitamin E levels as well as other systemic factors which may be related to lipid peroxidation in the family that we describe.

Birth Defects: Original Article Series, Volume 18, Number 6, pages 281–296

MATERIALS AND METHODS

Eight members of a family spanning three generations underwent complete eye examinations including stereo color fundus photography and stereo fluorescein angiography (Fig. 1). With the exception of a few drusen found in one member of the third generation (III-2) this generation (III-1, III-2, III-3) showed no abnormalities. One additional member of the family, II-9, sister of the proband, living in Alaska, last had a complete eye examination in 1961 and had a visual acuity of 20/20 OU, was myopic, and had a normal appearing fundus.

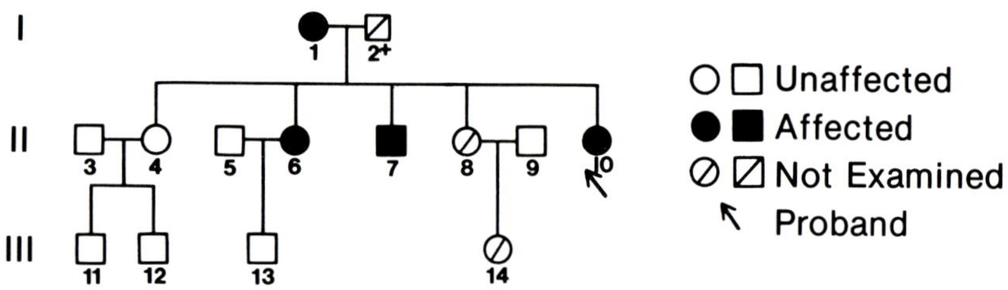

Fig. 1 Pedigree of family with macular dystrophy—circles represent females and squares males.

Five members of the family (I-1, II-4, II-6, II-7 and II-10) underwent visual function testing which included Goldmann visual fields, electroretinography, electro-oculography, and the Farnsworth-Munsell 100-hue test. Electroretinograms were recorded using a standard protocol which has been described in greater detail elsewhere (Jones et al. 1977a). Both light and dark adapted responses were obtained using the Grass PS-2 photostimulator at its maximum intensity (I=16). Responses to 30 Hz flicker in the light adapted state were recorded. In addition, responses to red and blue stimuli were recorded during the dark adapted portion of the test. Electro-oculograms were recorded using a standard protocol which has been reported in greater detail elsewhere (Jones, Stevens, and Gould 1977b). The Farnsworth-Munsell 100-Hue test was administered to each eye separately at a test distance of approximately 25 cm under the illumination of a Macbeth easel lamp.

Twenty-four hour urines were collected the day prior to the exam and quantitative amino acid analyses were performed on a Beckman 120B Amino Acid Analyzer. Fasting blood was collected and serum triglycerides, cholesterol, and high density lipoprotein levels were determined using Dow Diagnostic kits. Serum free fatty acids were determined by ^{63}Ni radiochemical assay (Ho 1970). Total plasma tocopherols were determined spectrophotometrically using a modification of the method described by Bieri (1969). Plasma zinc was determined by atomic absorption spectrophotometry, (Perkins-Elmer 1971). Whole blood selenium was analyzed fluorometrically after wet digestion (Oh, Ganther and Hoekstra 1974). Whole blood glutathione peroxidase levels were determined using the method described by Lloyd-Still and Ganther (1980). Plasma zinc, whole blood selenium and glutathione peroxidase levels were also determined in non-family member controls. Red blood fragility testing were done using the method described by Parpart et al. (1947).

Case Reports

Case 1 - The proband, a 29-year-old white female (II-10), was found to have pale atrophic lesions of the macular area of both eyes during a routine eye examination in January 1981. She had been told of "retinal scars" during a previous eye examination in 1969. She had no ocular symptoms. She reported no history of consanguinity in her family. At examination in January 1981, corrected visual acuity was R.E.: 20/20 with a -5.00 sphere correction and L.E.: 20/20 with a -6.25 +0.25 x 5° correction. A circumscribed zone of retinal pigment epithelial atrophy, about one disc area in size, was present in each macula (Fig. 2). There were hyperpigmented and drusen-like changes present within the atrophic area. A few drusen were located outside of the atrophic area in each macula (Fig. 2). Optic discs, retinal blood vessels, and peripheral retinae were normal. Goldmann visual fields were normal when tested with I2e test stimulus. Stereoscopic fluorescein angiography revealed hyper-fluorescence consistent with a "window defect" in the retinal pigment epithelium corresponding to the atrophic lesions in the macular area (Fig. 2). A few other focal areas of hyper-fluorescence, consistent with drusen, were noted in both maculae. Electroretinography (Fig. 3) and

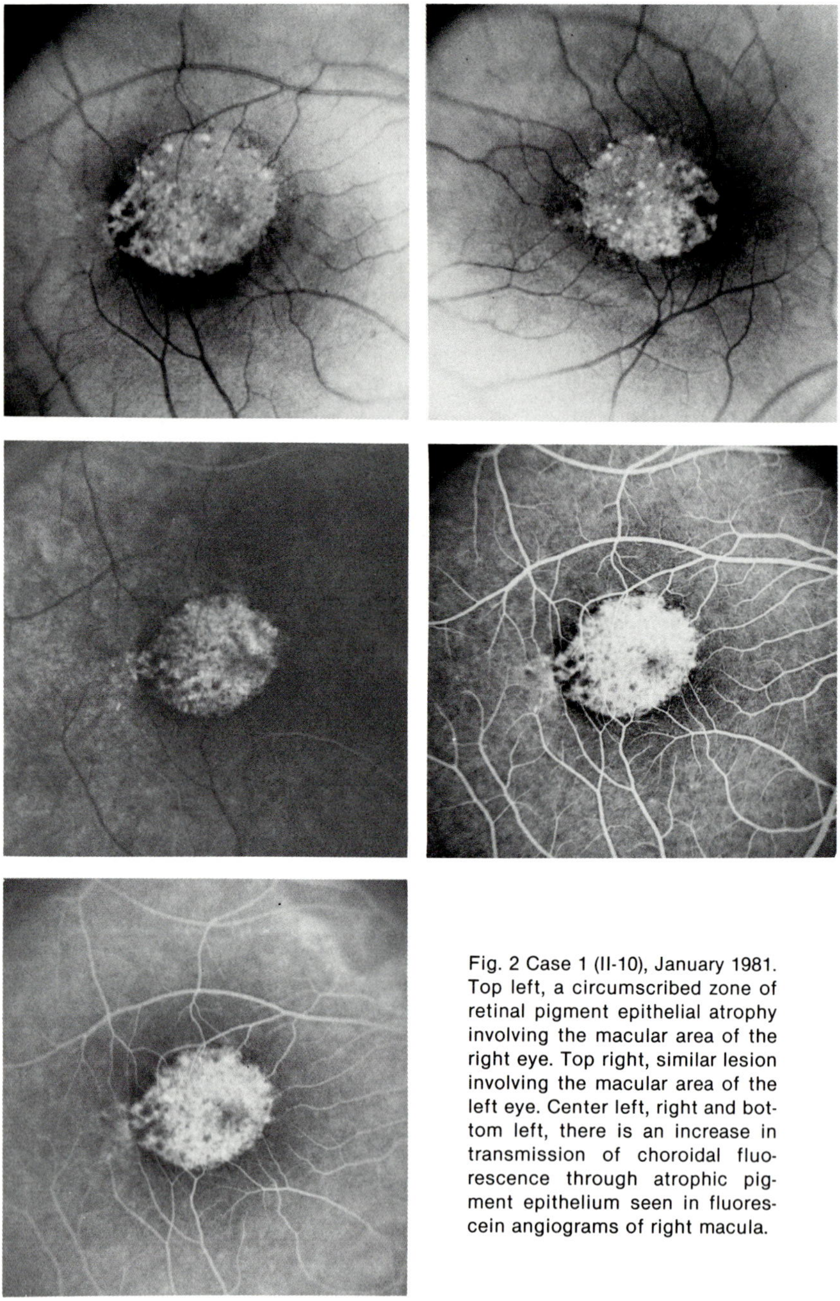

Fig. 2 Case 1 (II-10), January 1981. Top left, a circumscribed zone of retinal pigment epithelial atrophy involving the macular area of the right eye. Top right, similar lesion involving the macular area of the left eye. Center left, right and bottom left, there is an increase in transmission of choroidal fluorescence through atrophic pigment epithelium seen in fluorescein angiograms of right macula.

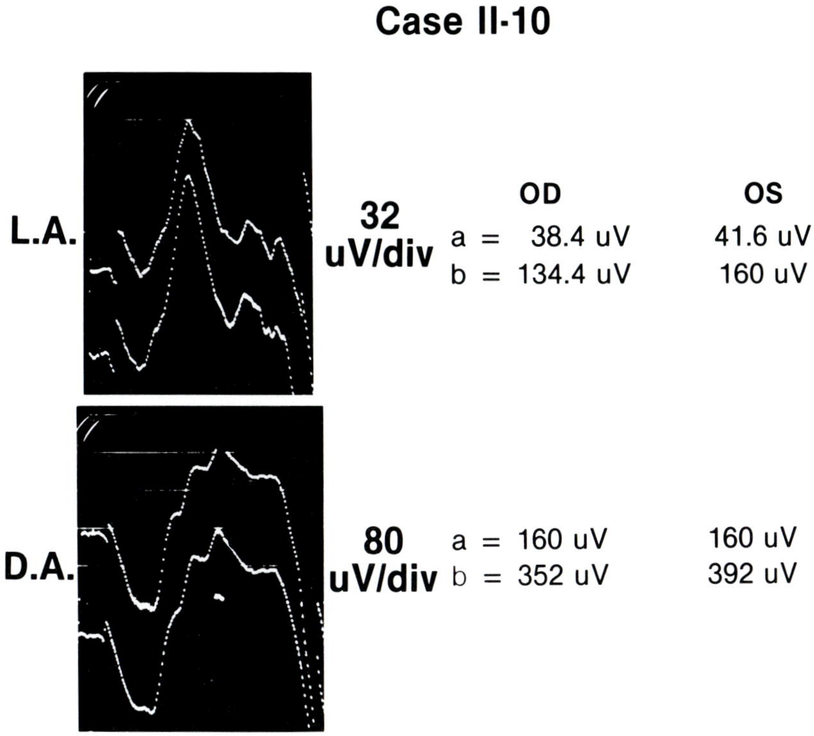

Fig. 3 Case 1 (II-10). Light and dark adapted electroretinograms, I = 16.

electro-oculography (Table) were normal. Color vision as tested on the Farnsworth-Munsell 100-Hue test was normal in each eye with a total error score of 85. Twenty-four hour urine analysis for quantitative amino acid determinations was normal. Fasting serum triglyceride, cholesterol, high density lipoprotein, free fatty acid and total lipid levels were all normal. Total plasma β-carotene and tocopherol levels were normal. The plasma zinc was similar to that of the controls. Whole blood selenium, glutathione peroxidase and red blood cell fragility studies were normal. These blood and urine studies were also found to be normal in all other members of the family studied (Cases I-1, II-4, II-6, II-7).

Electro-oculogram

	OD Lp/Dt	OS Lp/Dt
Case 1 (II-10)	2.48	2.47
Case 2 (II-1)	2.62	1.95
Case 3 (II-7)	2.65	2.60
Case 4 (II-6)	2.37	2.67
Normal	$\geq$1.95	

Case 2 - A 59-year-old woman, the proband's mother (I-1) had a chief complaint of severe loss of vision in both eyes first noted in November 1960 at 38 years of age. At that time, ophthalmologic examination revealed a best corrected visual acuity of 20/200 in each eye. She was found to have a pigmented disciform scar with subretinal and intraretinal hemorrhages present in the scar in the right macular area. A pigmented scar which "projected into the vitreous" of the left macular area was described. These scars were present within an area of atrophy of the retinal pigment epithelium. In the intervening period between 1960 to 1973 she was noted to have retinal hemorrhages in both maculae and developed more widespread choroidal atrophy of the posterior retina. Her mother was of Norwegian-German descent and her father of English-Scottish descent. Her two siblings and their six children were said to have normal vision but were unavailable for further examination.

At examination in January 1981, her visual acuity was R.E.: 20/200 with -6.75 +2.25 x 80° correction and L.E.: 20/125 with a -5.75 +2.00 x 70° correction. A raised disciform scar about one disc area in size was present

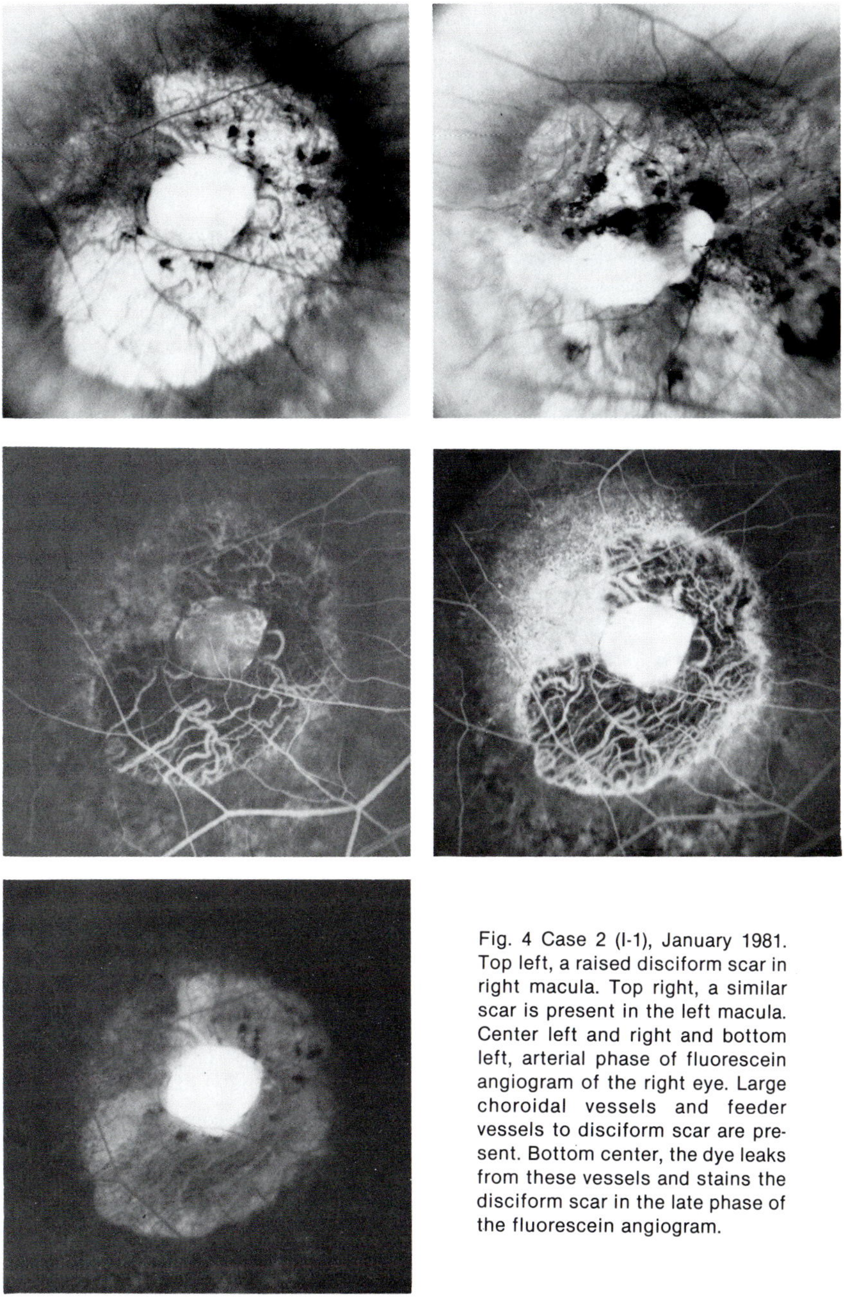

Fig. 4 Case 2 (I-1), January 1981. Top left, a raised disciform scar in right macula. Top right, a similar scar is present in the left macula. Center left and right and bottom left, arterial phase of fluorescein angiogram of the right eye. Large choroidal vessels and feeder vessels to disciform scar are present. Bottom center, the dye leaks from these vessels and stains the disciform scar in the late phase of the fluorescein angiogram.

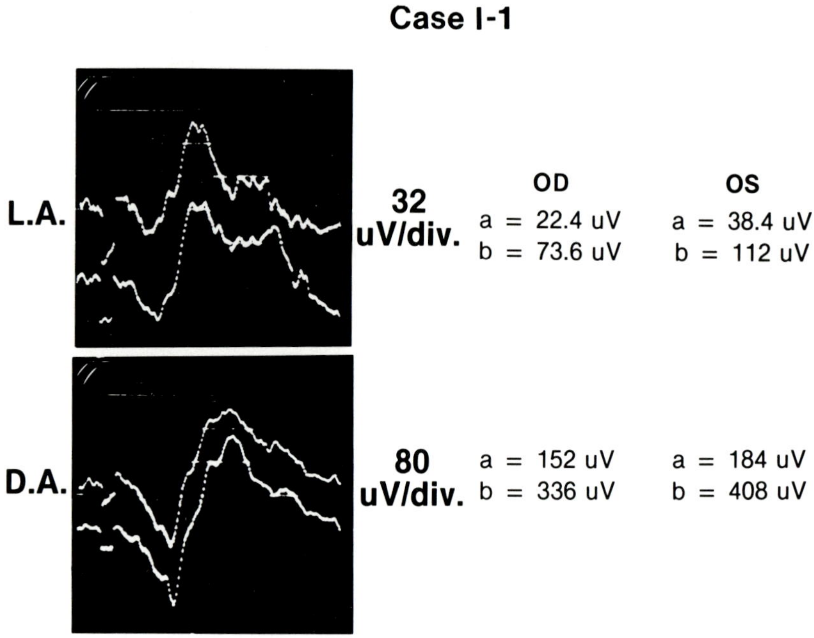

Fig. 5. Case 2 (I-1). Light and dark adapted electroretinograms, I = 16.

within a nine disc area of choroidal atrophy in the right macular area (Fig. 4). A few focal areas of hyperpigmentation were present in the posterior pole. A similar scar was present in a larger area of choroidal atrophy in the left macula (Fig. 4). Optic discs, retinal blood vessels and peripheral retinae were normal. Goldmann visual fields revealed a central scotoma on testing with a I4e test stimulus. Stereoscopic fluorescein angiography of the right eye demonstrated subretinal new vessels within the disciform scar (Fig. 4). Atrophy of the retinal pigment epithelium and choriocapillaris was present and only the larger choroidal vessels perfused (Fig. 4). With the exception of a slightly below normal a-wave in the light-adapted state, electroretinography was normal (Fig. 5). Electro-oculography light-peak to dark-trough ratios were R.E. 2.62, L.E. 1.95 which were normal; however, the interocular difference of 0.67 was considered abnormal

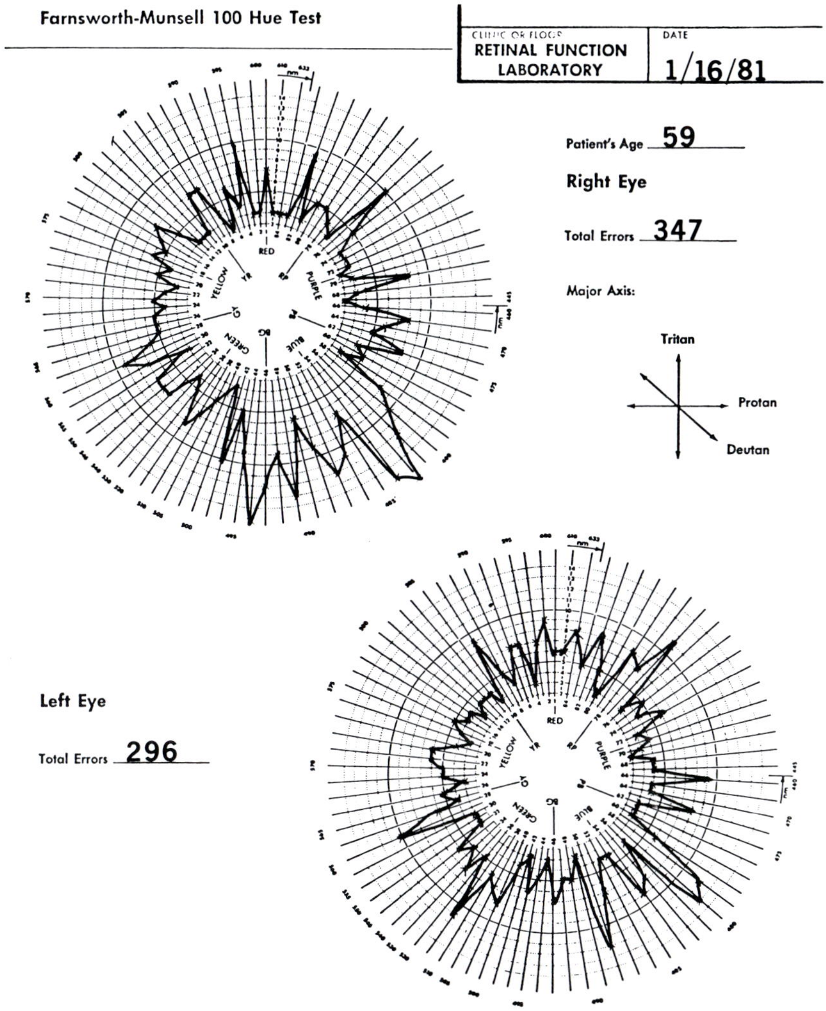

Fig. 6 Case 2 (I-1), Farnsworth-Munsell 100 Hue Test.

(normal interocular difference in our laboratory is 0.35 (Jones, Stevens, and Gould 1977) (Table). Color vision as tested on the Farnsworth-Munsell 100-Hue test was abnormal in each eye with an error score of 349 in the right eye and 296 in the left eye (normal for age 50-59 = 164) (Verriest 1963) and a non-specific axis (Fig. 6).

Case 3 - A 25-year-old male, the brother of the proband (II-7) was asymptomatic. His visual acuity was R.E. 20/16 with a -1.00 sphere and L.E. 20/20 with a -1.75 sphere correction. Bilateral central retinal pigment epithelium defects similar to that found in the proband, involving a zone about 3/4 disc area were present (Fig. 7). A few drusen-like lesions were present within and outside the atrophic areas. Optic dics, retinal blood vessels and peripheral retinae were normal. Stereoscopic fluorescein angiography revealed early hyperfluorescence, consistent with the central area of retinal pigment atrophy. The choroidal vasculature appeared intact. Goldmann visual fields were normal on testing with a I2e test stimulus. Electro-oculography, electroretinography, and Farnsworth-Munsell 100-Hue tests were all normal.

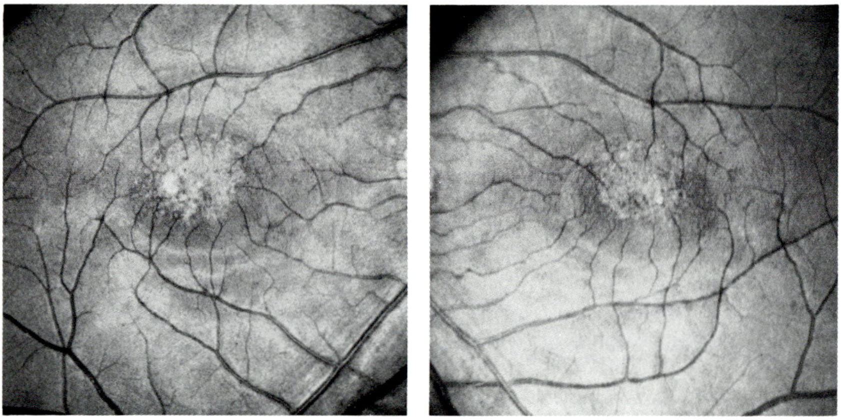

Fig. 7 Case 3 (II-7), January 1981. Left, right macula. Right, left macula. Retinal pigment epithelial atrophy involving both maculae is present.

Case 4 - A 37-year-old female, the sister of the proband (II-6) was asymptomatic. She was first examined in May 1961 and found to have normal visual acuity associated with atrophy of the pigment epithelium. Her visual acuity was R.E. 20/20 with a -7.50 +2.00 x 102° correction and L.E. 20/16 with a -6.50 +1.75 x 75° correction. She demonstrated bilateral central retinal pigment epithelium defects about 1 disc area in size associated with a few drusen (Fig. 8). Drusen of the optic nerve head were present in the left eye. The retinal vessels and the peripheral retinae were normal. Stereoscopic fluorescein angiography revealed hyperfluorescent "window defects" similar to her other affected siblings. All retinal function studies were normal.

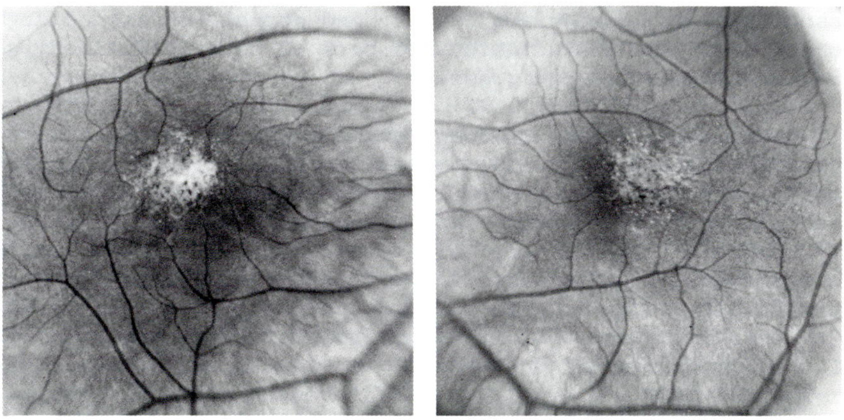

Fig. 8 Case 4 (II-6). January 1981. Left, right macula. Right, left macula. Retinal pigment epithelial atrophy involving both maculae is present.

DISCUSSION

Two generations of one family, a mother and 3 of her children, were affected by a bilateral symmetrical atrophy of the retinal pigment epithelium in the macular area. The pattern of inheritance is suggestive of autosomal dominance. Except for the mother, members of this family were asymptomatic and had good visual acuity and all retinal function studies were normal. All affected members of this family were myopic. The normal electroretinography and electro-oculography findings in members of this family are consistent with an abnormality limited to the macular area. The normal visual acuity and central color vision in members of the

OPTIC AND OTIC NEUROLOGIC ABNORMALITIES IN OCULOCUTANEOUS AND OCULAR ALBINISM

Carl J. Witkop, Jr.[1], Barrie Jay[2], Donnell Creel[3], R.W. Guillery[4]
16-262 HSUA, U-MN, Mpls, MN USA 55455[1], Moorfields Eye Hospital, London UK[2], VA Hospital, Salt Lake City, UT USA[3], Univ. Chicago, Chicago, IL USA[4]

INTRODUCTION

Albinism comprises a heterogeneous group of heritable disorders of the melanin pigment system. All forms of albinism are characterized by hypoplasia of the fovea, photophobia, nystagmus and decreased visual acuity in addition to absent or decreased melanotic pigment in skin, hair, and eyes (oculocutaneous albinism, OCA) or eye (ocular albinism, OA)(Witkop, Quevedo, Fitzpatrick, 1982). In *albinoidism*, there is hypomelanism of dermal and ocular tissues, but these patients do not have nystagmus or decreased visual acuity.

Ten disorders have been identified in humans with these clinical features of OCA and four with the features of OA (Witkop, Quevedo, Fitzpatrick, 1982) (Table 1).

Table 1

CLASSIFICATION OF INHERITED HYPOPIGMENTED CONDITIONS IN MAN

I. ALBINISM: Hypopigmentation with nystagmus and photophobia
   A. OCULOCUTANEOUS ALBINISM (OCA)
      1. Hairbulb Tyrosine Test Negative
         a. Tyrosinase-negative (Ty-neg) OCA [AR]
      2. Hairbulb Tyrosine Test Positive
         a. Tyrosinase-positive (Ty-pos) OCA [AR]
         b. OCA - Hemorrhagic diathesis, Hermansky-Pudlak Syndrome (HP) [AR]

Birth Defects: Original Article Series, Volume 18, Number 6, pages 299–318

Table 1, Cont'd.

c. Beguez Cesar-Chediak-Higashi (CH) Syndrome [AR]
d. Hypopigmentation - Microphthalmia (Cross Syndrome) [AR]
e. Brown OCA [AR]
f. Rufous OCA [AR]
g. Autosomal Dominant OCA
h. OCA with Black Lock and Congenital Sensorineural Deafness [AR]

3. Hairbulb Tyrosine Test Variable
a. Yellow Mutant (ym) OCA (Nance)[AR]

B. OCULAR ALBINISM (OA)
1. X-linked (Nettleship) [XOAN]
2. X-linked (Forsius-Eriksson) [XOAF]
3. Autosomal Recessive (Witkop) [AROA]
4. Ocular albinism, lentigines-deafness (Lewis) [AD]

All of the types of OCA except autosomal dominant OCA are inherited as autosomal recessive traits and in all except the black locks-albinism-deafness syndrome, melanocytes are present in the hypopigmented skin, hair, and eyes. They are absent in white skin and hair in BADS. These disorders can be distinguished from one another on the basis of clinical and biochemical criteria (Witkop, 1979; Witkop, et al., 1973; Witkop, et al., 1972; King and Witkop, 1976; King, et al., 1980), as well as by their genetic characteristics as determined by matings between albinos of different genotypes which in the double heterozygote complement each other and are nonallelic (Witkop, et al., 1970; Trevor-Roper, 1952, 1963; Jaeger and Jay, 1981) or show allelism (Hu, et al., 1980). Thus, the classic description of OCA as an autosomal recessive trait due to a defect in a single enzyme, tyrosinase (Garrod, 1908), must be modified to include a number of distinct genetic diseases, most of which have normal tyrosinase activity (King and Witkop, 1976, King, et al., 1978) and structural characteristics (Townsend, et al., 1981) of the enzyme.

Studies of the visual neuronal tracts in hypomelanotic animals and man have led to some emerging hypotheses concerning the role of pigment in embryogenesis. We wish to discuss some concepts and the evidence for the development of these hypotheses:

1. All types of hypomelanotic disorders manifesting nystagmus and decreased visual acuity have anomalous optic neuronal tracts, while those conditions lacking nystagmus do not.
2. Melanin pigment has a role in determining normal neuronal routing to the brain.
3. When pigment is lacking in the developing optic cup, the optic tracts tend to cross at the chiasm forming an abnormal visual system arrangement.
4. The role of pigment in the inner ear is similar to that in the optic system, so if lacking during development, decussation defects will be present in the otic tracts.
5. There is a central brain component to the nystagmus seen in all forms of albinism and that hypoplasia of the fovea alone is not the only factor in nystagmus.
6. There is a predicted anomalous relationship between the development of the abducens nucleus and the medial superior olive in albinos and in some of their allelic and non-allelic genotypes.

OPTIC TRACT DEFECTS IN ALBINOS

Retinogeniculate Defects

Classically, in vertebrates with laterally placed eyes and panoramic vision, most fish, amphibians, reptiles, and birds (Polyak, 1957), there is a complete decussation of optic fibers at the chiasma. Phylogenetically, as eyes develop stereoscopic vision and shift to a frontal position, the proportion of optic fibers which originates in the temporal retina and does not decussate increases (rat, 10 percent; dog and horse, 20 percent; cat, 30-40 percent) (Polyak, 1957; Creel and Giolli, 1972; Hayhow, et al., 1960). Primates and humans have from 45-50 percent uncrossed fibers (Kupfer, et al., 1967). Recent evidence indicates that the classic view is incorrect in detail and in many vertebrates retinofugal fibers do not segregate in the optic chiasm in a uniform way. While diencephalic centers together with their cortical targets tend to view only the contralateral hemifield, mesencephalic centers do not follow the classical pattern, except in primates (Guillery, 1982).

Initially anatomic and electrophysiologic studies of the retinogeniculate projections of albino animals showed that most fibers from the temporal retina, which in normally pigmented animals course to the same side of the brain as in the eye of origin, cross to the opposite side in albinos (Lund, 1965; Creel and Sheridan, 1966; Giolli and Guthrie,

1969; Guillery, 1969, 1971; Creel, 1971; Guillery, et al., 1971; Sanderson, 1972; Giolli and Creel, 1973; Guillery and Kaas, 1973; Guillery, et al., 1973; Sanderson, et al., 1974). These anatomic abnormalities in the albino optic neuronal pathway result in behavioral (Creel and Sheridan, 1966) and electrophysiologic abnormalities (Creel and Giolli, 1972; Montero, et al., 1968; Creel, et al., 1970). The defect is independent of species and was initially demonstrated in various animals with mutations at the *c*-locus (tyrosinase locus); in the albino (*c/c*) guinea pig (Creel and Giolli, 1972; Giolli and Creel, 1973), rat (Lund, 1965; Creel and Sheridan, 1966, Montero, et al., 1968; Creel, et al., 1970; Guillery, et al., 1971; Cunningham and Lund, 1971), rabbit (Giolli and Guthrie, 1969, 1971; Sanderson, 1972), mink (Sanderson, 1972; Sanderson, et al., 1974), ferret (Guillery, 1971, Siamese (c^{s}/c^{s}) cat (Guillery, 1969; Creel, 1971, 1971a; Guillery and Kaas, 1971; Kaas and Guillery, 1974), and chinchilla (c^{ch}/c^{ch}) white tiger.

It was postulated initially that the neuronal defect resulted from a nonpigmentary function of the enzyme tyrosinase, defective (deficient) in these animals. However, the defect is not confined to animals with mutations at the *c*-locus regulating tyrosinase. This was demonstrated by Creel and collaborators (Creel, et al., 1974; Creel, et al., 1979) in various types of human albinos. Monocularly stimulated, visually evoked potentials recorded from occipital leads over the right and left visual cortices give approximately symmetric responses in normal humans, reflecting the underlying approximately symmetric division of the optic tract. Creel et al. (1974, 1979) demonstrated asymmetric monocularly stimulated responses with reduction in the ipsilateral recordings in ty-pos, ym, brown, and HPS albinos, as well as in ty-neg human albinos (Figure 1). Of these types of albinism in humans, only the ty-neg OCA is possibly a homologue of *c*-locus albinism in animals. Since ty-neg and ty-pos albinism and HPS and ty-pos albinism are not allelic (Witkop, et al., 1961, Witkop, et al., 1970; Witkop, et al., 1982), and since ty-pos, brown and HPS melanocytes have tyrosinase activity varying from low normal to three times normal levels (King and Witkop, 1976; King, et al., 1978, 1980), Witkop et al. (1974) and Creel et al. (1974, 1979) postulated that the optic defect is associated with any defect which results in absence of pigment in the developing optic cup regardless of the underlying genetic mechanism. Sanderson and coworkers (1974) tested mink with a variety of genes con-

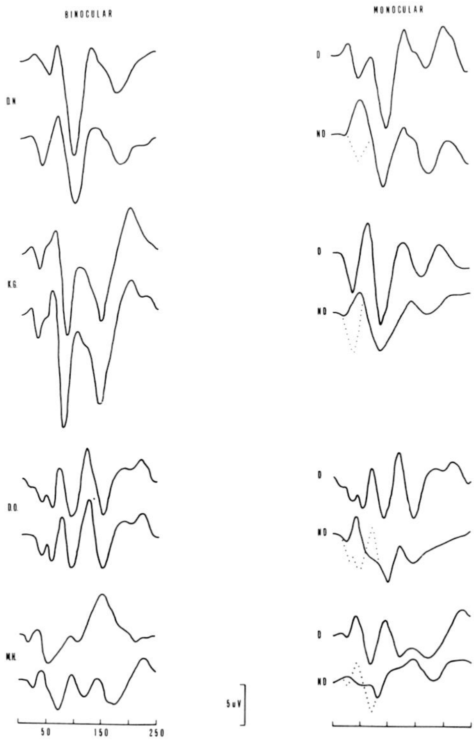

Fig. 1. Visually evoked potentials recorded from both hemispheres (O_1 - A_1 and O_2 - A_2) of four albino subjects under conditions of binocular and monocular illumination. Monocularly evoked potentials recorded from the hemisphere receiving the decussated optic fibers (D) can be directly compared to evoked potentials recorded from the hemispheres receiving nondecussated optic fibers (ND). Components missing from the ND evoked potential are indicated by dotted lines. Hori-

zontal time base is 250 milliseconds. Negative is up. After Creel, et al., 1974.

trolling pigment at different loci and demonstrated that any gene resulting in hypopigmentation of the fundi was associated with the optic defect.

Visually evoked potential studies of patients with generalized skin and hair pigmentation but with both the X-linked form of ocular albinism [XOAN](Nettleship, 1909; Falls, 1951) or autosomal recessive ocular albinism [AROA](Witkop, et al., 1978; O'Donnell, et al., 1978) also have asymmetric monocularly stimulated responses indicative of a decussation defect (Creel, et al., 1978)(Figure 2).

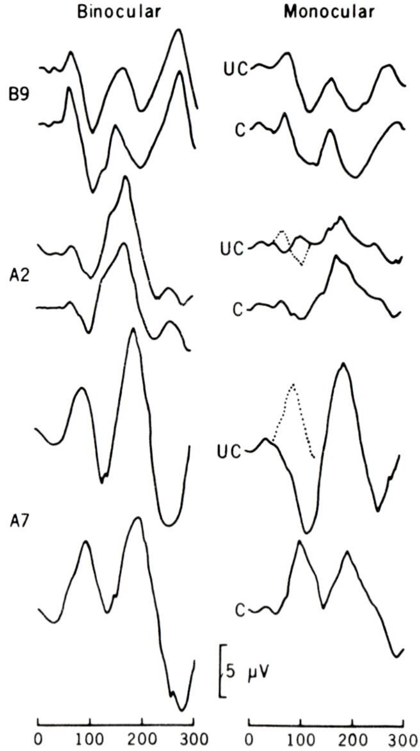

Fig. 2. Visually evoked potentials recorded

from both hemispheres (O_1-A_1 and O_2-A_2) of a brown-eyed subject (B9) and two ocular albinos (A2 and A7) under conditions of binocular and monocular illumination. Monocularly evoked potentials recorded from the hemisphere receiving the uncrossed (UC) optic fibers can be compared to evoked potentials recorded from the hemisphere receiving the crossed (C) optic fibers. Components missing from the UC evoked potential are indicated by dotted lines. Horizontal time base, 300 msec; negative is up. After Creel, et al., 1978.

Anatomic studies of albino human (Guillery, et al., 1975) and albino primate brains (Gross and Hickey, 1980) showed evidence for a disorganization of the retinogeniculate tracts. Anatomic investigations to date of three brains from human albinos (ty-pos & ty-neg) showed defects in the size, the orientation, and the layered segments of the lateral geniculate nuclei. Grossly, lateral geniculate nuclei appeared absent; the characteristic swelling did not show because the nucleus was rotated rostrolaterally about 30° to the frontal plane within the brain tissue, and the lateral tip was elevated. Abnormal fusions were found in the parvocellular layers, and only a single magnocellular layer was found in most sections (Fig. 3). The defects in human albino brains were essentially similar to those found in an albino monkey (Gross and Hickey, 1980).

Albino animals and humans with all types of OCA (ty-neg, ty-pos, ym, HPS, brown) and OA (XOAN, AROA) tested to date (Creel, et al., 1974; Guillery, et al., 1975; Creel, et al., 1978; Taylor, 1978; Coleman, et al., 1979; Creel, et al., 1979; King, et al., 1980) have abnormal optic neuronal pathways, however, the proportion of neurons rearranged in albinos varies and approximately 10 to 15 percent of animals and humans do not show evidence for a major rearrangement (Creel, et al., 1974, 1978). Evidence from Siamese cats suggests that temporal retina adjacent to nasal retina is most often anomalous (Kaas and Guillery, 1973; Guillery and Kaas, 1974). As a result of the decussation defect most human albinos lack the internal mechanism for binocular vision.

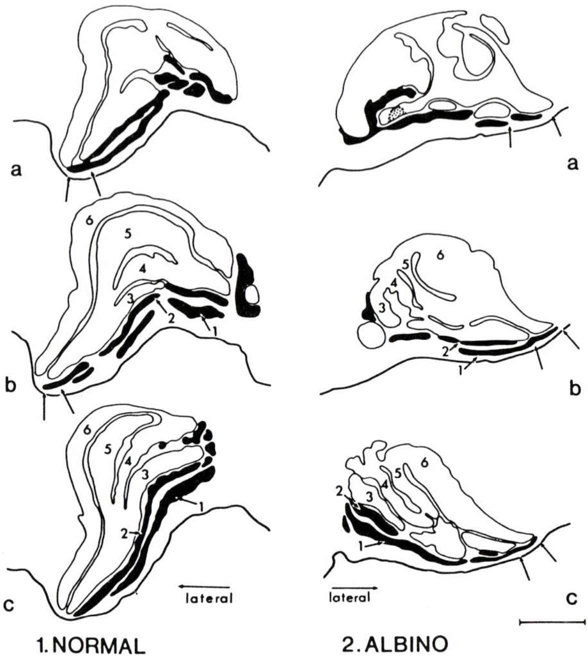

Figs. 3-1 and 3-2. Frontal sections taken at comparable levels through the lateral geniculate nuclei of a normal (1) and an albino brain (2). The most rostral sections (level a) pass through the zone in which the six-layered and the four-layered segments are fusing. The magnocellular layers are shown in black and the conventional numbering is indicated where 6 layers are evident. The bilaminar part of the nucleus is indicated by unlabelled arrows. Notice that the lateral part of the nucleus lies to the left in 3-1 and to the right in 3-2. Scale = 2 mm, After Guillery, et al., 1975.

The details of how pigment is involved in the development of the optic system is unknown, however the present evidence indicates that pigment in the optic cup is necessary for the specification of optic neurons to normal brain targets, and for the development of a normal fovea, a relationship anticipated by Ida Mann as early as 1937 (Mann, 1937).

Geniculocortical Defects

Evidence that the geniculocortical tracts are also anomalous in albinos was suggested by studies on Siamese (a *c*-locus mutation) cats, electrophysiologically by Hubel and Wiesel (1971), and also shown anatomically by Guillery and Kaas (1971) and Kaas and Guillery (1973). Guillery (1974) and Guillery and coworkers (1974) reasoned that given the initial decussation defect of the retinogeniculate pathway and normal connections from the lateral geniculate nucleus to the cortex, there would be a disruption of the order of the visual field segments, an inversion of a portion of the visual field as a reversal of normal such that there would be an ascending sequence in one layer of the cortex and a descending sequence in the same layer, and a noncorrespondence or mismatching of two adjacent layers (Figure 4). Partial compensation for these abnormalities was achieved in two ways in cats. In "Midwestern" cats, the input to the cortex from the A_1 layer of the lateral geniculate nucleus (normally temporal retinal nondecussated input) was suppressed. In "Boston" cats a rerouting of axons occurred, reversing the order of the misdirected mid-half-field segments (Figure 5). While both patterns partially correct the order of the field projection in the cortex, both patterns are essentially incompatible with a binocular visual mechanism.

Evidence that human albinos may have similar patterns in the geniculocortical tracts was presented by Carroll and associates (Carroll, et al., 1980, 1980a). Utilizing visually evoked potentials simultaneously recorded from multiple electrodes over the visual cortex area, two patterns of response were found suggestive of a "Boston" or "Midwestern" model. Reference to Figure 5 shows the underlying difference in the cortical rearrangements in the "Midwestern" and "Boston" patterns upon which they based their experimental design. In the "Midwestern" pattern the vertical meridian here represented by the border of field 9 remains at the 17-18 border in the cortex, while in the "Boston" pattern, it is shifted and

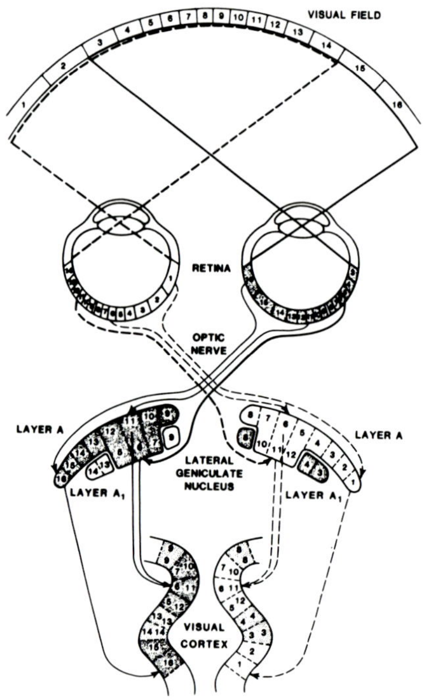

Fig. 4. Schematic representation of abnormal pathways (heavy arrows) to the lateral geniculate nuclei in the Siamese cat. If the connections from the lateral geniculate were normal, then the effects shown in the visual cortex would be expected. Projections from the two layers of the lateral geniculate would conflict so that neural activity at a single point in the cortex would be interpreted as stimuli in two parts of the visual field, such as in segments Nos. 5 & 12. After Guillery, 1974.

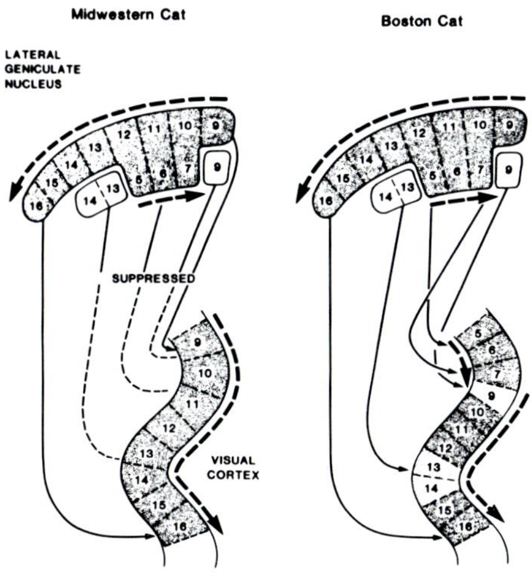

Fig. 5. Schematic representation of two types of patterns in the geniculo-cortical projections in Siamese cats which compensate for the disrupted projections in the lateral geniculate nucleus, illustrated here for the left side of the brain. In a "Midwestern" cat the input to the cortex from layer A is largely suppressed, eliminating the misdirected segments 5-7. Thus, the misdirected part of the visual field, although projected to the wrong cortex, "reads" correctly as a more or less continuous picture of the outside world. After Guillery, 1974.

additional components, here represented by 5-7, are inserted. Further, in the "Midwestern" pattern the abnormal input (5-7, Fig. 5), which overlies the mirror-symmetrical points of the temporal half-field and so has an identical position in relation to the occipital pole, has a reduced number of neurons responsive to nasal hemifield stimuli (Kaas and Guillery,

Utilizing the $\overline{P100}$ component of monocular visually evoked potentials which they suggest originate in cortical areas 17 and 18, they found two patterns of response in albinos suggestive of either a "Midwestern" (Group b, Figure 6) or a "Boston" (Group c, Figure 6) pattern. The particular type of pattern was not associated with a particular type of ty-pos or ty-neg OC albinism, or type of ocular albinism, but both patterns were found in various mutants.

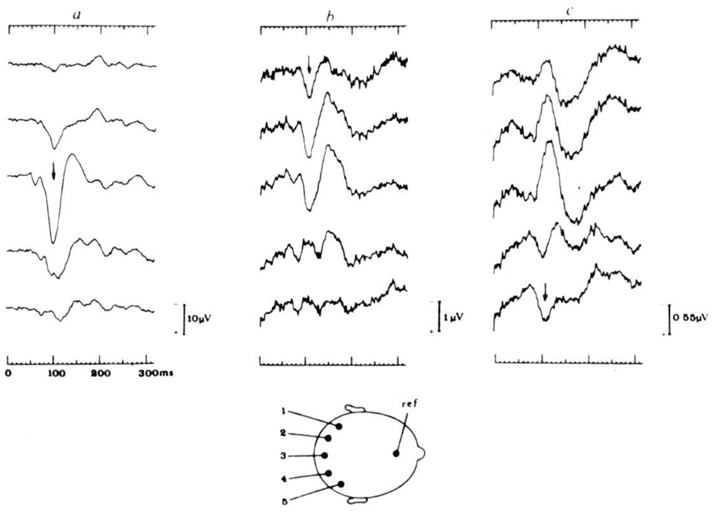

Fig. 6. Left eye whole-field (16 deg radius) VEPs from: *a*, a normal subject; *b*, the grand average of the 5 albino subjects with a $\overline{P100}$ (arrow) distribution ipsilateral to the stimulated left eye and *c*, the grand average of the 9 albino subjects with a contralateral $\overline{P100}$ (arrow) distribution. Note in the normal subject the larger amplitude and symmetrical distribution of the $\overline{P100}$ about the midline. The midline electrode of the transverse chain of 5 is situated 5 cm above the anion. After Carroll, et al., 1980.

Cooper et al., (1978) presented evidence that both patterns may co-exist in the same animal. Extending this work in Siamese cats, Cooper and Blasdel (1980) examined the visual field map in the region of the 17/18 border, and they suggest that the two patterns, "Boston" and "Midwestern" may represent ends of a continuum. They suggest that geniculocortical axons carrying aberrant ipsilateral field information in a given Siamese cat contains fibers directed by both mechanisms. Thus, although individual aberrant fibers within a single cat may fall into two distinct patterns on the basis of cortical termination, there could be a continuous variation between cats in the degree to which one or the other mechanism predominates within the total population of aberrant geniculocortical afferent fibers.

Optokinetic Defects

Collewijn et al., (1977) found that in albino rabbits restricting visual contrast to the anterior sector of the visual field, this sector being binocular in pigmented rabbits and somewhat homologous to the temporal retina in man, resulted in dramatically unstable eye position. When the target was moved, horizontal optokinetic eye movements were inverted and the direction of pursuit by the eye was opposite to that of the stimulus. They postulated that the optokinetic inversion could be causally associated with nystagmus in mammals, particularly cats and man, in which large proportions of temporal neurons remain ipsilateral in normal pigmented subjects but are rerouted to the contralateral side in the albino.

OTIC NEUROLOGIC DEFECTS IN ALBINISM

The auditory system in mammals, while more complex, is somewhat analogous to the optic system in that pigment is normally found in the inner ear (Wolff, 1931) and that there are both decussated and nondecussated neuronal paths in the brain. The amount of pigment in the inner ear is correlated directly with the amount of pigment in the iris (Bonaccorsi, 1965) and is lacking in albinos (Wolff, 1931). Evidence that an analogous decussation defect may exist in the auditory system of human ty-neg, ty-pos and HPS albinos was presented by Creel et al., (1980). Brainstem auditory evoked potentials in human albinos indicated a significant hemispheric asymmetry symptomatic of differences between decussated and nondecussated auditory pathways approximately at the level of the superior olivary nuclei, and most likely the medial superior olive (Figure 7).

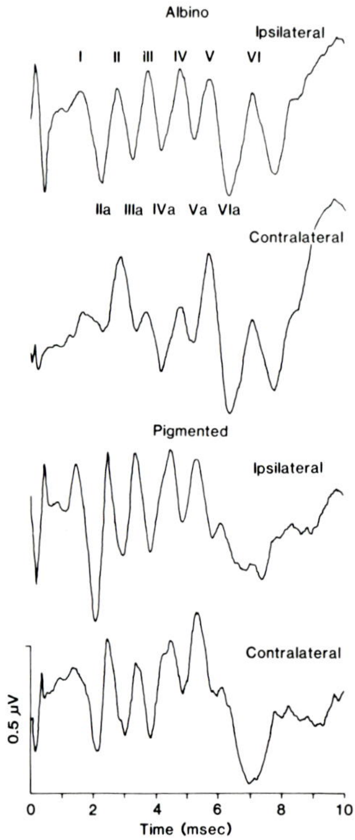

Fig. 7. Brainstem auditory evoked potentials recorded from hemispheres ipsilateral and contralateral to the stimulated ear in a human ty-neg albino and pigmented subject showing over 50 per cent attenuation of component III in the contralateral potential in the albino. The medial superior olive is most likely the primary generator of component III. After Creel, et al., 1980.

Garber, et al.(in press) tested age and sex matched pigmented subjects and ty-neg, ty-pos and HPS albinos and found that albino subjects performed significantly differently in a dichotic hearing test than pigmented subjects compatible with a postulated decussation defect in the auditory tract.

OPTIC-OTIC BRAINSTEM CONSIDERATIONS AND THEIR POSSIBLE ROLE IN NYSTAGMUS

There is a strong correlation in many species between the size of the medial superior olive and the size of the abducens nucleus that innervates the lateral rectus muscle of the eye (Harrison and Howe, 1974). The ratio of the size of the olive to the abducens nucleus varies markedly between animals with predominantly rod or predominantly cone foveae (Harrison and Howe, 1974), but also reflects differences between animals with panoramic vision and less developed temporal retinae versus those with binocular vision and well developed temporal retinae. The medial superior olive has been regarded as "a visual auditory system, having evolved as an adjunct to vision" (Irving and Harrison, 1967). On the basis of these considerations, Creel et al. (1980) proposed that the development of the abducens nucleus may be anomalous in albino mammals, as has been found in Duane retraction syndrome with strabismus (Jay and Hoyt, 1980; Hotchkiss, et al., 1980). If these considerations are correct, then when combined with the findings by Collewijn, et al. (1977) on optokinetic inversion in albino rabbits, they suggest that a brainstem component may be involved in the nystagmus and strabismus seen in albinos, rather than simple hypoplasia of the fovea alone. It should be noted that animals with poorly defined foveae such as the pigmented ground squirrel and rabbit do not have nystagmus, but the albino does.

SUMMARY

Six hypotheses were presented based upon recent investigations of the central nervous system anomalies in albinos.

All types of conditions with oculocutaneous and ocular hypopigmentation in man and animals with nystagmus tested to date have shown either electrophysiologic or anatomic evidence for a decussation defect in the optic tract. Patients without nystagmus but with hypopigmented fundi do not. Thus nystagmus is an important clinical sign for distinguishing forms of albinism from other hypopigmented eye disorders.

Current evidence strongly supports a role of pigment in determining neuronal brain target specification both in the optic cup and inner ear. When it is lacking in the developing eye, regardless of the underlying genetic defect, optic tracts tend to revert to crossed arrangements as found in a panoramic visual system. Further, the decussation defect is similar in all of the animal and human albinos tested. The overwhelming evidence finds the decussation defect associated with lack of pigment rather than with any specific enzyme defect. Initially it was believed that the fawn hooded rat was an exception to the emerging generalization that the decussation defect was associated with a lack of fundal pigment, as this animal has reduced ipsilateral tracts and the adult animal has pigmented fundi (Lund, 1965). However, fundal pigment is lacking at birth and does not develop until after the major portion of the postnatal specification time for the final optic neuronal arrangement is past. Evidence from VEP and functional studies of human albino's auditory system give evidence of a decussation anomaly at the superior olive. Animal studies now in progress suggest even greater differences than those presented for the defect in humans.

We have suggested that a brain component is present in generating nystagmus (and strabismus) in albinos possibly through anomalous development of the abducens nucleus controlling the lateral rectus muscle.

REFERENCES

Bonaccorsi P (1965). Il colore dell'iride come "test" di valutazione qualitativa, nell'uomo, della concentrazione de melanina nella stria vascolare. Annali Laringol, Otol, Rinol, Faringol 64:725.

Carroll WM, Jay BS, McDonald WI, Halliday AM (1980). Two distinct patterns of visual evoked response asymmetry in human albinism. Nature 286:604.

Carroll WM, Jay BS, McDonald WI, Halliday AM (1980a). Pattern evoked potentials in human albinism. J Neurol Sci 48:265.

Coleman J, Sydnor CF, Wolbarsht ML, Bessler M (1979). Abnormal visual pathways in human albinos studied with visually evoked potentials. Exp Neurol 65:667.

Collewijn H, Winterson BJ, Dubois MFW (1977). Optokinetic eye movement in albino rabbits: Inversion in anterior

visual field. Science 199:1351.
Cooper ML, Blasdel GG (1980). Regional variation in the representation of the visual field in the visual cortex of the Siamese cat. J Compar Neurol 193:237.
Cooper ML, Blasdel GG, Pettigrew JD (1978). Evidence in the Siamese cat for the simultaneous expression of Boston and Midwestern patterns. Assoc Res Vision Ophthalmol Abst 216.
Creel DJ (1971). Differences of ipsilateral and contralateral visually evoked responses in the cat: Strains compared. J Comp Physiol Psychol 77:161.
Creel DJ (1971a). Visual system anomaly associated with albinism in the cat. Nature (London) 231:465.
Creel DJ, Dustman RE, Beck EC (1970). Differences in visually evoked responses in albino versus hooded rats. Exp Neurol 29:298.
Creel D, Garber SR, King RA, Witkop CJJr (1980). Auditory brainstem anomalies in human albinos. Science 209:1253.
Creel DJ, Giolli RA (1972). Retinogeniculostriate projections in guinea pigs: Albino and pigmented strains compared. Exp Neurol 36:411.
Creel D, King RA, Witkop CJJr, Okoro AN (1979). Visual system anomalies in human albinos. In Klaus SN (ed): "Pigment Cell. Pathophysiology of Melanocytes," New Haven CT: S Karger, pp 21-27.
Creel D, O'Donnell FEJr, Witkop CJJr (1978). Visual system anomalies in human ocular albinos. Science 201:931.
Creel DJ, Sheridan CL (1966). Monocular acquisition and interocular transfer in albino rats with unilateral striate ablations. Psychonomic Sci 6:89.
Creel D, Witkop CJJr, King RA (1974). Asymmetric visually evoked potentials in human albinos. Evidence for visual system anomalies. Invest Ophthalmol 13:430.
Cunningham TJ, Lund RD (1971). Laminar patterns in the dorsal division of the lateral geniculate nucleus of the rat. Brain Res 34:394.
Falls HF (1951). Sex-linked ocular albinism displaying typical fundus changes in female heterozygote. Am J Ophthalmol 34:41.
Garber SR, Turner CW, Creel D, Witkop CJJr (in press). Auditory system abnormalities in human albinos. Ear Hearing.
Garrod AE (1908). Inborn errors of metabolism, Croonian Lectures, Lecture I. Lancet 2:1.
Giolli RA, Creel DJ (1973). The primary optic projections in pigmented and albino guinea pigs: An experimental

degeneration study. Brain Res 55:25.
Giolli RA, Guthrie MD (1969). The primary optic projections in the rabbit: An experimental degeneration study. J Comp Neurol 136:99.
Giolli RA, Guthrie MD (1971). Organization of subcortical projections of visual areas I and II in the rabbit: An experimental degeneration study. J Comp Neurol 142:351.
Gross KJ, Hickey TL (1980). Abnormal laminar patterns in the lateral geniculate nucleus of an albino monkey. Brain Res 190:231.
Guillery RW (1969). An abnormal retinogeniculate projection in Siamese cats. Brain Res 14:739.
Guillery RW (1971). An abnormal retinogeniculate projection in the albino ferret (*Mustela furo*). Brain Res 33:482.
Guillery RW (1974). Visual pathways in albinos. Sci Am 230.
Guillery RW (1982). The optic chiasm of the vertebrate brain. Cont Sensory Physiol (in press).
Guillery RW, Casagrande VA, Oberdorfer MD (1974). Congenitally abnormal vision in Siamese cats. Nature 252:195.
Guillery RW, Kaas JH (1971). A study of normal and congenitally abnormal retinogeniculate projections in cats. J Comp Neurol 143:73.
Guillery RW, Kaas JH (1973). Genetic abnormality of the visual pathways in a "white" tiger. Science 180:1287.
Guillery RW, Okoro AN, Witkop CJJr (1975). Abnornal visual pathways in the brain of a human albino. Brain Res 96:373.
Guillery RW, Scott GL, Cattanach BM, Deol MS (1973). Genetic mechanisms determining the central visual pathways of mice. Science 179:1014.
Guillery RW, Sitthi Amorn C, Eighmy BB (1971). Mutants with abnormal visual pathways: An explanation of anomalous geniculate laminae. Science 174:831.
Harrison JM, Howe ME (1974). Auditory system. Anatomy, Physiology (Ear). In Keidel W, Neff W (eds): "Handbook of Sensory Physiology, Vol 5," New York: Springer-Verlag, pp 284-336.
Hayhow WR, Webb C, Jervie A (1960). The accessory optic fiber system of the rat. J Comp Neurol 115:187.
Hotchkiss MG, Miller NR, Clark AW, Green WR (1980). Bilateral Duane's retraction syndrome. A clinical-pathologic case report. Arch Ophthalmol 98:870.
Hu F, Hanifin JM, Prescott GH, Tongue AC (1980). Yellow mutant albinism: Cytochemical, ultrastructural, and genetic characterization suggesting multiple allelism. Am J. Hum Genet 32:387.
Hubel DH, Wiesel TN (1971). Aberrant visual projections

in the Siamese cat. J Physiol 218:33.
Irving R, Harrison JM (1967). The superior olivary complex and audition: A comparative study. J Comp Neurol 130:77.
Jaeger C, Jay B (1981). X-linked ocular albinism. A family containing a manifesting heterozygote, and an affected male married to a female with autosomal recessive ocular albinism. Hum Genet 56:299.
Jay WM, Hoyt CS (1980). Abnormal brain stem auditory-evoked potentials in Stilling-Türk-Duane syndrome. Am J Ophthalmol 89:814.
Kaas JH, Guillery RW (1973). The transfer of abnormal visual field representation from the dorsal-lateral geniculate nucleus to the visual cortex in Siamese cats. Brain Res 59:61.
King RA, Creel D, Cervenka J, Okoro AN, Witkop CJJr (1980). Albinism in Nigeria with delineation of new recessive oculocutaneous type. Clin Genet 17:259.
King RA, Olds DP, Witkop CJJr (1978). Characterization of human hairbulb tyrosinase: Properties of normal and albino enzyme. J Invest Dermatol 71:136.
King RA, Witkop CJJr (1976). Hairbulb tyrosinase activity in oculocutaneous albinism. Nature 263:69.
Kupfer C, Chumbley L, Downer JC (1967). Quantitative histology of optic nerve, optic tract, and lateral geniculate nucleus of man. J Anat 101:393.
Lund RD (1965). Uncrossed visual pathways of hooded and albino rats. Science 149:1506.
Mann I (1937). "Developmental Abnormalities of the Eye." Cambridge: Cambridge University Press, p 155.
Montero VM, Brugge JF, Beitel RE (1968). Relation of the visual field to the lateral geniculate body of the albino rat. J Neurophysiol 31:221.
Nettleship E (1909). On some hereditary diseases of the eye. Trans Ophthalmol Soc U K 29:59.
O'Donnell FE, King RA, Green WR, Witkop CJJr (1978). Autosomal recessively inherited ocular albinism. Arch Ophthalmol 96:1621.
Polyak S (1957). In Klüver H (ed): "The Vertebrate Visual System," Chicago: University of Chicago Press.
Sanderson KJ (1972). Normal and abnormal retinogeniculate pathways in rabbits and mink. Anat Rec 172:398.
Sanderson KJ, Guillery RW, Shackleford RM (1974). Congenitally abnormal visual pathways in mink *(Mustela vison)* with reduced retinal pigment. J Comp Neurol 154:225.
Taylor WOG (1978). Eldrige-Green Lecture, 1978. Visual

disabilities of oculocutaneous albinism and their alleviation. Trans Ophthalmol Soc U K 98:423.

Townsend D, Witkop CJJr, Mattson J (1981). Tyrosinase subcellular distribution and kinetic parameters in wild type and *c*-locus mutant C57BL/6J mice. J Exp Zool 216:113.

Trevor-Roper PD (1952). Marriage of two complete albinos with normally pigmented offspring. Br J Ophthalmol 36: 107.

Trevor-Roper PD (1963). Albinism. Proc R Soc Med, Sec Ophthalmol 56:21.

Witkop CJJr (1979). Depigmentations of the general and oral tissues and their genetic foundations. Ala J Med Sci 16:331.

Witkop CJJr, Hill CW, Desnick SJ, Thies JK, Thorn H, Jenkins M, White JG (1973). Ophthalmologic, biochemical, platelet and ultrastructural defects in the various types of oculocutaneous albinism. J Invest Dermatol 60:443.

Witkop CJJr, Nance WE, Rawls RF, White JG (1970). Autosomal recessive oculocutaneous albinism in man: Evidence for genetic heterogeneity. Am J Hum Genet 22:55.

Witkop CJJr, Quevedo WCJr, Fitzpatrick TB (1978). Albinism. In Stanbury JB, Wyngaarden JB, Fredrickson DS (eds): "The Metabolic Basis of Inherited Disease, 4th Ed.," New York: McGraw-Hill, pp 283-316.

Witkop CJJr, Quevedo WCJr, Fitzpatrick TB (1982). Albinism. In Stanbury JB, Wyngaarden JB, Fredrickson DS (eds): "The Metabolic Basis of Inherited Disease, 5th Ed.," New York: McGraw-Hill.

Witkop CJJr, Van Scott EJ, Jacoby GA (1961). Evidence for two forms of autosomal recessive albinism in man. In "Proceedings of the Second International Congress of Human Genetics," Rome: Institute Gregor Mendel, pp 1064-1065.

Witkop CJJr, White JG, King RA (1974). Oculocutaneous albinism. In Nyhan L (ed): "Heritable Disorders of Amino Acid Metabolism," New York: Wiley, pp 177-261.

Witkop CJJr, White JG, Nance WE, Umber RE (1972). Mutations in the melanin pigment system in man resulting in features of oculocutaneous albinism. In Riley V (ed): "Pigmentation: Its Genesis and Biologic Control," New York: Appleton-Century-Crofts, pp 359-377.

Wolff D (1931). Melanin in the inner ear. Arch Otolaryngol. 14:195.

ALBINISM IN ENGLAND

Barrie Jay, MD, FRCS[1], Carl J Witkop, DDS, MS[2], and Richard A King, MD[2]
[1]Moorfields Eye Hospital, London, England,
[2]University of Minnesota, Minneapolis, MN, USA

Albinism may be defined as congenital heritable hypomelanosis involving the eye, skin and hair (oculocutaneous albinism - OCA), or apparently limited to the eye (ocular albinism - OA). Nystagmus, photophobia and reduced visual acuity occur in all forms of albinism; in their absence hypomelanosis should be termed albinoidism or cutaneous hypopigmentation (Witkop, 1979a). Both oculocutaneous and ocular albinism are heterogeneous groups of disorders which may be subdivided on anatomical, genetic or biochemical grounds.

Oculocutaneous albinism has been divided into tyrosinase-negative (ty-neg) and tyrosinase positive (ty-pos) forms (Witkop et al, 1963; Witkop, 1971) on the basis of the hair-bulb incubation test (Kugelman and Van Scott, 1961), and these two forms result from the presence of two non-allelic autosomal genes (Witkop et al, 1970; Nance et al, 1971). Further heterogeneity within this group has been demonstrated by the delineation of a number of other forms of albinism (yellow mutant, brown OCA, rufous OCA, autosomal dominant OCA) and by the description of syndromes comprising OCA in association with other systemic anomalies (Hermansky-Pudlak, Chediak-Higashi, Cross, OCA with black lock and congenital deafness) (Witkop, 1979a).

The classical form of X-linked ocular albinism (Nettleship, 1909) has been shown to be characterised by the presence of giant melanosomes in the skin of both caucasians and negroes (O'Donnell et al, 1976; O'Donnell et al, 1978a; Garner and Jay, 1980), and macromelanosomes have also been

Birth Defects: Original Article Series, Volume 18, Number 6, pages 319-325

nystagmus and no obvious translucency of his irides.

Pedigree 1595

In this family the father has X-linked ocular albinism, as has his brother; the mother has tyrosinase-negative oculocutaneous albinism. Their 18-month-old son has normal eyes with no nystagmus and no obvious iris translucency.

Pedigree 2079

In this third family the father also has X-linked ocular albinism, as has his brother; the mother has yellow-mutant oculocutaneous albinism. They have 2 daughters aged 9 and 6 years respectively. The older has a visual acuity of 6/9 part in one eye and 6/18 in the other, the second eye having strabismic amblyopia. Her blue irides are moderately translucent, she has no nystagmus, but her fundi show the characteristic changes of the heterozygous state of XOAN. The younger daughter has a visual acuity of at least 6/18. She has a consecutive divergent strabismus, blue irides that are moderately translucent, no nystagmus, but the characteristic fundus changes similar to her sister.

DISCUSSION

Many of the patients in this series were referred for genetic counselling; a number were referred in order to have a definitive diagnosis established. While it cannot be claimed that the distribution of the different genetic forms in this series is truly representative of the population of albinos in England, it does give an indication of the frequencies of these different forms presenting in a large ophthalmic hospital draining an appreciable percentage of the population of south-east England.

The two common forms of oculocutaneous albinism (ty-neg and ty-pos) were equally represented in this series and accounted for nearly 70% of all albinos seen in London. As the majority of patients in this series were caucasian, the equal frequencies of the two common forms of OCA was not surprising, being similar to that found in caucasians in North America, and in contrast to the greater frequency of ty-pos over ty-neg OCA in North American negroes (Witkop, 1979a).

It is instructive that the 2 examples of the Hermansky-Pudlak syndrome remained incorrectly diagnosed for several years, despite giving a history of haemorrhagic episodes. These 2 patients, aged 35 and 55 years, had no evidence of pulmonary fibrosis or ulcerative colitis and appear to present a milder clinical picture than that commonly seen in similar patients of East Indian or Puerto Rican origin. Patients with any form of albinism, and particularly those with a history of mild bleeding, should have platelet aggregation studies followed, if abnormal, by electron microscopic studies of their platelets. In the Hermansky-Pudlak syndrome there is an almost complete absence of electron dense bodies in platelets. It is important to establish the diagnosis as these patients are prone to develop severe haemorrhagic episodes after the ingestion of aspirin or aspirin-like drugs, and may require transfusions of normal platelets prior to surgery (Witkop, 1979b).

It may be surprising at first sight that a definitive diagnosis was not reached in 36 patients. A number of patients, however, are infants or young children with white or very blond hair and in this group it is often impossible to differentiate between ty-neg, ty-pos and ym OCA, or between OCA and AROA. In older patients, as well, it is sometimes difficult to distinguish between ty-pos OCA and AROA and there appears to be a gradation of phenotypic appearance between these two conditions, if indeed they are separate entities. In a population with a high proportion of blue-eyed blonds, it is often impossible to diagnose XOAN clinically in the absence of an obligate heterozygote; in such cases the diagnosis can only be made by demonstrating the presence of macromelanosomes in a biopsy of the skin. In addition, there is a small group of patients who cannot be classified into any of the known types of albinism.

There are still relatively few reports in the literature of the results of the mating between two individuals with different forms of albinism. The original couple reported by Trevor-Roper (1952) were shown to have tyrosinase-negative and tyrosinase-positive oculocutaneous albinism (Witkop et al, 1970), as were the negro couple described by Nance and his colleagues (1971). The normal offspring of these 2 marriages were evidence that the genes for ty-neg OCA and ty-pos OCA are non-allelic. There is presumptive evidence from another pedigree that the genes for ty-neg OCA and ym OCA are allelic (Hu et al, 1980). In the 3 families reported here the fathers had X-linked ocular albinism while the mothers had different forms of autosomal albinism. In 2 of these 3 families (pedigrees 516 and 1595) the offspring were normal, except for one daughter who, being an obligate heterozygote, had the fundus changes characteristic of the heterozygous state of XOAN. In the third family (pedigree 2079) the 2 daughters had, in addition to the typical fundus changes of the heterozygous state of XOAN, moderately translucent irides, strabismus, and possibly slightly reduced visual acuities. There is no good evidence, however, that these minor abnormalities resulted from the additive effects of the 2 non-allelic genes for albinism; similar changes have been observed in the blue-eyed offspring of tyrosinase-negative oculocutaneous albinos, where the offspring must be assumed to be heterozygotes for the ty-neg OCA gene.

There is still much we have to learn about albinism in man. Increases in our knowledge will result from clinical and genetic studies, but far greater increases will stem from laboratory studies which will eventually unravel the mysteries that are at present cloaked in the term 'albinism'.

REFERENCES

Frenk E, Lattion F (1982). The melanin pigmentary disorder in a family with Hermansky-Pudlak syndrome. J Invest Dermatol, in press.

Garner A, Jay B (1980). Macromelanosomes in X-linked ocular albinism. Histopathology 4:243.

Hu F, Hanifin JM, Prescott GH, Tongue AC (1980). Yellow mutant albinism: cytochemical, ultrastructural, and genetic characterization suggesting multiple allelism. Am J Hum Genet 32:387.

Jaeger C, Jay B (1980). X-linked ocular albinism. A family containing a manifesting heterozygote, and an affected male married to a female with autosomal recessive ocular albinism. Hum Genet 56:299.

Kugelman TP, Van Scott EJ (1961). Tyrosinase activity in melanocytes of human albinos. J Invest Dermatol 37:73.

Nance WE, Witkop CJ, Rawles RF (1971). Genetic and biochemical evidence for two forms of oculocutaneous albinism in man. Birth Defects 7(3):125.

Nettleship E (1909). On some hereditary diseases of the eye. Trans Ophthalmol Soc UK 29:LVII.

O'Donnell FE Jr, Green WR, Fleischman JA, Hambrick GW (1978a). X-linked ocular albinism in blacks. Ocular albinism cum pigmento. Arch Ophthalmol 96:1189.

O'Donnell FE Jr, Hambrick GW Jr, Green WR, Iliff WJ, Stone DL (1976). X-linked ocular albinism: an oculocutaneous macromelanosomal disorder. Arch Ophthalmol 94:1883.

O'Donnell FE Jr, King RA, Green WR, Witkop CJ Jr (1978b). Autosomal recessively inherited ocular albinism. A new form of ocular albinism affecting females as severely as males. Arch Ophthalmol 96:1621.

Trevor-Roper PD (1952). Marriage of two complete albinos with normally pigmented offspring. Br J Ophthalmol 36:107.

Witkop CJ Jr (1971). Albinism. In Hirschhorn K, Harris H (eds): "Advances in Human Genetics," vol 2, New York: Plenum Press, p 61.

Witkop CJ (1979a). Depigmentation of the general and oral tissues and their genetic foundation. Ala J Med Sci 16:331.

Witkop CJ (1979b). Albinism: hematologic-storage disease, susceptibility to skin cancer, and optic neuronal defects shared in all types of oculocutaneous and ocular albinism. Ala J Med Sci 16:327.

Witkop CJ Jr, Nance WE, Rawles RF, White JG (1970). Autosomal recessive oculocutaneous albinism in man: evidence for genetic heterogeneity. Am J Hum Genet 22:55.

Witkop CJ, Van Scott EJ, Jacoby GA (1963). Evidence for two forms of autosomal recessive albinism in man. In "Proceedings of the 2nd International Congress of Human Genetics," Rome:Instituto Gregorio Mendel, p 1064.

OCULAR FINDINGS IN CHEDIAK-HIGASHI DISEASE: A light and electron microscopic study of two patients

J. Libert[1], P. Dhermy[2], F. Van Hoof[3], J. L. Dufier[4], and G. Cornu[5].

1, 3, 5: Brussels, Belgium; 2, 4: Paris, France.

1: Service d'Ophtalmologie, Hopital St-Pierre, 322, rue Haute, B-1000 BRUSSELS, BELGIUM.

Chédiak-Higashi disease is a rare autosomal recessive syndrome, characterized by partial oculo-cutaneous albinism, frequent pyogenic infections and intermittent febrile episodes, leading to death at an early age. A lymphoma-like phase, also called accelerated phase, may sometimes develop with widespread lymphoid and histiocytic infiltration, pancytopenia, lymphadenopathy, hepato-splenomegaly and hemorragic syndrome (Blume and Wolff 1972). A similar disorder has been described in mink, mice, cattle and whale.

The diagnosis of the disease is based on the recognition of giant granules in leukocytes (the Chédiak anomaly), but abnormal inclusions are widespread and can be observed in skin, tyroid, gastric mucosa, pancreas, liver, kidney and liver cells (Donohue and Bain 1957, Sung et al 1969). They have been demonstrated to represent varieties of lysosomes (White 1966). Abnormalities of melanosome formation, accounting for the pseudo-albinism, are probably related to the same physiopathological mechanism but, despite many investigations, the basic defect remains unknown.

Very few microscopic studies of the eyes have been performed in Chédiak-Higashi disease (Spencer and Hogan 1960, Brégeat et al 1966, Johnson et al 1966, Bedoya et al 1969). Electron microscopic studies have been reported in mouse eyes (Robinson et al 1975, 1978) and only one in man (BenEzra et al 1980). In the present paper, we describe the ultrastructural lesions in two unrelated children affected with the disease, with a special attention to the melanin malformation and the dysgenesis of the

Birth Defects: Original Article Series, Volume 18, Number 6, pages 327–344

photoreceptors.

CASE REPORTS

Case 1, a boy, was the product of the first pregnancy of non-consanguineous parents. At the age of two months, oculocutaneous albinism, severe hepato-splenomegaly with pancytopenia and recurrent severe infections suggested the diagnosis of Chédiak-Higashi disease. This was confirmed by the recognition of typical giant granules in the leukocytes and abnormalities of hair melanosomes.

Despite massive antibiotherapy, corticotherapy and many transfusions, the child died at the age of three months in a septicemic syndrome. A complete autopsy was performed a few hours after death and revealed lesions related to a bacterial and mycotic infection as well as a widespread lysosomal storage process that was especially evident in liver and reticuloendothelial cells (Janne et al 1980).

Case 2, a girl, was the second child of non-consanguineous parents. Her older brother is healthy. From her first year, she suffered from repeated infectious episodes. She had fair and almost grey hair, her skin presented numerous achromic dots, her irises were blue and a marked photophobia was evident. The diagnosis was made at the age of three years on a clinical basis and was confirmed by the observation of the Chédiak anomaly in leukocytes.

A marked degradation of her general condition occurred when she was five years old, with febrile episodes and appearance of hepato-splenomegaly, polyadenopathies, anemia and hemorragic syndrome. She became drowsy and cachectic, and died at the age of 6 years in bacterial and fungal septicemia. General autopsic examination showed a pseudo-lymphomatous lymphocytic infiltration of the bone-marrow, the lymphatic ganglions, the liver and the pancreas. Great lysosomal inclusions were found by electron microscopical examination of alveolar macrophages and hepatocytes (Hurteaux 1979).

MATERIAL AND METHODS

Ocular tissues from both patients were obtained within two hours after death. They were prepared for light and electron microscopic examination following routine procedures. Hematein-eosin-safran, Giemsa and Fontana techniques were used on sections of the paraffin blocks. Semi-thin sections of Epon-embedded material were stained with toluidine blue. Ultrathin sections were stained with uranyl acetate and lead citrate, and were examined with a Philips EM 300 electron microscope (Laboratory of Electron Microscopy, Hotel Dieu, Paris - Prof. Y. Pouliquen, and Laboratory of Ophthalmology, University of Brussels - Prof. P. Danis).

OCULAR PATHOLOGY

Light Microscopy

In each case, the cornea and conjunctiva appeared to be normal. The irises were transparent, with occasional pigmented cells in the stroma and a few giant melanin granules in the posterior epithelium (Figure 1 a). The lack of pigmentation left evident the pupillomotor muscle fibers, which are usually masked. The ciliary and retinal pigment epithelium was also depigmented. Many cells were completely devoid of melanin granules. Others contained rare melanosomes, whose dimensions were widely variable and often reached several microns (Figures 1 c, d).

In the first case, the ciliary body and the choroid were diffusely infiltrated with round or oval shaped cells, resembling histiocytes. These cells contained many dense inclusions of different sizes (Figure 1 b) and it was often difficult to differentiate them from melanocytes. In the second case, on the contrary, the lymphocyte infiltration was less prominent and the melanocytes of the stroma seemed almost normally pigmented. Specimens of each case, stained with the Giemsa technique, showed the characteristic purple inclusions (the Chédiak anomaly) in the leukocytes of the choroid vessels.

The retina of the first case was artifactuously detached in the portion embedded in paraffin, but did not display striking abnormalities. It remained in place in the second case and appeared normal (Figure 1 c), with a good differentiation of the macular architecture. On the contrary, in specimens of the first case embedded in Epon, the retina kept normal contact with the pigment epithelium and semi-thin sections evidenced a marked dystrophic process of the photoreceptors, which appeared irregular, convoluted or fragmented (Figure 1 d). Moreover, the intercellular matrix was infiltrated with large macrophage-like cells, containing dense inclusions. The other retinal structures and the optic nerves were normal.

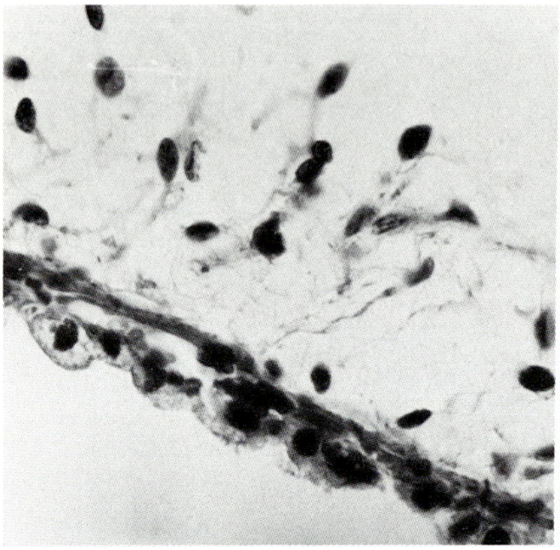

Figure 1 a

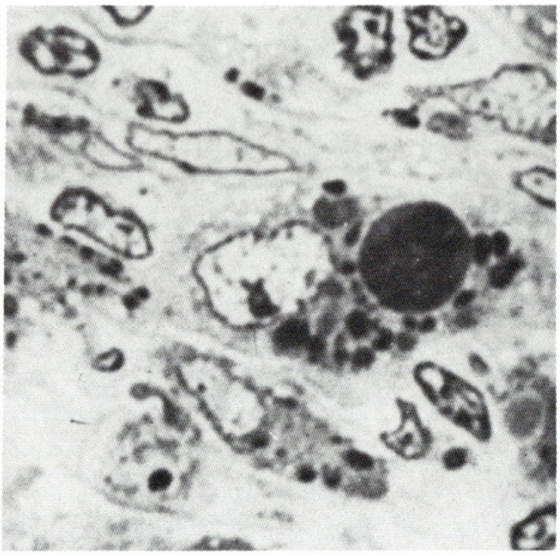

Figure 1 b

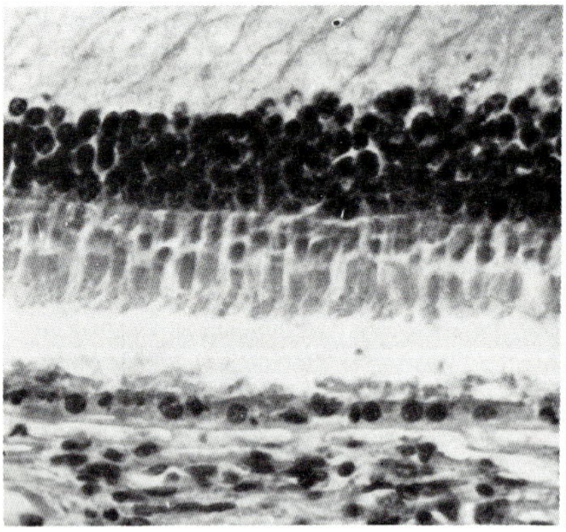

Figure 1 c

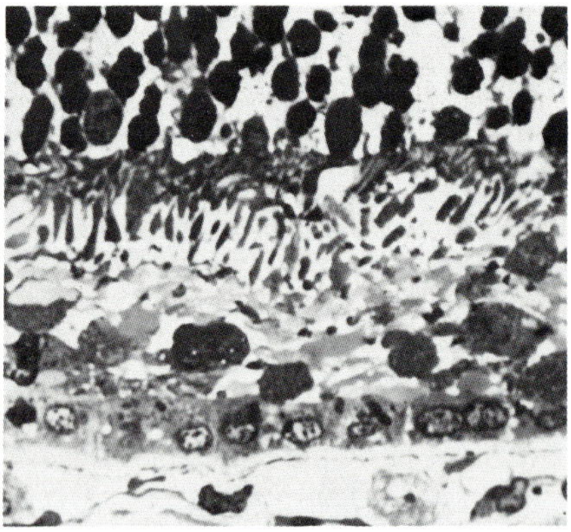

Figure 1 d

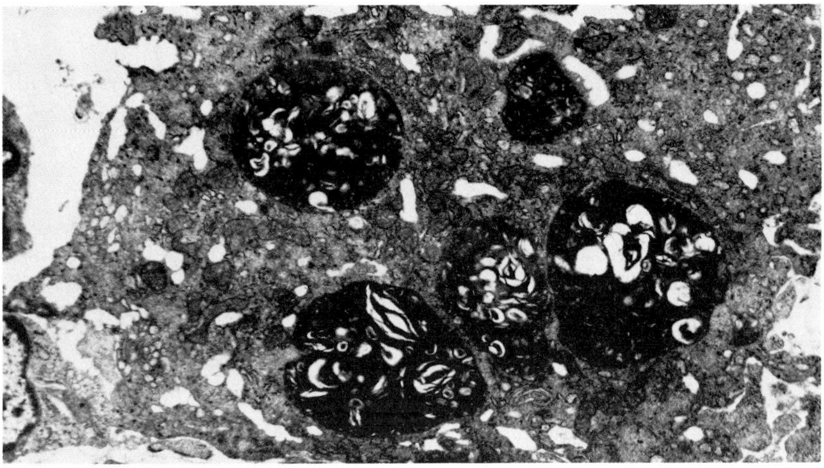

Figure 2 (X 7,000)

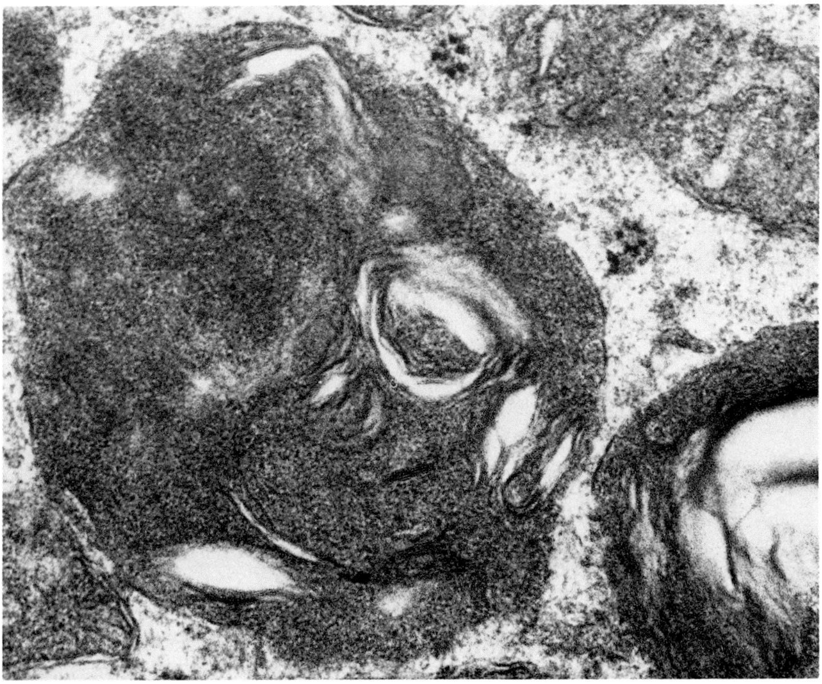

Figure 3 (X 70,000)

Electron Microscopy

Case 1. Abnormal histiocytes were observed in the conjunctival stroma and in the irises. They were especially numerous in the ciliary body and infiltrated diffusely the choroid. These cells were filled with dense membrane-bound inclusions, whose dimensions were comprized between 0.2 and 3 microns. At high magnification, these inclusions contained a compact finely granular material associated with irregular lamellar structures, with parallel or whorled arrangement (Figure 2, 3). Several fibers of the oculumotor and ciliary muscles presented the same storage process (Figure 4). On the contrary, corneal and conjunctival epithelial cells, keratocytes, sclerocytes, capillary endothelial cells as well as axons and Schwann cells of sensory nerves remained unaffected.

Only rare pigment wearing cells were recognizable in the irises, the ciliary body and the choroidal stroma. The melanocytes were exceptional and contained regular, spindle shaped

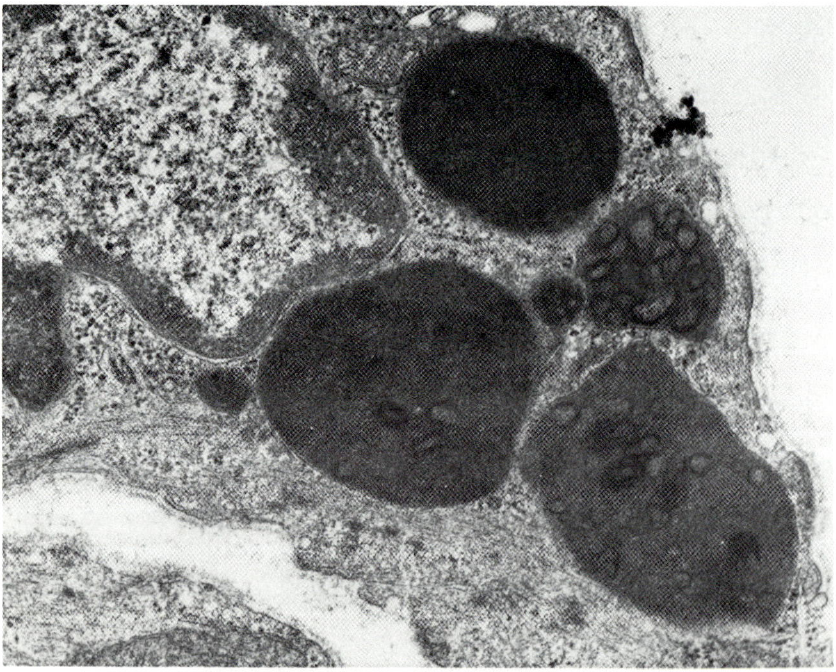

Figure 4 (X 30,000)

melanosomes with normal size. The other pigmented cells were macrophages presenting large inclusions with polylobulated contours, which contained several free melanin granules clumped together within a finely granular matrix. These large inclusions, whose dimensions may reach 5 microns, represent typical secondary lysosomes, with melanin residues and lipofuscin-like material.

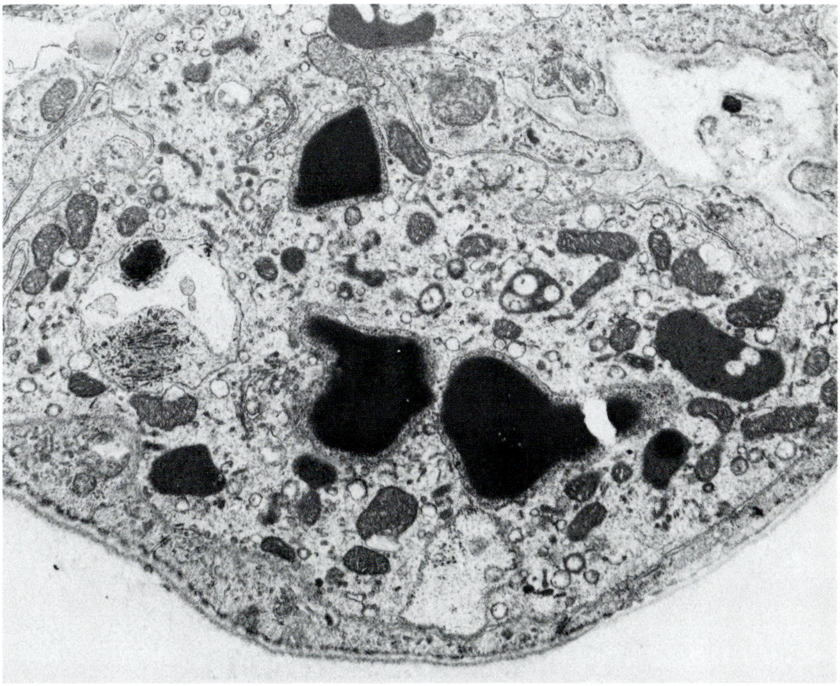

Figure 5 (X 6,600)

The pigment epithelium of the irises, the ciliary body and the retina presented striking abnormalities. Most of the cells were completely depigmented and even did not contain any immature melanosome. Some of them showed large complex inclusions with granular and lamellar material resembling those described in histiocytes. Some presented large secondary lysosomes with dark irregular melanin granules complexed with a lipofuscin-like material. Some others, finally, displayed dense formations, very abnormal by their sizes (0.5 - 5 microns) and by their shapes, as their profiles were round, oval or often

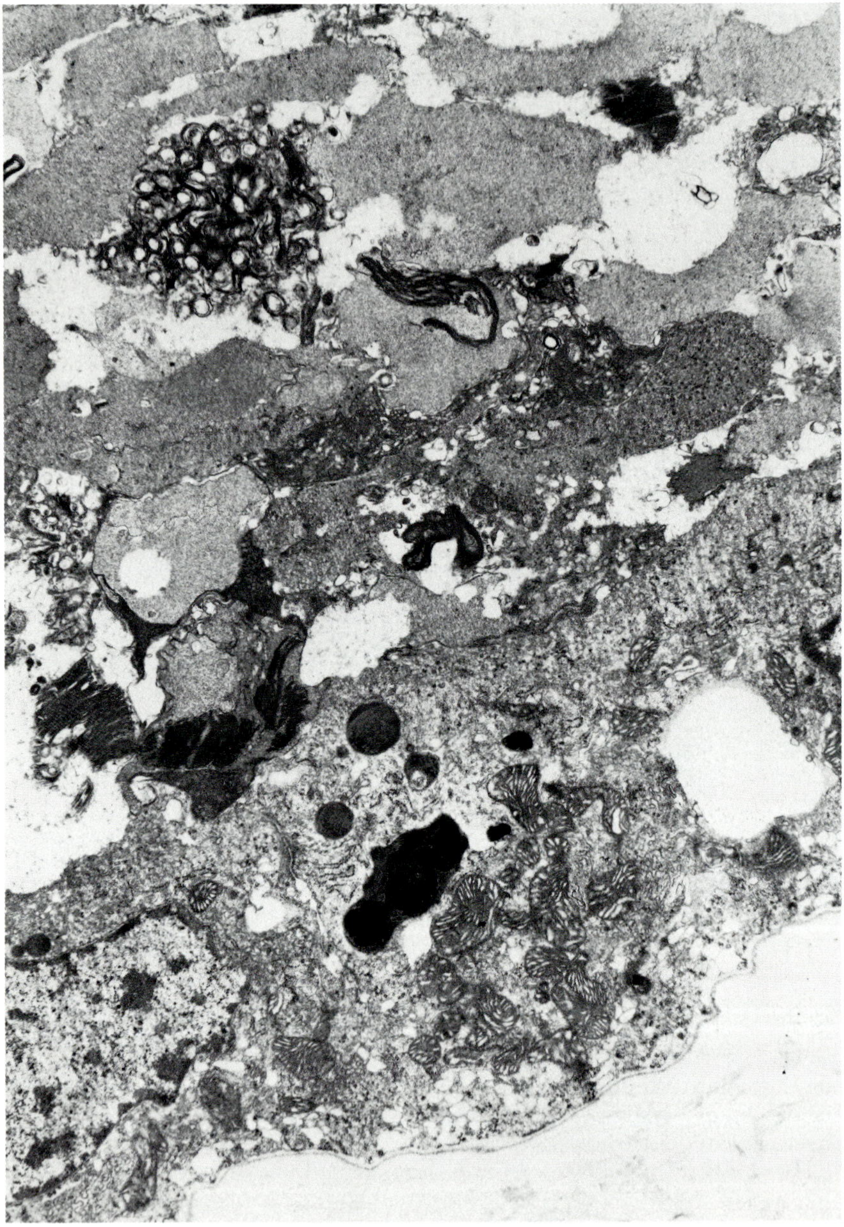

Figure 6 (X 8,000)

polygonal. These latter formations were also limited by a single membrane and contained a very dense and homogenous material, in which no structure could be disclosed even at the highest magnification and illumination power of the microscope. The greatest inclusions of this type were observed in the posterior epithelium of the iris and presented artifactual holes in their center, resulting from the embedding and cutting procedures (Figure 5).

The inner portion of the retina had well preserved structures. In particular, the ganglion cells had their usual appearance and did not show any lysosomal overloading. On the contrary, striking abnormalities were evident in the outer segments of the photoreceptors, confirming the lesions observed by light microscopy. Their inner portions were short and poor in mitochondria. Their outer portions appeared as undifferentiated cytoplasmic processes, which contained a granular homogenous matrix, some glycogen particles, several free ribosomes, and some fragments of smooth or rough endoplasmic reticulum. Occasionally, irregular lamellar architectures were evident, lying free in the distal portion of the cytoplasm but no well structurated rod or cone could be disclosed (Figure 6). The inter-photoreceptor spaces were infiltrated with macrophages, which presented the same dense pleiomorphic inclusions as the uveal histiocytes. They also displayed membrane bound inclusions, whose content resembled the irregular lamellar structures observed in the dysmorphic cytoplasm of the photoreceptors.

Case 2. Attention was focused in this case on the fine structure of the material observed in histiocytes and in pigmented cells. Unfortunately, the retina was not available for electron microscopy.

The choroid was infiltrated with lymphocyte-like cells, which presented round large inclusions surrounded by several smaller ones. All were limited by a single membrane and contained the same dense amorphous material (Figure 7). Heterogenous giant inclusions were observed in histiocytes. Some of these had a central dense homogenous core surrounded by a compact granular material. Others contained a lamellar matrix. Several normal melanocytes were also observed with regular melanin granules.

Important lesions were evident in the retinal pigment epithelium. The cells did not show any normal elementary mela-

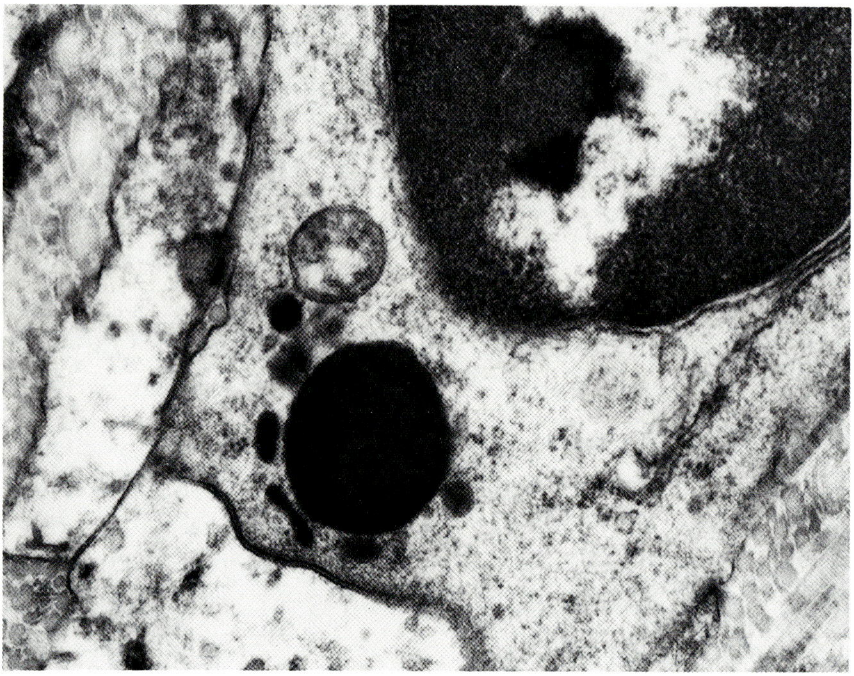

Figure 7 (X 30,000)

nosomes. On the contrary, they displayed three types of dysmorphic inclusions which were all limited by a single membrane. Inclusions of the first type were very large, had an ovoid shape and contained a giant spindle with more or less dense melanin deposits. Inclusions of the second type had a polycyclic contour and contained more or less fully melanized ovoids complexed with a dense lipofuscin-like material. They had all characters of secondary lysosomes and their dimensions were often very large (4 - 5 microns). They occupied then large portions of the cytoplasmic profiles (Figure 8). Inclusions of the third type were smaller, round shaped, and contained a very dense center with angular contours, surrounded by a lipofuscin-like material. Their dimensions were comprized between 1 and 2 microns. They were often grouped in the apical portion of the cells (Figure 9).

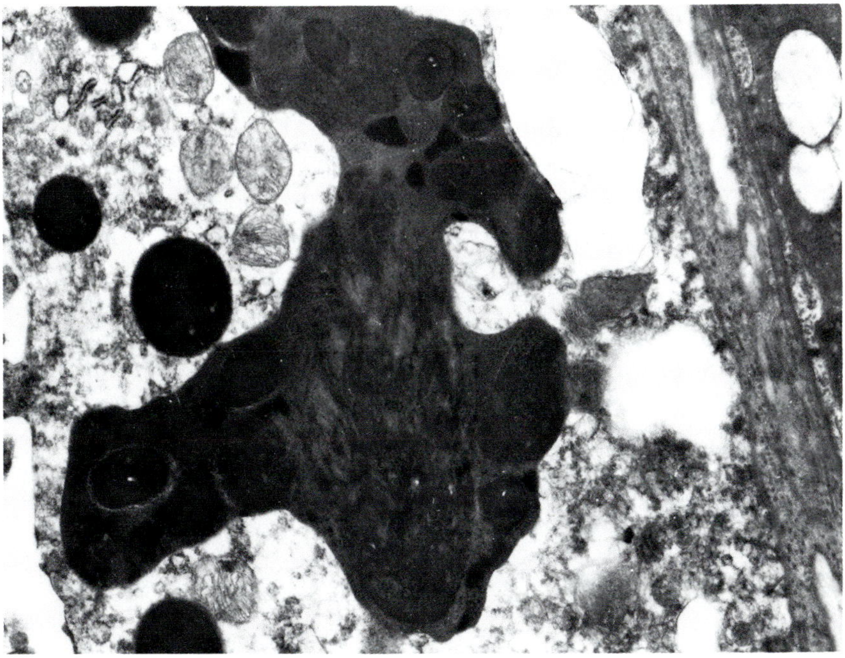

Figure 8 (X 16,000)

DISCUSSION

The two patients reported in the present study showed the typical clinical features of Chédiak-Higashi syndrome, with oculo-cutaneous albinism, history of repeated severe infections and the presence of pathognomonic cytological abnormalities. Although the clinical course was different, two distinct periods may be separated in the history of our patients, as in the classical reports (Blume and Wolff 1972). The first one is characterized by successive infectious episodes, whereas the second one is complicated by hematologic problems, with hepato-splenomegaly and pancytopenia. Both cases died from septicemia and there was obviously no lymphomatous transformation, in contrast with several descriptions of accelerated blood malignancy (Blume and Wolff 1972). Indeed, the general architecture of the lymphatic ganglions was well preserved and no malignant cell could be disclosed.

One child seemed to suffer from a more severe form of the disease, since he died at three months, while the second one survived to the age of six years. This clinical heterogeneity is not unusual in the course of the disorder and might depend on the severity of intercurrent infections, or on the precocity in the appearance of the hematological complications (Blume and Wolff 1972). Alternatively, it might also correspond to a genetic heterogeneity, a concept which is now classical in most of the lysosomal storage diseases (Sandhoff and Christomanou 1979).

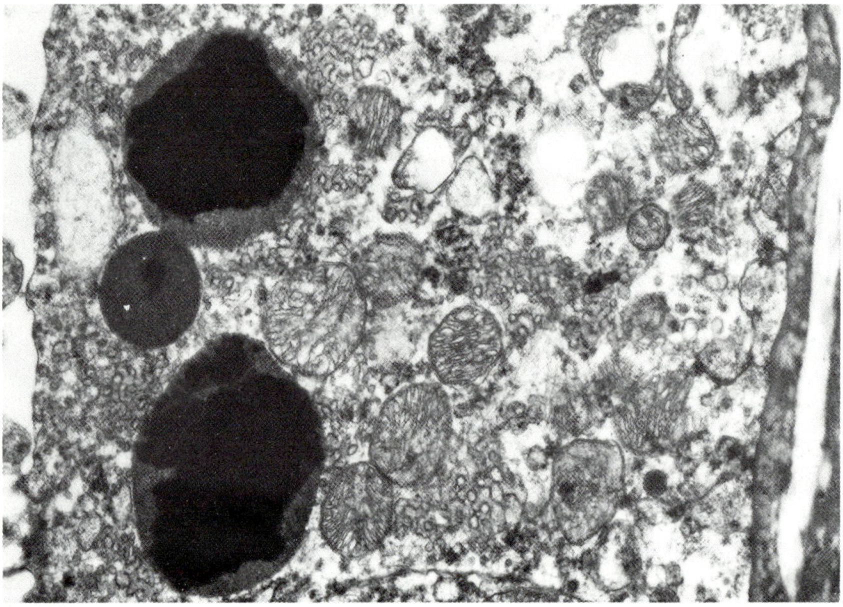

Figure 9 (X 16,000)

The more prominent feature, observed by light microscopy in the eyes of our patients, is the almost complete absence of normal melanosomes in usually pigmented cells, as uveal melanocytes and iridal, ciliary or retinal pigment epithelium. This disturbance of melanogenesis is part of the generalized pigment dilution (Windhorst et al 1968). It has been already reported in Chédiak-Higashi patients' eyes and accounts for the ocular pseudo-albinism (Spencer and Hogan 1960, Brégeat et al 1966, Johnson et al 1966, Bedoya et al 1969).

A few melanin granules are present however at electron microscopy. Normal melanosomes, with typical filamentous structures and normal sizes, are exceptional, and we were unable to find any premelanosome or immature melanosome, even in the first patient where they should be numerous because of his young age. The majority of the pigmented organelles are very abnormal in their sizes, their shapes and their fine structure. Three main types may be considered. The first type corresponds to great membrane-bound formations, whose dimensions are comprized between 1 and 2 microns and in which a spindle architecture is sometimes recognizable. They closely resemble the single melanosomes of unusual sizes but normal substructures described in the skin of Chédiak-Higashi patients (Zelickson et al 1967). A second type is represented by giant membrane-bound inclusions with polycyclic contours, whose dimensions may reach 5 microns. Their content is characterized by the presence of a dense granular material, resembling lipofuscin, in which are packed together several melanin ovoids of variable dimensions and showing unequal degrees of maturity (Figure 8). These formations are considered to correspond to polyphagosomes, containing normal melanosomes or macromelanosomes, which have lost their own limiting membrane and show different stages of degeneration. Similar heterogenous inclusions have been described in the pigment epithelium of beige mice and have been proven to be lysosomes by the demonstration of their acid phosphatase activity (Robison et al 1975, 1978). Their distribution is not restricted to the eyes; they have been found in the skin and hair of our patients and are classical in the literature (Windhorst et al 1968, Zelickson et al 1967). This abnormal packaging of melanin granules within giant lysosomes is believed to arise from the multiple fusion of elementary melanosomes (Robison et al 1975, 1976). Alternatively, an accelerated rate of autophagy might induce the sequestration of cytoplasmic portions which contain melanosomes. The catabolism of the incorporated material will then be more or less complete, leaving free melanin granules within the dense undigested lipofuscin-like material of large secondary lysosomes.

The third kind of pigmented formation is composed of very dark inclusions of great size with a round, oval or polyedric profile, which are observed in the iris and cilary body epithelium of the first case and in the retinal pigment epithelium of the second case (Figures 5 and 9). The core of these inclusions is dense and homogenous. In the second case, a peripheral fringe often appears that resembles the granular structure of lipofuscin. The center of the greatest ones is often disrupted by the cutting of thin sections (Figure 5). This probably results from their density, which did not allow sufficient fixation and impregnation during the embedding procedures. These inclusions are totally different from the macromelanosomes and the polyphagosomes described before, by their amorphous appearance even at the highest magnification and resolution power of the electron microscope. They are probably abnormal melanin formations, because they are found in theoretically pigmented cells and because they are as dark as the center of fully mature normal melanosomes. They are not classically reported in Chédiak-Higashi patients and resemble rather closely the abnormal pigment grains resulting from other disturbances of melanogenesis, as neurofibromatosis, the nevus spillus and X-linked ocular albinism (Jimbow et al 1967, Konrad et al 1974, O'Donnel et al 1976, 1978). In these conditions too, giant melanosomes are essentially non-filamentous in nature and melanin seems to precipitate in the absence of the spindle-shaped skeleton which characterizes normal human melanosomes.

The pigmentary dilution observed in the eyes of the patients then results directly from the abnormal melanogenesis and from the structural defects, which induce the formation of macromelanosomes, polyphagosomes and giant amorphous melanin inclusions. The very small number of well-formed melanosomes and the aggregation of the remaining granules inhibit the normal dispersion of melanin throughout the cells and account for the ocular pseudo-albinism, as it explains the skin abnormalities classically described (Windhorst et al 1968, Zelickson et al 1967).

In addition to the pigmentation abnormalities, a widespread storage process is also evident in many ocular structures, as muscle fibers, histiocytes and lymphocytes of the conjunctiva and the uvea. These cells display numerous membrane-bound inclusions, which contain pleiomorphic lamellar structures associated with a variable proportion of granular material. At electron microscopy, they appear to be totally similar to the typical Chédiak inclusions of the leukocytes and to the storage lysosomes observed in the liver and the lung of our patients. They have been proven to represent varieties of lysosomes by the demonstration of their acid phosphatase and peroxidase activities (White 1966). Their formation is independent of melanogenesis, since they are principally found in nonpigmented cells, but seems rather to be related to the pathogenesis of the lysosomal dysfunction. Their ultrastructural appearance suggests the storage of complex lipids. Their pleiomorphism recalls some characteristics of the material accumulated in Niemann-Pick disease (Libert and Danis 1979) and in lysosomal storage induced by amphiphilic drugs (Lüllmann et al 1975) or aminoglycoside antibiotics (Libert et al 1979), and suggests the presence of phospholipids. This hypothesis, already proposed on a biochemical basis (Kanfer et al 1968), will be the subject of further studies.

One must point out that the retinal tissue itself failed to reveal any storage lysosome. This was unexpected, especially for the ganglion cells, as brain neurons are classically involved (Sung et al 1969). However, the only child whose retina could be obtained for electron microscopic examination died at a very early stage of the disease and it is possible that abnormalities would have developed with a longer survival.

Finally, very important alterations of the photoreceptors were evidenced in our first case, with the presence of an undifferentiated cytoplasm, instead of the superposition of regular disks in outer segments. Unfortunately, an electron microscopic study could not be performed on the second case for comparison. Light microscopic evidence would have suggest the normality of the retina of this patient, but the low resolution power and the artefacts related to the technique may lead to many false interpretations. Clinical descriptions, with the classical low vision and nystagmus, as well as electroretinographic studies (Sabatino and Scialfa 1966) have proposed a tapeto-retinal degeneration as part of Chédiak-Higashi disease. Our electron microscopic findings confirm this hypothesis.

The pathologic photoreceptors of our first case closely resemble those described in Leber's congenital amaurosis (Mizuno et al 1977). They are believed to correspond to a lack of differentiation rather than to a true degenerative process, because they share many ultrastructural features with the fetal neurosensory retina (Yamada and Ishikawa 1966). Indeed, this latter is composed of short and amorphous cytoplasmic portions, containing few ribosomes and mitochondria, which progress slowly from the outer limiting desmosome line in the direction of the pigment epithelium. In these undifferentiated processes will appear later the classical outer segment structures by successive superposition of disks (Yamada and Ishikawa 1966). In Chédiak-Higashi disease, the photoreceptor elements seem to fail to differentiate during the prenatal development. The infiltration of the region by macrophage-like cells suggests the beginning of a reactive mechanism, similar to what occurs in retinitis pigmentosa. The complete absence of phagosomes within pigment epithelial cells does not allow us to consider the hypothesis that a defect in the catabolism of the shedded disks might initiate the troubles in the maintenance of the photoreceptor structures, as it has been suggested by the electron microscopic studies of albino-beige mice (Robison and Kuwabara 1978). On the contrary, our observation might be the unique pathological condition, among lysosomal storage disorders, in which a defect in the differentiation of normal disks seems to be at the origin of a retinitis pigmentosa-like degeneration. In all other conditions recognized until now, such as mucopolysaccharidoses and ceroid-lipofuscinoses, the overloading of the pigment epithelial cells by undigested material appears to be the initial phenomenon

CONCLUSION

Light and electron microscopic studies of the eyes of two patients affected with Chédiak-Higashi disease revealed a severe disturbance of melanogenesis, with pseudo-albinism and appearence of macromelanosomes, polyphagosomes and giant amorphous melanine grains. A widespread storage process was also evidenced within large lysosomes with pleiomorphic content. Finally, profound malformations of the photoreceptors suggested a failure in the differentiation of the neurosensory retina during the prenatal development.

ACKNOWLEDGEMENTS

We thank Dr Griscelli and Dr Delforge, who referred the patients to us. This study was supported by grants of the Belgian Fonds de la Recherche Scientifique Médicale N° 3-4542-79.

REFERENCES

Bedoya V, Grimley PM, Duque O (1969). Chédiak-Higashi syndrome. Arch Pathol 88:340.
BenEzra D, Mengistu F, Cividalli G, Weizman Z, Merin S, Auerbach E (1980). Chédiak-Higashi syndrome. Ocular findings. J Pediatr Ophthalmol Strabismus 17:68.
Blume RS, Wolff SM (1972). The Chédiak-Higashi syndrome: Studies in four patients and review of the literature. Medecine 51:247.

Brégeat P, Dhermy P, Hamard H (1966). Manifestations oculaires du syndrome de Chédiak-Higashi. Arch Ophtal 26:661.
Donohue WL, Bain HW (1957). Chédiak-Higashi syndrome. Pediatrics 20:416.
Hurteaux P (1979). Aspect ophtalmologique de la maladie de Chédiak-Higashi. Thesis Paris.
Janne C, Van Hoof F, Libert J, Cordier A, Cornu G (1980). La maladie de Chédiak-Higashi. Journées Annuelles de Pédiatrie, Brussels.
Jimbow K, Szabo G, Fitzpatrick TB (1967). Ultrastructure of giant pigment granules (macromelanosomes) in the cutaneous pigmented macules of neurofibromatosis. J Invest Derm 61:300.
Johnson DL, Jacobson R, Toyama R, Monahan RH (1966). Histopathology of eyes in Chédiak-Higashi syndrome. Arch Ophthal 75:84.
Kanfer JN, Blume RA, Yankee RA, Wolff SM (1968). Alterations of sphingolipids metabolism in leukocytes of patients with the Chédiak-Higashi syndrome. New Engl J Med 279:410.
Konrad K, Wolff K, Honigsmann H (1974). Giant melanosome: A model of deranged melanosome melanogenesis. J Ultrastruct Res 48:102.
Libert J, Danis P (1979). Differential diagnosis of type A, B and C Niemann-Pick disease by conjunctival biopsy. J Submicr Cytol 11:143.
Libert J, Ketelbant-Balasse P, Van Hoof F, Aubert-Tulkens G, Tulkens P (1979). Cellular toxicity of gentamicin. Am J Ophthal 87:405.
Lüllmann H, Lüllmann-Rauch R, Wasserman O (1975). Drug-induced phospholipidoses. Crit Rev Toxicol 4:185.
Mizuno K, Takel Y, Sears ML, Peterson WS, Carr RE, Jampol LM (1977). Leber's congenital amaurosis. Am J Ophthal 83:32.
O'Donnel FE, Hambrick GW, Green WR, Iliff WJ, Stone DL (1976). X-Linked ocular albinism - An oculucutaneous macromelanosomal disorder. Arch Ophthal 94:1883.
O'Donnel FE, Green WR, Fleischman JA, Hambrick GW (1978). X-Linked ocular albinism in blacks. Arch Ophthal 96:1189.
Robison WG, Kuwabara T, Cogan DG (1975). Lysosomes and melanin granules of the retinal pigment epithelium in a mouse model of Chédiak-Higashi syndrome. Invest Ophthal 14:312.
Robison WG, Kuwabara T (1976). Light-induced alterations of retinal pigment epithelium in black, albino and beige mice. Exp Eye Res 22:549.
Robison WG, Kuwabara T (1978). A new, albino-beige mouse: Giant granules in retinal pigment epithelium. Invest Ophthal Visual Sci 17:365.
Sabtino D, Scialfa A (1966). Un caso di syndrome di Greguez-Steinbrick-Chédiak-Higashi con grave compromissione dell elettro retinogramma. Ann Ottal Clin Occulist 92:793.

Sandhoff K, Christomanou H (1979). Biochemistry and genetics of gangliosidoses. Hum Genet 50:9.
Spencer WH, Hogan MJ (1960). Ocular manifestations of Chédiak-Higashi syndrome. Amer J Ophthal 50:1197.
Sung JH, Meyers JP, Stadlan EM, Cowen D, Wolf A (1969). Neuropathological changes in Chédiak-Higashi disease. J Neuropath Exp Neurol 28:86.
White JG (1966). The Chédiak-Higashi syndrome: A possible lysosomal disease. Blood 28:143.
Windhorst DB, Zelickson AS, Good RA (1968). A human pigmentary dilution based on a heritable subcellular structural defect - The Chédiak-Higashi syndrome. J Invest Derm 50:9.
Yamada E, Ishikawa T (1965). Some observations on the submicroscopic morphogenesis of human retina. In Rohen JW (ed): "Eye Structures," Stuttgart:Schattauer-Verlag, p 5.
Zelickson AS, Windhorst DB, White JG, Good RA (1967). The Chédiak-Higashi syndrome: Formation of giant melanosomes and the basis of hypopigmentation. J Invest Derm 49:575.

Lysosomal Storage Disease

TORTUOSITIES OF RETINAL AND CONJUNCTIVAL VESSELS IN LYSOSOMAL STORAGE DISEASES

J. Libert and D. Toussaint.

Université Libre de Bruxelles.

Service d'Ophtalmologie, Hopital St-Pierre,
322, rue Haute, B-1000 Brussels, Belgium.

Vascular abnormalities of the eyes are frequently reported in lysosomal storage diseases. They may appear as fusiform or saccular microaneurisms in the bulbar conjunctiva and as venous tortuosities in the retina. They also may develop in the skin and the mucosae, figuring telangiectatic lesions or even typical angiokeratoma.

These abnormalities are classical in Fabry's disease (Spaeth and Frost 1965), but have also been described in fucosidosis (Snyder et al 1976), mucolipidosis type 2 (Loonen et al 1974, Suzuki et al 1977), GMI gangliosidosis (Boniuk et al 1976) and in a new disease with still unknown enzyme defect (Tondeur et al 1981).

In Fabry's disease, they have been said to be either primary or secondary to systemic hypertension or renal disease (Franceschetti 1976). Personal observations suggested that they might be related to histopathological lesions in Fabry's disease and in fucosidosis (Libert et al 1976). In the present study, a comparison of the ultrastructural alterations of blood vessel walls in a wide series of lysosomal storage diseases supports this latter hypothesis.

MATERIAL AND METHODS

Conjunctival biopsies were performed for diagnostic purpose in about 200 patients affected with lysosomal storage diseases. Retinal tissues could be obtained at autopsy in some of them, representing many of the different pathological

Birth Defects: Original Article Series, Volume 18, Number 6, pages 347–358

One of our patients affected with the dysmorphic type of mucolipidosis I (sialidosis type 2) had been first diagnosed as an adult case of GMI gangliosidosis (Loonen et al 1974, Koster et al 1976) and later recognized as a sialidosis patient (Lowden and O'Brien 1979). At 23 years of age, he had a coarse face and presented a pyramidal, cerebellar and mental retardation syndrome. Hemangiomas were evident on the skin of the periombilical region and on the eyelids. Several capillary microaneurisms were observed on the bulbar conjunctiva (figure 1 b) but a marked corneal clouding made impossible the examination of the fundus. The second patient was not reported to have vascular abnormalities at 22 years of age (Sogg et al 1980).

Both patients affected with GMI gangliosidosis had normal ocular vessels at the age of 9 months. One of them died shortly after our examination. The second one survived until the age 20 months and showed tortuosities of the conjunctival capillaries at that time.

Finally, two sibs have been proven to represent a new lysosomal storage disease with still unknown biochemical defect (Tondeur et al 1981). In addition to their general dysmorphic and neurological syndrome, their ocular examination remained normal in the first years. At the age of 3, however, the oldest one developed conjunctival aneurisms and vascular tortuosities of the fundus. Both children are still alive at the age of 2 and 4 respectively.

A careful examination of the eyes of the other patients listed in table 2 and 3 failed to reveal any vascular abnormality, either in the conjunctiva or in the retina.

HISTOPATHOLOGICAL DESCRIPTIONS

Since the conjunctival and retinal lesions have been extensively described in the literature, we will only focus our attention in the present paper on the ocular blood vessels (tables 2 and 3).

Vascular lesions of the conjunctiva were very prominent in mucolipidosis 1 type 2, fucosidosis, GMI gangliosidosis, Fabry's disease, type A Niemann-Pick disease, Pompe's disease and in Tondeur's patients. They were characterized by a huge storage process within the lysosomes of the blood capillary

TABLE 2. Blood Capillary Endothelial Lesions in the Conjunctiva and the Retina.

	Number of conjunctival biopsies	Blood capillary endothelium	Number of retinal studies	Blood capillary endothelium
Mucopolysaccharidoses				
MPS I H	12	–	4	–
MPS I S	5	–	2	–
MPS II	8	–	2	–
MPS III	10	±	2	–
MPS IV	2	–	0	
MPS VI	2	–	0	
Mucolipidoses				
ML I type 1	2	–	0	
ML I type 2	2	+++	0	
ML II	9	+	5	+
ML III	6	+	0	
ML IV	1	+	0	
New disease	2	+++	0	
Oligosaccharidoses				
Fucosidosis	4	+++	1	+++
Mannosidosis	5	+	0	

TABLE 3. Blood Capillary Endothelial Lesions in the Conjunctiva and the Retina.

	Number of conjunctival biopsies	Blood capillary endothelium	Number of retinal studies	Blood capillary endothelium
Sphingolipidoses				
GM1 gangl.	2	+++	1	+++
GM2 gangl.	9	±	3	±
Fabry	31	+++	1	+++
MLD	11	–	4	–
Mucosulf.	4	±	0	
Krabbe	4	–	1	–
NPD type A	9	+++	5	+++
type B	4	+	0	
type C	9	±	0	
Ceroid-lipofuscinoses				
Infantile	3	+	1	+
Late infant.	5	+	2	+
Juvenile	11	+	2	+
Adult	1	–	0	
Miscellaneous				
Pompe	3	++	1	++
Cystinosis	5	–	1	–

endothelial cells. The fine structure of the accumulated material was often specific for the disease such as in fucosidosis with the alternation of clear and dark inclusions, in Fabry's disease with very organized lamellar architectures, in Niemann-Pick disease with altered and whorled lipid structures and in Pompe's disease with the juxtaposition of innumerable small glycogen particles. On the contrary, in mucolipidosis I type 2, GMI gangliosidosis and in Tondeur's patients, the material had an aspecific fibrillo-granular appearance (figure 2).

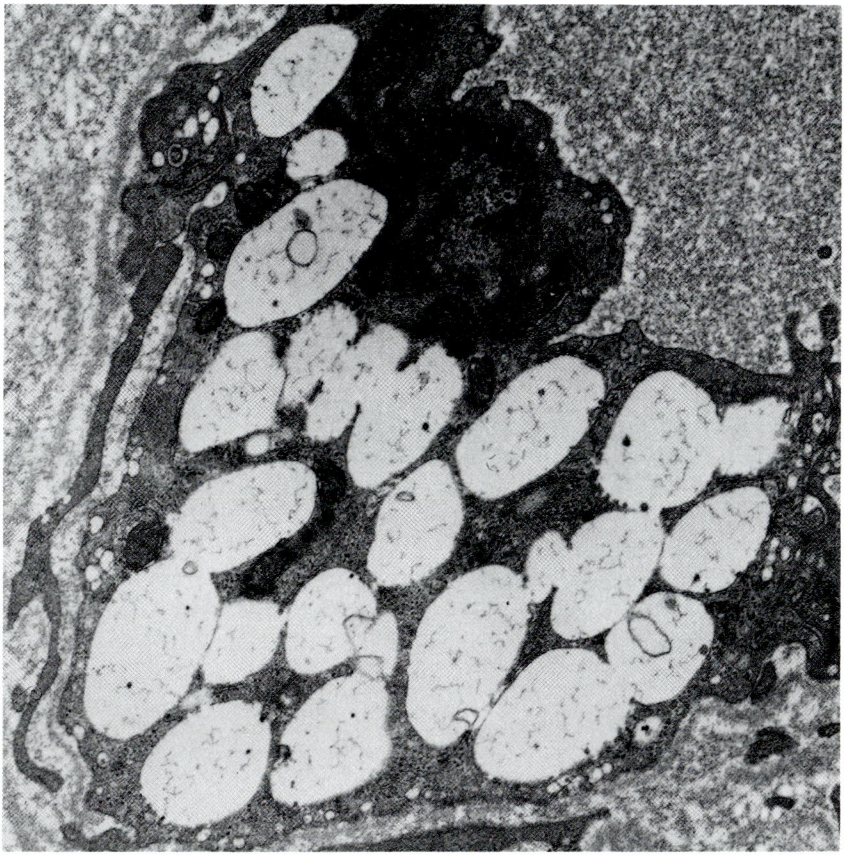

Figure 2. Accumulation of fibrillo-granular material within the lysosomes of conjunctival blood capillary endothelial cells in a patient affected with sialidosis type 2. X 23,000

The cyto-architecture of these endothelial cells was deeply transformed by the storage process. The cells were often ballooned and the distended lysosomes usually occupied more than half of the cytoplasm sections, leaving very little space for the nucleus and the other structures such as mitochondria, Golgi complex, endoplasmic reticulum, pinocytosis vacuoles, microfilaments and myofibrillary bundles.

In many other diseases, some storage lysosomes could be observed in the walls of conjunctival capillaries, but they were often isolated and never altered the general cytoplasmic organization. Finally, in several disorders, the blood capillary endothelium was completely spared, such as in most of the mucopolysaccharidoses, metachromatic leukodystrophy, Krabbe's disease, Kufs disease and cystinosis.

Retinal tissue could be examined in mucopolysaccharidoses, fucosidosis, mucolipidosis II, GMI and GM2 gangliosidoses, type A Niemann-Pick disease and in the neuronal ceroid-lipofuscinoses. Important alterations were observed in fucosidosis, GMI gangliosidosis and in type A Niemann-Pick, Fabry's and Pompe's disases. They consisted of images of a severe lysosomal storage process within the endothelial cells of the capillaries and veins (figure 3), that resembled closely the lesions described in the conjunctiva. Curiously, in many cases, the retinal arteries seemed less severely affected than the capillaries and veins. They even remained totally normal in our patient suffering from fucosidosis.

Very few inclusions were disclosed in vascular endothelial cells of patients affected with mucolipidosis II, GM2 gangliosidosis or ceroid-lipofuscinoses, whereas the vessels were unaffected in mucopolysaccharidoses, metachromatic leukodystrophy, Krabbe's disease and cystinosis.

DISCUSSION

Vascular tortuosities are observed in patients affected with Fabry's disease, fucosidosis, GMI gangliosidosis or MLI (sialidosis) type 2 and in Tondeur's patients. They have never been disclosed in patients affected with other lysosomal storage diseases neither in our series nor in the literature. These pathological images involve the conjunctival capillaries and retinal veins, but it is interesting to note that the retinal arteries are always spared. Similar telangiectasies may appear in the skin and the mucosae. They even may develop into angiokeratoma corporis diffusum in Fabry's disease, sialidosis type 2 and fucosidosis.

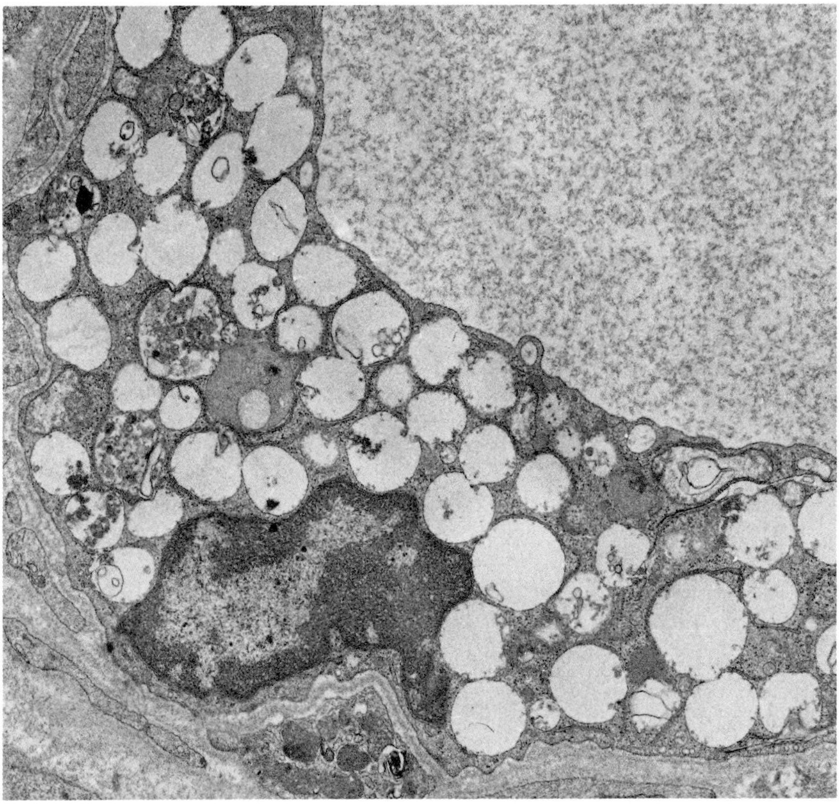

Figure 3. Severe lysosomal storage of a heterogenous material in capillary endothelial cells of a fucosidosis patient retina. X 5,000.

Vascular tortuosities are late and inconstant complications in our patients (table 1). They often appear in the last years of the course of the diseases and are not necessarily present in all affected subjects even at the moment of death. An extensive review of the literature in Fabry's disease indicates that about 50 % of affected males and 44 % of heterozygotes display obvious conjunctival lesions and that the frequency rises with the age of the patients (Franceschetti 1976). A similar observation has been made in fucosidosis and the presence of these abnormalities has even been proposed as means for the recognition of so-called protracted forms of the disease (Snyder et al 1976).

By electron microscopy, a considerable deformation of the endothelial cells of the capillaries and veins is evident in all diseases in which vascular tortuosities may develop. In the present paper, these lesions are described in conjunctival and retinal tissues, but they are part of a generalized process, since skin and liver biopsies of our patients, as well as general autopsy when it was possible, have shown the same abnormalities of vascular endothelial cells all over the body.

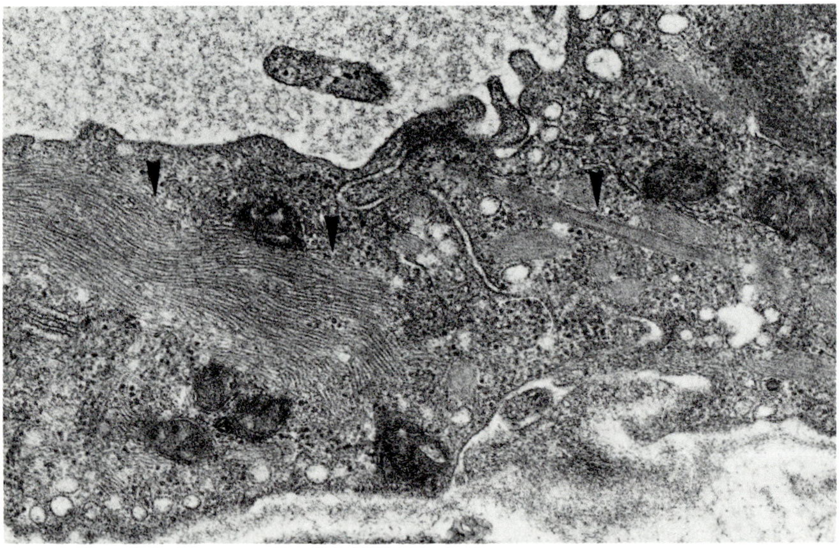

Figure 4. Fibrillary elements are numerous in the blood capillary endothelial cells of the conjunctiva in normal subjects. X 50,000.

These ultrastructural lesions are characterized by a huge storage process within lysosomes, whose volume often occupy more than half of the cytoplasm, leaving very little space for other organelles. More specifically, fibrillar elements, that are normally an important part of the architecture of the endothelial cells (figure 4), seem to be deeply disorganized and even totally absent. These degenerative changes must be responsible for a weak mechanical resistance of the vessel walls to blood pressure. If the disease has a prolonged evolution, this mechanical weakness will induce the characteristic tortuosities, dilatations and aneurisms after several years.

None of the patients, affected with diseases in which endothelial cells show mild histopathological lesions or are totally spared, ever presented any clinical vascular particularities. Curiously, however, patients affected with type A Niemann-Pick disease or with Pompe's disease never display aneurisms nor veinous tortuosities, although important alterations are evident in their vascular walls by electron microscopy. But both disease have a very accelerated course with an early death and the patients probably do not survive long enough to develop these clinical signs.

CONCLUSIONS

Histopathological studies of the conjunctiva and the retina in fucosidosis, mucolipidosis I, GMI gangliosidosis, Fabry's disease and a new disease with still unknown enzyme defect reveal an important overloading of the lysosomal system in the blood capillary and veins endothelial cells, with profound disorganization of the cyto-architecture of the vessel walls.

This process induces a loss of mechanical resistance against blood pressure and is responsible, with time, for the formation of the aneurism-like dilatations and venous tortuosities that are frequently described in these diseases.

ACKNOWLEDGMENTS

We thank all the physicians, who referred the patients to us for electron microscopic examination. This study was supported by a grant of the Belgian Fonds de la Recherche Scientifique Médicale N° 3-4542-79.

REFERENCES

Boniuk V, Ghosh M, Galin M A (1976). Conjunctival aye signs in GMI gangliosidosis. Birth Defects XII:543.

Franceschetti A T (1976). Fabry's disease: Ocular manifestations. Birth Defects XII:195.

Koster J F, Niermeijer M F, Loonen M C B, Galjaard H (1976). Beta-galactosidase deficiency in an adult. Clin Genet 9:427.

Libert J (1980). Diagnosis of lysosomal storage diseases by ultrastructural study of conjunctival biopsies. Pathol Ann 1:37.

Libert J, Tondeur M, Van Hoof F (1976). The use of conjunctival biopsy and enzyme analysis in tears for the diagnosis of homozygotes and heterozygotes with Fabry disease. Birth Defects XII:221.

Libert J, Van Hoof F, Tondeur M (1976). Fucosidosis: Ultrastructural study of conjunctiva and skin, and enzyme analysis of tears. Invest Ophthalmo 15:626.

Loonen M C B, Lugt L V D, Francke C L (1974). Angiokeratoma corporis diffusum and lysosomal enzyme deficiency. Lancet 2:785.

Lowden J A, O'Brien J S (1979). Sialidosis: A review of human neuraminidase deficiency. Am J Hum Genet 31:1.

Snyder R D, Carlow T J, Ledman J, Wenger D A (1976). Ocular findings in fucosidosis. Birth Defects XII:241.

Sogg R L, Steinman L, Rathjen B, Tharp B R, O'Brien J S (1980). Cherry-red spot myoclonus syndrome. In press.

Spaeth G L, Frost P (1965). Fabry's disease. Its ocular manifestations. Arch Ophthalmol 74:760.

Suzuki Y, Nakamura N, Fukuoka K, Shimada Y, Uono M (1977). Beta-galactosidase deficiency in juvenile and adult patients. Hum Genet 36:219.

Tondeur M, Libert J, Vamos-Hurwitz E, Van Hoof F, Thomas G H (1981). A new lysosomal storage disease. In press.

MUCOLIPIDOSIS I

Gerhard W. Cibis*', Ramesh C. Tripathi+, David J. Harris#
*University of Kansas, 'Children's Mercy Hospital, +University of Chicago,#Children's Mercy Hospital
*Kansas City, Ks., 'Kansas City, Mo.,+Chicago, Il.
#Kansas City, MO.

The term "mucolipidosis" describes storage diseases combining clinical findings of both mucopolysaccharidoses and lipidoses without mucopolysacchariduria. Some of the disorders in this group such as: Fucosidosis, Mannosidosis, GM_1 Gangliosidosis and Aspartyglycosaminuria have been chemically characterized by identification of specific enzyme deficiency or storage material. Others, such as I cell diseases, ML-III(pseudo-Hurler polydystrophy) and ML-IV remain chemically less well defined.

Mucolipidosis I as first described by Spranger et al (1968) includes Hurler like facies, skeletal dysplasia, cherry red macula, progressive ataxia, myoclonic epilepsy, mental retardation and death in childhood. Subsequent demonstration of a profound acid neuraminidase deficiency in ML-I patients (Cantz et al 1977) placed them into a group of phenotypically diverse primary acid neuraminidase deficient disease. These include sialidosis, (Durand et al 1977) the cherry red spot myoclonus syndrome, (Rapin et al 1978) the Goldberg-Cotlier syndrome(Goldberg et al 1971) and nephrosialidosis (Maroteaux et al 1978).

The exact clinical, biochemical and genetic relationship of these phenotypically diverse disorders is unclear. Two classifications have arisen. Lowden and O'Brien (1979) divide the neuraminidase disorders into two types both called sialidosis. Type I, normosomatic, presents at age 8-15 years with decreasing vision, cherry red spots, normal growth, intellect and appearance. These include the cherry red spot myoclonus syndrome patients.

Birth Defects: Original Article Series, Volume 18, Number 6, pages 359-380

Type II, labeled dysmorphic, includes the Goldberg-Cotlier and ML-I patients. These have varing degrees of Hurleroid appearance and mucopolysaccharidotic radiographic changes. A juvenile (10.4 years $\pm$ 5.3 years and infantile (0-10 months) age of onset further subdivide the dysmorphic group.

Kelly et al (1981) use the term sialidosis only for the normosomatic group. The juvenile and infantile onset dysmorphic type they call Mucolipidosis I. They feel that the various case reports of the dysmorphic group including Goldberg-Cotlier are describing different periods in the evolution of the same disorder, but differing from the cherry red spot myoclonus syndrome where a significant residual neuraminidase activity remains.

We report the clinical and pathologic ophthalmic findings in two cases of ML-I. The first has systemic findings previously published by Kelly et al (1981).

A female infant was born to a non-consanguineous caucasian couple. The mother had had a first trimester spontaneous abortion. The father was 31, the mother was 38 years of age at the time of birth. Pregnancy was complicated by maternal hypertension, ankle swelling, Herpes type I infection and an upper respiratory infection. Birth weight was 2.8 kg., length 46 cm. A heart murmur was noted at birth.

At 27 days of age she was readmitted to the hospital because of the heart murmur, hepatosplenomegaly and cardiomegaly. There was a suggestion of frontal bossing and anteversion of the nostrils. The corneas were clear. There was vitreous haze with hypopigmentation around the disc. Otherwise, the fundus was normal. There was no corneal clouding or cataracts. Neurological examination was unremarkable. Marked vacuolization of lymphocytes was observed in the peripheral blood smear. The cetyltrimethylammonium chloride test for mucopolysacchariduria was negative. Radiographs of the vertebrae as well as bones of the hands and feet were normal. Skin fibroblasts from a biopsy taken at 11 months of age revealed absences of neuraminidase and increased sialic acid. All the other enzymes were normal.

At 21 months of age the patient was of the 25th percentile for length (73 cm) and head circumference (44 cm). She weighed 7.5 kg. (50th percentile). Facial features had coarsened considerably with more frontal bossing. (Fig. 1).

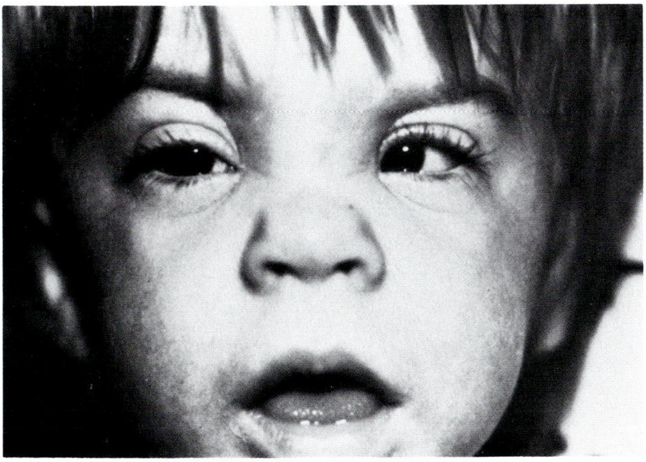

Fig. 1. Hurler like facies of patient. Note esotropia and telangiectasia like prominent skin vascular pattern.

Ophthalmic examination revealed corneal clouding deep stromal and epithelial. There were posterior sutural spoke like cataracts in both lenses (Fig. 2). Conjunctival vessels were uneven in caliber with saccular aneurysmal like

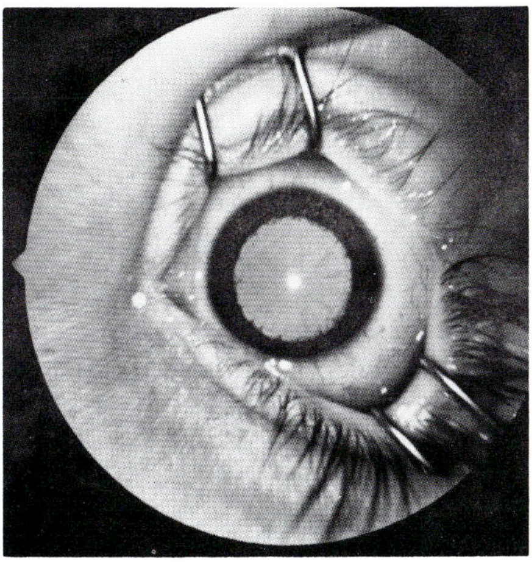

Fig. 2. Spoke like posterior sutural cataract photographed in retroillumination.

dilatations (Fig. 3). Retinal vessels, especially veins,

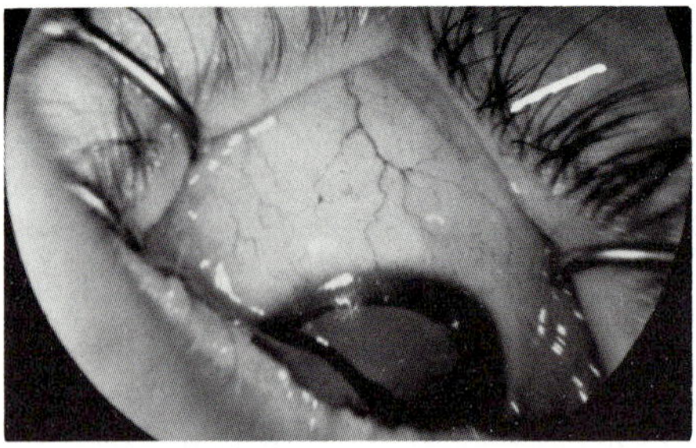

Fig. 3. Tortuous conjunctival vessels of uneven caliber with aneurysmal like dilatations.

had similar findings. (Fig. 4 & Fig. 5). There was no cherry red macula. Extraocular movements were normal with alternating esotropia. (Fig. 1). The patient had a severe hearing loss, was not sitting or standing but could roll over.

The skin had a prominent capillary vascular pattern. (Fig. 1). Radiographs showed cardiomegaly and broad ribs (Fig. 6), frontal bossing (Fig. 7), Hurler like changes of the phalanges (Fig. 8), lumbar kyphosis with inferior beaking of L2 (Fig. 9), remodling of the distal femurs, pelvis changes all consistent with a diagnosis of dysostosys multiplex.

At 24 months of age the patient was readmitted for treatment of cardiomegaly and ascites, without success. Wishing no further aggressive therapy the parents took her home where she died in the company of her parents and family pediatrician.

Both globes were enucleated within 4 hours of death and were fixed in 2.5 per cent buffered glutraldehyde and subsequently transferred to 10 per cent buffered formalin. On gross examination both globes measured 24 x 22 mm with normal corneal diameters. The globes were culloted and gross inspection appeared normal. One cullote was embedded in paraffin wax and sections stained with hematoxylin-eosin. Segments of conjunctiva, cornea, retina, sclera and choroid were post fixed in osmium tetroxide and embedded in epoxy-resins for transmission electron microscopy. Ultrathin sections were stained with uranyl acetate and lead citrate. "Thick" sections were stained with methaline blue for light

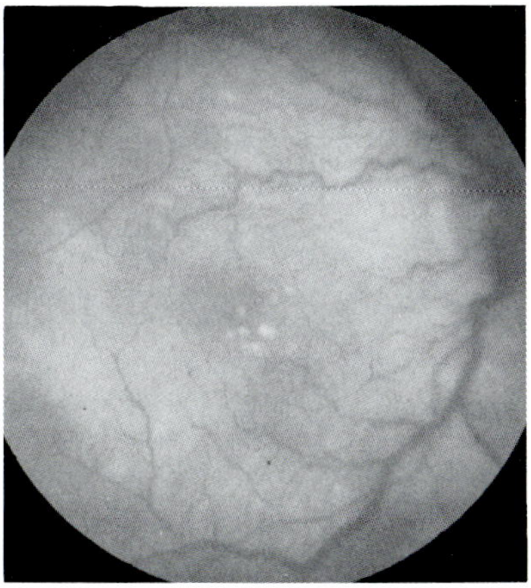

Fig. 4. Fundus right eye shows no cherry red spot, tortuous retinal veins and capillaries of uneven caliber with saccular aneurysmal like dilatations similar to those seen in conjunctival vessels. (Fig. 3). Quality of photographic detail is blurred due to corneal clouding.

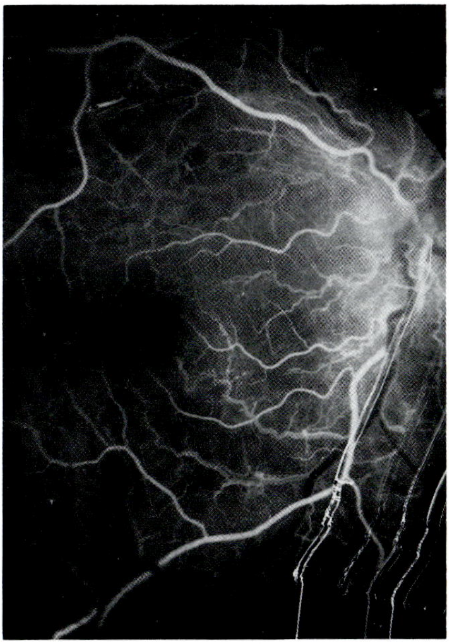

Fig. 5. Arterial phase fluorescein angiogram right eye showing uneven vessel diameters. Later phase photos deteriorated in quality due to rapid extravasation of fluorescein into the vitreous.

Light Microscopy: Routine wax sections for H+E staining light microscopy appeared normal. High power light microscopy of "thick" sections epon embedded material stained with methaline blue showed vacuoles in the corneal epithelium and stromal keratocytes. (Fig. 10). Retinal ganglion cells and

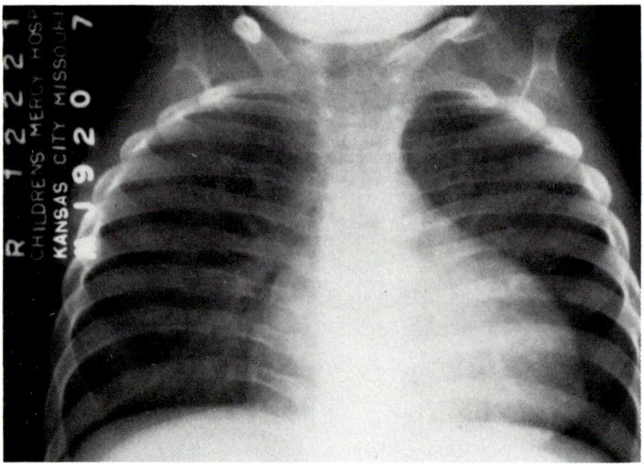

Fig. 6. Chest x-ray showing widened oar like ribs typical of the Hurler phenotype and cardiomegaly.

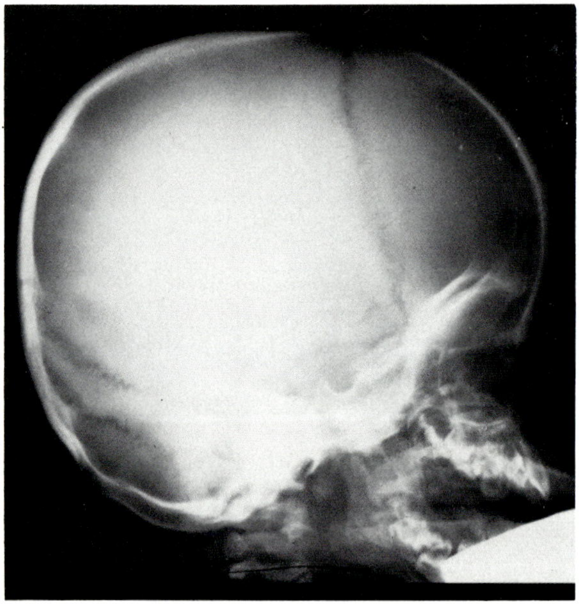

Fig. 7. X-ray of the skull shows a large head with prominent frontal bossing.

inner and outer nuclear layers appeared normal. Bowman's membrane was intact.

Electron Microscopy: Single unit membrane bound clear inclusions containing fine fibrillogranular material with

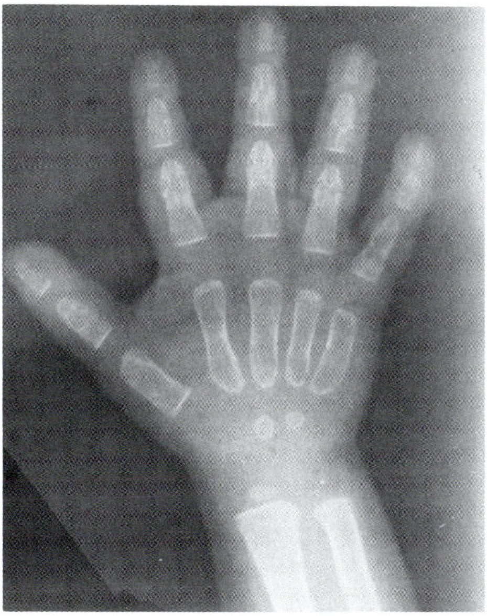

Fig. 8. Hand radiograph shows abnormal tubular bones with thin cortices, widened medullary cavities, and a coarse trabecular pattern all typical findings in the Hurler phenotype.

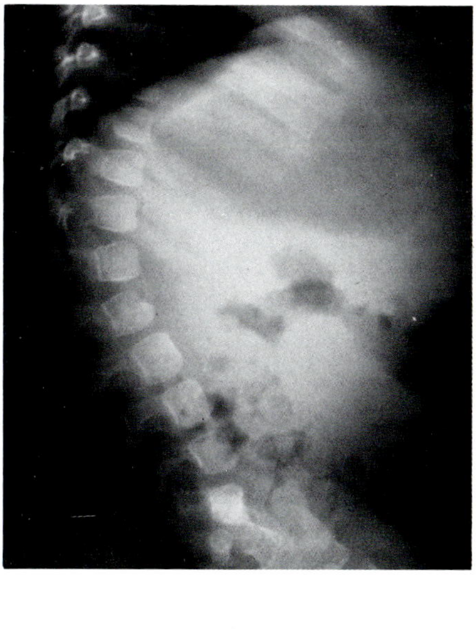

Fig. 9. The spine has a gibbus deformity with beaking of the body of L-2.

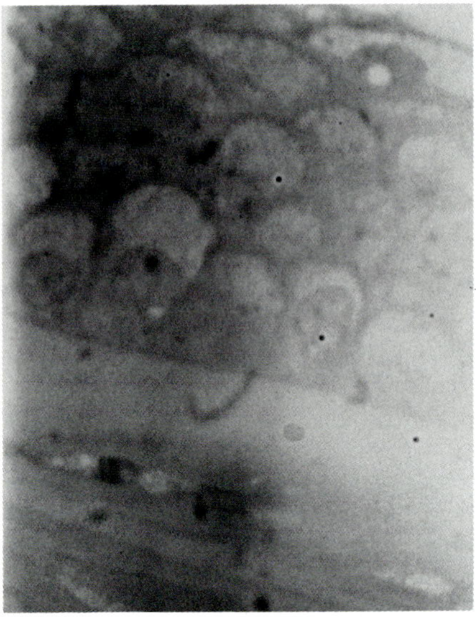

Fig. 10. Epon embedded "thick" section light micrograph of corneal stroma and epithelium. Vacuoles can be seen in all epithelial layers and stromal keratocytes. Bowman's membrane is intact.

occasional membranous lamellar bodies were the dominant pathologic feature. They were present in conjunctival and corneal epithelium (Fig. 11 & Fig. 12), corneal (Fig. 13 & Fig. 14) and conjunctival keratocytes and in the endothelial cells of conjunctival and retinal vessles. (Fig. 15). These inclusions were least prominent but present in all retinal nuclear layers. (Fig. 16). None were seen in the retinal pigment epithelium, sclerocytes or choroidal melanocytes. Membranous lamellar inclusions were rare and when present were usually in small clumps within a vacuole. (Fig. 12). Except for lamellar inclusions the vacuoles were generally clear with some residual fibrillogranular material similar to that seen in mucopolysaccharidoses and other mucolipidosis. In the cornea some fibrillogranular material was present extracellularly along corneal stromal keratocytes apparently extruded from breaks in the cell membrane. (Fig. 14). There was no significant distortion of stromal collagen lamellae by this extracellular material. (Fig. 13).

The second patient was born to a mother who had had multiple miscarriages and finally received depoprogesterone to sustain this pregnancy. The child is spastic, with cerebral palsy, unable to walk and has abnormal muscle movements. He cannot speak but his I.Q. appears normal. Systemic investigation and biochemical analysis have not pinpointed a diagnosis. Test for mucopolysacchariduria were negative.

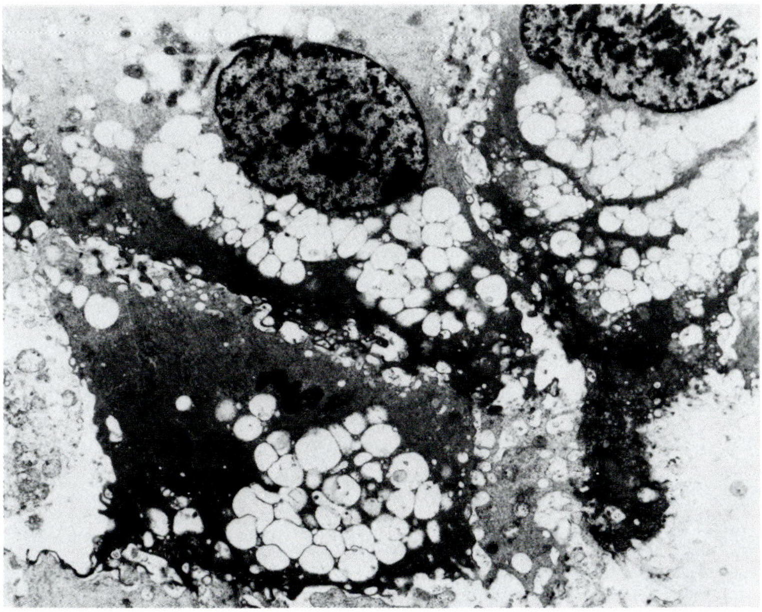

Fig. 11. Conjunctival epithelium showing clear vesicles with some fibrillogranular material and occasional lamellar bodies (8,000 x).

Ophthalmologically, bilateral corneal clouding was noted since early infancy. Slit-lamp examination recorded at 7 years of age revealed a central epithelial haze that appeared as bedewing and extended almost to the limbus. The cornea was not vascularized. Clinically the patient is diagnosed as ML-I. At the age of 7½ years, the severity of the corneal opacities necessitated a lamellar keratoplasty in the right eye. Some 10 months after the initial graft, a lamellar graft was performed in the other eye. The recurrance of the opacification in the epithelium and corneal stroma of the right eye necessitated an 8 mm perforating keratoplasty two years after the initial graft.

Portions of both corneal lamellar discs and the full thickness disc from the right eye were fixed in formaldehyde for conventional light microscopy and in glutaraldehyde

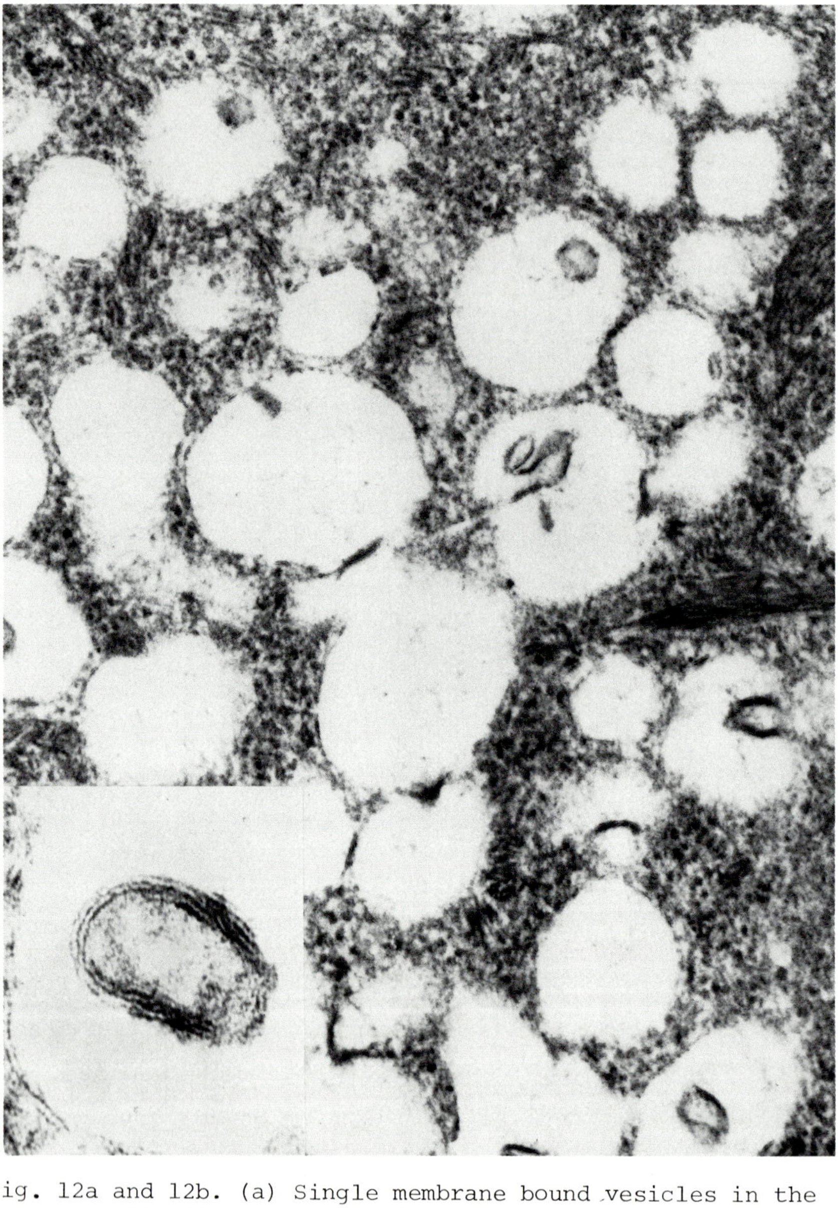

Fig. 12a and 12b. (a) Single membrane bound vesicles in the corneal epithelium with occasional lamellar bodies (52,000 x). (b) Shows lamellar inclusion at triple magnification (331,000 x).

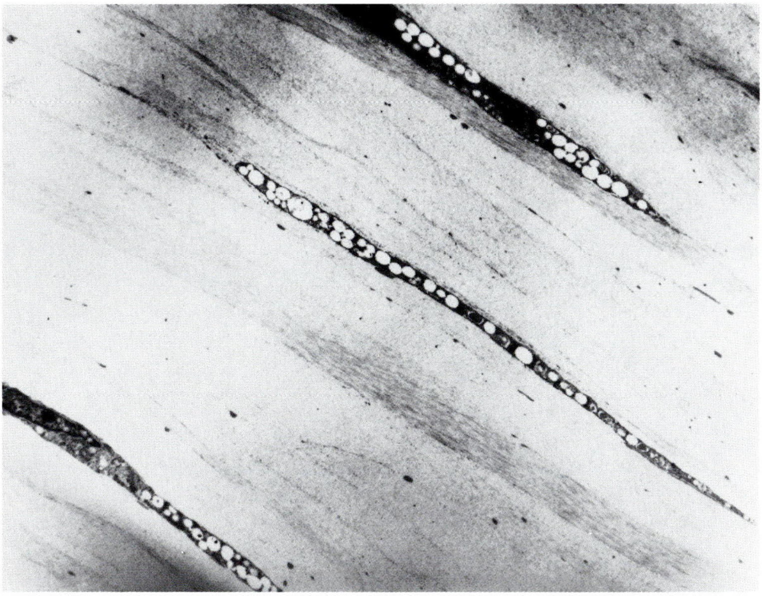

Fig. 13. Keratocytes of corneal stroma with single membrane bound vesicles. Membranous lamellar bodies are more rare than in corneal and conjunctival epithelium (Fig. 11 & Fig. 12) (5,000 x).

followed by osmium tetroxide for transmission electron microscopy. Virtually identical morphologic changes were seen in all three corneal specimens.

In all specimens, the corneal epithelium was moderately irregular with some loss of polarity of cells in the basal layer. The individual ballooned epithelial cells had somewhat eccentric nuclei and contained numerous cytoplasmic vacuolar configurations, most marked in the intermediate and superficial epithelial cell layers. The vacuolar configurations stained moderatley positive with alcian blue and periodic acid Schiff. Frozen sections stained with oil red O showed a few oil red O-positive granules in the vacuolar configurations. The basal cells appeared less vacuolated but contained an alcian blue and PAS-positive material mainly confined to the supranuclear region of the cells.

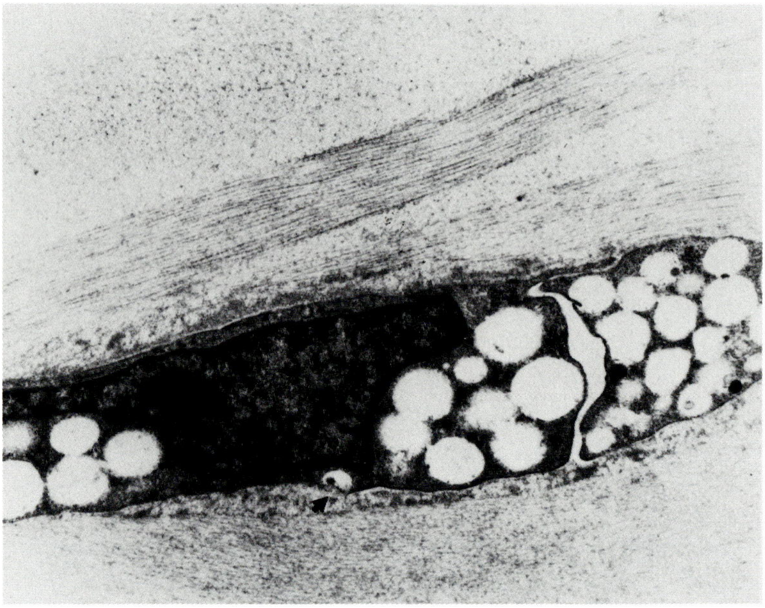

Fig. 14. Corneal keratocyte with vesicle and extracellular fibrillogranular material apparently extruded from breaks in the cell membrane (arrow) (20,000 x).

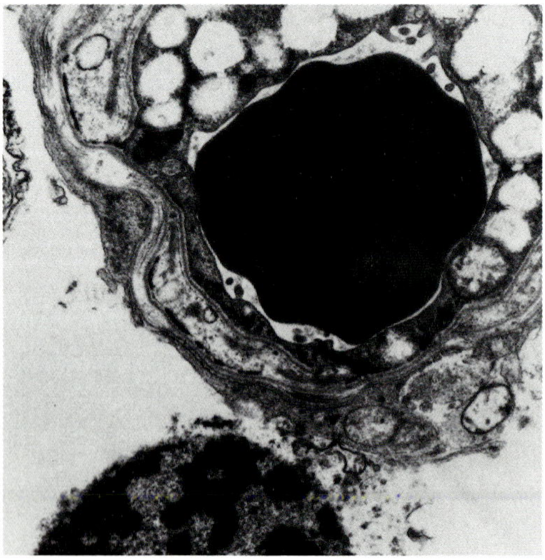

Fig. 15. Clear single membrane bound vesicles in the endothelial cells of a retinal blood vessel (19,500 x).

The basement membrane and Bowman's zone of the stroma were unremarkable. In the remainder of the stroma, particularly the superficial layers, variable staining with alcian blue and periodic acid Schiff was seen in and around some vacuolated keratocytes.

Semi-thin (1-2 um) sections stained with toluidine blue generally confirmed the findings of conventional light microscopy (Fig. 17). Additionally, it revealed irregularity in the staining of the epithelial cells.

Ultrathin (50-80 nm) sections stained with uranyl acetate and lead citrate showed that the vacuolar configurations in the cytoplasm of the epithelial cells were unit-membrane bound and were arranged singly or in clusters. Their content varied from electron-optically empty to electron-lucent granulo-amorphous material and many contained irregular electron-dense, membranous bodies (Fig. 18). At higher magnification, the membranous bodies showed lamellar profiles. Depending upon the plane section,some inclusions presented a

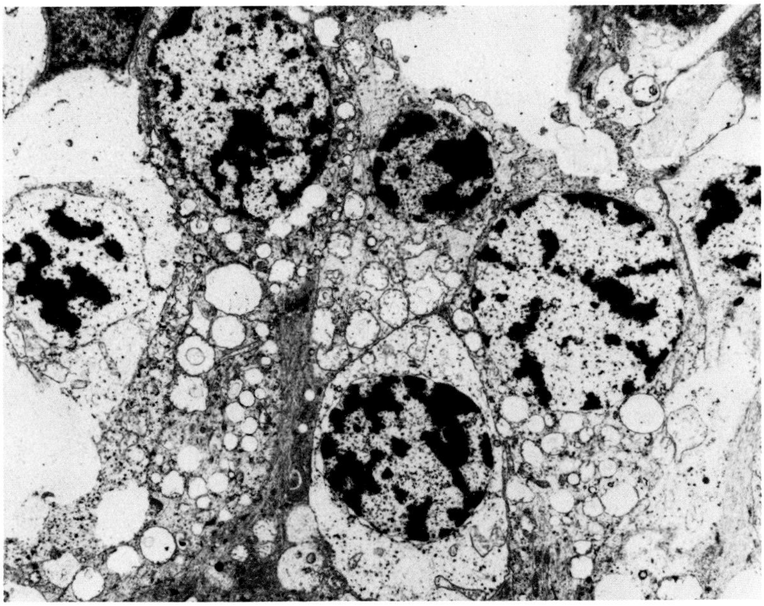

Fig. 16. Storage vesicles in the retina and inner nuclear layer.

disc-like arrangement with a remarkable concentric arrangement of the membranous lamellae. The individual lamellae measured approximately 5 nm in cross-sectional thickness, separated by about 7 nm clear interval (Fig. 19a & b) in the basal epithelial cells, the cytoplasmic vacuolar configurations were relatively small and discrete and were largely occupied by whorl-like membranous bodies (Fig. 20). In the keratocytes of the corneal stroma, the vacuolar configurations were largely electron-optically empty; occasionally, the vacuolar inclusions attained giant profile.

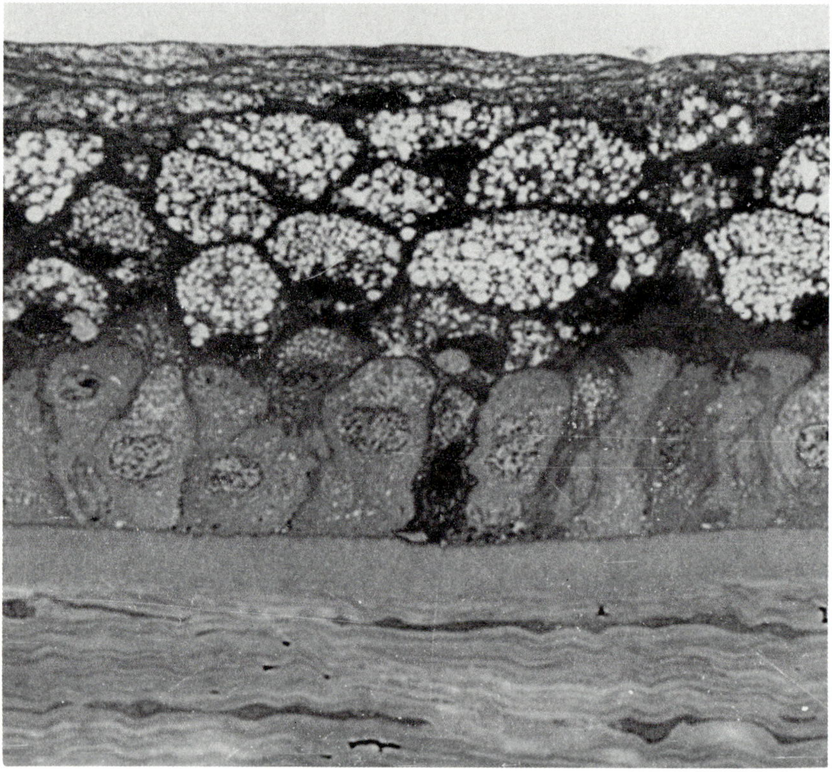

Fig. 17. Light micrograph of epoxy-resin embedded, 1 um section of the cornea showing "vacuolated" corneal epithelium with prominent involvement of the middle epithelial layers. Bowman's membrane is intact. Toluidine blue, (1320 x).

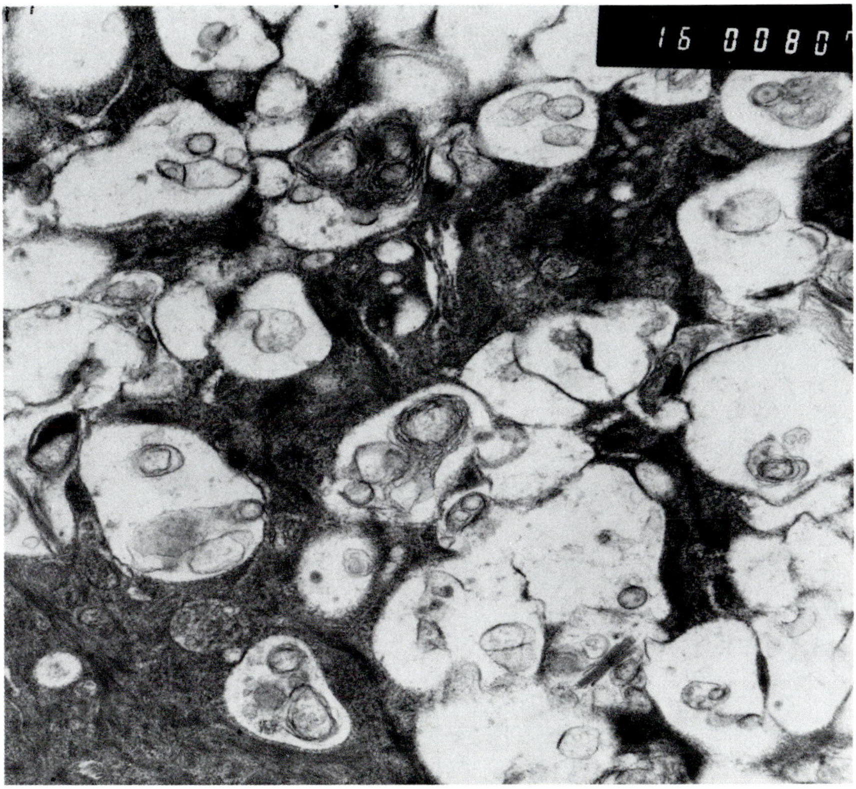

Fig. 18. Electron micrograph of the middle layer of the epithelium showing numerous membrane-bound vesicles containing electron-lucent flocculent or fine granulo-amorphous material and a variable amount of electron-dense membranous bodies. Some vesicles have coalesced together. Uranyl acetate and lead citrate. (33,000 x).

DISCUSSION

The clinical and histopathologic ophthalmic findings in both cases are a unique combination of mucopolysaccharidoses and sphingolipidoses related features justifying the chemically unspecific and therefore at times maligned term mucolipidosis. Clinically, there was corneal clouding typical

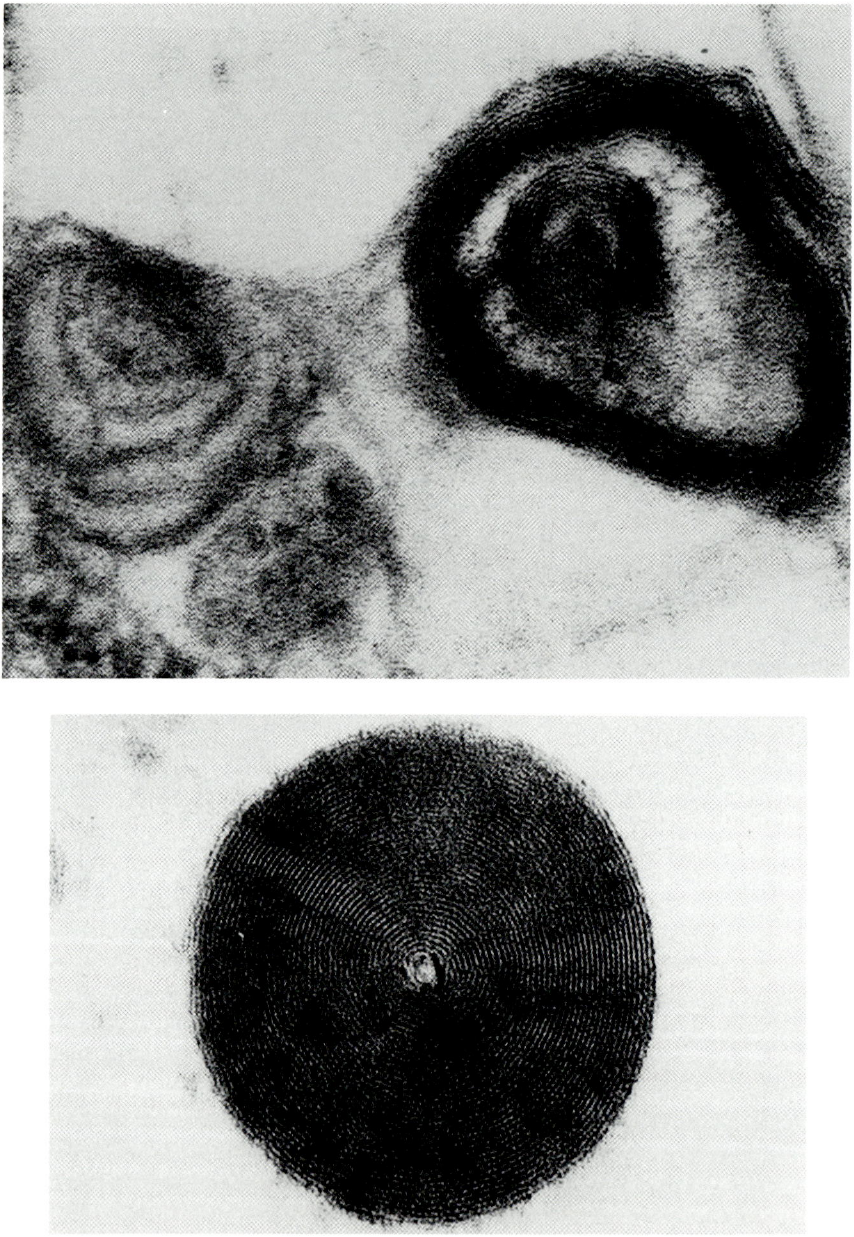

Fig. 19a & b. Higher magnification of the membranous inclusions in the vesicles of the epithelial cells. These inclusions present varied profiles. The individual lamellae are approximately 5 nm in thickness and when concentrically arranged are separated from each other with a clear interval of about 7 nm. Uranyl acetate and lead citrate.(a)(220,000 x) (b)(270,000 x)

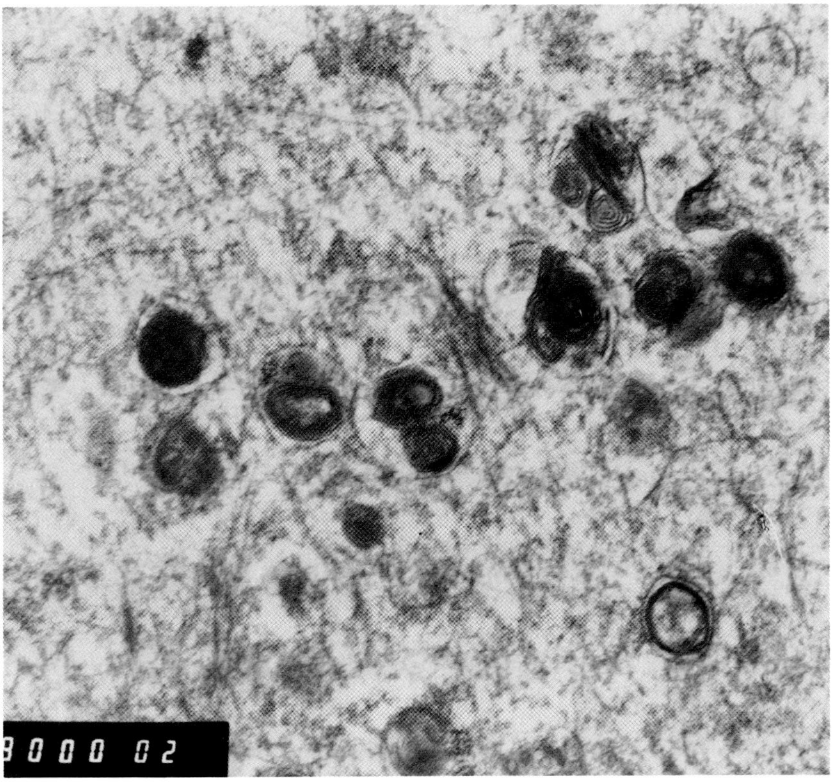

Fig. 20. Electron micrograph of the supranuclear region of the basal cells showing membranous inclusions contained by membrane bound, discrete vesicles. Note the predominance of myelinated bodies with little granuloamorphous material within the vesicles. Compare with Fig.18. Uranyl acetate and lead citrate. (40,000 x)

of mucopolysaccharidoses along with in case one cataracts and tortuous conjunctival and retinal vessels classically associated with Fabry's disease,(Franceschetti 1976) a sphingolipidosis. Similar retinal and conjunctival vascular changes are reported in the mucolipidoses; Fucosidosis, (Snyder et al 1976) (Liebert 1976) and GM_1 Gangliosidosis (Boniuk et al 1976). Spoke like cataracts thought to be pathognomonic for Fabry's disease (Spaeth 1965; Frost 1965) have been reported in Mannosidosis (Murphree et al 1976) and now ML-I.

Histopathologically, the inclusion vacuoles which are the pathologic hallmark of our cases most closely resemble those seen with the mucopolysaccharidoses (Kenyon 1974) with lamellar bodies typical of sphingolipidoses being rare. Lamellar bodies are characteristic of complex lipids, presumably glycolipids the major storage component in the sphingolipidoses and a minor storage component in the mucopolysaccharidoses (Kenyon 1974). They have also been found to varying degrees in other cases of mucolipidoses (Maroteaux et al 1978; Liebert 1976; Liebert et al 1977; Emery et al 1971; Merin et al 1976; Merin et al 1975; Kenyon et al 1979; Le Sec et al 1978; Liebert 1976; Kenyon 1976) some of which such as ML-II are a consequence of multiple enzyme activity. In other such as GM_1 Gangliosidosis the deficiency of a single enzyme (β-galactosidase) leads to the storage of two different substances a ganglioside and a mucopolysaccharide. Whether in this case the storage of two materials is primary therefore justifying the term mucolipidosis or secondary as in the mucopolysaccharidoses is unknown. The predominance of inclusions in blood vessels endothelial cells accounts for the retinal and conjunctival vascular torturosity in case one as it does in Fabry's disease (Franceschetti 1976; Kenyon 1974). In this case however, the vacuoles are clear, presumably containing oligosaccharides. In Fabry's disease they are membranous lamellar bodies, presumably lipid. Blood vessel endothelial cell inclusions similar to the ones in case one have been reported in Fucosidosis (Liebert 1976) and Mannosidosis (Liebert 1976; Kenyon 1976).

Light and electron microscopic studies of the corneal buttons in case two show the predominant pathology to be located in the epithelial rather than in the mesenchymally derived keratocytes. The involvement of the grafted cornea within one year reflects the severity and systemic nature of the disorder. Since MPL I is known to involve the epithelium of the conjunctiva, a total removal of the corneal epithelium would be of limited value since conjunctival epithelial cells which eventually replace the denuded corneal epithelium also share the defect. Similarly, it would appear that the remaining defective host keratocytes eventually invade the grafted corneal stroma to cause opacification.

In the basal epithelial cells membranous whorls largely occupy the unit bound membrane vacuoles. These gradually enlarge in the wing and superficial layers to contain amorphous granular material and therefore relatively fewer membranous inclusions. This suggests that the membranous inclusions are a primary storage substance.

With limited histopathological material available for the various diseases and the phenotypic diversity associated with isolated lysosomal enzyme deficiencies it is difficult to determine what features in any one case are diagnostic. In Mucolipidosis II (I cell disease) the corneal and conjunctival epithelium is often normal (Liebert et al 1977). In GM_1 Gangliosidosis, (Emery et al 1971) Mucolipidosis IV (Merin et al 1976; Kenyon et al 1979) and in our cases the epithelium is markedly involved. The stromal keratocytes were heavily affected as in the mucopolysaccharidoses and GM_1 Gangliosidosis. Unlike those cases Bowman's layer is intact in both our cases and there is no lamellar distortion. Such clinical features may be time dependent and had the patient one survived long enough, could have developed. Cherry red spots are a hallmark of acid neuraminidase deficient patients. Patient one is among the most severly affected for age reported. It is therefore possible that had she not had the cardiac and renal failure that contributed to her early death, the cherry red spot may have developed at a later date. This would be compatiable with Kelly et als (1981) viewpoint, that the juvenile and infantile onset dysmorphic type including the Goldberg-Cotlier syndrome are describing different periods in the evolution of the same disorder.

The great diversity of phenotypic expression in the acid neuraminidase deficiencies is typical of lysosomal storage diseases and comparable to the Hurler-Scheie phenotypes seen with α-L-iduronidase deficiency. Such phenotypic diversity has been postulated to result from allelic mutations of an enzyme active on several substrates (O'Brien 1975). This can give a variety of enzymes with variable patterns of activity towards different substrates. Neuraminic acid in the oligosaccharide chain of glycoprotein is bound by 2,3 and 2,6 linkage. It also occurs in monosialylated and polysialylated forms of gangliosides and is found in keratan sulfate. Allelic mutations of acid neuraminidase could well lead to different patterns of substrate accumulation and therefore variable phenotypic expression. The greater degree of residual enzyme activites seen with the cherry red spot myoclonus syndrome combined with a variable rate of metabolic turnover of such substrates dependent upon age could also account for the phenotypic differences.

There is evidence for at least three complementation groups within the acid neuraminidase disorders (Swallow et al 1981). Complementation analysis by somatic cell hybridization producing heterokaryons show the Lowden & O'Brien (1979) type I patient without skeletal findings to be pure acid neuraminidase deficients (Swallow et al 1981). The type II group into which our patient one falls includes deficients in both acid neuraminidase only and acid neuraminidase and $_{B}$-galactosidase. In our case one as well as the other two cases reported by Kelly et al (1981), $_{B}$-galactosidase activity in cultured fibroblast was normal. Despite this biochemical similarity of Kelly's cases there was a great deal of phenotypic variability. All these cases were not related and are therefore not necessarily homozygous for the same allele. While histopathologic biochemical evidence in our cases indicates the storage of oligosaccharides which presumably are the major storage compound in Mucolipidosis I the cherry red spot of the macula in cases other than our own suggest a concomitant storage of gangliosides. It is evident that numerous detailed biochemical, clinical and histopathologic reports are needed for classification of this disease complex.

Boniuk V, Gosh M, Galin M (1976). Conjunctival eye signs in GM_1 type I Gangliosidosis in The Eye and Inborn Errors of Metabolism. Bergsma D, Bron A, Cotlier E (eds.) National Foundation March of Dimes, Ser. XII #3. p. 543-549.

Cantz M, Gehler J, Spranger J (1977). Mucolipidosis I. Increased sialic acid content and deficiency of an -N-acetylneuraminidase in cultured fibroblasts. Biochem Biophs Res. Commun 74:732-738.

Durand P, Gatti R, Cavalieri S, Borrone C, Tondeur M, Michalski JC, Strecker G (1977). Sialidosis (ML-I). Helv. Paediat Acta. 32:391-400.

Emery J, Green W, Wyllie R, Howell R (1971). GM_1Gangliosidosis. Arch Ophth. 85:177-187.

Franceschetti A, Th. (1976). Fabry's Disease: Ocular Manifestations in The Eye and Inborn Errors of Metabolism, pages 195-208.

Goldberg MF, Cotlier E, Fichenscher LG, Kenyon K, Ennt R, Borowsky SA (1971). Macular cherry red spot corneal clouding and $_B$-galactosidase deficiency. Arch Intern Med 128:387-398.

Kelly T, Bartosheska L, Harris DJ, McLauley R, Feingold M, Schott G (1981). Mucolipidosis I (Acid Neuraminidase Deficiency). Am J Dis Child 135:703-708.

Kenyon K (1974). Ocular Ultrastructure of Inherited Metabolic Disease: in Genetic and Metabolic Eye Disease. Goldberg M (ed). p. 139-185.

Kenyon K, Maumenee I, Green R, Liebert J, Hiatt R (1979). Mucolipidosis IV. Arch Ophth 97:1106-1111.

Le Sec G, Stanescu R, Lyon G (1978). Un noveau type de sialidose avec atteinte Renale: La Nephrosialidose II etude anatomique. Arch Frac Pe'diat 35:830-844.

Liebert J (1976). Discussion remarks p. 255-256 in The Eye and Inborn Error of Metabolism.

Liebert J, Van Hoof F, Farriaux JP, Toussaint D (1977). Ocular Findings in I-cell Disease (Mucolipidosis Type II). AJO 83:617-628.

Liebert J, Kenyon K (1976). Discussion remarks in The Eye and Inborn Errors of Metabolism p. 329-334.

Lowden J, O'Brien JS (1979). Sialidosis: A Review of Human Neuraminidase Deficiency. Am J of Hum Genet 31:1-18.

Maroteaux P, Humbel R, Strecker G, Michalski JC, Mande R (1978). Un noveau type de sialidose avec atteinte renale La nephrosialidose. Arch Frac Pe'diat 35:819-829.

Merin S, Nemet P, Livni N, Lazar M (1976). The cornea in Mucolipidosis IV. J of Ped Ophth 13:289-295.

Merin S, Livni N, Berman ER, Yatziv S (1975). Mucolipidosis

IV: Ocular, Systemic and Ultrastructural findings. Inv Ophth 14:437-448.

Murphree A, Becudet A, Palmer E, Nichols B (1976). Cataract in Mannosidosis: in The Eye and Inborn Error Metabolism p.319-325.

O'Brien JS (1975). Molecular genetics of $GM:_B$-galactosidase. Clin Genet 8:303-313.

Rapin I, Goldfischer S, Katzman R, Engel J, O'Brien JS (1978) The cherry red spot myoclonus syndrome. Ann Neurol 3: 234-242.

Snyder R, Carlow T, Ledman D (1976). Ocular Findings in Fucosidosis: The Eye and Inborn Error of Metabolism p. 241-251.

Spaeth G, Frost P (1965). Fabry's Disease. It's Ocular Manifestations. Arch Ophth 74:760-769.

Spranger JW, Wiedemann HR, Tolksdorf M, Grancob E, Caesar R (1968). Lipomucopolysacharidoses. Z. Kinderheilk 103: 285-290.

Swallow D, Hogeveen A, Verheijen F, Galjaard H (1981). Complementation analysis of human sialidase deficiency using natural substrates. Ann Hum Genet 45:105-112.

TWO BROTHERS WITH PRESUMED MUCOLIPIDOSIS IV[1]

Johan Zwaan, M.D., Ph.D.[2] and Kenneth R. Kenyon, M.D.

Pediatric Service and Cornea Service of the Massachusetts Eye and Ear Infirmary, Morphology Unit and Cornea Research Department of the Eye Research Institute of the Retina Foundation, and the Department of Ophthalmology, Harvard Medical School, Boston, Massachusetts, 02114, USA

The mucolipidoses were first recognized as a separate group of genetic lysosomal storage diseases about a decade ago (Spranger and Wiedemann 1970). In some aspects they resemble the mucopolysaccharidoses, in others the lipidoses. Patients afflicted with these diseases show variable psychomotor and mental retardation and they may exhibit facial and skeletal abnormalities. They have no abnormal mucopolysacchariduria. Biopsies of various tissues have shown abnormal lysosomal inclusion bodies suggesting storage of acid mucopolysaccharide as well as glycolipids (see review by Legum, Schorr and Berman 1976).

The most recently recognized type of mucolipidosis is mucolipidosis IV, which was first reported in a 2 month old infant presenting with bilateral corneal clouding (Berman, Livni, Shapira, Merin and Levij 1974). Since then seven additional cases have been described (Merin, Livni, Berman and Yatziv 1975; Newell, Matalon and Meyer 1975; Merin, Nemet, Livni and Lazar 1976; Tellez-Nagel, Rapin, Iwamoto, Johnson, Norton and Nitowsky 1976; Kenyon, Maumenee,

[1]Supported in part by NEI Research Grant EY-03158, NEI Academic Investigator Award 00156, the Research to Prevent Blindness James S. Adams Research Award, and Grant-in-Aid from Fight for Sight, Inc., New York City.
[2]Send reprint requests to Dr. J. Zwaan, Dept. of Ophthalmology, Mass. Eye and Ear Infirmary, Boston, MA 02114, USA.

Birth Defects: Original Article Series, Volume 18, Number 6, pages 381-390

Green, Libert and Hiatt 1979). These patients were clinically characterized by corneal clouding and psychomotor retardation with an absence of gross skeletal or facial deformities. Seven of the patients were of Ashkenazi Jewish origin, while in one the origin was not specified. Histochemical and electron microscopic studies have been carried out on a variety of biopsy material from these patients. Abnormal accumulation of acid mucopolysaccharide and complex lipid was found but the storage material was not further characterized, although both mucopolysaccharide and gangliosides accumulate in cultured fibroblasts (Bach, Cohen, Kohn 1975; Bach, Zeigler, Kohn, Cohen 1977). Activities of most acid hydrolases in fibroblasts or leukocytes have been within the normal range, but recently it has been suggested that the specific defect in mucolipidosis IV is a reduced activity of lysosomal ganglioside sialidase (Bach, Zeigler, Schaap and Kohn 1979).

Recently we have seen two brothers, 21 and 18 years old, who show many features of mucolipidosis IV, in particular typical ultrastructural abnormalities of the conjunctiva. Even though some clinical findings and the origin of the patients are not entirely typical compared to those in previously reported cases of mucolipidosis IV, we believe that they in fact represent two additional examples of this rare metabolic disorder.

CASE HISTORIES

The first patient was born on February 22, 1960. Although the baby appeared normal at birth, within a few months it became clear that motor development was grossly delayed. At age 13 months patient underwent detailed evaluation. His head circumference was 44 cm, below the third percentile. Moderate hepatosplenomegaly was found. Profound hypotony was present and the boy was unable to lift his head. Babinski reflexes were bilaterally positive. Eye examination was normal. Laboratory studies were non-revealing. Skeletal survey showed microcephaly and a bone age of 6 months as compared to a chronological age of 13 months but no other abnormalities. No diagnosis was made. At age 22 months patient was institutionalized. In 1977 corneal opacification and pale optic nerve were noted, as well as a pigmentary retinopathy. No response to light or threat could be elicited. The pupils reacted only sluggishly to light. There was marked hypertonic quadriparesis. Severe kyphoscoliosis and pectus carinatum were present. The level of a variety of acid hydrolases in leukocytes was within the normal range. Urinalysis showed a weakly positive Berry spot test and an elevated urinary chondroitin sulfate was found. No diagnosis was made at that time, but in 1981, with the clinical picture essentially unchanged, a conjunctival biopsy was performed and processed according to routine methods (Kenyon, Maumenee, Green, Libert and Hiatt 1979; Kenyon 1980), which yielded a tissue diagnosis.

The second case is a younger brother of the first patient, born on January 21, 1963. Patient's abnormalities, first noted by his mother at about 4 months, and the subsequent clinical course were remarkably similar to his brother's and will not be elaborated here. Clinical laboratory findings were also very similar. A conjunctival biopsy was done here as well. Figure 1 shows the appearance of this patient.

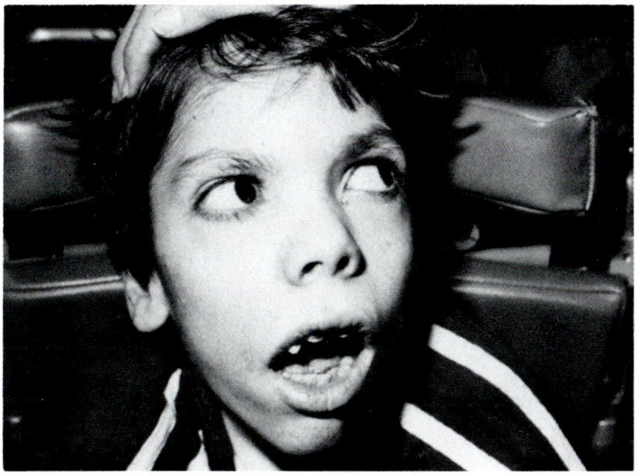

Fig. 1. The facial features of Case 2. Severe microcephaly, a large mouth and low-set large ears are present, but otherwise no unusual features are noticeable.

The family history was negative for mental retardation, neurological disease or other systemic disease. Other than refractive errors there are no known eye abnormalities in the family. Both parents were Hungarian Roman Catholics. There was no consanguinity. There is one normal female sibling and one normal female half-sib from a previous marriage of the mother as well as two half-sibs from a later marriage. The father of the boys is deceased.

ULTRASTRUCTURAL FINDINGS

Biopsy specimens of bulbar conjunctiva from both patients were processed for electron microscopy. Light microscopy was done on semithin sections stained with paraphenylenediamine

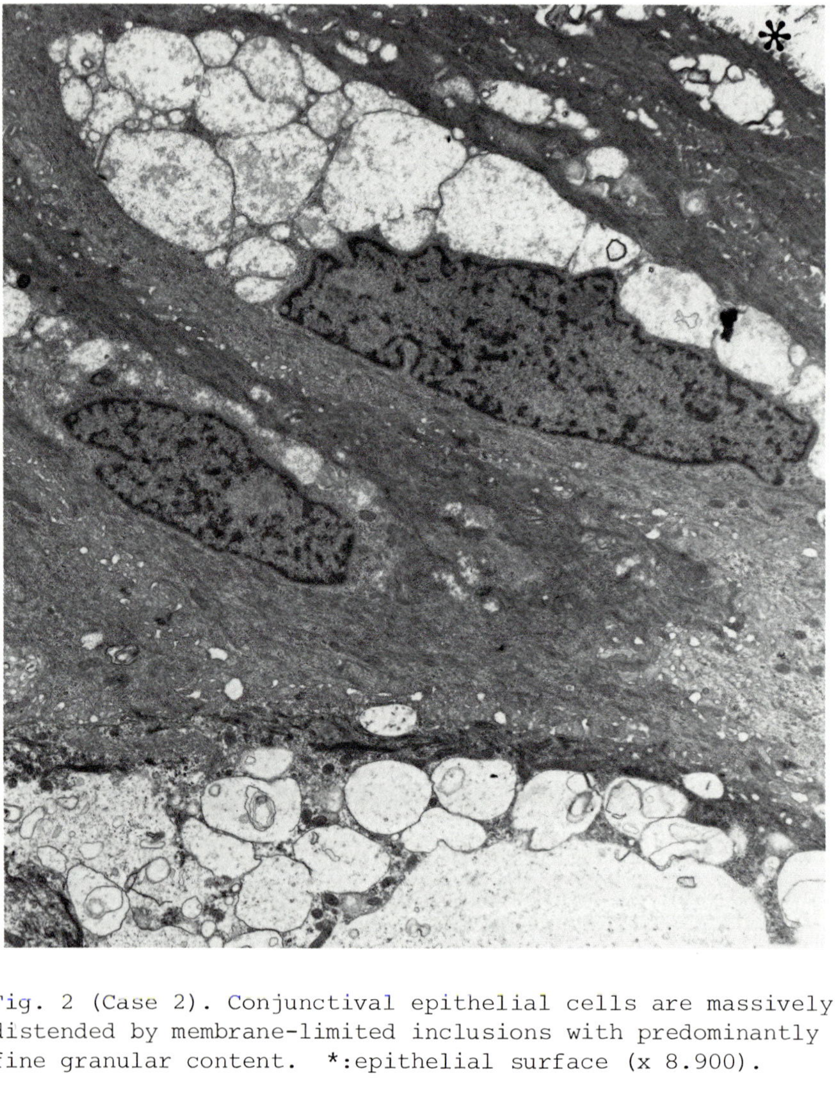

Fig. 2 (Case 2). Conjunctival epithelial cells are massively distended by membrane-limited inclusions with predominantly fine granular content. *:epithelial surface (x 8.900).

(Kenyon, Maumenee, Green, Libert and Hiatt 1979).

The conjunctival epithelium in both cases showed striking abnormalities even at the light microscope level. The superficial and intermediate epithelial cell layers were massively engorged with vacuoles, which with the transmission electron microscope were found to have a fine granular content consistent with the presence of acid mucopolysaccharide (Figure 2). The stromal connective tissue cells were less impressively involved by the storage phenomenon and ultrastructurally the material accumulated within the intracellular organelles, presumably lysosomes, consisted of concentric membranous lamellar whorls thought to represent complex phospholipids (Figure 3).

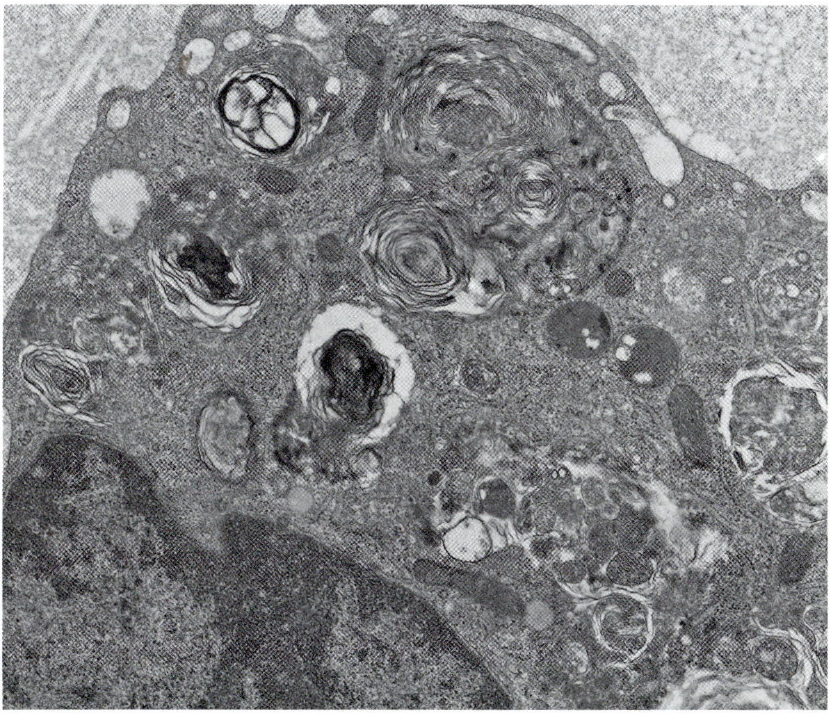

Fig. 3 (Case 2). Conjunctival stromal cells contain lysosome-like bodies filled with complex lipids arranged as concentric membranous lamellae (x 18,700).

The tissue macrophages, leukocytes and the endothelial cells of capillaries and lymphatics were also less severely affected. All, however, showed extensive single-membrane

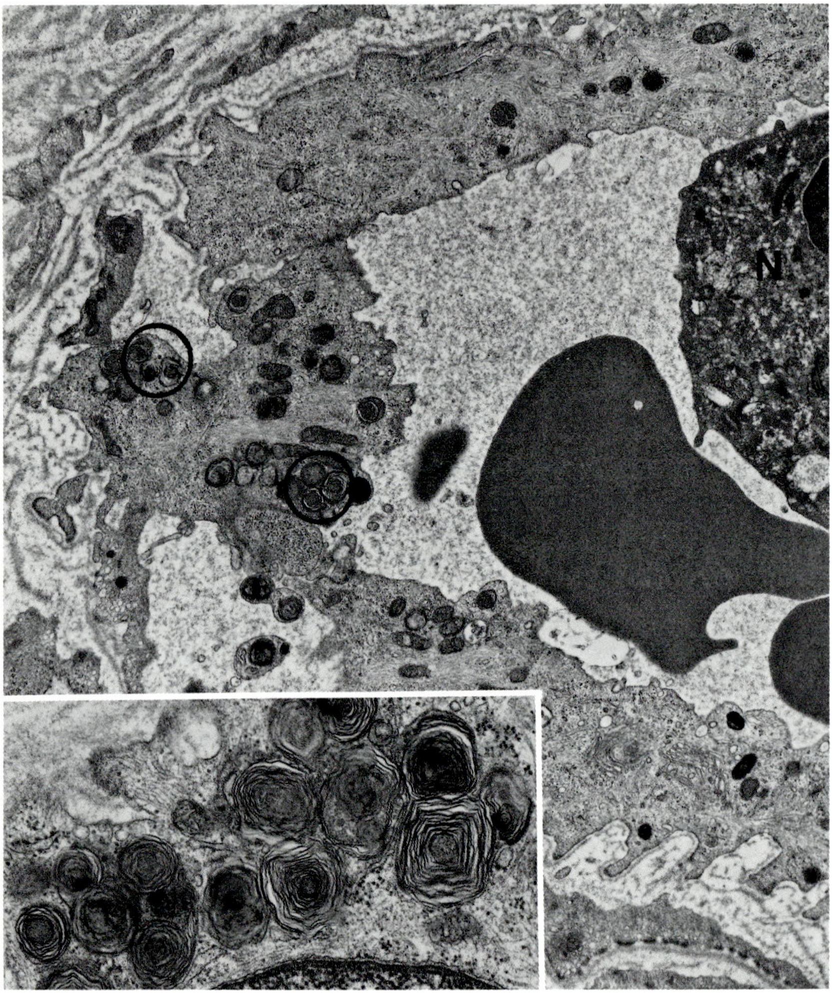

Fig. 4 (Case 1). Conjunctival capillary shows numerous inclusions (circled) within endothelial cells. A polymorphonuclear neutrophil(N) within the vascular lumen contains abnormal granular material (x 10,600). The inset shows, at higher magnification, the membranous lamellar character of the intralysosomal accumulations within the capillary endothelial cells (x 27,100).

limited vacuoles with membranous lamellar inclusions (Figure 4). Similar intracytoplasmic bodies were seen in the epithelial cells but those containing fibrillogranular material were much more numerous.

DISCUSSION

The diagnosis of mucolipidosis IV was suggested in our two patients by the combination of severe corneal clouding and mental and neurological retardation. Although kyphoscoliosis and other skeletal abnormalities were found in both brothers, these were thought to be secondary to long-standing spastic quadriparesis and immobility rather than a primary expression of the metabolic defect. Indeed, at an early age skeletal X-rays were unremarkable except for the presence of microcephaly and bone age retardation.

There are some clinical differences between these two patients and the ones reported previously, the significance of which is unclear at this time. Most patients were of Ashkenazi Jewish descent (Berman, Livni, Shapira, Merin and Levij 1974; Merin, Livni, Berman and Yatziv 1975; Merin, Nemet, Livni and Lazar 1976; Tellez-Nagel, Rapin, Iwamoto, Johnson, Norton and Nitowsky 1976; Kenyon, Maumenee, Green, Libert and Hiatt 1979), while the parents of our two patients were Hungarian and allegedly of non-Jewish extraction. Corneal clouding was a prominent presenting sign at a very early age in all patients. Psychomotor retardation was usually mild in the first months of life, although progressive. In contrast, our patients showed profound psychomotor retardation very shortly after birth and eye examinations were stated to be normal. Corneal opacification was not noted until the two brothers were in their mid-teens. This may be a true difference or the corneal abnormality may simply not have been noted earlier due to the institutionalized setting in which the boys were raised. Other differences are the moderate hepatosplenomegaly found early and the recent finding of mucopolysacchariduria with elevation of urinary chondroitin sulfate, both of which have been absent in the other patients. These findings may indicate that we are dealing with a variant of mucolipidosis IV, or they may represent minor variations due to differences in genetic background and in the age at which the patients were studied. Clarification of this will have to await the outcome of further biochemical studies.

and skin. Arch Ophthal 97:1106.
Kohn G, Livni N, Beyth Y (1975).Prenatal diagnosis of mucolipidosis IV by electron microscopy. Pediatr Res 9:314.
Legum CP, Schorr S, Berman ER (1976).The genetic mucopolysaccharidoses and mucolipidoses: review and comment. Advances Pediatr 22:305.
Merin S, Livni N, Berman ER, Yatziv S (1975).Mucolipidosis IV. Ocular,systemic and ultrastructural findings.Invest Ophthal 14:437.
Merin S, Nemet P, Livni N, Lazar M (1976). The cornea in mucolipidosis IV. J Pediatr Ophthal 13:289.
Newell FW, Matalon R, Meyer S (1975).A new mucolipidosis with psychomotor retardation,corneal clouding and retinal degeneration. Amer J Ophthal 80:440.
Spranger JW, Wiedemann HR (1970).The genetic mucolipidoses. Diagnosis and differential diagnosis.Humangenetik 9:113.
Tellez-Nagel I, Rapin I, Iwamoto I, Johnson AB, Norton WT, Nitowsky H (1976).Mucolipidosis IV: Clinical,ultrastructural, histochemical, and chemical studies of a case,including a brain biopsy. Arch Neurol 33:828.

A MILD VARIANT OF MUCOLIPIDOSIS TYPE 4 (ML4)

B.D. Lake, P.J. Milla, D.S.I. Taylor,
Elisabeth P. Young
Departments of Histopathology, Child
Health, Ophthalmology and Chemical
Pathology

Hospital for Sick Children and
Institute of Child Health
Great Ormond Street
London WC1N U.K.

INTRODUCTION

Mucolipidosis type 4 (ML4) is a relatively recently recognized disorder (Berman et al 1974) which is characterized by corneal clouding and psychomotor retardation. Although the earlier cases (Berman et al 1974, Livni and Merin 1978, Kenyon et al 1979) occurred in children of parents of Ashkenazi-Jewish origin, later cases (Goutières et al 1979) showed no such genetic links. Of the children with ML4 seen at The Hospital for Sick Children two brothers were from the United Arab Emirates, and the case presented here was the first born child of an English mother and a Cape Coloured father.

Most cases have suffered from moderate to severe psychomotor retardation. Our 8½ year old patient showed improvement with a corneal graft and we feel that he has a mild form of ML4 with minimal retardation which is mainly caused by his poor vision.

CASE HISTORY

D.V. was born at term following a normal

Birth Defects: Original Article Series, Volume 18, Number 6, pages 391–404

earlier and shortly after this his vision seemed to deteriorate. His acuity was found to be 6/60 and it became obvious that his grafted cornea was becoming cloudy and was involved in his basic disease process.

Reconsideration of the histology of the corneal graft suggested the possible diagnosis of ML4.

His vision continued to deteriorate and this was accompanied by a deterioration in his motor performance. He was therefore re-admitted for further assessment.

A visual evoked response and electroretinogram showed that the retinal response was now very poorly defined and was of low amplitude. The record suggested fairly gross loss of function of outer retinal receptor elements. The cortical response was still fairly well preserved.

His ataxia when walking was more noticeable but movements not guided by vision were unchanged, and he seemed to be making progress with his speech. However a psychological assessment showed that on the Williams scale he achieved a score at approximately the 4 year level at a chronological age of 7½ years. A skin biopsy was cultured and the fibroblasts examined.

MATERIAL AND METHODS

Light Microscopy: A portion of the removed corneal button was fixed in 4% phosphate buffered formaldehyde and processed into wax for routine sections.

Electron Microscopy: A portion of the corneal button, a conjunctival biopsy, cultured fibroblasts and a buffy coat of white blood cells were fixed in 2.7% glutaraldehyde in 0.1M cacodylate buffer pH7.4, osmicated and processed into Araldite. Ultra thin sections were stained with uranyl acetate and lead citrate.

Urinary Oligosaccharides: Unconcentrated urine from a random sample was applied to silica gel thin layer chromatography plates (Merck 5721) and developed in chloroform, methanol, water (70, 30, 5) or n-butanol, acetic acid, water (2, 1, 1) for 18 hours. Oligosaccharides were detected with diphenylamine, and sialyl residues were shown with the resorcinol reagent of Svennerholm (Lake and Goodwin 1976).

Neuraminidase (sialidase) Assay: Cultured fibroblasts were homogenized by hand and assayed within 2 hours of homogenization. Unhomogenized samples could be stored deep frozen for at least 2 years, but the enzyme was found to be unstable once the cells had been homogenized. The substrate, 4-methylumbelliferyl-N-acetyl-α-D-neuraminide, ammonium salt, was obtained from Koch-Light Laboratories Ltd, UK.

The incubation mixture consisted of 10 μl 0.4M sodium acetate buffer pH 4.2, 10 μl 4mM substrate in water, 10 μl homogenate containing up to 35 μg protein. Incubation at 25 ^{o}C was for 1-2 hours. The reaction was stopped by the addition of 2.47 ml 0.25M glycine-NaOH buffer pH 10.4 and the fluorescence read at 440 nm (excitation at 360 nm). Water was substituted for the homogenate in the blank. Protein was measured by the method of Lowry et al (1951).

RESULTS OF LABORATORY INVESTIGATIONS

The cells of the outer layers of the corneal epithelium showed marked vacuolation in contrast with the basal cells which appeared normal (Fig 1). The content of the vacuoles with PAS negative (Fig 2) but gave a positive reaction with Alcian Blue and colloidal iron (Fig 3) indicating acidic groupings. Stromal cells were not affected. Bowman's capsule and Descemets membrane were thinner than normal and vacuolation of the cells of Descemets membrane was found.

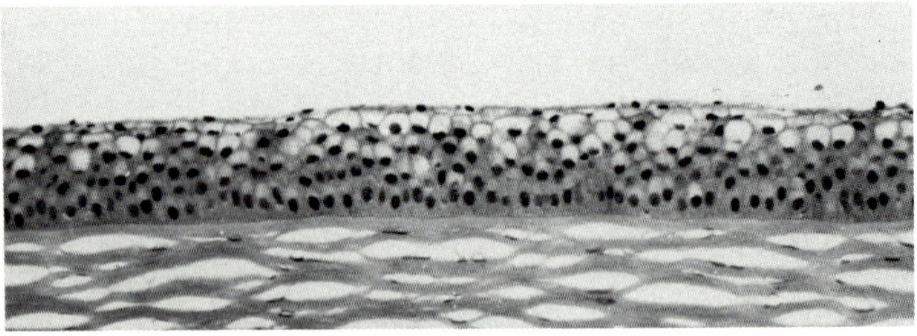

Figure 1 Corneal epithelium shows vacuolation of the superficial layers. Haematoxylin and eosin x 170

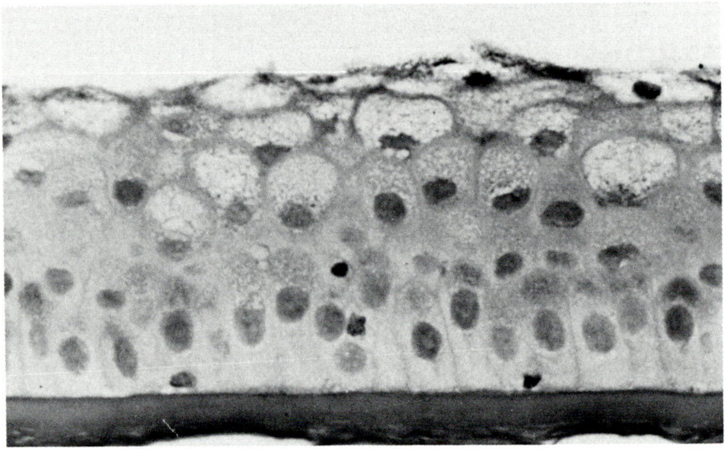

Figure 2 Only occasional PAS positive granules are present in the vacuolated corneal epithelium. PAS x 700

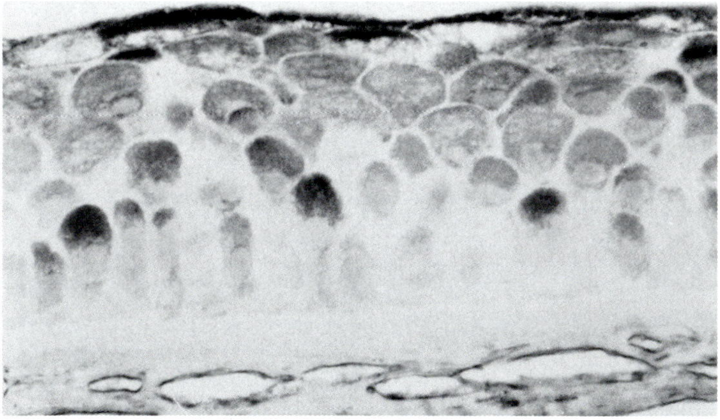

Figure 3 The vacuolated cells, and some in the deeper layers of the epithelium stain strongly with the colloidal iron reagent indicating the presence of an acidic substance. Colloidal iron x 700

Electron microscopy of the vacuolated superficial corneal cells showed mainly empty membrane bound vacuoles in which a few membranous lamellae could be seen (Fig 4). Epithelial cells of the conjunctiva contained numerous membranous cytoplasmic bodies (Fig 5). Similar MCB's and vacuoles were present in some fibroblasts of the conjunctival stroma.

Most lymphocytes were structurally normal and no vacuolation was seen by light microscopy. However membrane bound MCB's were found in occasional lymphocytes (Fig 6). Other blood cells appeared normal.

Cultured fibroblasts contained numerous densely osmiophilic inclusions measuring between 0.3 and 1.0 µm (Fig 7). The inclusions were membrane bound and contained tightly packed membranous cytoplasmic bodies (MCB's) (Fig 8).

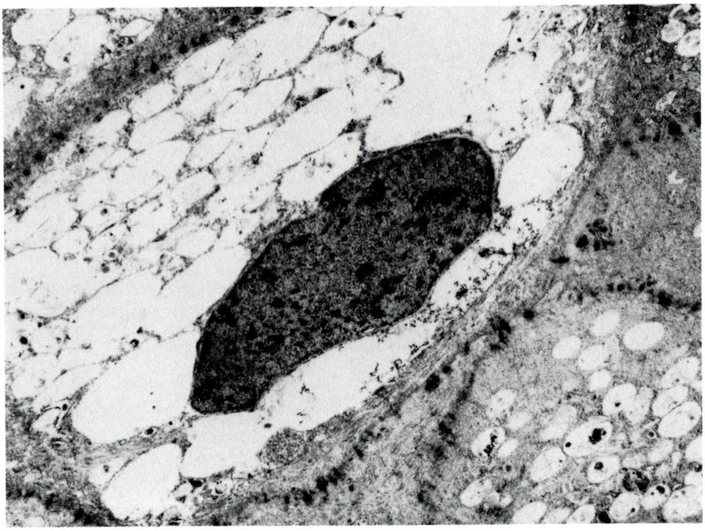

Figure 4 Electron photomicrograph of the vacuolated corneal epithelium showing membrane bound vacuoles containing only a few wispy lamellae. x 6750

Some inclusions appeared partly empty - possibly an artefactual result of sectioning. In many cells the rough endoplasmic reticulum was dilated and the lumen filled with a flocculent material (Fig 8). Golgi saccules were also dilated. The profusion of inclusions seen in this patient contrast markedly with the occasional MCB-like inclusions which were present in fibroblasts cultured from a patient with ML1.

Thin layer chromatography: Oligosaccharides detected with the diphenylamine spray were markedly increased at the origin, immediately above the origin and in a band with an Rf value of 0.28. A further band with an Rf value of 0.5 was also present. The pattern shows some similarities with ML1 but differs in the distribution of oligosaccharides at the origin (Fig 9). Sialyloligosaccharides detected by the resorcinol reagent (Fig 10) showed one band at the

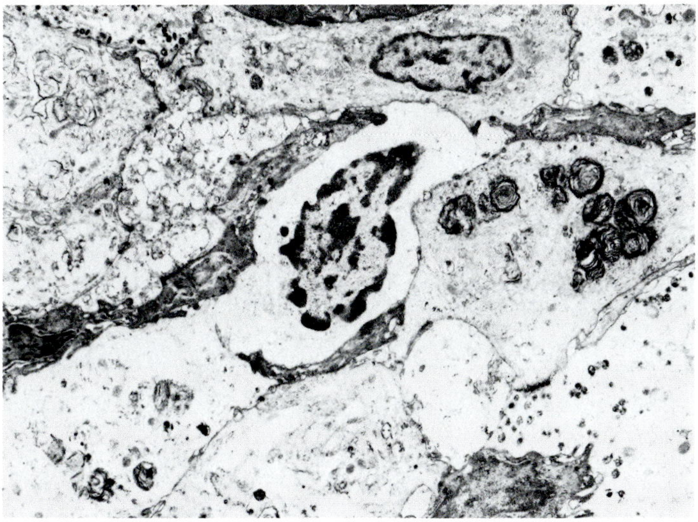

Figure 5 Electron photomicrograph of conjunctival epithelium containing several groups of membranous cytoplasmic bodies (MCB) x 6400

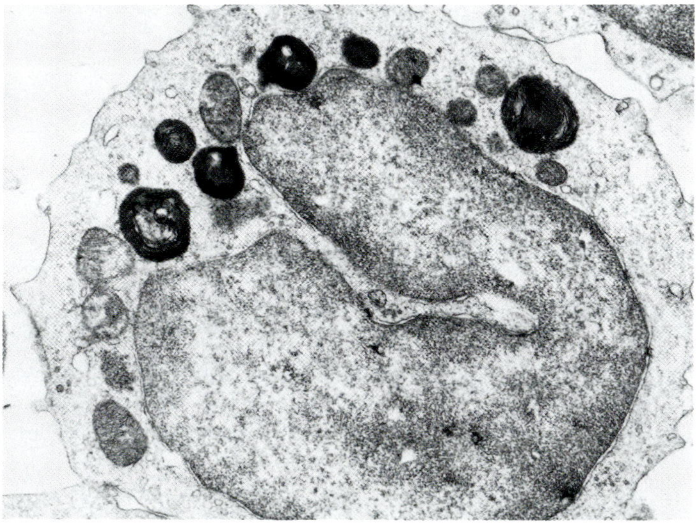

Figure 6 Some lymphocytes contain MCB's. No vacuolar changes are seen. x 17,500

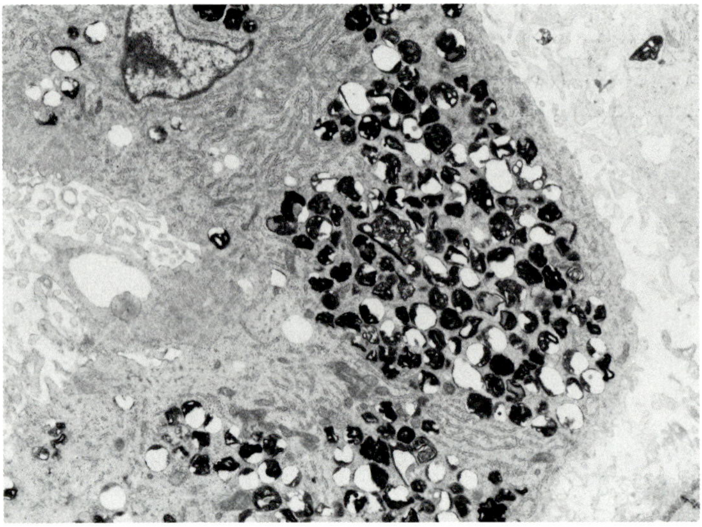

Figure 7 Cultured fibroblasts contain numerous electron dense inclusions measuring up to 1 μm in diameter x 6400

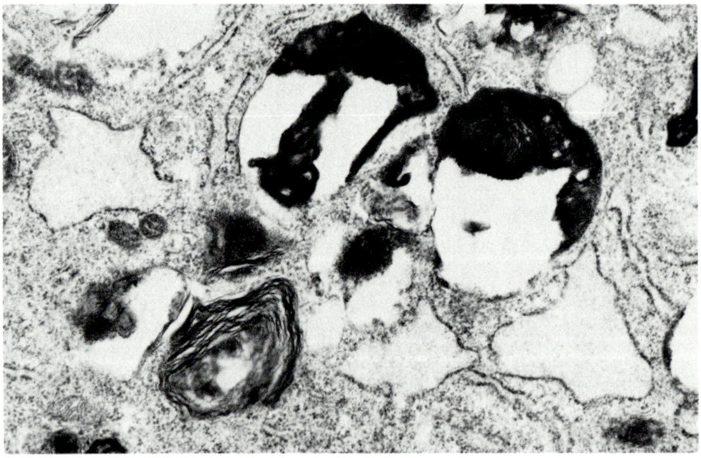

Figure 8 The dense inclusions in the cultured fibroblasts at higher magnification show as collections of MCB's. The endoplasmic reticulum is dilated and contains flocculent material. x 27,500

origin (o) and one band at C, 24 mm from the origin. In ML1 bands are present at O A and B. Normal controls, the patient and cases of ML1 showed bands above C, which were common to all.

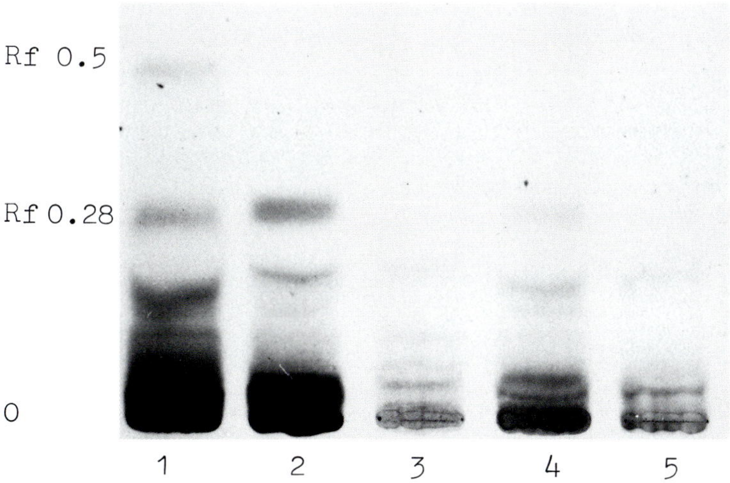

Figure 9 Thin layer chromatogram showing oligosaccharides in 30 µl urine; developed in chloroform, methanol, water (70, 30, 5): sprayed with diphenylamine.
Lane 1, patient DV; Lane 2, ML1 type 2; Lane 3, normal control; Lane 4, ML1 type 1; Lane 5, normal control. The pattern in the patient is similar to ML1, but the oligosaccharides close to the origin seem increased and to comprise several components.

Neuraminidase Assay

Normal controls	12.0 nmoles/mg protein/hr (range 7.8-17.5; N=14)
Patient DV	13.3 nmoles/mg protein/hr
ML1 (2 cases)	0.62, 0.89 nmoles/mg protein/hr.

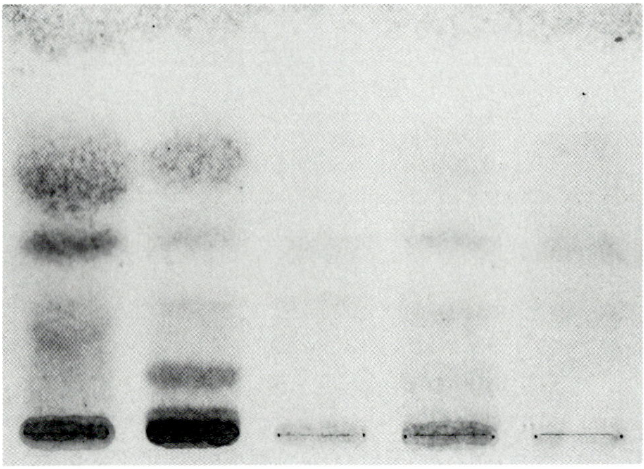

Figure 10 Thin layer chromatogram showing sialyloligosaccharides in 30 µl urine: developed in n-butanol, acetic acid, water (2, 1, 1): sprayed with resorcinol.
Lanes 1-5 as in figure 9.
ML1 patients show abnormal bands at O, A and B.
The ML4 patient shows abnormal bands at O and C only.

DISCUSSION

The clinical features of our patient are similar to but much milder than those previously described in patients with ML4. At the time of corneal graft he was not considered to show mental retardation and the diagnosis of a mucolipidosis was not entertained, until it became clear that the graft was becoming overgrown with abnormal epithelium. Re-evaluation of the corneal histology and electron microscopy of cornea, conjunctiva and cultured fibroblasts suggested a diagnosis of ML4.

Although others (Goutières et al 1979) could detect no urinary sialyloligosaccharides, our patient, patients with ML1 and controls all showed sialyloligosaccharide excretion. Patients with

ML1 and our patient showed different patterns, both of which could be distinguished from normal.

Sialic acid residues are widespread and can be found as part of many macromolecules, ranging from gangliosides found mainly in the brain but also present throughout the viscera, to acidic mucosubstances found in gut and exocrine glands. Sialic acid is also an integral part of immunoglobulins and blood group substances. Enzymes, concerned with hydrolysis of glycosidic bonds, generally have quite wide specificity; for example the deficiency of β-galactosidase activity results in the accumulation of a wide range of substances with a terminal β-galactose residue. In some instances there is clear substrate specificity and only one substance may be affected, as for example in galactocerebroside-β-galactosidase deficiency (Krabbe leucodystrophy).

Bach and his colleagues (1979) have described a deficiency of specific ganglioside sialidase in patients with ML4, A general sialidase deficiency has been shown in patients with the cherry red spot myoclonus syndrome (ML1 type 2) and in the severe type of ML1 (type 1). Most of the lysosomal storage disorders are expressed in at least two forms; e.g. the acute infantile and chronic adult forms of Gaucher's Disease and Niemann-Pick Disease and it would therefore not be surprising to encounter mild and severe forms of ML4.

In view of the ubiquitous nature of sialic acids we feel that many more varieties of mucolipidosis will be found.

In summary D.V. is now an 8½ year old boy who has severe visual and motor handicaps but a considerable proportion of his motor handicap and his delayed development is due to his visual defect. This may represent a milder variant of ML4 than cases hitherto described.

Acknowledgements: We thank Mrs. Virpi Smith for skilled technical work, and Mrs. Jean Mossman for culturing fibroblasts. We are grateful to

Professor O. H. Wolff for advice and encouragement.

REFERENCES

Bach G, Zeigler M, Schaap T, Kohn G (1979) Mucolipidosis type IV: Ganglioside sialidase deficiency. B. B. Res. Comm. 90:1341.

Berman ER, Livni N, Shapira E, Merin S, Levij IS (1974) Congenital corneal clouding with abnormal systemic storage bodies: a new variant of mucolipidosis. J. Pediat. 84:519.

Goutières F, Arsenio-Nunes M-L, Aicardi J (1979) Mucolipidosis IV Neuropadiatrie 10:321.

Kenyon KR, Maumenee IH, Green R, Libert J, Hiatt RL (1979) Mucolipidosis IV. Histopathology of conjunctiva cornea and skin. Arch Ophthalmol 97:1106.

Lake BD, Goodwin HJ (1976) Lipids. In Smith I, Seakins JWT (eds) Chromatographic and electrophoretic techniques. Volume 1 London Heinemann p345.

Livni N, Merin S (1978) Mucolipidosis IV. Ultrastructural diagnosis of a recently defined genetic disorder. Arch. Path. Lab. Med. 102:600.

Lowry OH, Rosebrough NJ, Farr AL, Randall RJ (1951) Protein measurement with the Folin reagent. J. Biol. Chem. 193:265.

CHEMICAL PATHOLOGY OF THE SIALIDOSES

Leonhard S. Wolfe, M.D., Ph.D.

Montreal Neurological Institute and Hospital

3801 University Street
Montréal, Québec, Canada H3A 2B4.

The mucolipidoses represent a group of recessively inherited lysosomal storage disorders which have clinical and pathological features of both the mucopolysaccharidoses and of the sphingolipidoses. There is however much heterogeneity in the clinical course, the degree of skeletal, facial and visceral changes and the severity of the neurological symptoms and dementia. In the last five years, there have been significant advances on the biochemical causes of these diseases. In Mucolipidosis II or I-cell disease and the clinically less severe Mucolipidosis III or Pseudo-Hurler Polydystrophy, the basic enzymatic defect has been shown to be due to deficient activity of uridine-5'-diphosphate-N-acetylglucosamine: glycoprotein N-acetylglucosaminylphosphotransferase (Reitman, Varki, Kornfeld, 1981; Hasilik, Waheed, von Figura, 1981). The function of this enzyme is in the processing of the glycoprotein side chains and the intracellular direction of glycosidases from the Golgi saccules to lysosomes by phosphorylation of α-linked mannose residues in the 6-position (Hasilik, Klein, Waheed, Strecker, von Figura, 1980; Reitman, Kornfeld, 1981). A deficiency of the enzyme leads to loss of intracellular glycosidases to the extracellular space and blood with inability to endocytose these enzymes since there is no mannose-6-phosphate on the plasma membrane glycoprotein receptors. The secreted enzymes also contain more sialic acid but the reasons for this are not entirely clear and, as a result, urinary sialyloligosacchariduria is present in I-cell disease.

Birth Defects: Original Article Series, Volume 18, Number 6, pages 405–409

Mucolipidosis IV which predominantly occurs in Jews of Ashkenazi origin has a prolonged clinical course characterized by congenital corneal opacities, retinal degeneration, athetosis and progressive motor and intellectual disability (Merin, Livni, Berman, Yatziv,1975; Tellez-Nagel, Rapin, Iwanoto, Johnson, Norton, Nitowsky, 1976). It appears due to a catalytically defective ganglioside α-N-acetyl neuraminidase to α-2→3 N-acetylneuraminic acid linkages to galactose in residues in G_{M1} and GD_{1a} gangliosides (Bach, Cohen, Kohn, 1975; Ben-Yoseph, Hahn, Nadler, 1981; Zeigler, Bach, 1981). α-N-acetyl neuraminidase activity in cultured fibroblasts to synthetic 4-methylumbelliferyl substrates is normal.

It is however in Mucolipidosis I or Sialidosis that the greatest phenotypic variability is seen. In the literature, many names have been given to clinical entities in this group: lipomucopolysaccharidosis, atypical mucopolysaccharidosis, macular corneal dystrophy, cherry red spot-myoclonus syndrome with or without dementia, Goldberg-Cotlier syndrome, G_{M1}-gangliosidosis variants type 3 and 4, adult β-galactosidase deficiency. Lowden and O'Brien in 1979 (Lowden, O'Brien, 1979) classified Mucolipidosis I into two broad categories, Sialidosis Type I Normosomatic Group and Sialidosis Type 2 Dysmorphic Group which was further subdivided into Juvenile and Infantile forms. The predominant clinical features in Type I are onset in early adolescence of decreasing visual acuity with cherry-red spots and progressive development of myoclonus epilepsy which becomes very severe and crippling and poorly controlled by anticonvulsant drugs. Intellectual capacity is only mildly affected. Biochemically, these patients have a marked loss of activity of the cryolabile enzyme α-N-acetylneuraminidase in leucocytes and fibroblast cell lines but the activity of other glycosidases including β-galactosidase is normal. In this $neur^{-}gal^{+}$ genotype the mutation is almost certainly at the locus for the enzyme α-neuraminidase primarily hydrolysing α2→6 linkages of N-acetylneuraminic acid in glycoproteins thus leading to accumu-lation in tissues and excretion in the urine of sialyloligosaccharides and sialylglycopeptides. In suspected cases biochemical diagnosis is relatively simple, namely screening of the urine for resorcinol positive oligosaccharides which if positive is followed by leukocyte or preferably fibroblast cell line activity of α-neuraminidase and β-galactosidase activity to the fluorogenic 4-methyl-umbelliferyl-glycoside substrates. At the Montreal Neurological Hospital, the urinary screening procedure consists of application of 25 μl of urine to two precoated silica gel G thin layer chromatographic plates, development twice in Butanol-Acetic Acid-water (2:1:1) followed by spraying one plate with the orcinol reagent as a general carbohydrate reactant and the other plate with the resorcinol reagent which shows specifically sialyloligosaccharides. It has become routine in our Hospital to screen urines of all patients with myoclonus epilepsy.

In Sialidosis type 2, clinically the children have a coarse facial appearance combined with other Hurleroid features and progressive loss of visual acuity, development of ataxia, often but not always myoclonus and intellectual deterioration. Cherry red spots may be present. Visceromegaly occurs only in the infantile onset patients. A marked sialyloligosacchariduria is present and the oligosaccharides contain N-acetylneuraminic acid in both $\alpha 2 \rightarrow 6$ and $\alpha 2 \rightarrow 3$ linkages. α-N-acetylneuraminidase activity in leukocytes and fibroblasts is deficient associated with a variable but markedly reduced activity of β-galactosidase as well (Lowden, O'Brien, 1979; Spranger,Gehler, Cantz, 1977; Ng Ying Kin, Wolfe, Watters, Pinsky, Lowden, 1978; Gravel, Lowden, Callahan, Wolfe, Ng Ying Kin, 1979). Recent studies of this $neur^{-}gal^{-}$ genotype by genetic complementation analysis and stability and turnover studies of the residual β-galactosidase activity strongly indicate that α-neuraminidase deficiency is not the primary biochemical disorder and cannot be used for carrier detection. Lysosomal enzymes in their pro-protein form are processed by peptide clipping to the mature enzymes. A defect in the late processing step for lysosomal α-neuraminidases and β-galactosidases resulting in increased susceptibility to degradation is suspected (Mueller, Shows, 1981; d'Azzo, Hoogeveen, van Diggelen, Reuser, Galjaard, 1981). Because of the very marked deficiency of β-galactosidase in patients in the infantile age group, this type of sialidosis has often been confused with G_{M1}gangliosidosis. For practical purposes, all suspected patients should have a TLC urine screen sprayed with both the orcinol and rescorcinol reagents and leukocyte assay for α-neuraminidase and β-galactosidase.

A further sialidosis phenotype has recently been described termed nephrosialidosis (Maroteaux, Humbel, Strecker, Michalski, Mande, 1978). In this disease a severe glomerular nephropathy is combined with dysmorphic facies, visceral storage, skeletal abnormalities and severe mental retardation. There is also marked storage of carbohydrate-containing material in sympathetic ganglia. Sialyloligosacchariduria and leukocyte $\alpha 2 \rightarrow 6$ neuraminidase deficiency are present with large elevations of β-galactosidase and β-hexosaminidase activities in leukocytes and fibroblast cell lines. How this condition relates to the dysmorphic sialidosis group biochemically is unclear.

Since phenotypic variability appears to be very common in Mucolipidosis I, the clinician should be alert to the possibility of this diagnosis in children with eye abnormalities, neurological and intellectual deficits with or without skeletal and visceral abnormalities. The urinary screening test is simple and inexpensive.

References

Bach G, Cohen MM, Kohn G (1975). Abnormal ganglioside accumulation in cultured fibroblasts from patients with Mucolipidosis IV. Biochem Biophys Res Commun 66:1483.

Ben-Yoseph Y, Hahn LC, Nadler HC (1981). Mucolipidosis IV: a Km defect in ganglioside neuraminidase. The 6th Internat Congr Human Genetics, p 77 Abstr.

d'Azzo A, Hoogeveen AT, van Diggelen OP, Reuser AJJ, Galjaard, H. (1981). Studies on the precursor form of β-galactosidase in combined β-galactosidase and α-neuraminidase deficiency. The 6th Internat Congr Human Genetics, p 90 Abstr.

Gravel RA, Lowden JA, Callahan JW, Wolfe LS, Ng Ying Kin NMK (1979). Infantile Sialidosis: A phenocopy of Type I G_{M1}-Gangliosidosis distinguished by Genetic Complementation and Urinary Oligosaccharides. Amer J Human Genet 31:669.

Hasilik A, Waheed A, von Figura K (1981). Enzymatic phosphorylation of lysosomal enzymes in the presence of UDP-N-acetylglucosamine. Absence of activity in I-cell fibroblasts. Biochem Biophys Res Commun 98:761.

Hasilik A, Klein U, Waheed A, Strecker G, von Figura K (1980). Phosphorylated oligosaccharides in lysosomal enzymes: Identification of α-N-Acetylglucosamine (1)phospho(6)mannose diester groups. Proc Natl Acad Sc USA 77:7074.

Lowden JA, O'Brien JS (1979). Sialidosis: a review of human neuraminidase deficiency. Amer J Human Genet 31:1.

Spranger J, Gehler J, Cantz M (1977). Mucolipidosis I - A Sialidosis. Amer J Med Genetics 1:21.

Maroteaux P, Humbel R, Strecker G, Michalski J-C, Mande R (1978). Un nouveau type de Sialidose avec atteinte renale: la nephrosialidose. Arch franç Pédiat 35:819.

Merin S, Livni N, Berman ER, Yatziv S (1975). Mucolipidosis IV: Ocular, systemic and ultrastructural findings. Invest Ophthal 14:437.

Mueller OT, Shows TG (1981). Genetic complementation analysis of human β-galactosidase and α-neuraminidase deficient mucolipidosis and other neuraminidase deficiencies. The 6th Internat Congr Human Genetics, p 84 Abstr.

Ng Ying Kin NMK, Wolfe LS, Watters G, Pinsky L, Lowden JA (1978). Sialyloligosaccharide excretion and neuraminidase deficiency in clinical phenotypes of sialidosis. Clin Res Vol 26:854A.

Reitman ML, Varki A, Kornfeld, S. (1981). Fibroblasts from Patients with I-cell Disease and Pseudo-Hurler Polydystrophy are Deficient in Uridine 5'-Diphosphate-N-Acetylglucosamine:Glycoprotein N-Acetylglucosaminyl-phosphotransferase Activity. J Clin Invest, 67:1574.

Reitman ML, Kornfeld S (1981). UDP-N- Acetylglucosamine: Glycoprotein N-acetylglucosamine-1-phosphotransferase. Proposed enzyme for the phosphorylation of the high mannose oligosaccharide units of lysosomal enzymes. J Biol Chem 256:4275.

Spranger J, Gehler J, Cantz M (1977). Mucolipidosis I - A Sialidosis. Amer J Med Genetics 1:21.

Tellez-Nagel E, Rapin I, Iwanoto T, Johnson AB, Norton WT, Nitowsky H (1976). Mucolipidosis IV: Clinical, Ultrastructural, Histochemical and Chemical Studies of a Case, Including Brain Biopsy. Arch Neurol 33:828.

Zeigler M, Bach G (1981). The nature of the sialidase deficiency in Mucolipidosis IV. The 6th Internat Congr Human Genetics, p 78 Abstr.

LIPID INCLUSIONS IN HUMAN OCULAR TISSUES *IN VITRO* INDUCED BY AMINOGLYCOSIDE ANTIBIOTICS

D.J.D'AMICO, K.R.KENYON, D.M.ALBERT, and L.HANNINEN

MASSACHUSETTS EYE AND EAR INFIRMARY, EYE RESEARCH INSTITUTE OF THE RETINA FOUNDATION, HOWE LABORATORY OF OPHTHALMOLOGY, HARVARD MEDICAL SCHOOL, BOSTON, MASSACHUSETTS, USA.

INTRODUCTION

Certain drugs induce an intralysosomal accumulation of polar lipids in experimental animals and in humans (Lullmann 1975). A characteristic feature of these drug-induced lipidoses is the presence of numerous cytoplasmic inclusions which typically display a lamellated or crystalloid appearance on ultrastructural examination. Multiple observations suggest that these inclusions result from drug-induced alteration in the lysosomal handling of polar lipids, and these abnormalities may serve as an experimental model of genetically transmitted lysosomal storage disorders such as Fabry's disease.

Ocular manifestations in drug-induced lipidoses range from the benign verticillate corneal deposits seen with chronic chloroquine or amiodarone administration (Pullhorn 1976, D'Amico 1981) to the devastating retinopathy after prolonged chloroquine usage (Ramsey 1972). Recently, subconjunctival injection of gentamicin has been shown to induce conjunctival lipidosis in humans and experimental animals (Libert,1979). The conjunctiva appeared grossly normal and evidence of drug effect was confined to the presence of typical inclusions on ultrastructural examina-

---

(Reprint requests: K.R.Kenyon, 20 Staniford St.,Boston, Massachusetts, 02114, USA)
(Supported in part by NIH Academic Investigator Award EY00156, the James S. Adams Research Award of Research to Prevent Blindness, and Fight For Sight, Inc., NYC (Kenyon))

Birth Defects: Original Article Series, Volume 18, Number 6, pages 411–420

tion of this tissue. Although presumably innocuous in the conjunctiva, lamellated inclusions have been extensively documented as a hallmark of the nephrotoxicity of aminoglycoside antibiotics (gentamicin, tobramicin, etc.) in animal models (Houghton 1978). Interestingly, the relatively lower lipidosis-inducing properties of tobramicin versus gentamicin in animal models have been related to the lower potential for clinical nephrotoxicity with tobramicin.

The present study examined the induction of lipidosis by aminoglycosides in tissue cultures of human conjunctiva and retinal pigment epithelium (RPE), and in cultures of bovine RPE.

METHODS

Human conjunctiva was obtained by simple biopsy at the time of routine cataract surgery in patients free of chronic drug use. Conjunctival specimens approximately one cubic millimeter in size were maintained at 37 degrees Centigrade as explants in RPMI 1640 medium supplemented with 5% fetal calf serum. Control specimens of conjunctiva were cultured in this medium without any antibiotics. Experimental specimens (from the same individual) were cultured in media identical to the controls except for the addition of 100 micrograms/ml of gentamicin, tobramicin, or streptomycin. Cultures were maintained for 10 to 28 days, and explants were fixed in Karnovsky's fixative and processed for light and transmission electron microscopy by routine techniques.

Cultures of RPE/choroid were prepared from human eyes obtained at autopsy, and from bovine eyes within six hours of slaughter. Under sterile technique, eyes were opened in an equatorial fashion just posterior to the rectus muscle insertions. The anterior segment, vitreous,and retina were discarded, and discs of RPE/choroid approximately 4 mm in diameter were obtained with a biopsy punch. These cultures were treated in an identical manner as the conjunctival cultures described above. Also as in the conjunctival studies, care was taken to ensure that controls were obtained from exactly the same eye in order to detect any lipid inclusions occuring in the tissues prior to being subjected to the experimental protocol.

RESULTS

Lipidosis was induced in cultures of human conjunctiva by each of the antibiotics tested. Figure 1 shows conjunctiva

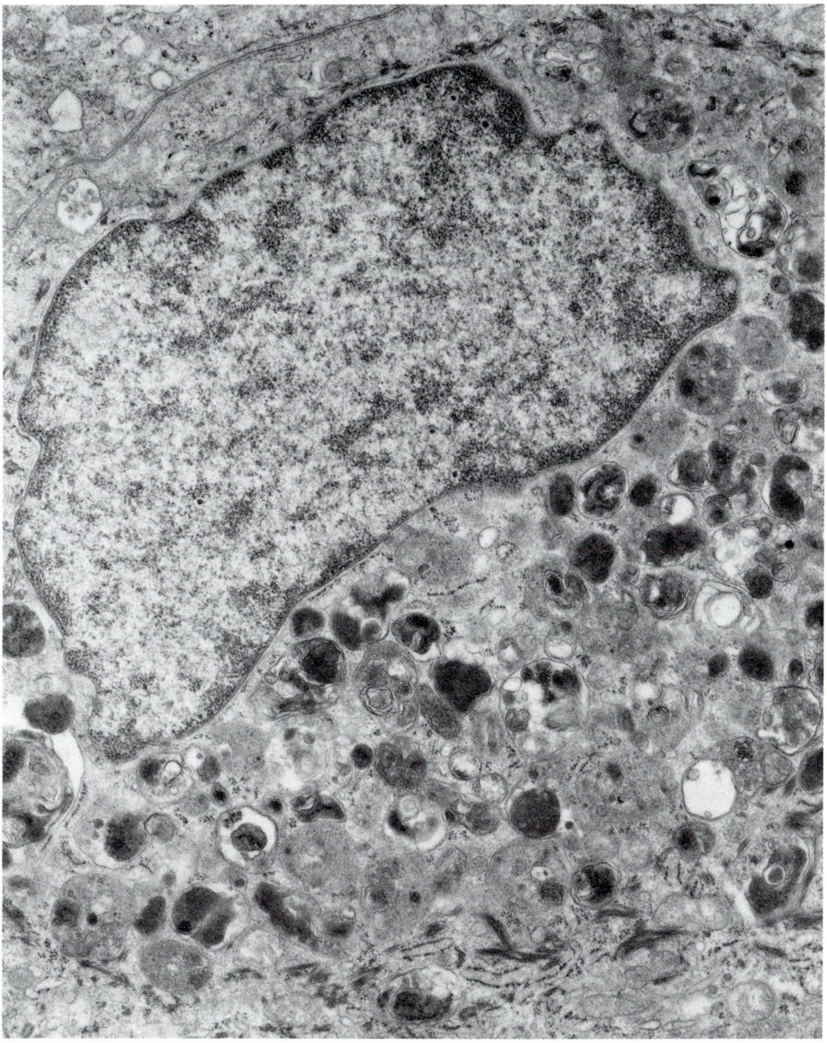

Fig. 1: Human conjunctiva, gentamicin medium, 22 days in vitro. Epithelial cells contain numerous, membrane-limited inclusions, approx. 0.3 to 1.0 u diameter, having pleomorphic electron-dense and membranous lamellar contents. (x18,700)

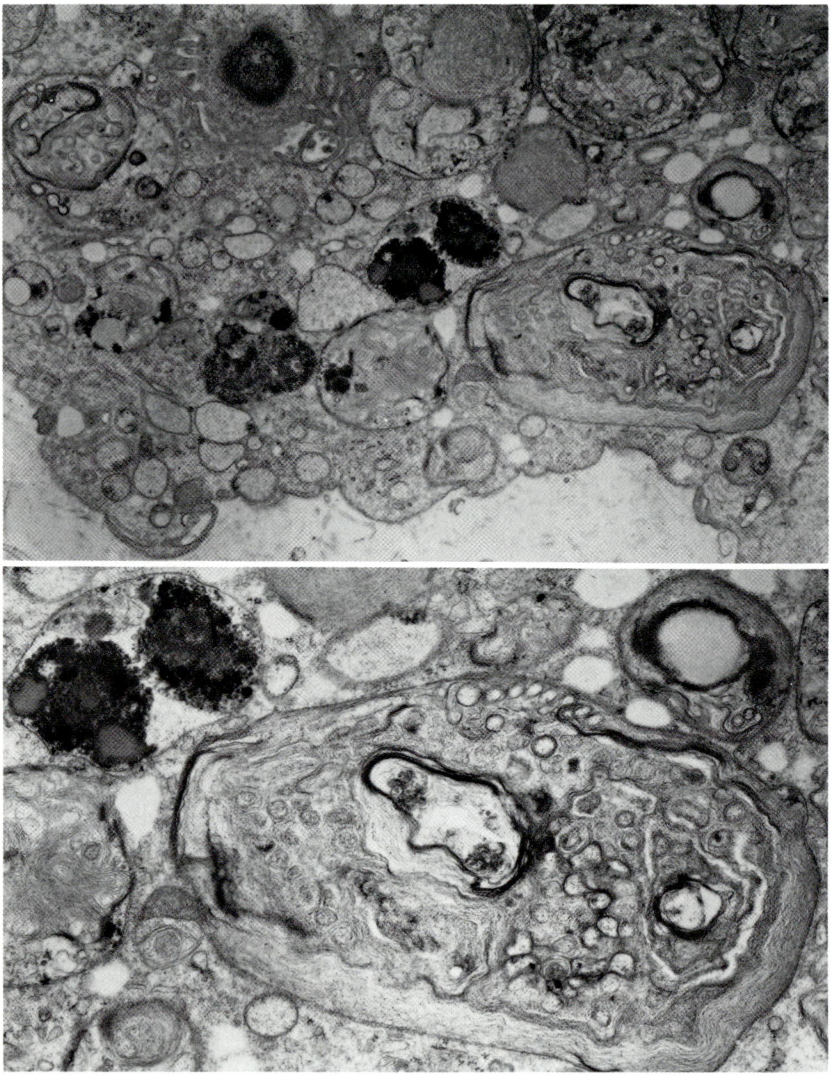

Fig. 2: Human conjunctiva, tobramycin media, 22 days in vitro. TOP: Stromal cells are ballooned by storage vacuoles as large as 7 u in diameter. No abnormal extracellular accumulations are evident (x8,000). BOTTOM: Higher magnification resolves concentric configuration of membranous lipid, plus electron-dense globular lipids (16,700).

maintained in gentamicin-containing medium for 22 days. The inclusions display both lamellated and crystalloid patterns. Results were quite similar in cultures exposed to tobramicin, as seen in Fig. 2. However, streptomycin-induced inclusions (Fig. 3) are distinctly different, and display a more uniform, almost circular membrane filled with amorphous osmophilia. Inclusions were not observed in control conjunctiva.

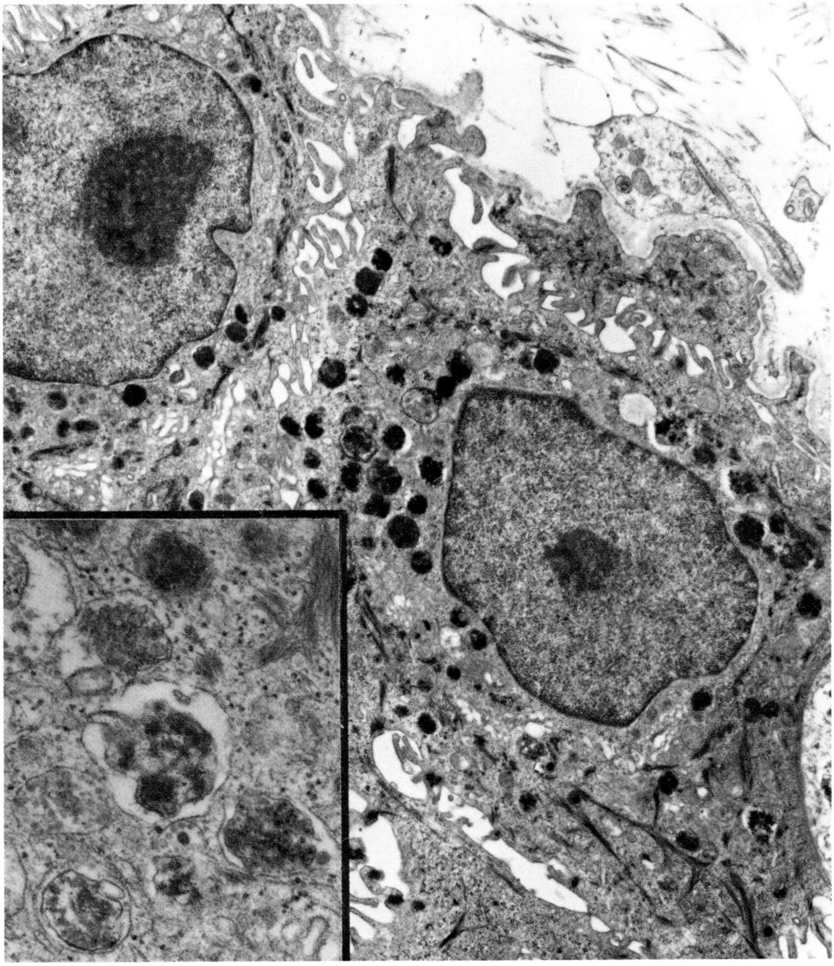

Fig. 3: Human conjunctiva, streptomycin media,22 days in vitro. Basal epithelial cells demonstrate multiple, small inclusions (less than 0.5 u diameter) (x8,900). Inset: Higher magnification reveals amorphous osmophilic pattern that is typical of streptomycin induced inclusions. (x43,400).

RPE/choroid cultures also developed lipidosis after exposure to aminoglycoside antibiotics. As shown in Fig. 4, bovine cultures exposed to tobramicin display choroidal connective tissue cells containing an abundance of lamellated inclusions that were not observed in control cultures. In Fig. 5, human RPE cells cultured for 15 days in gentamicin-containing medium display membrane-limited inclusions that frequently display a lamellated appearance peripherally and amorphous material centrally. These inclusions are easily distinguished from the prominent melanin granules.

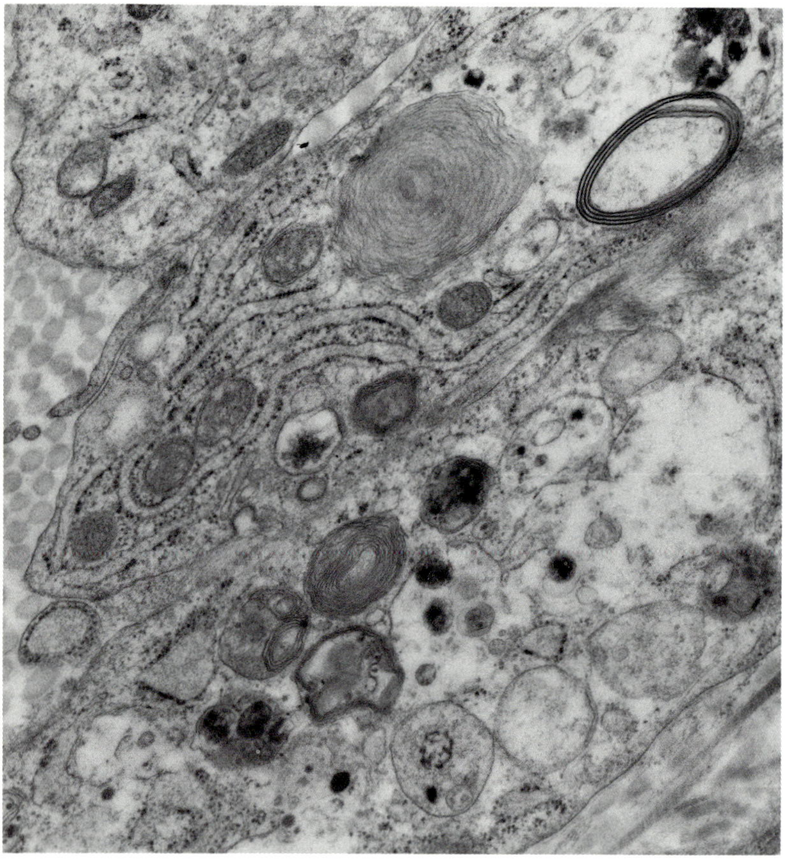

Fig. 4: Bovine RPE/choroid, tobramicin medium, 23 days in vitro. Choroidal connective tissue cells show concentric lamellar intracytoplasmic storage bodies (x27,100).

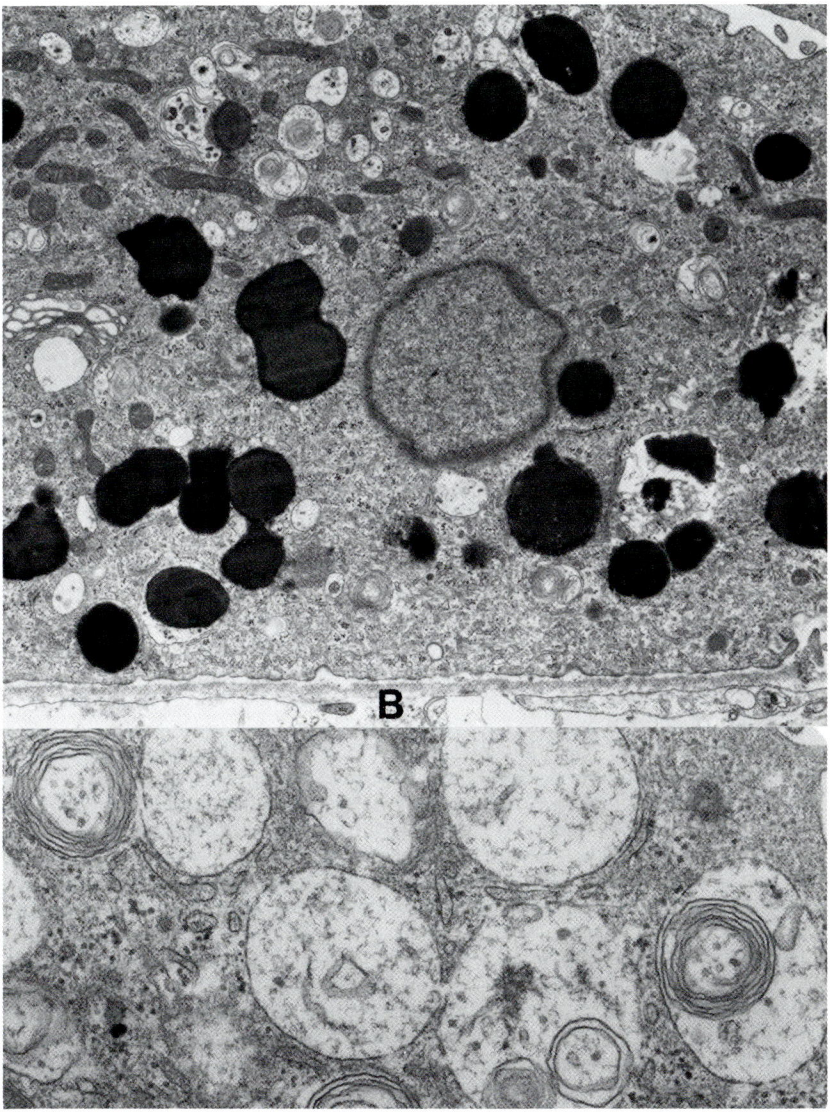

Fig. 5: Human RPE/choroid, gentamicin medium, 15 days in vitro. TOP: Pigment epithelial cells exhibit multiple membrane-limited inclusions with variable content, in addition to melanosomes. Bruch's membrane (B) is evident below (x12,600). BOTTOM: Higher magnification resolves concentric membranous lamellae, in addition to fine granular material, within inclusions (x45,000).

DISCUSSION

The present study documents the production of abnormal lysosomal inclusions by aminoglycoside antibiotics in tissue cultures of human and bovine ocular cells. These findings corroborate the aminoglycoside-induced lysosomal enzyme abnormalities in fibroblast cultures as reported previously (Tulkens 1978). With regard to gentamicin and tobramicin, the lamellated morphology of the inclusions corresponds well to the inclusions produced in the proximal tubular cells of the rat by aminoglycosides in studies of the nephrotoxicity of these compounds (Houghton 1978); however, the presently employed in vitro technique did not allow comparison of the relative lipidosis-inducing properties of the drugs. Also, the distinctly different inclusions resulting from streptomycin addition to the medium are quite similar to those first observed by Wersall in his study of the ototoxicity of this drug in the cat (Wersall 1962). Libert has presented evidence of gentamicin-induced lipidosis in human conjunctiva after subconjunctival injection of the drug (Libert 1979); the present study extends these findings to a tissue culture model and documents the production of aminoglycoside-induced inclusions in cultures of human and bovine RPE/choroid for the first time.

Aminoglycoside antibiotics are among the many agents that cause lipid inclusions in experimental animals and in man (Lullman 1975). Abnormal lysosomal accumulations of polar lipids, frequently with a lamellated or crystalloid morphology, are the hallmark of this process. Well-known examples of drug-induced lipidoses include: 1) the keratopathy seen with chronic chloroquine administration, and possibly the retinopathy and myopathy seen with chloroquine as well (Pullhorn 1976, Ramsey 1972, Rosenthal 1978), 2) the keratopathy with amiodarone usage (D'Amico 1981), 3) gentamicin nephrotoxicity (Houghton 1978), and 4) the ototoxicity of streptomycin (Wersall 1962). Although the direct relationship between the lipidosis and the specific pathology observed in the above mentioned settings is as yet unestablished, numerous observations document the alteration of lysosomal function and appearance as the earliest manifestation of drug effect. Lullmann and co-workers hypothesize (Lullmann 1975, 1978) that inclusions are formed when the inciting drug is transported into the lysosome where it is protonated in the acidic environment and complexed with polar lipids. These complexes are unable to rapidly exit the lysosome or be degraded, and lysosomal intoxication with presumed compromise of cellular function is the result. Accordingly, these drug-induced lipidoses are thought to result from a bulk interaction of drug and lipid, and the presumably nonspecific interference with lysosomal function must be contrasted with the specific lysosomal deficits seen in the inherited lysosomal storage disorders; these latter are thought to result from the genetically-transmitted abnormality of a specific intralysosomal enzyme. Fabry's disease is exemplary as its pathogenesis is related to the deficiency of ceramide trihexosidase, an alpha galactosidase. (Kenyon 1974). Nevertheless, striking parallels exist between features of certain drug-induced lipidoses and the inherited lysosomal disorders. The verticillate keratopathy of Fabry's disease is remarkably similar to the keratopathy of chloroquine or amiodarone usage (Francois 1968), and intralysosomal accumulations are seen in each of these conditions. The drug-induced lipidoses may provide an experimental model to study certain aspects of inherited lysosomal storage disorders.

With regard to aminoglycoside-induced lipidosis, it is important to emphasize that these antibiotics are frequently added to tissue culture media as a routine antibacterial prophylaxis in doses similar to those employed in the present study. In view of the production of lipidosis in ocular tissues in culture by gentamicin, tobramicin, and streptomycin, caution is suggested in the interpretation of morphologic or functional abnormalities in tissues in culture in which these antibiotics are media constituents.

REFERENCES

D'Amico DJ, Kenyon KR, Ruskin JN (1981). Amiodarone Keratopathy: Drug-induced Lipid Storage Disease. Arch. Ophthal. 99:257.

Francois J (1968). Cornea Verticillata. Bull. Soc. Belge. Ophtalmol. 150:656.

Houghton DC, Plamp CE, DeFehr JM, Bennett WM, Porter G, Gilbert D (1978). Gentamicin and Tobramicin Nephrotoxicity: A Morphologic and Functional Comparison in the Rat. Am. J. Pathol. 93:137.

Kenyon KR (1974). Ocular Ultrastructure of Inherited Metabolic Disease. In Goldberg MF (ed):"Genetic and Metabolic Eye Disease," Boston, Little Brown and Co, pp 139-185.
Libert J, Ketelbant-Balasse PE, VanHoof F, Aubert-Tulkens G, Tulkens P (1979). Cellular Toxicity of Gentamicin. Am. J. Ophthal. 87:405.
Lullmann H, Lullmann-Rauch R, Wasserman O (1975). Drug Induced Phospholipidoses. CRC Crit. Rev. Toxicol. 4:185.
Lullmann H, Lullmann-Rauch R, Wasserman O (1978). Lipidosis Induced by Amphiphilic Cationic Drugs. Biochem. Pharmacol. 27:1103.
Pullhorn G, Thiel HJ (1976). Das Ultrastrukturelle Bild der Chloroquin Keratopathie. Albrecht Von Graefes Arch. Klin. Exp. Ophthalmol. 201:89.
Ramsey MS, Fine BS (1972). Chloroquine Toxicity in the Human Eye. Am. J. Ophthal. 73:229.
Rosenthal AR, Kolb H, Bergsma D, Huxsoll D, Hopkins JL(1978). Chloroquine Retinopathy in the Rhesus Monkey. Invest. Ophthalmol. 17:1158.
Tulkens P, Trouet A (1978). The Uptake and Intracellular Accumulation of Aminoglycoside Antibiotics in Lysosomes of Cultured Rat Fibroblasts. Biochem. Pharmacol. 27:415.
Wersall J, Hawkins JE (1962). The Vestibular Sensory Epithelia in the Cat Labyrinth and their Reactions in Chronic Streptomycin Intoxication. Acta Oto-laryng. 54:1.

Corneal Storage Diseases and Dystrophies

FAMILIAL LECITHIN:CHOLESTEROL ACYLTRANSFERASE (LCAT) DEFICIENCY

Egil Gjone

Department of Medicine, University Hospital, Rikshospitalet, Oslo 1, Norway

INTRODUCTION

In normal human plasma, 70-75% of the circulating cholesterol is esterified to a long chain fatty acid. The enzyme responsible for the formation of the major part of the cholesteryl esters in plasma is lecithin:cholesterol acyltransferase (LCAT) produced in the liver and functioning in the circulating plasma.

LCAT catalyzes the formation of cholesteryl esters by promoting acyl group transfer from the lecithin to the unesterified cholesterol of plasma lipoproteins (Fig.1) preferentially on the high density lipoproteins (HDL). The cholesteryl esters formed by the LCAT reaction may be transferred to other plasma lipoproteins. According to John Glomset's theories, one of the main functions of this reaction is to regulate the homeostasis of free cholesterol in the body. Free cholesterol is a constituent of all cell and subcellular membranes.

Free cholesterol is taken up by plasma HDL, esterified by means of LCAT to cholesteryl ester and transported to the liver. Here it is transformed to bile acids and secreted into the bile stream. Thus, the HDL-LCAT system plays an important role as a renovation system in the body. This homeostasis influences both membrane lipoproteins and circulating plasma lipoproteins. Lack of LCAT may lead to various forms of cholesterol accumulation and deposition in a variety of cells and tissues.

Birth Defects: Original Article Series, Volume 18, Number 6, pages 423–432

LIPID DEPOSITS IN LCAT DEFICIENCY

In familial LCAT deficiency there is a storage of lipid materials in various tissues because of lack of the enzyme in plasma.

The erythrocyte lipid composition is abnormal, with target cell formation, anemia, and reduced erythrocyte life span. Phagocytosis of lipid material leads to formation of sea-blue histiocytes in bone marrow and spleen. Familial LCAT deficiency seems to be the only disease so far described in which all the patients studied reveal the presence of sea-blue histiocytes. Foam-cell formation occurs in bone marrow, kidney glomeruli, and kidney arteries. Early atherosclerosis occurs. Corneal opacities are present in all patients and fundus changes have been observed in two.

CORNEAL OPACITIES

We have studied the Norwegian patients and also the Swedish one with familial LCAT deficiency. All gave a history of corneal cloudiness from early childhood, except one. The anamnestic information did not specifically state that these changes were present at birth, although they may have been. They were, however, present before puberty in some patients, even before they started school at the age of seven. The corneal opacities did not usually cause any complaints. The visual acuity and fields were within normal limits in the early stage of the disease.

The opacities have a characteristic appearance which makes it rather easy to get a correct diagnosis. In addition to a lipoid arcus, which is always present, there are numerous minute, grayish dots in the entire stroma, giving the cornea a cloudy to misty appearance (Fig. 2). This cloudiness may be overlooked as both corneas are affected to the same extent. When the patient's cornea is compared with a normal one, the difference is fairly obvious.

The grayish dots are evenly distributed in all layers of the stroma, without affecting the Descemet membrane. Near to the limbal area the dots increase in numbers, forming a grayish, circular band which is separated from the limbus by a relatively clear zone of corneal tissue in most patients. The outer border of the arcus is somewhat irregular and blurred because of variations in the number of stromal dots (Fig. 3). In one patient crystals (presumably of cholesterol) were seen near the Descemet membrane just peripheral to the circular band.

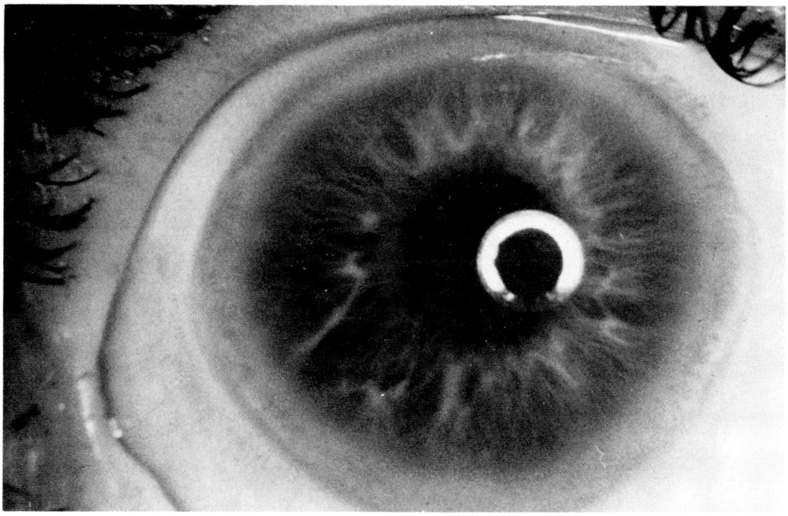

Fig. 2 Corneal appearance in Familial LCAT Deficiency

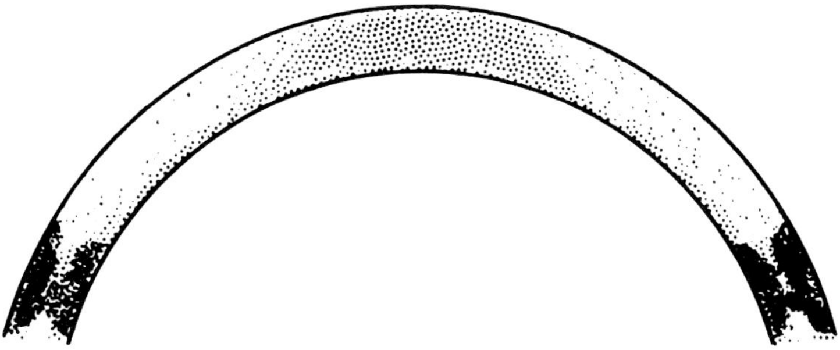

Fig. 3 Sketch of pattern of opacities in corneal stroma

FUNDUS CHANGES

In one of the Norwegian patients (a 55-year-old man) minor aneurysmic dilations in a retinal vein at the optic disk in one eye were seen. In the other eye a minute retinal hemorrhage was observed, and in both eyes a peripapillary mottled, atrophic area with pigmentary accumulations and ruptures of the Bruch membrane resembling those seen in angioid streaks were found.

Another patient (a 37-year-old woman) was on hemodialysis from April 1970 to January 1973, when a kidney transplantation was performed. She presented normal ophthalmoscopic findings until May 1971, when both disks showed blurred borders with several flameshaped hemorrhages at and near the optic disk. Exudates were not found, and the systemic blood pressure was normal. From July 1971 through January 1972 the disk margins were completely blurred with narrow vessels and a protrusion of 2-3 diopters. During these months a decrease in corneal indentation pulse amplitudes was recorded by dynamic tonometry, suggesting impairment of the ocular blood supply. In July 1972 the protrusion had disappeared and in December 1972 the left eye turned amaurotic after a period of functional loss. The disk looked pale and atrophic. The visual acuity in the other eye declined from 20/20 to 20/40 during the same period of time, with constriction of the visual field.

COMMENTS ON THE OCULAR FINDINGS

The corneal deposits in Familial LCAT Deficiency most probably consist of cholesterol or closely related lipid materials, even though histochemical studies or electron microscopy have not been carried out.

The ruptures of the Bruch membrane seen in our first patient may have been caused by a malfunction of this basal membrane-like structure because of deposits of lipid material, just as the retinal hemorrhages, disk protrusion, and vein dilations may indicate lesions in the vessel walls as well, with leakage of pathologic material into the surrounding nervous tissue or ischemia because of arterial obstruction. No definite conclusions may of course be drawn about these fundus changes and their specific relationship to Familial LCAT Deficiency, as they so far have been observed in only two patients.

LIPID DEPOSITS IN KIDNEYS

Proteinuria has been present in all patients described so far except one. Proteinuria is therefore a characteristic finding in patients with Familial LCAT Deficiency, and renal failure is the serious life-threatening complication. This disease should therefore be born in mind in all cases of familial renal disease. In 1967 we described foam cells in the glomerular tuft of the kidney in a needle biopsy from the first patient. Further studies of the lipid deposits in the kidneys have been performed by needle biopsy in other patients and from studies of the kidneys of a patient when bilateral nephrectomy was performed before kidney transplantation in January 1973. The kidneys were slightly enlarged, pale and appeared fatty with a firm, not adherent capsule. Light microscopic examination showed that the Bowman's capsule was thickened, the mesangium prominent, and foam cells were present in the glomerular tufts. Arterioles were observed with thickened intima and narrowing of the lumen. In the renal arteries and arterioles, subendothelial deposits of lipid material were observed. Fatty deposits with foam cells were seen in other wall layers. Lipid analysis in separated kidney glomeruli showed that the amount of cholesterol was markedly higher than normal, all of it as free cholesterol.

Electron microscopic examination revealed that the capillary lumina were partially filled with a meshwork of membranes and particles having an amorphous mottled structure. The capillary wall was abnormal; in some places there were prominent fenestrations whereas in other areas there was an absence of endothelium, irregular thickness of the basal membrane, and fusion of the foot processes. Membrane-limited particles were present in both the subendothelial and subepithelial regions. Pathological changes of this type in the kidney have not previously been reported and hence they seem to be unique for Familial LCAT Deficiency.

ATHEROSCLEROSIS

Patients with Familial LCAT Deficiency develop atherosclerosis. This may be deduced from descriptions of pathological changes in the renal arteries and arterioles that are compatible with early atherosclerotic changes. This view is further supported by autopsy findings from a 40 year-old patient which showed marked atherosclerosis in the aorta.

GENETICS

The family pattern strongly suggests an autosomal recessive mode of inheritance. The Norwegian form most likely is one mutational event occurring before the year 1700. Typing with different genetic marker systems indicates that genetic linkage exists between the alpha-haptoglobin gene and the LCAT gene. When genetic statistical methods are applied, it is usually recognized that a lod (log odds) score of 3 or more is sufficient to prove linkage. In our study, the lod score was about 3.4 at the recombination fraction of 0.00. This proves linkage and shows that the LCAT gene is located in close proximity to the alpha-haptoglobin locus, which is situated between the middle and terminal point of the long arm of chromosome 16. This is the first linkage group reported on this chromosome. Thus, it is highly probable that LCAT deficiency is a single genetic defect caused by the lack of LCAT activity in plasma.

REFERENCES

Bethell W, McCulloch Wj, Ghosh M (1975). Familial lecithin:cholesterol acyltransferase deficiency. Light and electron microscopic findings from two corneas. Canad J Ophthal 10:494.

Borysiewicz L & al. (1981) Personal communication.

Bron AF, Lloyd JK, Fosbrooke AS, Winder AF, Tripathi RC (1975). Primary lecithin:cholesterol acyltransferase deficiency disease. Lancet 1:928.

Chevet D, Ramee PL, Thomas R, Garre M, Alcindor LG (1976). Hereditary lecithin:cholesterol acyltransferase deficiency: Report of a new family with two afflicted sisters. Kidney Inter 10:185.

Frolich J, Godolphin WJ, Reeve CE, Evelyn K (1978). Familial LCAT deficiency. Report of two patients from a Canadian family of Italian and Swedish descent. Scand J Clin Lab Invest 38, Suppl 159:156.

Gjone E, Norum KR (1968). Familial serum-cholesterol

ester deficiency: Clinical study of a patient with a new syndrome. Acta Med Scand 183:107.
Gjone E, Skarbøvik AJ, Blomhoff JP, Teisberg P (1974). Familial lecithin:cholesterol acyltransferase deficiency: Report of a third Norwegian family with two afflicted members. Scand J Clin Lab Invest 33, Suppl 137:101.
Gjone E, Blomhoff JP, Skarbøvik AJ (1974). Possible association between an abnormal low density lipoprotein and nephropathy in lecithin:cholesterol acyltransferase deficiency. Clin Chim Acta 54:11.
Gjone E, Blomhoff JP, Holme R, Hovig T, Olaisen B, Skarbøvik AJ, Teisberg P (accepted for publication 1981). Familial LCAT deficiency: Report of a fourth family from Northwestern Norway. Acta Med Scand.
Gjone E, Norum KR, Glomset JA (1977). Familial LCAT deficiency. In 4th ed. Stanbury JB, Wyngaarden JB, Fredrickson DS (eds): "The Metabolic Basis of Inherited Disease", New York: McGraw-Hill, p 589.
Hamnstrøm B, Gjone E, Norum KR (1979). Familial plasma lecithin:cholesterol acyltransferase deficiency: Report of a Swedish family. Br Med J 2:283.
Iwamoto A, Naito C, Teramoto T, Katu H, Kaka M, Kariya T, Shimuzu T, Oka H, Oda T (1978). Familial lecithin:cholesterol acyltransferase deficiency complicated with unconjugated hyperbilirubinemia and peripheral neuropathy. The first reported case in the Far East. Acta Med Scand 204:219.
Norum KR, Gjone E (1967). Familial plasma lecithin: cholesterol acyltransferase deficiency. Biochemical study of a new inborn error of metabolism. Scand J Clin Lab Invest 20:231.
Norum KR, Børsting S, Grundt I (1970). Familial lecithin:cholesterol acyltransferase deficiency. Acta Med Scand 188:323.
Salmon S, Alcindor LG, Beugler I, Ayrault-Jarrier M, Infante R, Chevet D, Polonovski J (1976). Etude-immunoelectrophoretique des lipoproteines plasmatiques dans un cas de deficience familiale en lecithine-cholesterol acyltransferase. Clin Chim Acta 66:311.
Torsvik H, Gjone E, Norum KR (1968). Familial plasma cholesteryl ester deficiency: Clinical studies in a family. Acta Med Scand 183:387.
Utermann G, Schoenborn W, Langer KH, Dicker P (1972). Lipoproteins in LCAT deficiency. Humangenetik 16:295.

CORNEAL OPACIFICATION AND FAMILIAL DISORDERS AFFECTING PLASMA HIGH-DENSITY LIPOPROTEIN

A.F. Winder and L.K. Borysiewicz

Institute of Ophthalmology and Moorfields Eye Hospital, London EC1 & The Royal Postgraduate Medical School, London W12, England

INTRODUCTION

Diffuse bilateral opacification of the cornea is a feature of three familial dyslipoproteinemias - familial high-density lipoprotein (HDL) deficiency or Tangier disease, Fish-Eye disease, and lecithin : cholesterol acyltransferase (LCAT) deficiency (Schaefer, Zech, Schwartz, Brewer 1980 : Carlson, Philipson 1979 : Gjone 1981) and has been described in a further possibly familial variant of apolipoprotein A deficiency (Gustafson, McConathy, Alaupovic, Curry, Persson 1979). These disorders express various defects in the HDL/LCAT system in plasma, which affects lipoprotein synthesis and composition, and exchange and transfer of lipid between plasma and tissues. Analysis of corneal material has been performed for one case of LCAT deficiency and for two cases of Fish-Eye disease (Winder, Bron 1978 : Philipson 1982) and from these results it is possible that shared influences contribute to the opacification. These findings are discussed together with further data on a new case of LCAT deficiency with a presentation originally suggesting a diagnosis of Fish-Eye disease. It is evident that expression in this group of disorders can be modified by secondary influences, both local and systemic, and that corneal appearances can also be modified although some degree of opacification is eventually universal. It is proposed that these disorders have in common defective clearance of lipid from the cornea, consequent to various abnormalities of the HDL/LCAT system in plasma, the specific corneal appearances being modified by further non-genetic influences.

Birth Defects: Original Article Series, Volume 18, Number 6, pages 433–440

TANGIER DISEASE

Abnormalities in plasma characteristically include moderate elevation of triglyceride and reduction of total cholesterol and low-density lipoprotein (LDL). Apolipoprotein A and HDL are present in trace quantities only. The fundamental defect remains obscure. All components of normal HDL fractions are present, and LCAT activity appears effective in plasma since the proportion of cholesterol in esterified form is normal. The defect may therefore involve availability or assembly of HDL components, although accelerated catabolism of the apolipoprotein A_1 component has also been described (Schaefer, Blum, Levy, Jenkins, Alaupovic, Foster, Brewer 1978).

Lipid enriched with esterified cholesterol accumulates widely in tissues, mostly in foam cells. Studies on isolated cornea are not described, but the punctate and presumably lipid-rich deposit has a pan-stromal distribution accentuated peripherally, has affected all homozygotes age over 40 years and some younger patients, and may significantly affect vision (Schaefer, Zech, Schwartz, Brewer 1980). The marked accumulation of lipid in the tonsils may be facilitated by ambient coolness, maintaining the deposits below their relevant component phase-transition temperatures which owing to changes in composition may also be increased (Katz, Small, Brook, Lees 1977). This effect may also influence the pattern of corneal deposition, which can be accentuated in the medial and lateral quadrants (Spaeth 1971), that is, in the cooler regions of the cornea as is now confirmed by infrared thermography (Fielder, Winder, Cooke, Bowcock 1981).

VARIANT APOLIPOPROTEIN A DEFICIENCY

Dyslipoproteinemia and moderate diffuse opacification of the cornea was described in a female age 48 years by Gustafson, McConathy, Alaupovic, Curry and Persson (1979). Abnormalities in plasma include moderate hypertriglyceridemia without enrichment of the LDL fraction, normal range total cholesterol but marked reduction of the HDL apolipoprotein A fraction. Distribution of lipid in the lipoprotein classes of plasma was also abnormal, but the proportion of cholesterol present in ester form and thus presumably LCAT activity appeared normal. Various tissue deposits of lipid were noted, with foam cells, but the tonsils were not enlarged.

Expression in this patient may have been modified by associated hypothyroidism and its treatment, but a family study revealed minor lipoprotein abnormalities in other members, consistent with a genetic influence. On clinical and biochemical criteria this condition differs from other recognized disorders affecting the HDL/LCAT system in plasma.

FISH-EYE DISEASE

Ocular appearances in this disorder resemble those seen with boiled fish, and three cases in two families are described, possibly with dominant inheritance (Carlson, Philipson 1979 : Carlson 1979:: Philipson 1982). Abnormalities in plasma include hypertriglyceridemia with enrichment of the LDL fraction, normal range total cholesterol and proportion in esterified form presumably excluding any deficiency of LCAT activity in plasma, and much reduced levels of HDL. The corneal opacification significantly affected vision from about age 15 years, although cataracts later found at keratoplasty may also have contributed. Material from two corneas showed diffuse opacification affecting all layers except epithelium, and enrichment with phospholipid and cholesterol with a reduced proportion in esterified form (Philipson 1982). These corneal findings resemble those reported for LCAT deficiency (Winder, Bron 1978) and may indicate a functional LCAT deficiency of restricted distribution. Certainly the clinical and biochemical features of this disorder closely resemble in several respects those of authentic familial LCAT deficiency.

LCAT DEFICIENCY

This plasma enzyme operates in association with HDL as preferred substrate, facilitating transfer of lipid between tissues and plasma and between lipoprotein components. Major deficiency leads to abnormalities in all lipoprotein classes, reduction of the proportion of cholesterol present in esterified form, and in tissue deposits including foam cells. Most patients show moderate elevation in plasma of triglyceride and total cholesterol, with reduction of the apolipoprotein A fraction to about 30% of normal and absence of normal mature HDL components. Abnormal components including lipoprotein X are also found (Gjone 1981).

Corneal opacification is a feature of all known cases and may arise during childhood, although visual impairment is not marked unless additional problems such as trachoma also apply (Gjone 1981; Winder, Bron 1978). The punctate stromal deposit is accentuated peripherally and a clear zone may be present. Opacification is not apparently influenced by the pattern of dyslipoproteinemia and also developed in those few cases with marked hypocholesterolemia and subnormal levels of the LDL fraction (Gjone, Blomhoff, Skarbovic 1974; Bethell, McCulloch, Ghosh 1975; Winder, Bron 1978). One cornea has proceeded to microscopic and biochemical analysis. Inclusion bodies, some membrane-bound, were present with occasional myelin figures : the sample was enriched with phospholipid and the proportion of cholesterol present in esterified form was reduced (Winder, Bron 1978). Renal impairment is a common late feature, possibly associated with the presence of abnormal large molecular weight lipoprotein material in the low density fraction (LMLDL; Gjone, Blomhoff, Skarbovic 1974), although from recent observations this relationship is not close (Borysiewicz, Soutar, Evans, Rees, Thompson 1981).

LCAT DEFICIENCY SIMULATING FISH-EYE DISEASE

We have seen at presentation a female age 48 years of Irish extraction with chronic renal failure, on transfer to the Hammersmith Hospital, London in 1979, for possible renal transplantation. She was then observed to have a diffuse haze symmetrically affecting both corneas (Fig. 1), the fine punctate deposit extending through the full thickness of the stroma being accentuated peripherally but without a definite lucid interval, as shown in the accompanying figure. The epithelium was not involved. Visual acuity was not grossly deficient at 6/12 in each eye : the patient did not complain of reduced acuity and believed it had been stable for years. Clouding had also been recorded 19 years previously on treatment of a corneal abrasion, after which no further action was taken. This was then recorded as a fine, flocculent corneal dystrophy, affecting the full thickness of the stroma and particularly the superficial layers; visual acuity was 6/9 in each eye and there was no known family history. Toxemia had developed during pregnancies in 1960 and 1964, the proteinuria had increased in 1966 following a sore throat and subsequently renal function had progressively declined. The patient was known to have a long-standing fluctuating

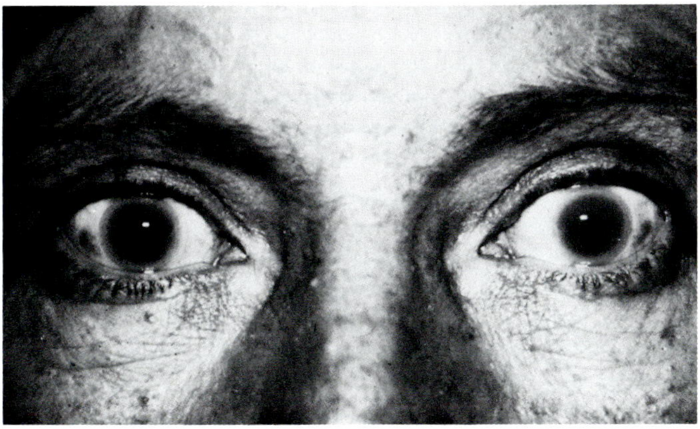

Fig. 1. Corneal appearances in LCAT deficiency simulating Fish-Eye disease

mixed type llb/IV hyperlipidemia, plasma lipids in 1966 being cholesterol 10.6 mM (nephrotic syndrome) and in 1977 triglycerides 21.0 mM, cholesterol 5.2 mM. On transfer in 1979 and shortly after peritoneal dialysis plasma lipids were triglycerides 3.4 mM, cholesterol 3.6 mM and increasing. HDL as cholesterol was reduced to less than 5 mg%, 0.13 mM. The LDL fraction in plasma was enriched with triglyceride and the proportion of cholesterol in plasma as ester form was reduced to about 40%, a level sufficient however on previous data to exclude familial LCAT deficiency. The patient believed that her two older sisters then alive and well and particularly her deceased father also had bilateral corneal clouding, and it was later appreciated that a twin brother had died age 36 years with renal failure and hypertension, his corneal status being unknown.

This patient therefore had bilateral, diffuse and long-standing opacification of the cornea, hypertriglyceridemia with enrichment of the LDL fraction, deficiency of HDL with evidence of LCAT activity, and significantly a family history of corneal abnormalities over two generations. These are the characteristics of Fish-Eye disease which had recently been described and the renal failure also present was reasonably presumed to be acquired. Subsequently however it was appreciated that she had been transfused shortly before transfer to correct anemia, a common feature of LCAT deficiency. Deficiency was established one month after transfusion, and the diagnosis was confirmed by a family study, the nature of any ophthalmological lesion in the deceased father remaining obscure. Renal biopsy revealed foam cells and inclusion bodies in the glomerular basement membrane, with additional changes consistent with immune-complex deposition. Interestingly, LMLDL was present in plasma from this patient and from her two older sisters who had no clinical problems, showing dissociation between the incidence of the LMLDL component and the extent of clinically significant renal damage. Development of such renal damage in familial LCAT deficiency appears to be more random than had previously been appreciated, and a case report emphasizing the renal aspect in this family has recently been presented (Borysiewicz, Soutar, Evans, Rees, Thompson 1981). Presentation was therefore modified by acquired influences - previous transfusion, renal damage and an overlay of secondary renal hyperlipoproteinemia. The residual LCAT activity inferred in plasma at presentation presumably derived from the transfusion as the subsequent decline did not suggest that intestinal LCAT enzyme had been released into plasma as a consequence of peritoneal dialysis.

DISCUSSION

Corneal opacification in these disorders is associated with marked deficiency of HDL in plasma, and established or presumed impairment of the LCAT reaction. Hypertriglyceridemia is also commonly present but levels of triglyceride and of very-low density lipoprotein in plasma tend to show an inverse relationship with HDL through uncertain mechanisms, and the association of corneal opacification with HDL deficiency is probably more significant. Pan-corneal opacification is also not a general feature of hypertriglyceridemia, although any corneal arcus present may perhaps be a little diffuse (Winder, Dodson, Galton 1980). It is not known if or how the presence in plasma of LDL enriched with triglyceride affects the corneal opacification. Various studies of corneal arcus indicate that insudation of lipoprotein from plasma into cornea is a continuous process broadly in balance with clearance. This balance may be upset as by increased insudation with hyperlipidemia or local vascular anomalies, or by more local factors such as temperature variation. It is of special interest that corneal opacification is also a feature of those cases of LCAT deficiency without major hyperlipidemia, and for which plasma levels of low density lipoprotein in particular are reduced below the normal range.

From these various observations we conclude that diffuse corneal opacification in the above disorders results from defective clearance rather than increased entry of lipid, consequent to defects in remobilization arising from major impairment of the HDL/LCAT system in plasma. The degree of corneal opacification and the balance between entry, accumulation and clearance is also influenced by secondary factors - damage by trachoma in our first LCAT case, perhaps major renal hyperlipoproteinemia in our second, and probably local temperature variation in Tangier disease. The nature of Fish-Eye disease and the contribution of any second factors other than cataracts to the clinical presentation remain to be determined. The pattern of lipid in cornea resembles that described for LCAT deficiency and some local deficiency may conceivably apply, although on present evidence enzyme activity of this type is not deficient in plasma. For all these disorders as for the normal cornea, any contribution of local synthesis to lipid accumulation has not yet been evaluated.

ACKNOWLEDGEMENTS

We thank Dr. Bo Philipson, Professor Egil Gjone and Dr. Gilbert Thompson for helpful advice and discussion.

REFERENCES

Bethell W, McCulloch C, Ghosh M (1975). Lecithin: cholesterol acyl transferase deficiency. Light and electron microscopic findings from two corneas. Canad J Ophthal 10: 494.

Borysiewicz LK, Soutar A, Evans DJ, Rees AJ, Thompson GR (1981). The relationship of renal abnormality to plasma lipoproteins in familial lecithin cholesterol transferase (LCAT) deficiency. Quart J Med 74: Autumn (in press).

Carlson LA (1979). A further case of fish-eye disease. Lancet ii : 1376.

Carlson LA, Philipson B (1979). Fish-eye disease. A new familial condition with massive corneal opacities and dyslipoproteinaemia. Lancet ii : 921.

Fielder AR, Winder AF, Cooke DE, Bowcock SA (1981). Arcus senilis and corneal temperature in man. In "The Cornea in Health and Disease" : VI Congress Europ Soc Ophthalmol London : Roy Soc Med and Academic Press, p. 1015.

Gjone E (1981). Familial lecithin: cholesterol acyltransferase deficiency - a new metabolic disease with renal involvement. Adv Nephrology 10 : 167.

Gjone E, Blomhoff JP, Skarbovik AJ (1974). Possible association between an abnormal low density lipoprotein and nephropathy in lecithin : cholesterol acyltransferase deficiency. Clin Chim Acta 54 : 11.

Gustafson A, McConathy W, Alaupovic P, Curry MD, Persson B (1979). Identification of lipoprotein families in a variant of human plasma apolipoprotein A deficiency. Skand J Clin Lab Invest 39 : 377.

Katz SS, Small DM, Brook JG, Lees RS (1977). The storage lipids in Tangier disease. J Clin Invest 59 : 1045.

Philipson BT (1982). Fish-Eye disease. This volume.

Schaefer EJ, Blum CB, Levy RI, Jenkins L, Alaupovic P, Foster DM, Brewer HB (1978). Metabolism of high density lipoprotein apolipoproteins in Tangier disease. New Engl J Med 299 : 519.

Schaefer EJ, Zech LA, Schwartz DE, Brewer HB (1980). Coronary heart disease prevalence and other clinical features in familial high-density lipoprotein deficiency (Tangier disease). Ann Intern Med 93 : 261.

Spaeth GL (1971). Ocular manifestations of the lipidoses. In Tasman W (ed.): "Retinal disease in children". New York: Harper and Row, p. 127.

Winder AF, Bron AJ (1978). Lecithin: cholesterol acyltransferase deficiency presenting as visual impairment, with hypocholesterolaemia and normal renal function. Skand J Clin Lab Invest 38 suppl 150 : 151.

Winder AF, Dodson PM, Galton DJ (1980). Ophthalmological complications of the hypertriglyceridaemias. Trans Ophthal Soc UK 100 : 119.

FISH EYE DISEASE

Bo T. Philipson M.D.

Dept.of Ophthalmology,Karolinska Hospital

104 01 Stockholm, Sweden

A new familial condition characterized by dyslipoproteinaemia and corneal clouding has recently been described by Carlson and Philipson (1979). This condition was called Fish eye disease (FED) due to the dense corneal opacification resembling a boiled fish eye. FED is distinctly different from other reported familial conditions, but has many similarities with Tangier disease (Fredrickson, Altrocchi, Avioli, Goodman and Goodman,1961) and LCAT dificiency (Norum and Gjone,1967). Three cases of FED have been studied to date, two sisters and one unrelated woman (Philipson, Carlson, Holmberg and Kock,1981).

CLINICAL COURSE

Corneal clouding first became evident near the end of the second decade of life in all cases studied, but none of the patients were aware of visual impairment initially. During the third decade, allthree women noticed a slight visual impairment at dusk and in bright sunlight. Visual acuity slowly deteriorated to about 0.4 (20/50) by age 60, and color discrimination was also impaired. The general health has remained good. In all cases of FED studied, the patients continued working until age 60 to 65 despite severe visual problems at dusk, during the dark winter months, or in poor illumination.

In the family of the two sisters studied (fig.1) these corneal opacities were present in the father as well as in a third sister who was killed in an accident at age 37. Almost identical opacities and dyslipoproteinemia between the index cases suggests a genetic transmission.

Birth Defects: Original Article Series, Volume 18, Number 6, pages 441–448

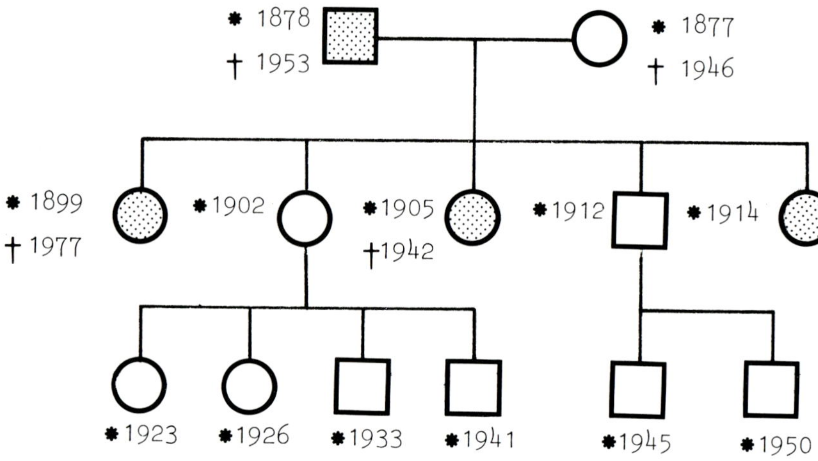

Figure 1 Family tree for the FED family. FED disease dotted symbols

Limited family medical histories, however, do not reveal the nature of genetic transmission, except to show that FED is not a sex-linked dominant trait.

SLITLAMP APPEARANCE

All FED patients were in the seventh decade of life when studied. In all cases, the corneae were symmetrically opaque to the extent that the irises could only be seen as an indistinct shadow (fig.2). Under magnification in the slit lamp, the corneal cloudiness appeared as small dot-like grey-white-yellow opacities forming a mosaic pattern. The opacities were present in all layers of the cornea except in the epithelium. The turbidity was relatively even over the corneal surface but seemed to be somewhat more opaque at the periphery. In the peripheral corneae of the two sisters, a thin superficial yellow ring was visible about 1mm from the limbus. Generally, in each case, corneal thickness was increased to about 0.7mm, the epithelium appeared normal,and the sensation was normal. The conjunctiva was unremarkable except for a more pronounced appearance of the blood vessels which may have been due to the slight yellow color. The intraocular pressure has been normal in all cases.

Figure 2

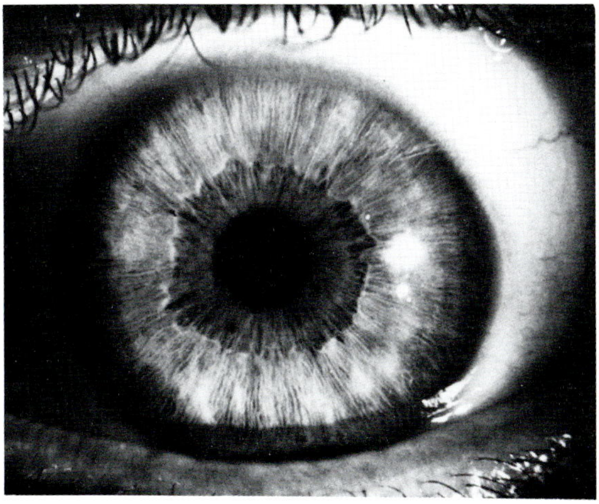

Normal cornea from the daughter, 37 years old, of a FED-patient

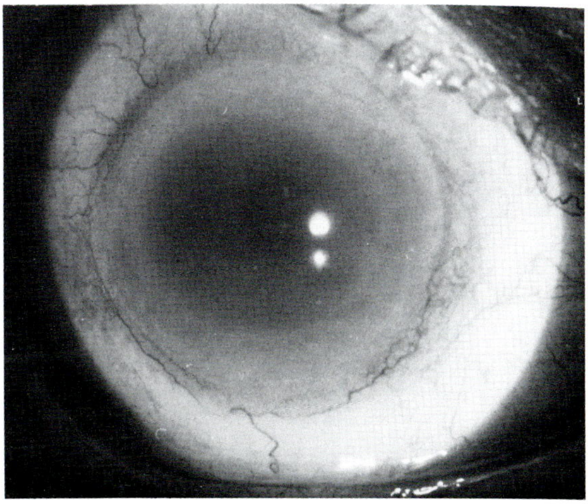

The cornea from a FED patient, 65 years old. The corneal cloudiness obscures the iris

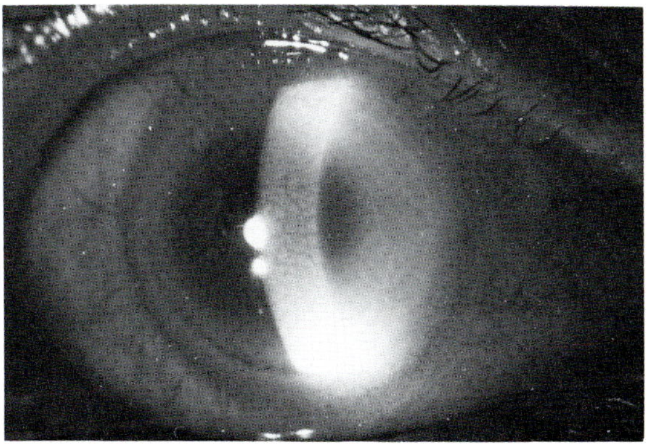

Slitlamp photo of the cornea from a FED patient, 71 years old. Note the dot-like opacities

CORNEAL TRANSPLANTATION

Presently, the only treatment of the visual impairment is corneal transplantation. In two cases, corneal grafting has been performed with no complications. A cortical cataract was visible in one case after trepanation of the cornea, and a cryoextraction of the lens was done. In both cases, the corneal graft has stayed clear; visual acuity and color discrimination have been improved. The fundus has been inspected ophthalmoscopically and with fluorescin angiography. Except for an uneven pigmentation of the maculae, the appearance has been normal for the age.

SERUM LIPOPROTEIN CHANGES

All the FED cases had very similar lipoprotein changes in the serum (Carlsson,1981). The main findings are summarized in Table 1. They are hypertriglyceridaemia, increased very low density lipoproteins (VLDL) with a normal cholesterol/ triglyceride ratio, a high triglyceride concentration in low density lipoproteins (LDL), and a cholesterol concentration in high density lipoproteins (HDL) reduced by 90% compared to controls.

Table 1
Median values for cholesterol (CH) and triglycerides (TG) in whole serum and in serum lipoproteins for three cases of FED and for 55 controls. Median mean (med), minimal (min) and maximal (max) values are given in mmol/l.

		VLDL		LDL		HDL		SERUM	
		CH	TG	CH	TG	CH	TG	CH	TG
FED	Min	0.81	0.86	4.00	1.46	0.10	0.05	5.07	2.68
	Med	1.67	3.30	4.99	2.03	0.18	0.07	6.48	5.61
	Max	2.26	4.40	6.52	3.32	0.42	0.16	8.82	7.32
Control	Min	0.02	0.20	1.89	0.14	1.14	0.13	4.25	0.59
	Med	0.30	0.56	3.94	0.33	1.84	0.24	6.39	1.20
	Max	0.87	1.35	7.37	1.11	2.94	0.43	9.40	2.28

PATHOLOGY

The corneal buttons from the two transplanted corneas were studied by histochemistry, microradiography and electron-microscopy. The epithelium, Descemete´s membrane, and the endothelium appeared normal by all methods. Bowmans layer was filled with abundant small vacuoles covering about 15% of the volume. The stroma contained, in addition, a high frequency of vacuoles with a diameter of up to 2 µm. The vacuoles were lined by a thin layer of osmiophilic material, and their content was amorphous. They did not appear to be associated with the keratocytes, but were located in between the collagen fibrills. The frequency of the vacuoles was variable with a tendancy toward the higher frequencies appearing in ill-defined circular regions having a diameter of approximately 0.5mm. This was constant throughout the depth of the cornea, occupying about 20 per cent of the stroma.

Methanol-chloroform extraction revealed a 15% decrease in dry mass compared to 3.4% decrease in the normal cornea. Chemical extraction indicated a strong increase (~100%) in cholesterol. Only 6% of the cholesterol was esterified compared to 68% in controls.

The vacuoles stained with the OTAN-method and the PAN-method indicating a cholesterol containing lipid material in the vacuoles. Free cholesterol is presumably accumulated to some extent in the vacuoles. The nature of the major part of the material in the vacuoles is not known, but it might be a proteolipid material.

CLINICOPATHOLOGIC CORRELATION

The vacuoles are responsible for the increased scatter of light which is observed as a clouding of the cornea. At the border between the normal stroma and the deposited material there must be refractive index differences causing scatter of light. The mosaic pattern of the opacities in the cornea might be explained by the higher frequency of vacuoles in regions about 0.5mm in diameter, interspaced with regions of less vacuoles. The absence of vacuoles with deposited material in the epithelium is probably due to its relatively rapid turn-over of cells. The accumulation of deposited material in Bowmans layer and in the stroma is very slow, as evidenced by the fact that the two corneal transplants have stayed biomicroscopically clear for at least one and three years, respectively.

DIFFERENTIAL DIAGNOSIS

Corneal opacities which are manifestations of systemic disease are generally not classified as dystrophies. Central crystalline corneal dystrophy of Schnyder is, however, a systemic disorder with hyperlipidemia (Grop ,1973). The corneae of older persons with this disease can be relatively opaque, and might then be hard to distinguish from the corneae in FED. Central crystalline corneal dystrophy is characterized by a dense corneal arcus and minute cholesterol crystals in the stroma, which causes a grey stromal haze. There are also round globules in the stroma which supposedly contain neutral fats, triglycerides and noncrystalline cholesterol. Although the globules of Schnyder's dystrophy resemble those seen in FED, crystals are never seen in the latter. Also, Schnyder's dystrophy opacities are central, not covering all the cornea. Furthermore, both the serum cholesterol and the triglycerides may be elevated in Schnyder's dystrophy, which often is accompanied by genu valgum (Luxenberg,1967).

Tangier disease and lecitin-cholesterol acyl-transferase (LCAT) deficiency are two familial conditions with corneal clouding and dyslipoproteinemia. Tangier disease has severe deficiency or absence of high density lipoproteins (HDL) in plasma and abnormal low density lipoproteins (LDL). Common clinical findings include enlarged yellow tonsils, hepatosplenomegaly and neuropathy. The dyslipoproteinemia of LCAT-deficiency is characterized by a reduction of cholesterol esters in the plasma lipoproteins due to the absence of the LCAT-enzyme and the very low density lipoproteins (VLDL), LDL and HDL to about 65%. The clinical findings are anemia, proteinuria and eventually chronic renal failure.

The corneal changes of Tangier disease and LCAT-deficiency are dot-like opacities throughout the stroma and covering the entire cornea, but much less dense than those seen in the older patients with FED. The visual impairment has been reported to be very small in Tangier disease and LCAT-deficiency (Herbert, Gotto and Fredrickson,1978; Hörven, Gjone and Egge, 1976).

Fish eye disease (FED) differs strikingly from both Tangier´s disease and LCAT deficiency; FED has none of the major clinical symptoms of either. In contrast to LCAT deficiency, the LCAT activity is normal in FED, and there is a normal content of cholesterol esters in the lipoproteins. The electrophoretic mobility of HDL is normal in FED but pathological in Tangier´s disease.

While the above conditions share certain characteristics with Fish eye disease, it is clear that FED is a uniquely separate disorder which may be distinguished from them.

REFERENCES

Carlson L.A., Philipson B. (1979) Fish-Eye Disease, a new familial condition with massive corneal opacities and dyslipoproteinaemia. The Lancet ii:921-923

Carlson L.A. (1981) Fish Eye Disease: a new familial condition with massive corneal opacities and dyslipoproteinaemia. Clinical and laboratory studies in two afflicted families. Eur J Clin Inv In press

Fredrickson D.S., Altrocchi P.H., Avioli L.V., Goodman D.S., Goodman H.C. (1961) Tangier Disease. Ann Intern Med 55: 1016-1020

Grop K. (1973) Clinical and histological findings in crystalline corneal dystrophy. Acta Ophthalmol 120:52-57

Herbert P.N., Gotto A.M., Fredrickson D.S. (1978) Familial lipoprotein deficiency. The Metabolic Basis of Inherited Disease, 4th edn New York: Mac Graw Hill Chapter 28 p.544

Hörven I., Gjone E., Egge K. (1976) Ocular manifestations in familial LCAT deficiency. Birth. Defects XII, 271-278

Luxenberg M. (1967) Hereditary crystalline dystrophy of the cornea. Am J Ophthalmol 63:507-511

Norum K.R., Gjone E. (1967) Familial plasma lecithin: cholesterol acyltransferase deficiency. Biochemical study of a new inborn error of metabolism. Scand J Clin Lab Invest 20: 231-237

Philipson B.T., Carlson L.A., Holmberg Å., Kock E. (1981) Ocular manifestations in fish eye disease, manus.

FACTORS INFLUENCING THE VARIABLE EXPRESSION OF XANTHELASMATA AND CORNEAL ARCUS IN FAMILIAL HYPERCHOLESTEROLAEMIA

A.F. Winder

Institute of Ophthalmology Moorfields Eye Hospital and the Lipid Clinic St. Bartholomew's Hospital, London EC1, England

INTRODUCTION

Heterozygous familial hypercholesterolaemia affects about 1 per 500 live births in Europe and north America, and homozygotes also rarely occur. In these disorders, defects in the cell surface receptor system for low-density lipoprotein (LDL) impair delivery of cholesterol to peripheral tissues, resulting in elevation of LDL in plasma consequent mainly to reduced fractional turnover (Goldstein, Brown 1977; Shepherd, Lorimer, Bicker, Packard, 1979). Levels of high density lipoprotein (HDL) in plasma are also generally depressed, and those of the triglyceride-rich very-low-density lipoprotein (VLDL) may be elevated in a type IIb pattern. Xanthelasmata and premature corneal arcus are common features of these disorders and may lead to presentation and diagnosis although there is wide individual variation in the incidence and rate of progression of these and other adventitious deposits. (Adlersberg, Parets 1949, Schatz 1969; Gagne, Moorjani, Brun, Toussaint, Lupien 1979). Most earlier studies on the effects of age on patterns of hyperlipidaemia for these familial disorders have shown that patterns for individuals are broadly constant from early life until diagnosis and treatment (Kwiterovich, Fredrickson, Levy 1974; Slack, Preece, Giles 1980). Thus analysis of these patterns in patients of different ages and with a range of expressions of xanthelasmata and corneal arcus may indicate systemic factors affecting this variable expression. This analysis has been performed, and since ophthalmological expression of the hyperlipoprotein-

Birth Defects: Original Article Series, Volume 18, Number 6, pages 449-462

patients age over 30 years at presentation and assessment or when xanthelasmata were first recorded before treatment. Data is shown in table 1. It was assumed that xanthelasmata first noted at presentation were of recent onset. These two groups with and without

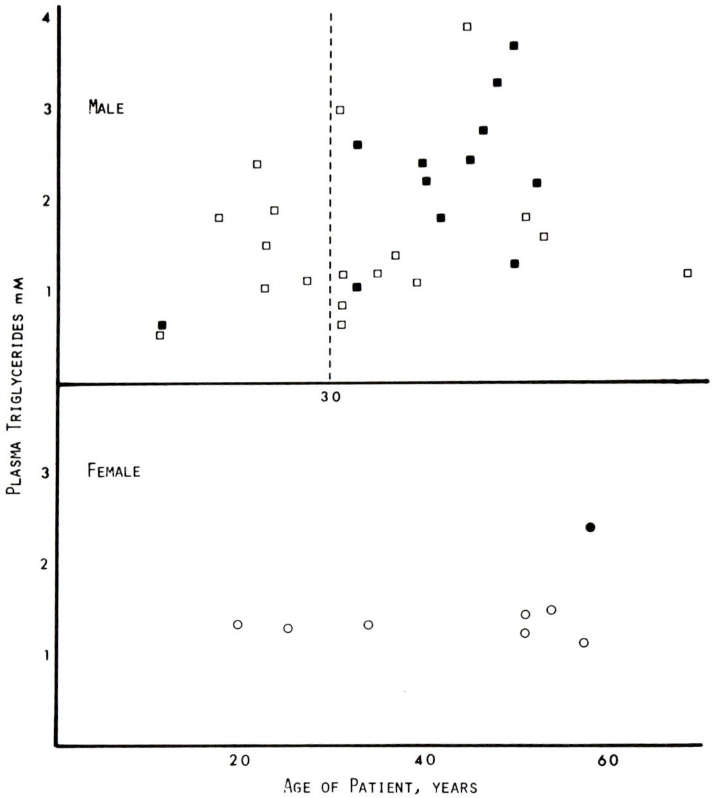

Figure 1. Incidence of xanthelasmata-shaded-in heterozygotes, showing data for age and fasting plasma triglycerides at presentation.

xanthelasmata fortuitously each contained 11 subjects and were well-matched for age. The two groups could not be fully resolved by discriminant analysis, largely owing to data obtained for patient 16. Some differences between the groups observed on comparison for individual variables is shown in table 2: owing to the small difference in mean

Table 2 Comparison between male heterozygotes age over 30 years with and without xanthelasmata

Variable	with	without	P.
Age	43.7 ± 6.6 (11)	41.4 ± 12.2 (11)	0.59
TG	2.33 ± 0.78(11)	1.63 ± 0.98 (11)	0.076
log TG	0.79 ± 0.38(11)	0.36 ± 0.52 (11)	0.036
chol (c)	10.05 ± 1.78(11)	8.96 ± 1.04 (11)	0.94
c x Age	436.4 ± 88.1 (11)	369.5 ± 107.2 (11)	0.25
HDLC	0.78 ± 0.12(6)	1.20 ± 0.19 (9)	<0.001
LDLC	8.22 ± 2.21(6)	7.32 ± 0.89 (8)	0.31
H/L	0.10 ± 0.03(6)	0.17 ± 0.04 (9)	0.004
log TG x Age	35.3 ± 18.4 (11)	15.8 ± 20.9 (11)	0.031

Data shown are mean, standard deviation and number of patients.

age the compound terms incorporating age were not additionally helpful in this analysis. Data for plasma triglyceride - but not for total - or HDL-cholesterol - was skewed and converted to logarithms for further determination of significance. The group without xanthelasmata had significantly higher levels in plasma of HDL (as cholesterol), higher HDL/LDL-cholesterol ratios and lower levels of triglycerides than the group with xanthelasmata. Plasma levels of total cholesterol were higher in the xanthelasma group but the difference was not significant.

Some data on the six homozygotes seen is shown in table 3. Xanthelasmata were the cause of presentation in patient E at age 1.5 years and were present on assessment at age 19.5 years. The other patients did not have and were not known to have had xanthelasmata, although

Table 3 Arcus grade and plasma lipids in six homozygotes, assessed at age stated. Patient E had xanthelasmata.

Patient	Age/Sex	Arcus	Chol mM	TG mM
A	5.3F	1	23.6	1.19
B	28.9F	0	16.1-11.4	2.0
C	15.3M	2	19.8	1.8
D	16.5M	2	20.1- 8.4	1.07
E	19.5M	2	18.0	1.85
F	26.7M	3	15.5- 8.7	0.9

all six patients had extensive cutaneous or other xanthomata. All except patient C had ischaemic heart disease and all but patient B had corneal arcus. Levels of cholesterol in plasma of patients B, D and F had been reduced to the mean lower values also shown by plasma exchange over periods of approximately 1, 2 and 3 years respectively. However the age-integrated exposure to hypercholesterolaemia was clearly greater for this group than for age-matched heterozygotes also considered, whereas exposure to hypertriglyceridaemia was not marked. Plasma levels of HDL were markedly depressed in all patients.

OBSERVATIONS FOR CORNEAL ARCUS

A detailed analysis of the relationship between age,

plasma cholesterol and extent of corneal arcus was restricted to the 19 male and 8 female heterozygotes assessed at presentation and before treatment. This data is presented as a scattergram in figure 2. All three patients without macroscopic arcus were aged below 25 years and both patients with a grade 4 arcus were aged over 57 years. However not all subjects below the age of 50 years had extensive arcus, and this variability was also shown

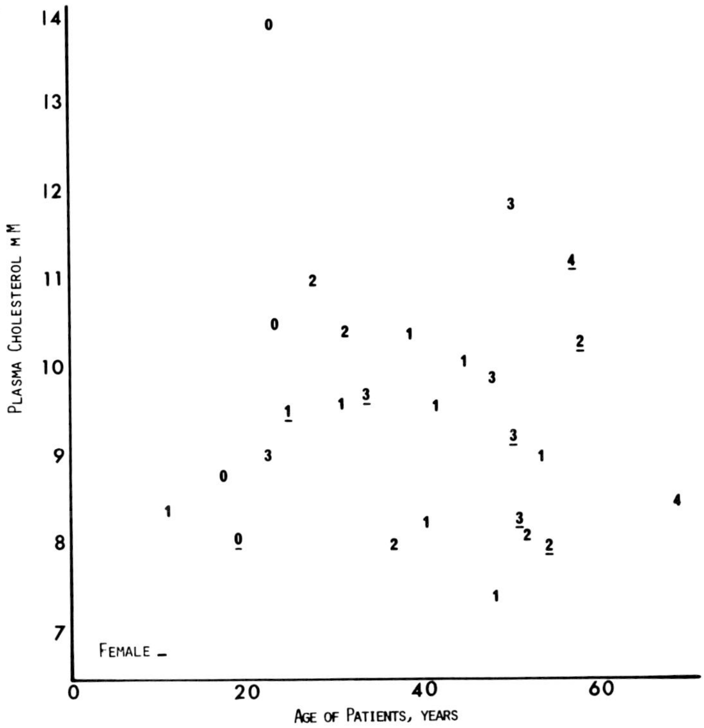

Figure 2. Degree of corneal arcus, fasting plasma cholesterol and age at presentation for heterozygotes.

for the 6 homozygotes as shown in table 3. Further statistical analysis of this data confirmed that the extent of corneal arcus correlated closely with age, for males alone or for both sexes combined (s <0.001). Significant correlations with arcus grade were not obtained with plasma triglyceride or total cholesterol, HDL- or LDL-cholesterol or with the HDL/LDL-cholesterol ratio. Correlations were obtained with these terms additionally incorporating age but these were invalid in view of the correlation with age alone. Thus the extent of arcus did not correlate with any of the systemic lipoprotein factors considered, and the wide individual variation within the general relationship with age also indicated that other possibly local influences were significant.

LOCAL INFLUENCES

Xanthelasmata

The lipid composition of xanthomata of recent origin resembles that of plasma and is influenced by changes in the pattern of dyslipoproteinaemia, but the deposit subsequently matures to more stable and saturated material. (Baes, van Gent, Pries 1968). Winder and Bruckdorfer (in preparation) have examined the range of thermal transition temperatures of lipid material from long-standing xanthomata. These transitions were observed to occur in a range progressing above local skin temperature, consonant with the chemical changes noted and exceeding the range observed for unmodified plasma lipid. These changes in chemical properties and consequently thermotropic phase behaviour may therefore contribute to the lack of mobilisation and refractory nature of long-standing deposits, as has been proposed on similar grounds for the lipid accumulating in the tonsils, cornea and other sites in patients with Tangier Disease (Katz, Small, Brooks, Lees 1977).

Corneal Arcus

Infra-red thermography of the human cornea has shown that the upper and lower limbal quadrants are 0.8-1°C warmer than the centre, which is about 3.6°C below core temperature. (Fielder, Winder, Cooke, Bowcock 1981). These observations are consistent with the original suggestion of Braendstrup (cited by Forsius 1954) that local temperature influenced the pattern of distribution of corneal arcus, presumably because insudation is more active in the warmer regions, and local temperature may also be a factor in the chronicity of corneal arcus once formed. We have not yet been able to directly determine the range of transition temperatures of arcus material in vitro because of problems of sensitivity, but chemical analysis of the deposit indicates that the pattern of acyl residues present is less unsaturated and of greater mean chain length than that of plasma. (Sheraidah, Winder, Fielder 1981). These changes would be expected to increase the range of transition temperatures and decrease ease of mobilisation of the deposit. Our attempts to determine whether variation in the extent of corneal arcus in patients heterozygous for familial hypercholesterolaemia is a function of individual variation in corneal thermographic profiles in vivo currently remain inconclusive.

Corneal temperature and local blood flow are interrelated, and limbal vascular anomalies produce changes in the anatomical pattern of corneal arcus. It is likely that insudation of lipoprotein material at the limbus is a continuous process, and that arcus arises as a delayed result of imbalance between insudation and remobilisation. We have observed marked unilateral arcus in association with contralateral carotid stenosis, and reduced intraocular pressure which may also favour insudation and imbalance as above (Fielder, Winder, Sheraidah, Cooke 1981). Homozygous patient E is of special interest in that when seen age 19.5 years he had lower segment arcus on both sides, with additional upper segment deposit on the left as shown in figure 3. He then also had marked bilateral carotid bruits, probably due to the carotid root narrowing characteristic of homozygous familial hypercholesterolaemia. However, he had been noted to have a carotid bruit on the right side only at age 5 years. Differential carotid stenosis and unequal ocular effects may therefore have contributed to the unequal distribution of arcus observed. Unfortunately the patient has since died during further aortic root surgery and thermographic studies and tonometry were not performed.

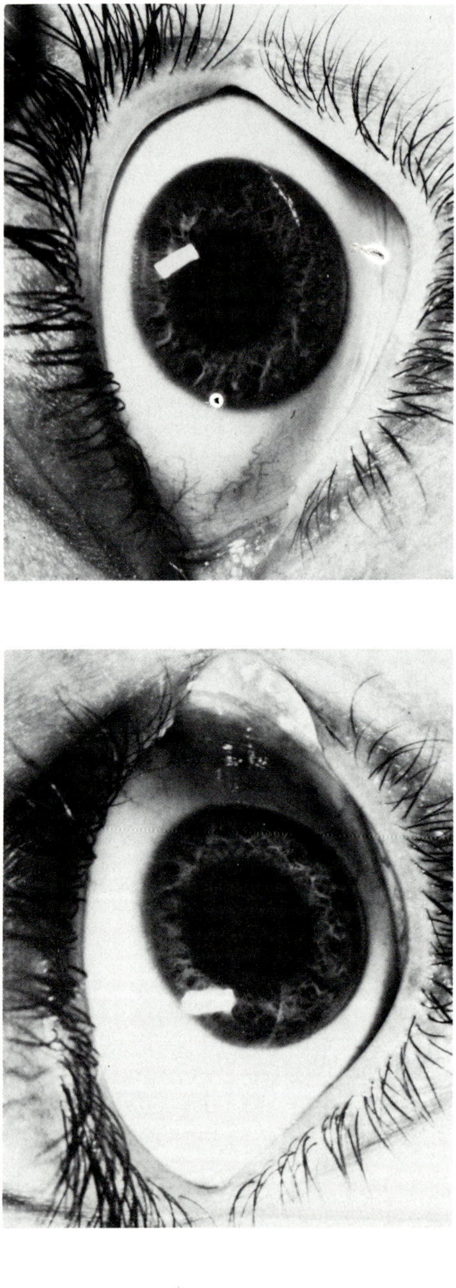

Figure 3. Differential corneal arcus in a homozygote age 19.5 years with unequal development of carotid stenosis

CONCLUSION

This study has shown that in the extreme case of familial hypercholesterolaemia the incidence of xanthelasmata but not of corneal arcus is affected by component variation within the pattern of hyperlipidaemia. The group of patients with xanthelasmata showed elevated levels in plasma of triglycerides and by implication of VLDL, and levels of HDL as cholesterol were reduced, in comparison with the xanthelasma-free group. The mean elevation of plasma cholesterol also seen was not significant. The two lipoproteins VLDL and HDL are known to be inversely related in familial hypercholesterolaemia, although the probably multiple causes of this relationship have not been precisely determined, and they may not be independent factors in the development of xanthelasmata. It may be however that hypertriglyceridaemia is the overrid -ing systemic aetiological factor and that the intra-cellular deposit is derived predominantly from VLDL. HDL may hinder this accumulation by effecting remobilisation of insudated material, as is proposed for atheromatous lesions (Gordon, Castelli, Hjortland, Kannel, Dawber 1977) and has been inferred from remobilisation of lipid observed in tissue culture (Stein, Glangeaud, Fainarn, Stein 1975). The indifferent relationship with the level of total cholesterol in plasma is emphasised by the observations on homozygotes. All six patients had major hypercholesterolaemia and reduced levels of HDL but levels of triglyceride in plasma were normal range or borderline and xanthelasmata arose in only one patient. Watanabe, Yoshimura, Wagasugi and colleagues have recently reported data obtained for 53 patients with xanthelasmata, including 5 male and 6 female patients with heterozygous familial hypercholesterolaemia. They found for this mixed group that levels of triglycerides in plasma and its distribution through the lipoprotein components were important variables, and that levels of total plasma cholesterol were also increased in the group with xanthelasmata in comparison with normal control subjects. The lack of correlation between an incidence of xanthelasmata and the distribution and extent of other adventitious lipid deposits has been widely noted and remains obscure.

The development of corneal arcus is closely related to the duration of hyperlipoproteinaemia, and thus to the patients' age, rather than to its extent or pattern. Since the incidence of corneal arcus is increased in association with various patterns of hyperlipidaemia this latter is an aetiological factor, and the relationship with age may indicate a permissive effect, the process becoming time- rather than dose-dependent above a threshold level of hyperlipaemia. Plasma levels of HDL in particular did not seem to influence the natural history of this extracellular deposit, in contrast to observations for the intracellular deposits of xanthelasmata. Expression may also be influenced by local factors, of which intraocular pressure, and local vascular perfusion perhaps affecting ocular temperature, insudation or remobilisation have been identified.

It seems reasonable to assume that similar influences apply to the development of both xanthelasmata and corneal arcus when they arise in association with familial hypercholesterolaemia or with less specific lipoprotein disorders when the inconstant systemic background in particular is generally difficult to evaluate. The above observations may clarify both these relationships and the diagnostic and prognostic significance of these two ophthalmological lesions.

ACKNOWLEDGEMENTS

The co-operation of Dr. D.J. Galton, Dr. G.R.Thompson and Dr. A.R. Fielder with clinical studies, Mrs. B. Payne and Dr. J. Stocks with laboratory data and Mr. H.C. Donovan with statistical analysis is greatly appreciated.

REFERENCES

Adlersberg D, Parets AD (1949). Genetic studies of 201 persons with hereditary hypercholesterolaemia (abstract) J Clin Invest 28:767.

Baes H, Van Gent CM, Pries C (1968). Lipid composition of various types of xanthoma. J Invest Dermatol 51:286.

Fielder AR, Winder AF, Cooke DE, Bowcock SA (1981). Arcus senilis and corneal temperature in man. In "The Cornea in Health and Disease": VI Congress Europ.Soc.Ophthalmol. London: Roy Soc Med and Academic Press, p. 1015.

Fielder AR, Winder AF, Sheraidah GAK, Cooke ED (1981). Problems with corneal arcus. Trans Ophthal Soc UK 101: in press.
Forsius H (1954). Arcus senilis. Acta Ophthalmol (Kbh) suppl. 42:1.
Friedenwald WT, Levy RI, Fredrickson DS (1972). Estimation of the concentration of low-density lipoprotein cholesterol in plasma, without use of the preparative ultracentrifuge. Clin Chem 18:499.
Gagne C, Moorjani S, Brun D, Toussaint M, Lupien P-J (1979). Heterozygous familial hypercholesterolaemia. Relationship between plasma lipids, lipoproteins, clinical manifestations and ischaemic heart disease in men and women. Atherosclerosis 34:13.
Goldstein JL, Brown MS (1977). The low density lipoprotein pathway and its relation to atherosclerosis. Ann Rev Biochem 46:897.
Gordon T, Castelli WP, Hjörtland MC, Kannel WB, Dawber TR (1977). High density lipoprotein as a protective factor against coronary heart disease. Amer J Med 62:707.
Katz SS, Small DM, Brook JG, Lees RS (1977). The storage lipids in Tangier disease. J Clin Invest 59:1045.
Kwiterovich PO, Fredrickson DS, Levy RI (1974). Familial hypercholesterolaemia (one form of familial type II hyperlipoproteinaemia). A study of its biochemical, genetic, and clinical presentation in childhood. J Clin Invest 53:1237.
Schatz IJ (1969). Classification of primary hyperlipaemia. Observations on 214 patients. J Amer Med Assoc[n] 210:701.
Shepherd J, Bicker S, Lorimer AR, Packard CJ (1979). Receptor-mediated low density lipoprotein catabolism in man. J Lipid Res 20:999.
Sheraidah GAK, Winder AF, Fielder AR (1981). Lipid-protein constituents of human corneal arcus. Atherosclerosis 40:91.
Slack J, Preece M, Giles P (1980). Identification of children who are heterozygotes for familial hyper-cholesterolaemia. In Gotto AM, Smith LC, Allen B (eds.): "Atherosclerosis V" New York:Springer, p.244.
Stein Y, Glangeaud MC, Fainarn M, Stein O (1975). The removal of cholesterol from aortic smooth muscle in culture and Landschutz ascites cells by fractions of human HD apolipoprotein.Biochem Biophys Acta 380:106.

Watanabe A, Yoshimura A, Wakasugi T, Tatami R, Ueda K, Ueda R, Haba T, Kametani T, Koizumi J, Ito S, Ohta M, Miyamoto S, Mabuchi H, Takeda R (1981). Serum lipids, lipoprotein lipids and coronary heart disease in patients with xanthelasmata palpebrarum. Atherosclerosis 38:283.

CURRENT CONCEPT OF MACULAR CORNEAL DYSTROPHY

Gordon K. Klintworth, M.D., Ph.D.

Duke University Medical Center

Durham, North Carolina 27710

Of the many well-defined inherited disorders of the cornea (see review by Klintworth 1980a) macular corneal dystrophy (MCD) is the most thoroughly investigated and this report summarizes the current status of our knowledge about MCD and highlights some observations on the disease.

In MCD clinical disease is limited to the cornea where whitish ill-defined opacities gradually accumulate within a hazy corneal stroma of both eyes in persons who are almost always otherwise healthy. The opaque spots usually first become evident in the central cornea at about puberty, but sometimes the cornea appears abnormal on slit-lamp examination during infancy and early childhood. In most cases the opacities become apparent to the eye of an observer without magnification before forty years of age. With time the opaque spots enlarge, become more numerous and confluent, and involve the peripheral cornea. In some cases the entire cornea eventually loses its transparency. Excrescences often form on the posterior surface of Descemet's membrane (cornea guttata) but, in contrast to Fuchs' dystrophy corneal edema with sub-epithelial bullae are not usually features. Visual acuity progressively diminishes as the cornea opacifies and eventually keratoplasty becomes necessary to restore vision, usually before the end of the fifth decade. Rarely, vision does not deteriorate until late in life. While most grafts remain transparent indefinitely following keratoplasty, the dystrophy recurs in the donor tissue on rare occasions sometimes within three years (Lorenzetti and Kaufman 1967; Morgan 1966; Klintworth 1981b; Robin et al., 1977). In recurrences that have been confirmed histologically the peripheral cornea is affected more extensively than the central cornea (Klintworth 1981b), probably as a result of the infiltration of the

Birth Defects: Original Article Series, Volume 18, Number 6, pages 463–477

corneas with MCD. Moreover, fibroblasts from normal individuals often accumulate similar material (Klintworth and Smith 1977). Assays of several degradative enzymes of glycosaminoglycans and glycoproteins in cultured fibroblasts from the cornea, skin or conjunctiva of persons with MCD have failed to disclose a consistent abnormality (Cotlier et al. 1973; Horwitz and Klintworth 1980), in contrast to many other inherited storage diseases. Especially noteworthy is the finding of normal amounts of several enzymes involved in keratan sulfate catabolism (galactose 6-sulfate sulfatase, N-acetylgalactosamine 6-sulfatase, β -D galactosidase, and N-acetylglucosamine 6-sulfatase) (Horwitz and Klintworth 1980). Unlike the inherited systemic mucopolysaccharidoses kinetic studies on cultured corneal fibroblasts using radioactive labelled precursors of glycosaminoglycans have also been without avail. Fibroblasts from patient's with MCD fail to accumulate ^{35}S-sulfate or ^{3}H-glucosamine labelled glycosaminoglycans (Klintworth 1977; Klintworth and Smith 1977). Moreover, they do not secrete excessive amounts of labelled macromolecules into the medium. After vital staining with acridine orange cultured skin and corneal fibroblasts from persons with MCD differ strikingly from similarly treated skin fibroblasts from patients with the systemic mucopolysaccharidoses, which take up the dye to accumulate it avidly in lysosomes containing stored glycosaminoglycans (Klintworth et al., 1979). An occasional cultured cell in MCD develops giant lysosomes but this abnormality is not characteristic of MCD, as once suggested (Francois et al. 1976), also occuring in poorly preserved normal cells as when cultural conditions are inadequate.

STUDIES USING ORGAN CULTURE

The incubation of portions of intact corneas in radioactive medium has provided the only consistent *in vitro* abnormality in MCD. When the technique of organ culture was first applied to the disease by Klintworth and Smith (1977) it was unexpectedly observed that a cornea with MCD produced less keratan sulfate than normal. Since then we have found organ cultures of corneas from 5 individuals with MCD to incorporate less ^{35}S-sulfate, and usually less ^{3}H-glucosamine into keratan sulfate I than normal corneas (Klintworth and Smith 1980). This observation has been confirmed independently by Hassell et al. (1980) in a study of 3 corneas from persons with MCD. Later it was discovered by serendipity that corneas with MCD synthesize excessive quantities of oligosaccharides that elute in characteristic positions from DEAE-Sephacel with a linear gradient of lithium chloride in front of the sulfated glycosaminoglycans (Klintworth and Smith, 1980). In further studies on ^{35}S-sulfate and ^{3}H-glucosamine labelled organ cultures of corneas from patients with MCD, the proteoglycans and glycoproteins have been extracted, isolated and analyzed. In such investigations notable deviations from the norm have been detected in all investigated organ cultures of corneas with MCD (Hassell et al. 1980; Klintworth and Smith 1981a,c). Corneal organ cultures from 5 different patients with MCD have not synthesized keratan sulfate proteoglycan, but have yielded instead a glycoprotein with unusually large oligosaccharide side chains and a lower molecular weight than keratan sulfate proteoglycan. A significant amount of this protein from corneas with MCD is degraded by mixed glycosidases, but keratan sulfate-ß-endogalactosidase has little effect on it (Hassell et al. 1980; Klintworth and Smith 1981a). Hassell et al. (1980) speculated that it might be a precursor of keratan sulfate proteoglycan and this hypothesis is supported by the observation that the abnormal glycoprotein extract of corneas with MCD reacts with a purified IgG antibody to the core protein of corneal keratan sulfate proteoglycan (monkey) as determined by the ELISA (enzyme linked immunosorbent assay) reaction (Hassell et al. 1981). Within the limits of the employed analytical techniques no major difference has been detected in the galactosaminoglycan proteoglycan (chondroitin sulfate proteoglycan) fraction of corneal organ cultures in MCD and normal controls.

While most organ cultures of corneas with MCD have synthesized a similar glycoprotein one specimen synthesized proteoglycans that eluted in the usual positions of keratan sulfate and galactosaminoglycan proteoglycans but produced an abnormal shoulder on the elution peak of the structural glycoproteins (Klintworth 1980b).

After a prolonged extraction in 4M and 8M guanidine hydrochloride (48 hours in each) the dystrophic keratocytes in corneas with MCD still contain abundant intracellular material with the histochemical and ultrastructural attributes of nonextracted corneas with MCD. The stored substance coincides with concentrations of non-extractable isotope as revealed by autoradiography (Klintworth and Smith 1981c) and transmission electron microscopy has revealed it to be situated at sites of disrupted cells that lack intact cell membranes (Klintworth and Smith 1981c).

ORIGIN OF STORAGE MATERIAL

It has long been suspected that corneal fibroblasts produce

their storage material. This view is supported by the transmission electron microscopic observation in MCD of a dilated endoplasmic reticulum (a site of synthesis of complex metabolites) in some corneal fibroblasts of surgically excised corneal tissue with MCD. While not conclusive a lack of morphologic evidence of phagocytosis argues against the ingestion of the stored material.

IDENTITY OF STORAGE MATERIAL

While the identity of the storage material in MCD remains uncertain it possesses several well-defined characteristics which pro vide clues to its nature. It is insoluble in lipid solvents and does not appear to be extractable with high concentrations of guanidine hydrochloride. The stored material reacts positively with periodic acid-Schiff, alcian blue, metachromatic dyes, and Mowry's modification of Hale's colloidal iron technique, but histochemical procedures that demonstrate lipid and protein are notably negative (Jones and Zimmerman, 1959, 1961; Klintworth and Vogel 1964; Garner 1969). These staining qualities are not significantly affected by enzymatic degradation with testicular hyaluronidase, chondroitin ABC lyase, chondroitin AC lyase, keratan sulfate endo-β-galactosidase and mixed exoglycosidases. By transmission electron microscopy the storage product's affinity for colloidal iron, periodic acid-Schiff-thiocarbohydrazide-silver proteinate and periodic acid-silver methenamine can be demonstrated (Klintworth and Vogel 1964; Klintworth and McCracken 1979). While antibodies to human corneal keratan sulfate proteoglycan are not yet available, Hassell et al. (1981) found the deposits in MCD to cross-react with antibodies to the core protein of monkey corneal keratan sulfate proteoglycan.

According to histochemical experience the affinity of the stored material for ferric ions at pH 2 suggests a substance rich in sulfate or phosphate groups (Pearse 1968), while the positive metachromasia points to the existence of free electronegative surface charges in the material. The periodic acid-Schiff positivity of the abnormal accumulations indicates that the compound does not diffuse away during tissue fixation and contains a significant number of "1,2-glycol" (-CHOH-CHOH-) groupings in unsubstituted form or its oxidation product (-CHOH-CO-) (Hotchkiss, 1948).

Because the histochemical findings point to a polysaccharide they need to be viewed in the light of corneal carbohydrate containing macromolecules (glycosaminoglycans, proteoglycans, glycoproteins and glycolipids). Glycosaminoglycans consist of numerous molecular species of varying degrees of sulfation and length. The normal cornea contains keratan sulfate, chondroitin-4-sulfate, chondroitin-6-sulfate and chondroitin, and under pathologic circumstances heparan sulfate, dermatan-4-sulfate, dermatan-6-sulfate, and hyaluronic acid are also synthesized in excessive quantities by this tissue. Some of these glycosaminoglycans occur within the same polymer. With the exception of hyaluronic acid, a constituent of the developing cornea, other glycosaminoglycans are normally bound covalently to protein forming proteoglycans. Corneal keratan sulfate (keratan sulfate I) accounts for about half of the sulfated glycosaminoglycans in the normal cornea and differs in structure from cartilaginous keratan sulfate (keratan sulfate II). Keratan sulfate I with its repeating unit of N-acetyllactosamine also contains fucose, sialic acid and mannose and has ester sulfate on N-acetylglucosamine and some galactose moieties. It is unique to the cornea and is believed to be linked to a protein core by an N-glycosylamine bond between N-acetylglucosamine of a mannose containing oligosaccharide and the amide group of asparagine as in other asparagine-linked glycoproteins (Klintworth 1977). Although human corneal proteoglycans have not been fully characterized much is known about these structural macromolecules from studies in other species. Recent characterizations of corneal proteoglycans have disclosed keratan sulfate to be the only polysaccharide component of one corneal proteoglycan (keratan sulfate proteoglycan), while chondroitin sulfate is a component of a different proteoglycan (Axelsson and Heinegard 1978; Hassell et al. 1979). Bovine keratan sulfate proteoglycan appears to be composed of monomers consisting of about 45% protein (molecular weight approximately 32,000), 30% keratan sulfate (present as 1-3 polymers) and 10-12% oligosaccharides (present as about 12 chains (each with a molecular weight of about 700-1000) (Axelsson and Heinegard 1978). Keratan sulfate proteoglycan in the rhesus monkey on the other hand contains more protein (74%) (molecular weight 40,000 to 70,000) and has one or two keratan sulfate side chains each with a molecular weight of 7,000 (Hassell et al. 1979).

Little is known about the composition of those corneal structural glycoproteins that lack attached glycosaminoglycans and knowledge about corneal glycolipids is virtually non-existent.

Of the polysaccharides synthesized by normal and pathologic corneas some (chondroitin-4-sulfate, chondroitin-6-sulfate, hyaluronic acid, dermatan-6-sulfate, and dermatan-4-sulfate) are unlikely candidates as the storage product because of the failure of certain enzymes (testicular hyaluronidase, chondroitin ABlyase, chondroitin ABC lyase) to degrade the stored material. Taken together with the biochemical attributes of the cornea, some histochemical features of the abnormal intra-and extracellular accumulations in MCD suggest keratan sulfate as the storage substance. Keratan sulfate, like the abnormal accumulations, has an affinity for alcian blue at low pH with magnesium chloride concentrations having a molarity of up to 0.8 (Garner 1969; Klintworth 1977). Moreover, of the glycosamingolycans keratan sulfate, which contains galactose rather than uronic acid, was the only one stated to give a positive periodic acid-Schiff reaction (Quintarelli 1968).

SIGNIFICANCE OF EXTRACELLULAR DEPOSITS

While extracellular accumulations within the corneal stroma may follow disintegration of affected cells, the deposits within Descemet's membrane clearly have a different origin and almost certainly reflect a functionally abnormal corneal endothelium. After the formation of this cellular monolayer and the beginning of the production of its basal lamina, Descemet's membranes continually thickens in an orderly manner throughout life as in the annual rings of a cross-section of a tree. Because it has no apparent turnover, the depth of abnormalities within it reflect their time of deposition, especially as one would expect large macromolecules to become entrapped in, and not pass through, Descemet's membrane. The abnormalities in Descemet's membrane in MCD presumably only become expressed after birth, because the most anterior portion of the membrane invariably appears normal by transmission electron microscopy. In some cases the layering of extracellular deposits within Descemet's membrane points to an intermittent postnatal expression of the metabolic defect.

SIGNIFICANCE OF ABNORMALITIES IN CORNEAL ORGAN CULTURES IN MACULAR CORNEAL DYSTROPHY

The relationship between the abnormalities found in organ cultures of corneas with MCD and the basic pathologic state remains uncertain. The finding that organ cultures of corneas with MCD not only synthesize less keratan sulfate and keratan sulfate proteoglycans that normal, but produce an abnormal glycoprotein and excessive amounts of certain oligosaccharides raises the issue of whether these substances are the storage material of MCD. While this remains an open question other observations in MCD suggest that some, if not all, observed metabolic differences between corneal organ cultures with MCD and controls may not reflect the fundamental defect in MCD. Since it is only possible to study corneal tissue late in the course of MCD, when keratoplasty becomes necessary to improve vision, the abnormalities in organ cultures may mirror an altered metabolic state of corneal fibroblasts caused by their excessive intracellular accumulation. At such times the keratocytes are invariably stuffed with their characteristic intracellular storage material. In all likelihood this storage product influences the synthetic activity of affected cells, especially since certain glycosaminoglycans are known to influence the synthesis of other related compounds (Funderburgh and Chandler 1978). It is conceivable that excessive quantities of a keratan sulfate-like molecule within corneal fibroblasts inhibit keratan sulfate and keratan sulfate proteoglycan synthesis by a feedback mechanism and that affected cells then synthesize increased amounts of oligosaccharides and one or more glycoprotein. Such an interpretation would account for: (1) differences between different corneas with MCD, (2) the apparent non-susceptibility of the stored material to enzymes that degrade the glycoprotein and oligosaccharides which organ cultures of corneas with MCD produce, (3) the non-extractibility of the storage product of MCD by prolonged incubation in high concentrations of guanidine hydrochloride using conditions that extract the abnormal glycoprotein. Some differences between affected corneas, however, may be due to heterogeneity in MCD, especially since accumulated clinical and genealogical data suggest that the disease is not homogeneous (Klintworth, unpublished observations).

CURRENT STATUS OF CONCEPT THAT MACULAR CORNEAL DYSTROPHY IS AN INHERITED DISORDER OF KERATAN SULFATE CATABOLISM

For many years MCD, which is analogous to the systemic mucopolysaccharidoses in several respects, has been suspected of being a localized storage disease of glycosaminoglycans (mucopolysaccharides) (Klintworth and Vogel, 1964). Most of the morphologic, histopathologic, and tissue culture data on MCD is consistent with the notion that the dystrophy is a storage disorder of keratan sulfate I caused by an inherited deficiency of a degradative enzyme. Involvement of the corneal endothelium is also in keeping with this view as this cellular monolayer can synthesize some keratan sulfate *in vitro* (Yue et al., 1976). That MCD may not be a storage disease of corneal keratan sulfate, as once thought, but of another carbohydrate containing macromolecule is raised by several observations: (1) the failure to detect a storage disease in cell culture, (2) the failure to detect defective activity of enzymes involved with keratan sulfate catabolism, (3) the storage material is not conspicuously degraded by keratan sulfate β-endogalactosidase, (4) the storage material reacts significantly with periodic acid-Schiff unlike purified keratan sulfate (Klintworth and Smith 1981c), (5) organ cultures of corneas with MCD synthesize less keratan sulfate and keratan sulfate proteoglycan than normal corneas do (Klintworth and Smith 1977, 1981a and c;Hassell et al. 1980), and (6) organ cultures of corneas with MCD incorporate excessive amounts of labeled glucosamine into oligosacharides and abnormal glycoproteins (Klintworth and Smith 1977, 1981 a and b; Hassell et al. 1980), and (7) the extracellular deposits in Descemet's membrane indicate an abnormal extracellular product and (8) the detection of a storage disease in hypothalamic neurons of one patient with MCD suggests that the disorder may affect metabolic pathways other than keratan sulfate.

By themselves some of these observations do not negate the hypothesis that MCD is a genetically determined storage disease due to a defective enzyme that is essential for the catabolism of corneal keratan sulfate. For example, keratocytes from individuals with an inherited disorder of keratan sulfate I catabolism would not be expected to store keratan sulfate 1 in culture, because confluent cultures of corneal fibroblasts of man, and other species, normally produce insignificant amounts of keratan sulfate 1 in culture (Conrad and Dorfman 1974; Klintworth and Smith, 1976,1981b). Also, despite unrewarding results in attempts to detect defective enzymes it should be stressed that bonds between different moieties in glycosaminoglycans, and other carbohydrate-containing compounds, normally become cleaved by enzymes in a specific order. Not only is the sequence of enzymatic degradation of keratan sulfate poorly understood, but most of the necessary enzymes remain unidentified. The periodic acid-Schiff positivity of the storage material and its failure to be degraded by keratan sulfate β-endogalactosidase in tissue sections of corneas with MCD are the strongest arguments against the storage material being normal keratan sulfate. Because corneal organ cultures from patients with MCD synthesize an abnormal glycoprotein, while not producing keratan sulfate proteoglycan, and evidence that keratan sulfate is normally synthesized through a glycoprotein intermediate (Hart and Lennarz 1978) prompted Hassell et al. (1980) to propose that MCD may be an inborn error of corneal keratan sulfate proteoglycan maturation. While it is conceivable that the abnormal glycoprotein observed with the organ cultures in MCD is a

Figure 1. Transmission electron micrograph of fibrillary intracellular storage substance within keratocyte of cornea with MCD. X14,000

Figure 2. Descemet's membrane in MCD with honeycombed appearance within part of its structure (arrows). The corneal endothelium (E) contains abnormal intracytoplasmic accumulations. X15,000

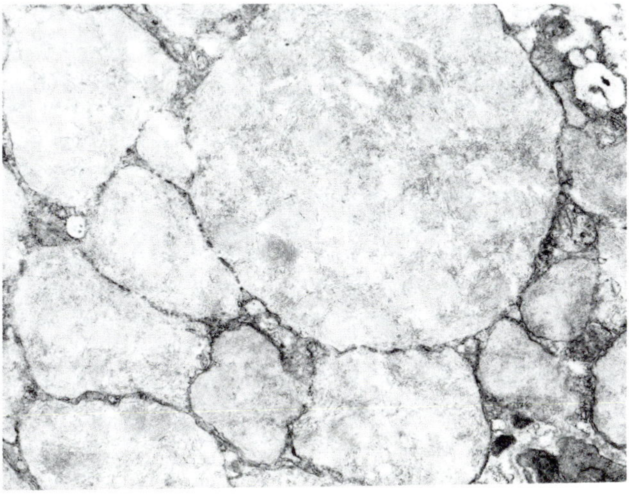

1

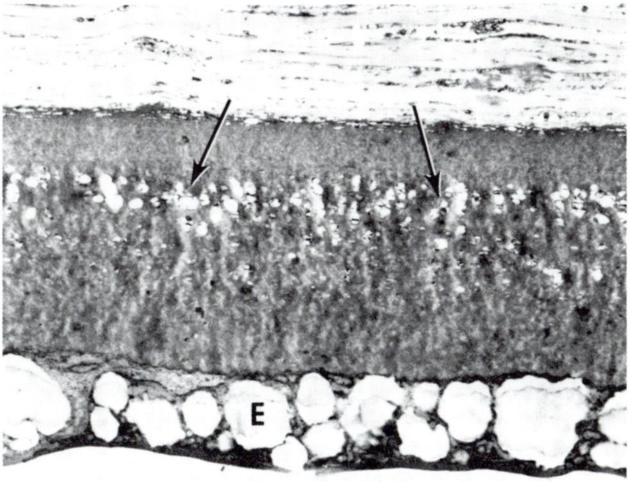

2

precursor of keratan sulfate proteoglycan, the theory fails to explain several observations: (1) Why should the corneal fibroblasts store a precursor of keratan sulfate proteoglycan? One would not expect the intracellular accumulation of compounds due to a defect in synthetic pathways because of the inherent ability of cells to degrade compounds that they synthesize. Well-established inherited storage diseases result from a defect in the catabolism of the stored material and none are known to be due to a block in the synthesis of a metabolic product. (2) Why are the intracellular accumulations not digested by enzymes that degrade the abnormal glycoprotein, which organ cultures of MCD corneas produce? (3) Protein is not a significant component of the storage material in MCD according to histochemical analyses. (4) Why is the storage product not extracted from corneas with high concentrations of guanidine hydrochloride even when cell membranes are disrupted?

CONCLUSION

Despite much work the basic metabolic defect in MCD remains elusive and while the storage material has yet to be identified with certainty current data indicates a carbohydrate rich molecule and an abnormal keratan sulfate remains a possible suspect. Further investigations on corneal tissue from patients with MCD and on normal corneas will hopefully help to establish the nature of the storage substance, as well as determine the basic metabolic defect, and answer remaining questions about this inborn error of metabolism.

ACKNOWLEDGMENTS

Supported in part by research grant 1 RO1-EY00146 from the National Institutes of Health.

REFERENCES

1. Axelsson I, Heinegard D (1978). Characterization of the keratan sulphate proteoglycans from bovine corneal stroma. Biochem J 169:517.
2. Conrad GW, Dorfman A (1974). Synthesis of sulfated mucopolysaccharides by chick corneal fibroblasts in vitro. Exp Eye Res 18:421.
3. Cotlier E, Yamashiroya H, and Hughes WF (1973). Unpublished observation.

4. Francois J, Victoria-Troncosco V, Maudgal PC, Victoria-Ihler A. (1976) Study of lysosomes by vital stains in normal keratocytes and keratocytes from macular dystrophy of the cornea. Invest Ophthalmol 15:599-605.
5. Funderburgh J, Chandler J: Glycosaminoglycans of cultured stromal keratocytes - responsiveness to the extracellular matrix. Invest Ophthalmol Vis Sci 17(Suppl):210, 1978.
6. Garner A (1969). Histochemistry of corneal macular dystrophy. Invest Ophthalmol 8:475.
7. Hart GW, Lennarz WJ (1978). Effects of tunicamycin on the biosynthesis of glycosaminoglycans by embryonic chick cornea. J Biol Chem 253:5795.
8. Hassell JR, Newsome DA, Hascall VC (1979). Characterization and biosynthesis of proteoglycans of corneal stroma from rhesus monkey. J Biol Chem 254:12346.
9. Hassell JR, Newsome DA, Krachmer J, Rodrigues MM (1980). Macular corneal dystrophy: failure to synthesize a mature keratan sulfate proteoglycan. Proc Nat Acad Sci USA 77:3705.
10. Hassell JR, Newsome DA, Nakazawa K, Rodriques M, Krachmer J (1981). Deposits in macular corneal dystrophy contain abnormal proteoglycans. Invest Ophthalmol Vis Sci 20(suppl) 115.
11. Horwitz AL, Klintworth GK (1980). Unpublished observations.
12. Hotchkiss RD (1948). A microchemical reaction resulting in the staining of polysaccharide structures in fixed tissue sections. Arch Biochem 16:131-141.
13. Jones ST, Zimmerman LE (1959). Macular dystrophy of the cornea (Groenouw type II): clinicopathologic report of two cases with comments concerning its differential diagnosis from lattice dystrophy (Biber-Haab-Dimmer). Am J Ophthalmol 47:1.
14. Jones ST, Zimmerman LE (1961). Histopathologic differentiation of granular, macular and lattice dystrophies of the cornea. Am J Ophthalmol 51:394.
15. Klintworth GK (1977). The cornea-structure and macromolecules in health and disease: A review. Am J Pathol 89:719.
16. Klintworth GK (1980a). Corneal dystrophies, In Nicholson D (ed.). "Ophthalmic Pathology Update", New York: Masson Publishing, p. 23.
17. Klintworth GK (1980b). Research into the pathogenesis of macular corneal dystrophy. Trans Ophthalmol Soc U.K. 100:180.
18. Klintworth GK (1981a). Macular corneal dystrophy: a localiz-

ed mucopolysaccharidosis? In Daentl DL (ed.). "Clinical, Structural and Biochemical Advances in Hereditary Eye Disorders", Alan R. Liss, in press.

19. Klintworth GK (1981b). Unpublished observations.
20 Klintworth GK (1982). Disorders of glycosaminoglycans (mucopolysaccharides) and proteoglycans. In Garner A, and Klintworth GK (eds.), "Pathobiology of Ocular Disease", Volume B, Chapter 30, New York: Marcel Dekker, Inc., p.863.
21. Klintworth GK, Hawkins HK, Smith CF (1979). Acridine orange particles in cultured fibroblasts: a comparative study of macular corneal dystrophy, systemic mucopolysaccharidoses types I-H and II and normal controls. Arch Pathol Lab Med 103:297.
22. Klintworth GK, McCracken JS (1979). Corneal diseases, In Johannessen JV (ed.) "Electron Microscopy in Human Medicine", Volume 6, Part 3, Chapter 5, New York: McGraw-Hill, p. 239.
23. Klintworth GK, Smith CF (1976). A comparative study of extracellular sulfated glycosaminoglycans synthesized by rabbit corneal fibroblasts in organ and confluent cultures. Lab Invest 35:258.
24. Klintworth GK, Smith CF (1977). Macular corneal dystrophy: studies of sulfated glycosaminoglycans in corneal explant and confluent stromal cell cultures. Amer J Pathol. 89:167.
25. Klintworth GK, Smith CF (1980). Abnormal product of corneal explants from patients with macular dystrophy. Amer J Pathol 101:143-158.
26. Klintworth GK, Smith CF (1981a). Additional observations on corneal organ cultures in MCD. Invest Ophthalmol Vis Sci 20 (suppl): 115,
27. Klintworth GK, Smith CF (1981b). Difference between the glycosaminoglycans synthesized by corneal and cutaneous fibroblasts in culture. Lab Invest 44:553.
28. Klintworth GK, Smith, CF (1981c). Analyses of the proteoglycans and glycoproteins synthesized by corneal organ cultures with macular dystrophy. In preparation.
29. Klintworth GK, Vogel FS (1964). Macular corneal dystrophy: an inherited acid mucopolysaccharide storage disease of the corneal fibroblast. Amer J Path 45:565.
30. Lorenzetti DWC, Kaufman HE (1967). Macular and lattice dystrophies and their recurrences after keratoplasty. Trans Am Acad Ophthalmol Otolaryngol 71:112.
31. Morgan G (1966). Macular dystrophy of the cornea. Brit J Ophthalmol 50:57.
32. Pearse AGE (1968). "Histochemistry: Theoretical and Appli-

ed" (Third edition), volume 1. Boston: Little Brown and Company, p.350.
33. Quintarelli G (1968). Methods for the histochemical identification of acid mucopolysaccharides: a critical evaluation. In Quintarelli G (ed): "Chemical Physiology of Mucopolysaccharides. International Symposium on The Chemical Physiology of Mucopolysaccharides, Milan, Boston: Little, Brown and Co., p. 199.
34. Robin AL, Green WR, Lapsa TP, Hoover RE, Kelley JS (1977). Recurrence of macular corneal dystrophy after lamellar keratoplasty. Am J Ophthalmol 84:457.
35. Teng CC (1966). Macular dystrophy of the cornea. A histochemical and electron microscopic study. Am J Ophthalmol 62:436.
36. Yue BYJT, Baum JL, Silbert JE (1976). The synthesis of glycosaminoglycans by cultures of rabbit corneal endothelial and stromal cells. Biochem J 158:567.

POSTERIOR POLYMORPHOUS CORNEAL DYSTROPHY: RECENT DEVELOPMENTS

Merlyn M. Rodrigues, Tung-tien Sun
Jay Krachmer, David Newsome
Clinical Brahch, National Eye Institute, NIH
Bethesda, MD; Johns Hopkins Medical School,
Baltimore, MD; University of Iowa, Iowa City, IA

Posterior polymorphous dystropy (PPMD) has been recognized as an autosomal dominant heritable disease with distinct clinical and histologic features. Clinically, the posterior cornea usually shows bilateral vesicular areas of thickening, ridges and sheets or irregularly shaped opacities (Fig. 1) (Cibis, Krachmer, Phelps and Weingeist, 1977). Within families, the corneal involvement can vary from a few isolated vesicle-like lesions to total corneal decompensation with edema and band keratopathy. Unusual clinical variants characterized by ring-shaped corneal clouding have been described (Witschel, Sundmacher, Theopold and Jaeger, 1980). Iridocorneal adhesions varying from tiny lesions seen only on gonioscopy to large broad based adhesions and glaucoma occur less frequently (Cibis, Krachmer, Phelps and Weingeist, 1976). Electron microscopy of edematous corneal buttons from patients with PPMD has revealed one to two layers of epithelial-like cells lining the posterior surface of an abnormal Descemet's membrane (Boruchoff and Kuwabara, 1971; Tripathi, Casey and Wise, 1974; Rodrigues, Waring, Laibson and Weinreb, 1975; Waring, Rodrigues and Laibson, 1978; Polack, Bourne, Forstot and Yamaguchi, 1980; Rodrigues, Sun, Krachmer and Newsome, 1980). In this paper we review recent findings that the epithelial-like cells contain keratin proteins (Rodrigues, Sun, Krachmer and Newsome, 1980) a marker for epithelial cells (Sun and Green, 1977, 1978; Sun, Shih and Green, 1979; Franke, Schmid and Osborne, 1978; Franke, Appelhans and Schmid 1979). We also review the *in vitro* characteristics of cells of the posterior cornea in PPMD which display features of epithelial rather than of

Birth Defects: Original Article Series, Volume 18, Number 6, pages 479–491

irregularity of the corneal endothelium and epithelium. The corneal endothelium was either a monolayer or a double layer of cells lining the posterior surface of Descemet's membrane (Fig. 2 inset). Descemet's membrane displayed a multilayered appearance and was irregular in thickness. The stromal collagen and the stromacytes were unremarkable.

2. Antikeratin staining: Indirect immunofluorescent staining of the PPMD corneal endothelial tissue with guinea pig antisera against total human epidermal keratins and individual purified human keratins (MW 65K, 63K, 55K and 46K) (Sun and Vidrich, 1981), as well as a mouse monoclonal antibody specific for several low molecular weight human epidermal keratins (Woodcock-Mitchell, and Sun, 1981) revealed staining of the epithelial-like cells on the posterior corneal layer that corresponded to areas of epithelial-like cells demonstrated by scanning and transmission electron microscopy. (Rodrigues, Sun, Krachmer and Newsome, 1980).

3. Scanning electron microscopy: Scanning electron microscopy of the corneal endothelium in all specimens revealed areas of epithelial-like cells intermixed with endothelial-like cells (Rodrigues, Sun, Krachmer, and Newsome, 1980), The endothelial-like cells were characterized by a polygonal appearance of fairly uniform cells with the usual junctional complexes, while the epithelial-like cells were much larger and squamoid in appearance with numerous microvillus projections (Fig. 3). In areas away from the defect the epithelium displayed the usual appearance except for edema.

4. Transmission electron microscopy: Numerous studies by transmission electron microscopy demonstrated multilaminar Descemet's membrane (Fig. 2) with a stratified appearance of the posterior corneal layers that appeared epithelial-like (Waring, Rodrigues and Laibson, 1978) and displayed numerous desmosomal junctional complexes and 8-10 nm diameter cytoplasmic filaments. They also displayed numerous microvillus projections facing the anterior chamber. The stroma showed evidence of edema.

B. Cell Cultures:

1. Phase-contrast: Cells grown in explant cultures of Descemet's membrane from patients with PPMD displayed *in vitro* characteristics more typical of epithelium than of corneal endothelium. (Fig. 4).

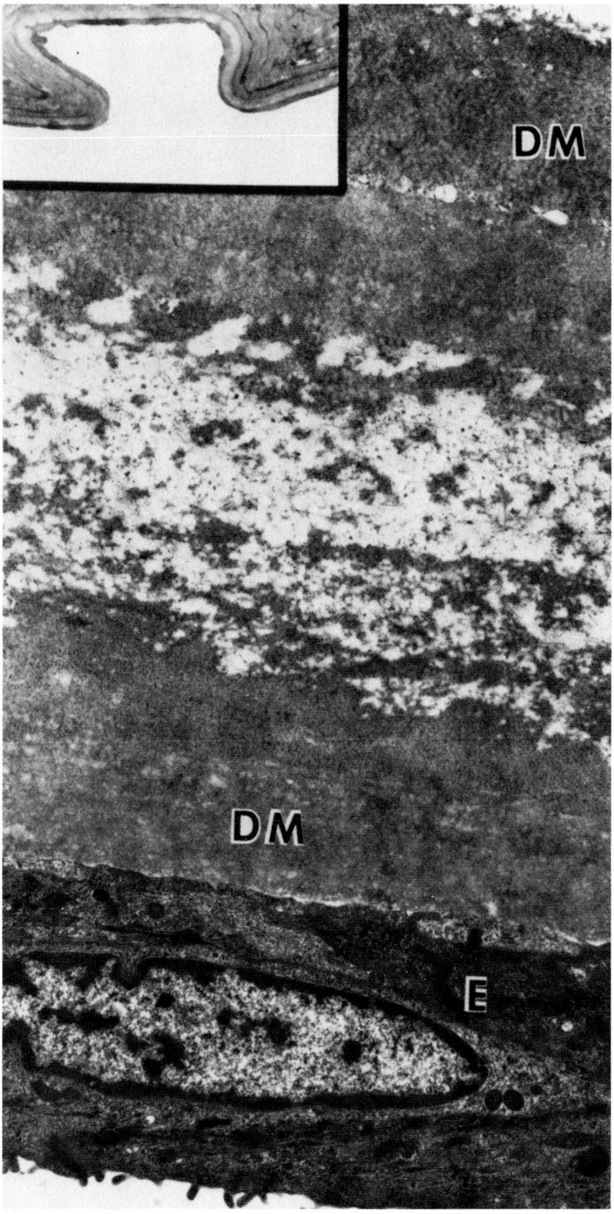

Fig. 2. Transmission electron micrograph of PPMD shows multi-laminar Descemet's membrane (DM) with areas of abnormal posterior banding. The endothelial cells (E) display microvillus projections facing the anterior chamber as well as desmosomal junctions (X12,900). Inset shows the posterior cornea lined by an irregular layer of cells (Toluidine blue, X500).

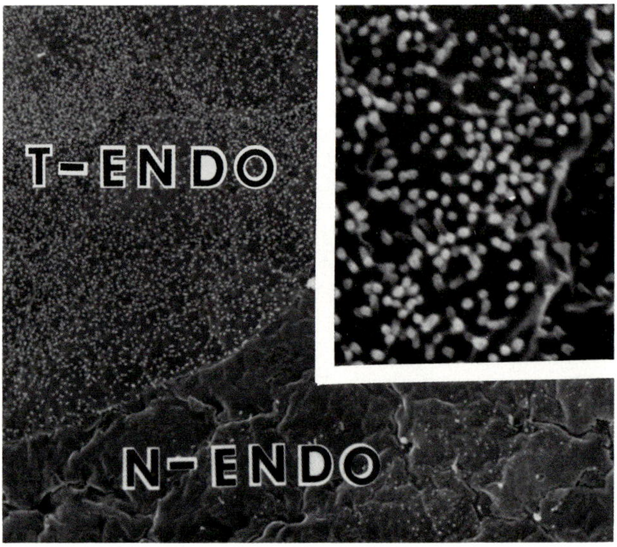

Fig. 3. Scanning electron micrograph of corneal tissue with PPMD showing large flat transformed endothelial cells (T-ENDO) with an epithelial-like appearance adjacent to normal endothelial cells (N-ENDO) (2200). Inset shows microvillus projections of T-ENDO cells at higher magnification (X11,000).

The time of appearance of outgrowth after explantation of Descemet's membrane from the PPMD specimens was unusual in comparison with normal endothelial outgrowth; it is faster by two to three days and thus more like control epithelial explants. In PPMD specimens, cells appeared on the dishes within 24-48 hours. In cases of controls, epithelial outgrowth began in 24 to 48 hours but endothelial cells usually required four to six days to appear on the dish (Rodrigues, Newsome, Krachmer and Sun, 1981).

2. Indirect immunofluorescent staining: Indirect immunofluorescent staining of corneal "endothelial" cells cultured from a patient with PPMD with antisera against total keratins revealed a mixed cell population with cytoplasmic filamentous fluorescence only in epithelial-like cells (Fig. 5).

3. Scanning electron microscopy: Scanning electron microscopy of the cell cultures revealed mostly epithelial-like cells arranged in groups or monolayers. These cells

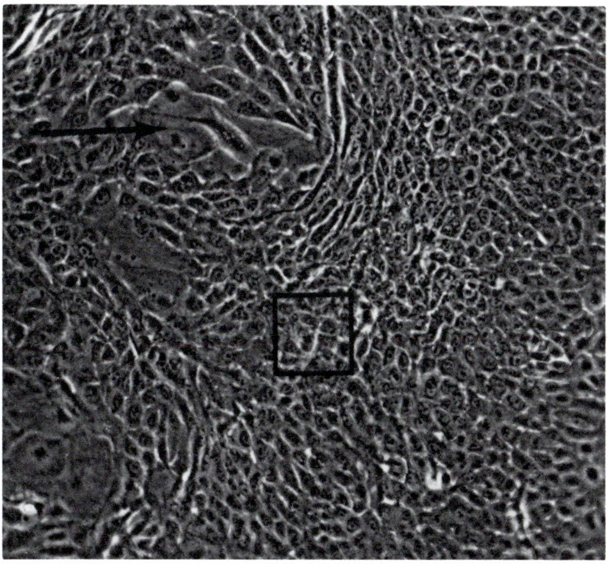

Fig. 4. Phase contrast microscopy of primary outgrowth from explant of Descemet's membrane 5 days in vitro. Epithelial-like cells (box) are polygonal with sharp borders. Occasional endothelial-like cells (arrow) are present at the periphery (X120).

appeared large, flat and squamoid with myriad microvillus projections (Rodrigues, Newsome, Krachmer, and Sun, 1981).

4. Transmission electron microscopy: Cell cultures revealed a stratified pattern with 2-3 layers of cells that were attached by desmosomal junctions and displayed numerous apical microvillus projections, prominent Golgi and smooth endoplasmic reticulum and moderate numbers of mitochondria (Rodrigues, Newsome, Krachmer, and Sun, 1981). These cells also showed 8-10 nm cytoplasmic filaments that were similar to normal corneal epithelial cells in culture; occasional fibroblast-like cells with prominent dilated rough endoplasmic reticulum were also present.

DISCUSSION:

The detailed classic clinical features of PPMD have been

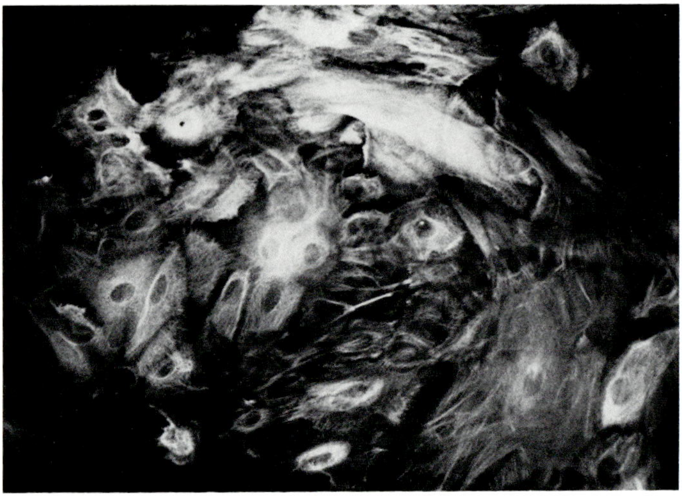

Fig. 5A

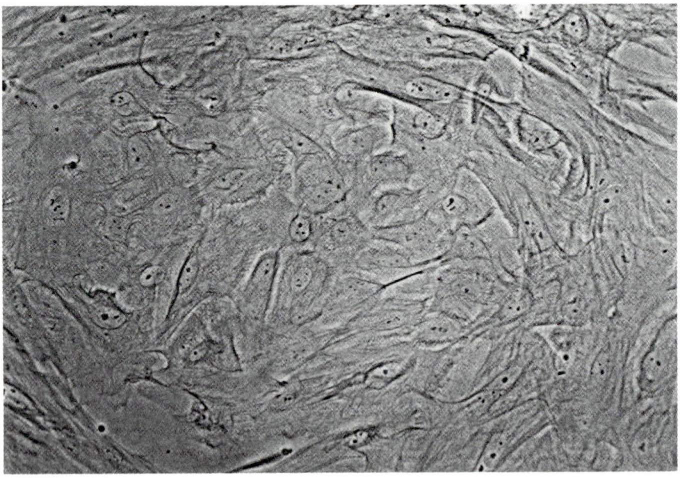

Fig. 5B

well documented (Grayson, 1974: Cibis, Krachmer, Phelps and

Fig. 5A. Indirect immunofluorescent staining of PPMD corneal endothelial cell culture with antiserum against total human epidermal keratin. Cytoplasmic fluorescence and desmosomal junctions of epithelial-like cells in A. (X220).

Fig. 5B. In B the same field viewed with phase contrast shows a mixed cell population composed of epithelial-like cells corresponding to those stained in A as well as unstained peripheral cells corresponding to endothelial cells (X220).

Weingeist, 1976; Cibis, Krachmer, Phelps and Weingeist, 1977). The precise age of onset is difficult to determine since most patients remain asymptomatic. Corneal edema has been observed at birth or early infancy (Cibis, Krachmer, Phelps, Weingeist, 1977) and is suggestive of a possible congenital disorder. In our cases requiring keratoplasty, the endothelial disease was difficult to visualize because of varying degrees of epithelial edema, stromal edema and band keratopathy in one case. Broad iridocorneal adhesions and glaucoma were present in two of our cases. Clinical and histological variants of PPMD have been described. A recent study reported varying clinical involvement in three members of a family with PPMD; the father showed endothelial blister-like lesions while his daughter and grandson had ring-shaped corneal clouding which progressed to severe edema. Histologically, the posterior cornea was lined by epithelial-like cells (Witschel, Sundmacher, Theopold and Jaeger, 1980). Another variant of PPMD characterized by congenital diffuse corneal clouding has been reported as hereditary corneal edema (Kanai, Waltman, Polack and Kaufman 1971).

Electron microscopy of tissue specimens has generally been on corneal buttons obtained at penetrating keratoplasty from advanced symptomatic patients with corneal edema. These cases have usually shown a multilaminar appearance of Descemet's membrane with a normal anterior 110 banded layer and a thin posterior layer composed of basement membrane-like material and fusiform bundles of 55-110 nm banded collagen. The epithelial-like cells lining the posterior surface of Descemet's membrane are characterized by numerous microvillus projections facing the anterior chamber, desmosomal junctions, 10 nm filaments and scant mitochondria (Boruchoff and Kuwabara, 1971; Tripathi, Casey and Wise 1974;

Rodrigues, Waring, Laibson, 1978; Polack, Bourne, Forstot and Yamaguchi, 1980; Witschel, Sundmacher, Theopold and Jaeger, 1980). Although the epithelial-like cells on the posterior corneal surface appear typical of advanced PPMD, occasional variants have been described. In a case without corneal edema, posterior epithelial-like cells were not detected (Johnson and Brown, 1978). Another patient showed excrescences of Descemet's membrane with degenerated endothelium (Hanselmayer, 1972). In another report of hereditary deep dystrophy of the cornea, Descemet's membrane displayed guttate excrescences and stromal calcific deposits were present (Hogan and Bietti, 1969). The latter case probably represents a corneal endothelial and stromal disease other than PPMD since the posterior cornea showed no fibroblast-like or epithelial-like alterations.

The differential diagnosis of PPMD includes the spectrum of entities comprising the iridocorneal endothelial syndrome (Chandler's syndrome, essential iris atrophy and the iris nevus syndrome) (Eagle, Font, Yanoff and Fine, 1979; Rodrigues, Streeten and Spaeth, 1978; Shields, 1979) and Rieger's syndrome. In the iridocorneal endothelial syndrome, there is unilateral involvement affecting young to middle-aged women (Phelps, Krachmer, Cibis and Weingeist, 1980) and the corneal endothelial cells do not stain with antibodies to human epidermal keratin as in PPMD (Rodrigues, Newsome, Krachmer and Sun, 1980). Riegers syndrome is characterized by finer strands that attach from the iris to cornea in contrast to the broader iridocorneal adhesions in PPMD (Cibis, Krachmer, Phelps, and Weingeist, 1976). In Rieger's anomaly systemic abnormalities such as maxillary hypoplasia, deafness and dental defects frequently occur whereas such changes have not been described with PPMD except for a patient with associated microdontia (Grayson, 1974).

Immunofluorescent staining of the cornea with antibodies to human total epidermal keratin has been useful in demonstrating that the epithelial-like cells of the posterior cornea in PPMD contain keratin proteins (Rodrigues, Sun, Krachmer, and Newsome, 1980). The corneal endothelial cells of normal human corneas. Fuchs' dystrophy, interstitial keratitis, Chandler's syndrome, and congenital corneal endothelial dystrophy did not stain with antibodies to total epidermal keratin (Rodrigues, Newsome, Krachmer, and Sun, 1981. Recently we have found that the PPMD corneal endothelial cells also stained with antibodies to individual keratins (anti-65K, anti-63K, anti-55K and anti-46K as well as with a monoclonal antibody to keratins.

The cell cultures of corneal endothelium of PPMD expressed essentially the same *in vitro* characteristics observed *in vivo* in tissue specimens (Rodrigues, Newsome, Krachmer and Sun, 1981). In contrast to the pure population of endothelial cells cultured from normal human corneal endothelium, in PPMD the cell population showed two distinct cell types, some resembling epithelial-like cells while others were typical of corneal endothelium. Scanning and transmission electron microscopy of these epithelial-like cells in cultures of the corneal endothelium in PPMD showed stratification, desmosomal cell projections, microvillus projections and 8 nm cytoplasmic filaments (Rodrigues, Newsome, Krachmer, Sun, 1981). In addition, these cells stained with antibodies to total epidermal keratin.

The pathogenesis of the unusual epithelial-like cells on the posterior cornea in PPMD is uncertain but could represent transdifferentiation of embryonal cells (Okada, 1981) or an abnormal differentiation of certain cells of neural crest origin, such as the corneal endothelial cells in the avian eye (Johnson, Noden, Hazelton, Coulombre, 1979, Kupfer, 1978).

ACKNOWLEDGEMENT:

We thank Joseph Hackett and Patricia Donohoo for their assistance.

REFERENCES:

Boruchoff A, Kuwabara T (1976). Electron microscopy of posterior polymorphous degeneration. An ultrastructural and clinical report. Am J Ophthalmol 72:879.

Cibis GW, Krachmer JH, Phelps CD, Weingeist TA (1976). Iridocorneal adhesions in posterior polymorphous dystrophy. Trans Am Acad Ophthalmol Otolaryngol 81:770.

Cibis GW, Krachmer JH, Phelps CD, Weingeist TA (1977) The clinical spectrum of posterior polymorphous dystrophy. Arch Ophthalmol 95:1529.

Eagle RC, Font RL, Yanoff M, Fine BS (1979). Proliferative endotheliopathy with iris abnormalities. The iridocorneal endothelial syndrome. Arch Ophthalmol 97:2104.

Franke WW, Schmid E, Osborn M, et al. (1978) Different

intermediate sized filaments distinguished by immunofluorescence microscopy. Proc Natl Acad Sci USA 75:5034.
Franke WW, Appelhans B, Schmid E, et al (1979). Identification and characterization of epithelial cells in mammalian tissues by immunofluorescence microscopy using antibodies to prekeratin. Differentiation 15:7.
Grayson M (1974). The nature of hereditary deep dystrophy of the cornea: Its association with iris and anterior chamber dysgenesis. Trans Am Ophthalmol Soc 72:879.
Hanselmayer H (1972). Zur histopathologie der hinteren polymorphen Hornhautdystrophie nach Schlichting II. Ultrastructurelle befunde une pathophysiogische bemer Kugan. Albrecht von Graefes Arch Klin Ophthalmol 185:53.
Hogan MJ, Bietti G (1969). Hereditary deep dystrophy of the cornea (polymorphous) Am J Ophthalmol 68:777.
Johnson BL, Brown SI (1978). Posterior polymorphous dystrophy: a light and electron microscopic study. Br J Ophthalmol 62:89.
Johnston MC, Noden BM, Hazelton RD, Coulombre AJ (1979). Origin of avian ocular and periocular tissues. Exp Eye Res 29:27.
Kanai A, Waltman S, Polack FM, Kaufman HE (1971). Electron microscopic study of hereditary corneal edema. Invest Ophthalmol Vis Sci 10:89.
Kupfer C (1978). A new hypothesis on anterior chamber developmental anomalies associated with glaucoma. Trans Ophthalmol Soc UK 98:213
Okada TS (1981). Phenotypic expression of embryonic neural retinal cells in cell culture. Vis Res 21:83.
Polack FM, Bourne WM, Forstot SL, Yamaguchi T (1980). Scanning electron microscopy of posterior polymorphous corneal dystrophy. Am J Ophthalmol 89:575.
Rodrigues MM, Waring GO, Laibson RP, Weinreb S (1975). Endothelial alterations in congenital corneal dystrophies. Am J Ophthalmol 80:678.
Rodrigues MM, Sun T-T, Krachmer J, Newsome D (1980). Epithelialization of the corneal endothelium in posterior polymorphous dystrophy. Invest Ophthalmol 19:832.
Rodrigues MM, Newsome DA, Krachmer JH, Sun T-T (1981). Posterior polymorphous dystrophy of the cornea: cell culture studies. Exp Eye Res. In press.
Rodrigues MM, Phelps CB, Krachmer JH, Weingeist TA (1980). Glaucoma due to endothelialization of the anterior chamber angle. A comparison of posterior polymorphous dystrophy of the cornea and Chandler's sydrome. Arch Ophthalmol 98:688.

Rodrigues MM, Streeten BW, Spaeth GL (1978). Chandler's syndrome as a variant of essential iris atrophy. A clinicopathologic study. Arch Ophthalmol 96:643.
Shields MB (1979). Progressive essential iris atrophy, Chandler's syndrome and the iris nevus (Cogan-Reese) syndrome: A spectrum of disease. Surv Ophthalmol 24:3.
Sun T-T, Green H (1977). Cultured epithelial cells of cornea, conjunctiva and skin: Absence of marked intrinsic divergence of their differentiated states. Nature 269:489.
Sun T-T, Green H (1978). Immunofluorescent staining of keratin fibers in cultured cells. Cell 14:469.
Sun T-T, Shih C, Green H (1979). Keratin cytoskeletons in epithelial cells of internal organs. Proc Natl Acad Sci 96:2813.
Sun T-T, Vidrich A (1981). Keratin filaments of corneal epithelial cells. Vis Res 21:55.
Tripathi R, Casey T, Wise G (1974). Hereditary posterior polymorphous dystrophy. An ultrastructural and clinical report. Trans Ophthalmol Soc UK 94:211-225.
Waring GO, Rodrigues MM, Laibson PR (1978). Corneal dystrophies II. Endothelial dystrophies. Surv Ophthalmol 23:147.
Witschel H, Sundmacher R, Theopold H, Jaeger W (1980). Posterior polymorphous dystrophy of the cornea (Schlichting). An unusual clinical variant. Albrecht von Graefes Arch Klin Ophthalmol 214:15.
Woodcock-Mitchell K, Sun T-T (1981). Selective immunohistochemical staining of basal cells of normal epidermis by a monoclonal antibody to low molecular weight keratins. Submitted.

HEREDITARY MUCOEPITHELIAL DYSPLASIA, A DISEASE OF GAP JUNCTION AND DESMOSOME FORMATION

Carl J. Witkop, Jr.[1], James G. White[1], and George O. Waring[2]
University of Minnesota[1], Emory University[2]
16-262 Health Sciences Unit A, 515 Delaware St. SE, Minneapolis, MN 55455[1], Emory University Clinic, 1365 Clifton Road, NE, Atlanta, GA 30308[2]

INTRODUCTION

Hereditary mucoepithelial dysplasia (Witkop, et al., 1978, 1979) is a recently recognized autosomal dominantly inherited genodermatosis which has been observed in three kindreds. One of the affected kindreds was described initially by Okamoto, et al. (1977) as a chronic mucocutaneous candidiasis syndrome. Examination of material from this kindred, however, confirmed the identity of the disorder in this family with those subsequently seen, the *Candida* most likely being an adventitious organism in the propositus. The condition is a panepithelial defect affecting conjunctival, corneal, oral, nasal, cervical, vaginal, urethral, anal, and bladder mucosae. Patients develop cataracts, follicular keratoses, non-scarring alopecia, repeated bouts of pneumonia, interstitial fibrocystic lung disease resembling the Hamman-Rich syndrome (Hamman and Rich, 1944), spontaneous pneumothorax, and a terminal cor pulmonale (Witkop, et al, 1979).

The first manifestations of the disorder appear in early infancy as severe photophobia, tearing, and nystagmus. By one year of age, orificial mucosae develop flat, fiery red plaques which persist throughout life and involve the conjunctival, oral, nasal, vaginal, cervical, urethral and anal mucosae. Beginning in the second to fourth year of life, repeated bouts of upper-respiratory infections interspersed with a chronic rhinorrhea frequently progress to five or more annual episodes of pneumonia. These episodes of pneumonia are often accompanied by loss of hair resulting in non-scarring alopecia and coarse scanty scalp hair, diarrhea, melena,

Birth Defects: Original Article Series, Volume 18, Number 6, pages 493-511

enuresis, pyuria, and hematuria. Non-vesicular, follicular papules develop on unexposed skin and persist throughout life. Corneal scarring and posterior subcapsular cataracts are noted from five to seven years of age, and most patients are legally blind by seven to nine years of age. Restrictive, interstitial, fibrocystic lung disease accompanied by frequent episodes of spontaneous pneumothorax characterize the major problems of the second and third decades. All known affected deceased kindred members have died with restrictive lung disease, clubbing of the fingers and cor pulmonale.

Affected women have had repeated abnormal vaginal and cervical PAP smears, and red, "erosive" lesions of these areas which have been treated unsuccessfully by cryosurgery and conization.

Affected males have had repeated operations for urethral obstruction.

Hematologically, patients have had a low grade chronic eosinophilia from 9 to 29 percent.

Biopsies from skin; oral, cervical and corneal mucosae; as well as cytologic smears from conjunctival, nasal, oral, vaginal, cervical, urethral, and bladder mucosae have shown similar histologic and cytologic features. Histologically, the number of cells in the epithelial layer is reduced. There is a lack of development of intercellular attachments (dyshesion, Reed and Clark, 1971). Basal and parabasal cells are vacuolated. Numerous round eosinophilic, refractile, dyskeratotic cells resembling the corp ronds of Darier disease are found in biopsies and smears. There is a lack of epithelial cell maturation with reduced cornification and keratinization. Mucosal cells show vacuolization of the cytoplasm, strand-shaped inclusions and individual cell dyskeratosis.

Ultrastructural features of mucosal cells from all tissues examined are similar. Numerous cells show intracellular cytoplasmic vacuoles, a paucity of keratohyalin granules, cytoplasmic inclusions of wheat-sheaf-like bundles of filaments, strands and undulating bands resembling isolated gap junctional material (Witkop, 1980), reduced number of desmosomes, and cell junctions, and enlarged intercellular spaces filled with a homogenous, lightly radiodense material.

We describe here the ocular features of this disorder.

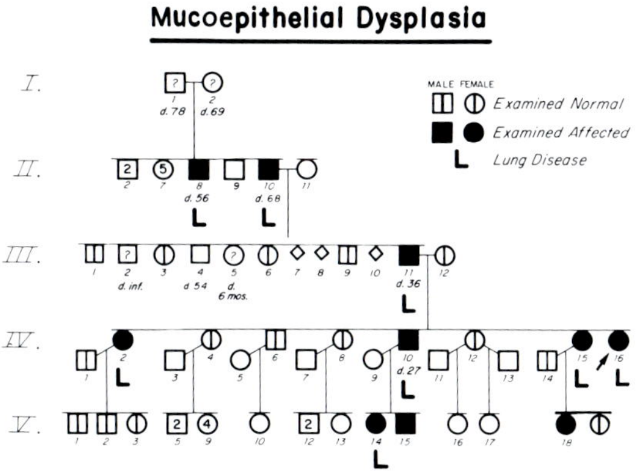

Fig. 1

CASE PRESENTATIONS

V-18 (Fig. 1) was 3 years, 6 months of age at the time of this examination. At 6 months gestation, her mother who was also affected, had an episode of pneumonia in which she lost all of her hair, and had an ocular herpes simplex infection which rendered her blind until the week following a full term uneventful delivery. At 3 days of age, the child developed extensive staphylococcal pustules of the skin of her abdomen and chest. Crops of pustules recurred every 2 to 3 months until the present time, involving the skin of her torso and axilla which responded to antibiotic and Mycolog therapy. At 3 months of age she was hospitalized for 3 days with a high fever, diarrhea and melena diagnosed as a viral gastroenteritis. By 6 months of age, she had developed severe photophobia, tearing and nystagmus, a continuous rhinorrhea and fiery red periorificial lesions of the nose, mouth, urethra, anus and vagina. She was diagnosed as having multiple allergies after an eosinophilia was noted and testing showed she reacted to a wide spectrum of soaps, plastics, creams, flowers and grass. She lost scalp hair which is now scanty.

At 1 1/2 years the patient was examined by these investigators as a part of a familial study of the disorder (Witkop, et al., 1978, 1979). At that time she had severe esotropia, tearing, blepharospasm, photophobia, horizontal nystagmus, red, periorificial mucosae involving nose, lips, oral vestibule, cheek, hard and soft palate, pharynx, and conjunctivae. She had a beefy red scrotal tongue. She had a copious serous rhinorrhea from which coagulase negative *Staphylococci* and *Corynebacteria* were isolated. PAP stained smears from oral tissues and urinary sediment show cellular abnormalities described previously. Ocular examination showed superficial vascularization of the cornea from 3 to 6 o'clock with microcystic lesions in the corneal epithelium. A vascular pannus in the left eye extended from 10 to 12 o'clock and was accompanied by epithelial microcysts in this area.

The patient was re-examined at age 3½ years at Emory University Ophthalmology Clinic. The right eye had a superficial pannus for 360 degrees. Superiorly, two thumbnail-shaped patches of subepithelial vascularized scar tissue were present. Splotchy areas throughout the entire cornea of white scarred tissue and faint vascularization were present.

The left eye had a superior pannus formation with moderately dense subepithelial opacities and vascularization that extended about 3 mm into the cornea from approximately 10 o'clock to 3 o'clock (Fig. 2). The remainder of the cornea was avascular but with mild punctate keratopathy. Fine focal intraepithelial whitish opacities were present in both eyes below a roughened hazy, opacified corneal epithelium. A mild posterior subcapsular cataract was present.

In both eyes, there were no iris abnormalities and the anterior chamber was deep and clear. A cup-disc ratio of 0.1 was noted with normal pink color. The macula was clear and vessels were seen past the equator. The right eye was slightly hyperopic. Applanation tensions under Halothane anesthesia for both eyes were 2 mm of mercury and the corneal diameter was 12.0 mm. Scotopic and photopic responses at all stimuli intensities in the electroretinogram were depressed. Responses within normal values of 133% in the right eye and 130% were found in the electrooculogram. Photopic and scotopic adaptation curves were both normal as was color vision. Visual acuities in the right eye were not recorded because of intense reflex blepharospasm. The acuity of the left eye was 6/30 as determined by Allan pictures.

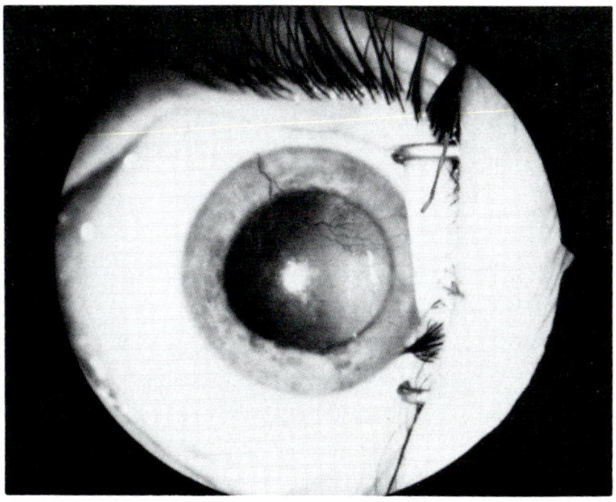

Fig. 2. Pannus formation in the left eye of V-18 at 3½ yrs. of age.

A biopsy of the conjunctiva of the inferiolateral fornix and oral and urinary cytologic material were obtained from the patient. Smears of the oral, vaginal, and cervical mucosae and urinary sediment were obtained from the mother as well as biopsies of the oral, cervical and vaginal mucosae. Material was fixed and prepared for light and electron microscopy utilizing standard procedures.

IV-10 was born of a full term pregnancy from an unaffected mother. His father had mucoepithelial dysplasia. In the neonatal period, he was noted to have severe photophobia and tearing, and left esotropia. He was hospitalized for otitis media at 2 weeks of age, and for measles at 6 months of age during which he developed a continuous rhinorrhea which persisted throughout life. By 1½ years of age he had developed erythematous periorificial mucosal lesions of his nose and anus. He was hospitalized at 2½ years for severe photophobia, tearing and nystagmus and was found to have bilateral keratoconjunctivitis with corneal vascularization, bronchopneumonia and anemia. Readmission 4 months later for the same complaint revealed in addition to the aforementioned findings, fiery red conjunctivae, heaping of the corneal epithelium at the limbus, vascularized opacified corneas (which yielded sterile cultures) flat red mucosal lesions of the mouth, nose, lips, gingivae, palate, pharynx, urethra and anus. He had red retracted eardrums and alopecia. Treatment for avitaminosis A was ineffective. Cortisone eye drops were ineffective. He was hospitalized for several bouts of pneumonia during which he lost all of his hair. By 3 years, 2 months he had developed a generalized perifolliculitis of his skin. By 5 years he could only distinguish fingers at 3 feet. At 6 years, 2 months he was admitted to a psychiatric unit with the complaint that he could not read or write. Both lenses were found to be opaque. At 8 years his eye lesions were treated with beta radiation without noticeable improvement. Five hospital admissions and three outpatient admissions documented at least eight episodes of pneumonia, the last associated with a spontaneous pneumothorax at 11 years of age. He had progressive fibrosis of the lungs, bronchial pneumonia and emphysema. A second spontaneous pneumothorax occurred at 16 years, 3 months of age accompanied by diarrhea, melena, loss of hair, enuresis, and pneumonia. A cataract extraction on his right eye was performed at a local hospital at 17 years. A partial right right lamellar keratoplasty was performed. The graft, infected with *Pseudomonas aeruginosa* and coagulase positive *Staphylococci* became opaque. The histologic report on the excised cornea noted degenerative corneal epithelium, pannus and stromal edema (Fig. 3A).

Six months later, a right partial lamellar corneal graft also failed and he developed an enophthalmitis. One month later, he developed a 35% left pneumothorax. The following month, a penetrating corneal graft of his right eye failed. Cultures were sterile. At 18 years, the cataract in his left eye was extracted followed by prolapse of his iris requiring surgical repair. His right eye had a scarred ectatic anterior segment. After 3 more episodes of spontaneous pneumothorax, a left upper lobectomy found a meaty nonexpansive lung with bronchiectasis, organizing pneumonia, interstitial fibrosis, and numerous cysts and blebs on the pleural of the lung.

After this episode the patient moved to California where he met his prospective wife through a program for the blind. Prior to their marriage, they requested genetic counseling, as she had congenital anophthalmia. They were informed that they would not have affected children as "his defect will cancel out yours". Subsequently they had two children affected with mucoepithelial dysplasia. After several more bouts of spontaneous pneumothorax and pneumonia a left thoracotomy was performed with talc insufflation. He developed cyanosis and clubbed fingers. He died at 27 years of cor pulmonale.

The original blocks and H & E stained slides of the cornea from the patient were obtained and the blocks recut and stained with H & E and PAP stains.

RESULTS

Histologic features of the conjunctiva of patient V-18 were not unusual. Except for one cell with phagocytic vacuoles containing laminated bands of material, the only unusual feature seen ultrastructurally was a lack of desmosomes. Only four desmosomes were identified in only a single pair of keratinocytes, but as these structures are not plentiful in conjunctivae from this area, it is consistent with the findings in other mucosa in this disease but by itself not a diagnostic finding.

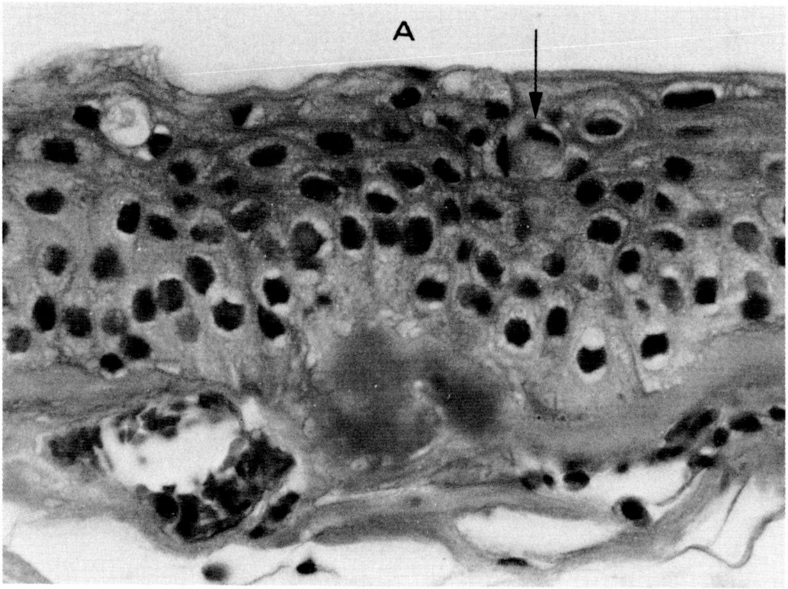

Fig. 3A. Patient IV-10, original cornea, shows edema and

vascularization of the stroma, disruption of Bowman's layer, loss of nuclear polarity of the basal cells, vacuolization and nuclear atypia of the epithelial cells and individual dyskeratotic cells (arrow), H & E stain. X192.

The original corneal button from patient IV-10 was abnormal throughout (Fig. 3A). The stroma was edematous. Small vessels were present throughout the anterior one third of the corneal stroma. In several places, Bowman's layer was splayed into the basal cell layer, disrupted in other areas, and varied in thickness. The epithelial layer varied from 2 to 8 cells thick. There was loss of nuclear polarity in the basal cells with most nuclei occupying the surface pole of the cell rather than the basement membrane pole. The cytoplasm of the basal cells contained numerous vacuoles. The polygonal cells were disoriented, contained both large and small vacuoles and pleomorphic nuclei with dark-staining clumps of chromatin. Wide intercellular clefts separate the superficial squamous cells from the underlying polygonal cells. There were numerous sharply rounded, rigid-appearing, eosinophilic staining, dyskeratotic cells in the mid and upper layers of the epithelium most prominently shown in the tissue sections stained with PAP stain. These were frequently surrounded by a more normal appearing cell forming a cell-in-cell appearing structure. These resemble the cell-in-cell bodies or corps rond seen in hereditary benign intraepithelial dyskeratosis and Darier's disease. The overall histologic features of the disorder resemble those described for the corneal lesions of keratosis follicularis spinulosa decalvans (Franceschetti, Jaccottet and Jadassohn, 1957), (Fig. 3B).

The donated cornea removed from IV-10 at his second lamellar keratoplasty showed essentially the same features in the epithelium noted in his cornea, with the exception of greater variation in the thickness of the epithelial layer which varied from 1 to 10 cells in thickness, and extensive fibrovascular infiltration in and posterior to Bowman's layer (Fig. 3C).

PAP stained smears from the conjunctival limbus showed cell-in-cell type dyskeratotic bodies, and cells with vacuolated cytoplasm and pleotropic nuclei. Strands of included material were found in some cells similar to those

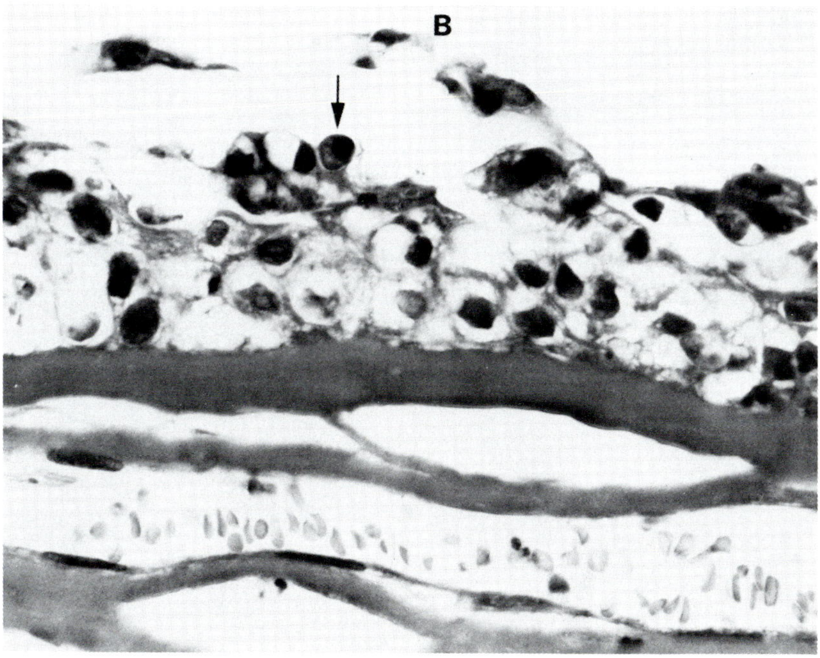

Fig. 3B. PAP stained original cornea, IV-10, shows abundant eosinophilic dyskeratotic cells (arrow) among vesiculated, dyshesive squamous cells. X100.

seen in oral, nasal, bladder, vaginal and cervical cells. These inclusions and vacuoles did not stain with Dane's keratin stain, Sudan black or Baker's phospholipid stain. Some vacuoles stained intensely with PAS; the reaction was reduced following diastase digestion.

The urinary, vaginal, cervical, gingival, and palatal mucosal cells of the mother of V-18 (IV-15) showed similar abnormalities in all tissues. Histologically there was a failure of maturation of epithelium with a lack of cornification and keratinization. The epithelia were thin with dyshesion of cells and exfoliation at the surface of immature well nucleated cells. Cytologically,cells showed anisocytosis, poikilocytosis, large paranuclear vacuoles, transcytoplasmic strands and aggregates of material, cytoplasmic polychromato-

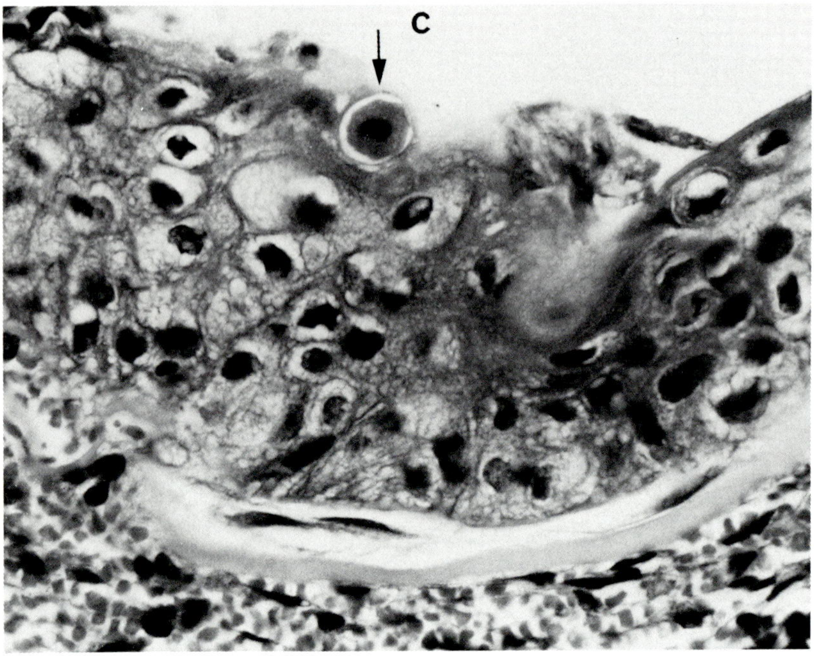

Fig. 3C. Donated corneal button removed from IV-10 placed during first lamellar keratoplasty shows the same changes in the epithelium and anterior stroma as seen in the patient's original cornea (Fig. 3A). H & E stain. X192.

philia, bizarre-shaped hyperchromatic nuclei and pseudopodia of cytoplasm. Many small round dyskeratotic cells and cell-in-cell structures were seen (Fig. 4).

Electron photomicrographs showed essentially identical features in all epithelia. The basement membrane was intact but frequently duplicated. Dilated intercellular spaces were filled with an amorphous material (Fig. 5). The number of desmosomes decreased progressively from the basal to the squamous layer so that many squamous cells had few identifiable attachments (Fig. 5, arrow). Gap junctions were also rare in these cells in contrast to their abundancy in normal tissues from these sites. Desmosomes that were present had a paucity of attached tonofilaments which are normally

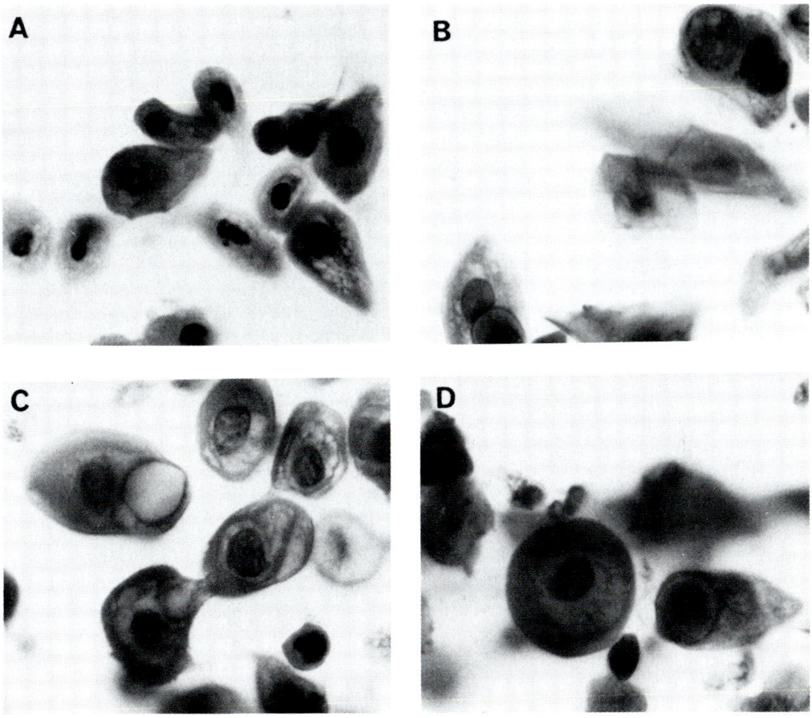

Fig. 4. Exfoliated cells from mucosal surfaces A. Limbal conjunctiva, B. Palate, C. Vagina, D. Bladder show similar features of vacuolated cells with hyperchromatic pleomorphic nuclei, poikilocytosis, anisocytosis, and round dyskeratotic cells. PAP. X480.

striking in oral epithelia. There were no keratohyalin granules in any cells. In most cells, a perinuclear or slightly eccentric band of cytoplasm contained numerous vacuoles filled with amorphous material, and autophagic vacuoles filled with cellular debris. Intermingled in the cytoplasm were wheat-sheaf-like bundles of filaments which individually were larger than the tonofilaments attached to desmosomes. Undulating strands which were bound by ribosomes adjacent to the nucleus but devoid of ribosome peripherally showed a defined structure. When adjacent to the nucleus and ribosomally bound, these bands had an internal diagonal periodicity of

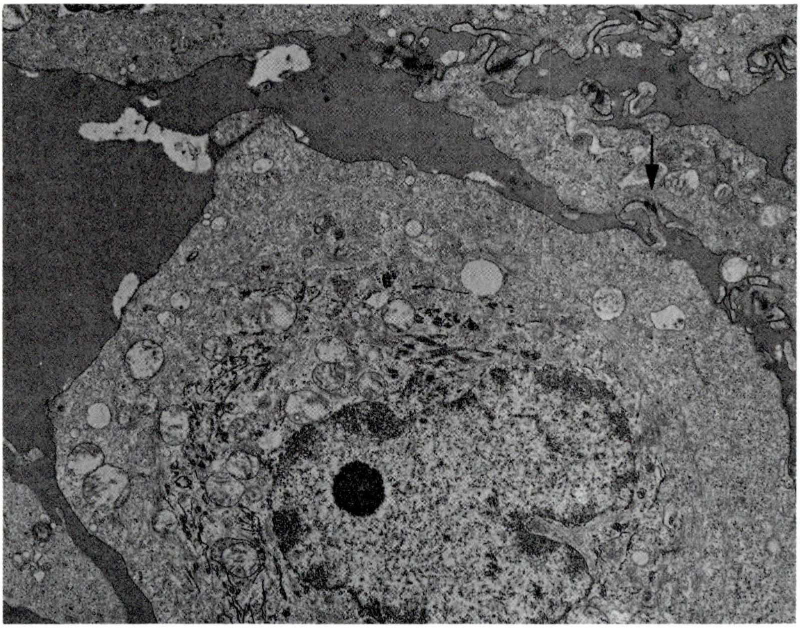

Fig. 5. Electron photomicrograph of gingival epithelium shows paucity of desmosomes (arrow), amorphous moderately electron-dense intercellular material, bands and aggregates of material as well as vacuoles distributed around the nucleus (original magnification X3,300).

about 2-3nm (Fig. 6). This periodicity is maintained as bordering ribosomes decreased in number and the bands assumed a trilamellar appearance (Fig. 7, arrow). Farther from the nucleus these trilamellar bands appear to fuse to become pentalamellar (Fig. 7). When no longer ribosomally bound, these bands may be associated with plaque-like structures with filaments which appear to interdigitate with the band (Fig. 8). At the periphery of the cell, the bands tend to aggregate into multiple layered bands (Fig. 9). These pentalamellar structures are of the same size and resemble morphologically gap junctions and the multiple bands resemble aggregates of isolated gap junctions (Goodenough, 1974, Witkop, 1980).

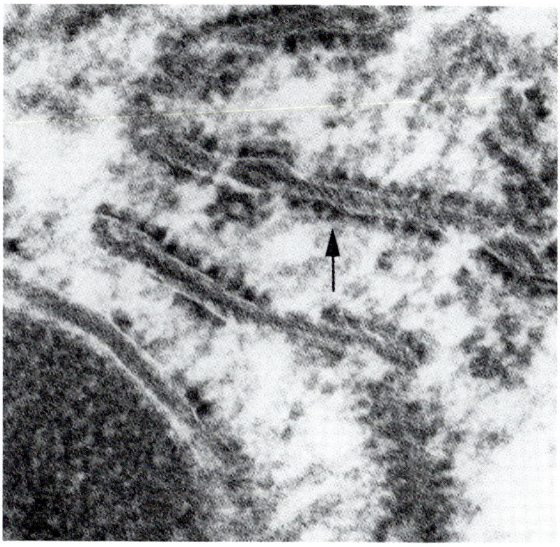

Fig. 6. Ribosomal-bound bands adjacent to nucleus have internal diagonal periodicity (arrow). Orig. magnification X180,000.

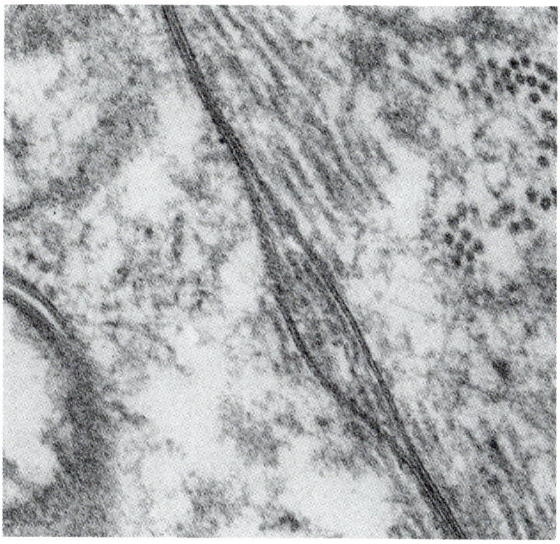

Fig. 7. Trilamellar bands tended to

fuse forming pentalamellar bands resembling gap junctional material. Original magnification X52,000.

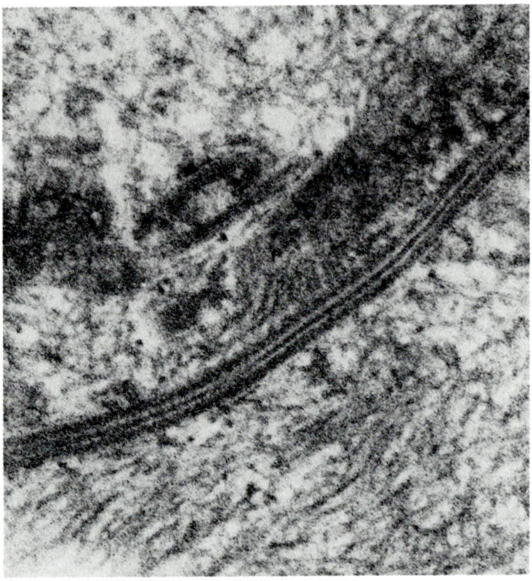

Fig. 8. Plaque-like structures with tonofilament-like attachments appear to interdigitate with the pentalamellar bands. Original magnification X52,000.

DISCUSSION

Hereditary mucoepithelial dysplasia has been observed in three kindreds by the authors and shows an autosomal dominant mode of transmission in each family. The ocular lesions are an early and prominant feature of the disorder. The dyshesive nature of the epithelial cell defect most likely accounts for the early corneal keratosis and subsequent pannus formation which produce the clinical features of severe photophobia, blepharospasm, tearing and nystagmus. Corneal opacification and the development of posterior subcapsular cataracts lead

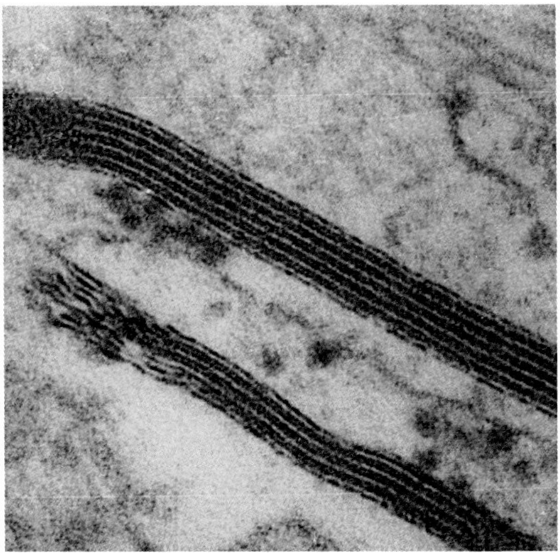

Fig. 9. Peripheral to the central perinuclear area pentalamellar bands appeared to fuse into multiple lamellar bands resembling the aggregation of gap junctional material *in vitro*. Original magnification X180,000.

to marked visual impairment by 5 to 7 years of age.

The histologic, cytologic and ultrastructural features of the ocular and other mucosal tissues suggest that junctions between cells are defective in formation. It is not known for certain whether the included bands of material are identical to gap junction material, although their morphologic resemblance is striking. Gap junctions and desmosomes are deficient in mucosal cells.

Compatible with an interpretation that this disorder involves gap junctions, is the development of cataracts from 3½ to 5 years of age. Gap junctions are found in high density in tissues that function under relatively anoxic, avascular conditions (Goodenough, Paul and Culbert, 1978). Lens is particularly rich in gap junctions which provide the only known mechanism for cellular interchange. It has been postulated that they have a major role in glycolysis in maintaining this tissue (Philipson, Hanninen and Balazs, 1975) and also cornea (Kreutziger, 1976). Theoretically, as this is a dominantly inherited disorder and affected patients are heterozygous, the normal gene should code for normal structured protein. Thus, these patients would be expected to have some normal connections. The fact that they do not have congenital cataracts, but develop them in childhood, suggests that the lens functions normally for a time but then develops premature cataracts. Against the interpretation that this is a disorder of gap junction formation, is the lack of significant clinical involvement of tissues known to be rich in gap junctions such as muscle and liver. Cells of these tissues however, lack desmosomes which are involved in this disease. It is possible that the formation of junctions are involved, but under different genetic control in ectodermal than in mesodermal tissue. Of more than passing interest is the suggestion made by Barnett and Szabo (1973) that gap junctions are necessary for the normal keratinization and cornification of mucosal epithelia. The findings in this disorder substantiate that interpretation.

Affected children have severe photophobia, and blepharospasm with associated tearing requiring examinations under anesthesia. The major external finding is diffuse conjunctival vascular dilatation, without specific papillary or follicular formation. The cornea displays a diffuse punctate epithelial keratopathy, without focal concentration. This feature probably produces the severe clinical photophobia. Gradually, in early childhood, a subepithelial pannus begins to form, which ultimately occupies the entire cornea at the level of Bowman's layer. Associated with the visual deprivation in infancy and childhood are nystagmus, strabismus, and amblyopia. Concomitantly, posterior subcapsular cataracts appear and visual impairment is severe in the first decade of life.

The first major problem is to establish a proper diagnosis. Because none of the ocular findings are specific for hereditary mucoepithelial dysplasia, an early precise diagnosis on ocular findings alone is difficult to make. Most helpful is the associated involvement of other mucosal surfaces, like mouth, vagina, and anus, and the family history that suggests autosomal dominant inheritance.

This disease must be distinguished from a number of similar ocular problems (O'Connor, 1980). Hereditary mucoepithelial dysplasia can be distinguished from atopic diseases like hay fever, vernal conjunctivitis, and atopic keratoconjunctivitis by the absence of seasonal exacerbations, lack of responsiveness to topical glucocorticoids and sodium chromoglycate, the vigorous growth of pannus, and the general absence of other atopic problems like asthma and eczema (although abnormalities of skin and the bronchopulmonary system may be misinterpreted as atopic disease). It can be distinguished from ocular involvement in Stevens Johnson syndrome by the absence of an initial severe systemic febrile illness (although these children are susceptible to multiple infections frequently treated with antibiotics that have been associated with erythema multiforme), the absence of the blister and target skin lesions, and the absence of severe conjunctival cicatrization and keratinization. Likewise, the disorder is distinguished from toxic epidermal necrolysis (Lyell's disease) by the absence of an acute bullous skin disease with a "scalded skin" appearance.

In the early stages, the disorder can be confused with chronic blepharokeratoconjunctivitis associated with staphylococcal exotoxins, producing an epithelial keratitis, marginal ulceration or phlyctenulosis. The absence of a history of hordeola, chalazia, and marginal blepharitis leads one from this diagnosis. Also absent are the focal white subepithelial marginal infiltrates separated from the limbus by a clear zone and the focal elevated vascularized nodules of phlyctenulosis. However, both diseases are associated with a chronic diffuse punctate epithelial keratopathy and gradually progressive pannus formation, although the pannus in staphylococcal eye disease is usually faint and flat, while that in hereditary mucoepithelial dysplasia is usually more elevated and thick. Staphylococcal disease usually has its onset in later childhood (except for purulent staphylococcal ophthalmia neonatorum), while hereditary mucoepithelial dysplasia begins in very early childhood. The disease will not be confused with ocular cicatricial pemphigoid, since that is a disease of older age.

Management of these patients is extremely frustrating, paralleling that of the children with ocular erythema multiforme (Stevens Johnson syndrome). Protection of the corneal epithelial surface is paramount, and the use of frequent topical artificial tears and ointments along with lateral

Connective Tissue Diseases of the Eye

THE EYE IN THE MARFAN SYNDROME

Irene H. Maumenee, M.D.

The Johns Hopkins Hospital, Wilmer Institute
Baltimore, Maryland 21205

PATIENTS AND METHODS

In patients with the Marfan syndrome, problems of diagnosis and management from an ocular and systemic point of view persist. In order to answer the question of possible correlation and thus predictive value as between the ocular and systemic findings and between individual ocular signs, I collected data on 160 consecutive patients with the Marfan syndrome. A variety of medical specialists refer between 150 and 200 patients annually for ocular evaluation to help with the diagnosis and management of presumed Marfan syndrome.

The diagnosis of the Marfan syndrome is based on four criteria: ocular, cardiovascular, and skeletal disease, and familial occurrence. In the present study all patients suspected of being affected received a thorough physical examination including measurements of body proportions, chest auscultation, chest x-ray, and echocardiogram as minimum aspects. In a patient with the classic Marfan syndrome the diagnosis is certain, and frequently three or four of the criteria are fulfilled. However, some mildly affected patients are seen in families, or sporadically, and in these a definite diagnosis may be quite difficult. No laboratory examination or test exists to confirm or negate this diagnosis. In mild cases, the presence of at least two of the clinical criteria was required to make the diagnosis. No patient with a questionable diagnosis was included in this study, nor was lens dislocation alone considered a sufficient criterion for inclusion, even if the family history was positive for lens dislocation. In order to determine which of

Birth Defects: Original Article Series, Volume 18, Number 6, pages 515–524

Maumenee IH (1981). The eye in the Marfan syndrome. Tr Ophthalmol Soc, in press.
Pyeritz RE, McKusick VA (1979). The Marfan syndrome: Diagnosis and management. New Engl J Med 300:772-777.

This study was supported in part by grant number EY 01773 from the National Eye Institute.

Parts of this paper have previously been included in a thesis for the American Ophthalmological Society as partial requirement for admission as a member, and the thesis is being published.

THE WAGNER-STICKLER SYNDROME

Ruth M. Liberfarb, M.D., Ph.D.
Tatsuo Hirose, M.D.
From Retina Associates and The
Eye Research Institute of
Retina Foundation, Boston, MA 02114

Based on our study of 70 affected persons in 22 families (Liberfarb et al., 1979 and 1981), we propose the designation of the Wagner-Stickler syndrome for the phenotype, the ocular features of which have been known as the Wagner syndrome by ophthalmologists (Wagner, 1938), whereas the ocular and nonocular (orofacial and skeletal) features have been known as the Stickler syndrome by geneticists (Stickler et al., 1965, Stickler and Pugh, 1967). We have determined the frequency of ocular and nonocular features in affected individuals and identified several ocular and nonocular features which are progressive. We have also established an approximate age of onset in the group with known retinal disease at diagnosis as compared to the age of onset in the asymptomatic group ascertained by family screening.

The Wagner-Stickler syndrome is a hereditary disorder with an autosomal dominant pattern of inheritance and with great variability in expressivity. The association of the features (ocular, orofacial, and skeletal) in this disorder suggests a basic underlying connective tissue disease.

To justify using the designation of this phenotype as the Wagner-Stickler syndrome it is helpful to consider the initial reports. Vitreoretinal degeneration, an ocular sign seen in several different and well delineated connective tissue disorders was first described (Wagner, 1938) in three generations of a Swiss family. The following ocular manifestations were noted in affected persons: vitreoretinal degeneration; vitreous bands; retinal pigmentation sometimes seen sheathing thin retinal arteries; chorioretinal atrophy;

Birth Defects: Original Article Series, Volume 18, Number 6, pages 525–538

presenile cataracts; myopia; astigmatism and strabismus. The family was restudied again after a number of years (Bohringer et al., 1960; and Ricci, 1960). In this family, poor vision was associated with myopia and cataracts. Although retinal detachment was not noted in any of the 28 members of the original family, retinal detachment has been the most common ocular feature to bring subsequent families to medical attention. Nonocular features were rarely noted in the early literature on the Wagner syndrome. Thus, the Wagner syndrome has been classified as a rare disorder with ocular manifestations only (Maumenee, 1979). Wagner himself (Wagner, 1938) did note hearing loss in one 17-year-old patient with ocular problems. More recently, nonocular features such as cleft palate, characteristic facies, and skeletal abnormalities have been noted (Jansen, 1962; Delaney et at., 1963; Alexander and Shea, 1965; Frandsen, 1966; Hagler and Crosswell, 1968; Van Balen and Falger, 1970; and Hirose et al., 1973). Because for the most part, these nonocular features can be quite subtle, it is understandable that these could have been overlooked by Wagner and others.

In the mid-1960s, Stickler and his associates described a connective tissue dysplasia they called hereditary progressive arthroophthalmopathy (Stickler et al., 1965; and Stickler and Pugh, 1967). Clinical characteristics included eye findings and joint problems associated with characteristic facial appearance, cleft palate, and hearing loss. Little attention was given to the eye findings, which were similar to those of the Wagner syndrome.

A number of authors have noted the similarity of phenotypic features of the Wagner and Stickler syndrome (Hall, 1974; Herrmann et al., 1975; Knobloch, 1975).

SUBJECTS AND METHODS

We examined 22 patients diagnosed by one of us (T.H.) on the basis of ocular findings as having the Wagner syndrome. We also examined 68 relatives of these index patients, 30 of whom had been previously diagnosed as having retinal problems.

Of the 90 persons examined, 39 were male, 51 were female, and all were white. Their ages ranged from 10 months to 74 years. These individuals underwent the following evaluation:

a complete medical history; a physical examination focusing on the nonocular abnormalities associated with the Stickler syndrome (2,3,4); and an ophthalmologic evaluation, including indirect ophthalmoscopy using scleral depression and a slit-lamp examination of the vitreous and the fundus with the Goldmann three mirror lens. Three patients whose ocular problems had been documented elsewhere had physical examinations only. A medical history was obtained to document the time when each abnormal feature was first noted.

The presence of some of the nonocular features such as maxillary hypoplasia, small chin, highly arched palate and depressed bridge of the nose was a subjective determination by the examiner (R.M.L.). The presence of arachnodactyly was determined by measuring the length of the metacarpals relative to the width from the anterior-posterior radiograph of the hand, using the method of Eldridge (5). Arm span was determined by measuring the distance between the tips of the middle fingers with the arms extended laterally. The upper to lower segment ratio was determined from a measurement from the top of the head to the upper edge of the symphysis pubis (upper segment) and the upper edge of the symphysis pubis to the floor when standing in bare feet.

Twenty-six affected individuals had radiographs of the hands and long bones. Thirty-seven affected individuals had audiograms.

Of the 90 persons examined, 70 were diagnosed as having the Wagner-Stickler syndrome. At the time of examination, 52 of the 70 affected persons knew that they had a retinal disorder (Group A); 18 (age 2-52 years) were asymptomatic (Group B). Fourteen of the asymptomatic persons had retinal changes of which they were unaware; four had no retinal abnormality but had other ocular and nonocular features of the syndrome. Twenty family members were found to be unaffected.

CASE REPORT

Two families have been described in detail (Liberfarb et al., 1979; Liberfarb et al., 1981) to illustrate the variability of the ocular and nonocular features of the Wagner-Sticker syndrome within a family. Members of one of these families are shown in Fig. 1-4.

detachments and cataract were among the earliest recognized ocular features.

Vitreous degeneration may occur before the second decade but was not noted in the limited number of patients examined in our study. Vitreous degeneration was noted frequently in patients after the first decade. Liquefaction, resulting in an optically empty appearance of the vitreous, was followed by fibrillar condensation of the gel and development of visible vitreous membranes, frequently noted in patients over age 20 years.

Chorioretinal degeneration without pigmentations appears in some patients examined under the age of 20 years. Deposition of pigmentation along blood vessels and equatorially progresses in frequency with advancing age.

Myopia, retinal breaks and detachments, astigmatism, cataracts and glaucoma are clearly progressive. Retinal detachments, cataracts and glaucoma, the problems most frequently bringing affected patients to ophthalmologists are rare in children, becoming more common in adolescents.

Of the nonocular features, hearing loss and arthritis were noted to be progressive. In general, patients under age 30 with sensorineural hearing loss were asymptomatic. Only some of the patients aged 30 to 50 years were aware of their hearing loss. All patients over age 50 were aware of some hearing loss.

Premature arthritis was diagnosed from history. Few patients under 30 complained of joint pain, stiffness, or swelling. Such complaints became more common with advancing years. Many of the patients over 50 reported having had such symptoms for over 20 years.

Table 2

Incidence of Features of the Wagner-Stickler Syndrome in 70 Affected Persons by Age

Feature	% (No.) 0-10 yrs (n=5)	11-20 yrs (n=25)	21-30 yrs (n=8)	31-50 yrs (n=21)	50 yrs (n=11)
Vitreous degeneration	0 (0/3)	80 (16/20)	86 (6/7)	94 (15/16)	90 (9/10)
Without visible membrane	0 (0/3)	45 (9/20)	0 (0/7)	13 (2/16)	20 (2/10)
With visible membrane	0 (0/3)	35 (7/20)	86 (6/7)	81 (13/16)	70 (7/10)
Chorioretinal degeneration	20	67 (16/24)	71 (5/7)	57 (4/7)	80 (8/10)
without pigmentation	20	33 (8/24)	14 (1/7)	14 (1/7)	10 (1/10)
with peri-vascular and/or equatorial	0	33 (8/24)	57 (4/7)	43 (4/7)	70 (7/10)
Myopia	40	76	75	80	92
Retinal breaks and detachments	20	64	75	75	92
Astigmatism	20	40	100	53	64
Cataract	20	40	38	50	83
Glaucoma	0	0	0	15	25
Sensorineural hearing loss		83 (10/12)	67 (4/6)	92 (12/13)	100 (8/8)
Premature arthritis	0	16	50	55	75

3. Penetrance of the Wagner-Stickler Phenotype

All the 22 index patients had affected relatives, which suggests that the spontaneous mutation rate is very low. Sixteen families had affected members in at least three generations. No persons appeared to transmit the mutant gene without having some phenotypic features.

Although it was common for relatives to have similar features, most families had not recognized that the ocular or nonocular features were inherited.

DISCUSSION

Since many of the facial and skeletal features are present before the onset of ocular problems, all relatives of affected persons regardless of age should be examined for these nonocular features. Those with the nonocular features should then be followed closely by an ophthalmologist in order to diagnose the eye problems as early as possible. Absence of the nonocular features in the young does not rule out the possibility that eye problems will develop in the future. Routine ophthalmological examinations probably into the third decade should be instituted before the diagnosis of the Wagner-Stickler syndrome can be ruled out.

We have dealt with many affected individuals whose interrelated features had not been recognized previously. We have also dealt with many families who had not been aware of the obvious inheritance of these problems. Our experience impressed us with the need for physicians apt to be caring for affected persons to be aware fo the Wagner-Stickler syndrome.

Such physicians include pediatricians, family practitioners, internists, ophthalmologists, obstetricians otolaryngologists, orthopedists, rheumatologists, geneticists and orthodontists. The Wagner-Stickler syndrome should be considered a diagnostic possibility in any newborn infant with cleft palate and small chin, and in all cases of dominantly inherited myopia, with or without retinal detachment and deafness, in dominantly inherited cleft palate and also in dominantly inherited mild spondyloepiphyseal dysplasia with or without joint laxity and slender tubular bones.

In order to bring about improved management of persons with the Wagner-Stickler syndrome, thereby improving the prognosis for preserving good vision, we recommend a management plan based on early diagnosis of those at risk, long-term monitoring of affected persons, timely intervention, genetic counseling and family screening of persons at risk.

REFERENCES

Alexander RL and Shea M (1965). Wagner's disease, Arch Ophthalmol 74: 310.

Bohringer HR, Dieterle P, and Landolt E (1960). Zur Klinik und Pathologie der Degeneration hyaloideo-retinalis hereditaria (Wagner), Ophthalmologica 139: 330.

Delaney WV, Podedworny W, and Havener WH (1965). Inherited retinal detachment, Arch Ophthalmol 69: 44.

Eldridge R (1964). The metacarpal index, Arch Int Med 113: 140.

Frandsen E (1966). Hereditary hyaloideoretinal degeneration (Wagner) in a Danish family, Acta Ophthalmol 44: 223.

Hagler WS and Crosswell HH(1968). Radial perivascular chorioretinal degeneration and retinal detachment, Trans Am Acad Ophthalmol Otolaryngol 72: 203.

Hall J (1974). Stickler syndrome presenting as a syndrome of cleft palate, myopia and blindness inherited as a dominant trait, Birth Defects X: 157.

Herrmann J, France TO, Spranger JW et al (1975). The Stickler syndrome (hereditary arthroophthalmopathy), Birth Defects XI: 76.

Hirose T, Lee KY, and Schepens CL (1973). Wagner's hereditary vitreoretinal degeneration and retinal detachment, Arch Opthal 89: 176.

Jansen LMMA (1962). Degeneratio hyaloideo-retinalis hereditaria, ophthalmologica 144: 458.

Knobloch WH (1975). Inherited hyaloideoretinopathy and skeletal dysplasia, Trans Am Ophthalmol Soc LXXIII: 417.

Liberfarb RM, Hirose T, and Holmes LB (1979). The Wagner-Stickler syndrome: a genetic study. Birth Defects XV: 145.

Liberfarb RM, Hirose T and Holmes LB (1981). The Wagner-Stickler syndrome: a study of 22 families. J Pediatr 99: 394.

Maumenee IH (1979). Vitreoretinal degeneration as a sign of generalized connective tissue diseases, Am J Ophthal 88: 432.

Ricci PA (1960). Clinique et transmission genetique des differentes formes de degenerescence vitreo-retinienne, Ophthalmologica 139: 338.

Stickler, GB, Belau PG, and Farrell FJ et al (1965). Hereditary progressive arthroophthalmolopathy, Mayo Clin Proc 40: 433.

Stickler GB and Pugh D (1967). Hereditary progressive arthro-ophthalmolopathy. II. Additional observations on vertebral abnormalities, a hearing defect and a report of a similar case. Mayo Clin Proc 42: 495.

Van Balen ATM and Falger ELF (1970). Hereditary hyaloideoretinal degeneration and palatoschisis, Arch Ophthalmol 44: 152.

Wagner H (1938). Ein bischer unbekanntes Erbleiden des Auges (Degeneratio hyaloideo-retinalis hereditaria) beobachtet im Kanton Zurich, Klin Monastbl Augenheilkd 100: 840.

OCULAR AND SYSTEMIC MANIFESTATIONS OF STICKLER'S SYNDROME: A PRELIMINARY REPORT

Thomas A. Weingeist, M.D., Ph.D. (a)
Vernon Hermsen, M.D. (a)
James W. Hanson, M.D. (b)
Robert M. Bumsted, M.D. (c)
Stuart L. Weinstein, M.D. (d)
William H. Olin, D.D.S. (e)

The University of Iowa   Iowa City, Iowa 52242

Supported in part by Grant RR59 from
Clinical Research Centers Branch, NIH

Are Wagner's disease and Stickler's syndrome separate entities or do they represent opposite ends of the spectrum of the same disorder? Wagner (Wagner 1938), a Swiss ophthalmologist, described the ocular findings of a large family with an autosomal dominant disorder. The condition which Wagner termed hereditary hyaloideoretinal degeneration was characterized by myopia, early cataract formation, liquefaction of the vitreous, retinal vascular and retinal pigmentary alterations. None of the patients in "Wagner's family" had extraocular abnormalities or developed a retinal detachment on follow-up examination (Bőhringer 1960; Ricci 1960; Ricci 1961).

Stickler et. al. (Stickler 1965; Stickler 1967) described an autosomal dominant condition which resembled Wagner's disease. The patients differed in that they usually had a high degree of myopia and retinal detachment was common. In addition, characteristic orofacial, skeletal and auditory abnormalities were noted which set hereditary progressive arthro-ophthalmopathy (Stickler's syndrome) apart from Wagner's disease. Since the publication of these classic papers, numerous authors have referred to these entities. Nevertheless, there is still confusion in the literature and uncertainty

Birth Defects: Original Article Series, Volume 18, Number 6, pages 539–560

among clinicians as to whether these two disorders are the same or different.

This is a preliminary report of a prospective, multi-specialty investigation of the ocular and systemic manifestations of Stickler's syndrome. More than 47 individuals from 12 families have been studied by members of the Departments of Ophthalmology (a), Pediatrics (b), Otolaryngology (c), Orthopedics (d), and Dentistry (e) in an effort to clearly define this entity, and to establish the incidence and the severity of various anomalies within this population. Sixteen individuals from this group have been thoroughly evaluated and represent the main data base for this continuing study.

METHODS

The protocol for this study was approved by the Committee on Human Research at The University of Iowa. Consent forms were signed by each subject or a responsible parent or guardian prior to inclusion in the study. Most subjects were admitted to the Clinical Research Center and evaluated during the course of 2 to 3 days. Many patients had been followed for 5 or more years prior to entering the study. With few exceptions, all affected individuals were completely evaluated by members of the five services involved in this investigation.

The propositus and family were interviewed and examined in order to establish a family pedigree. Whenever possible, members from two or three generations were interviewed at the same time in order to corroborate historical material. Particular attention was paid to information relating to orofacial anomalies, hearing loss, skeletal disorders and ocular problems; however, associated anomalies were also noted and investigated, if they appeared to be related to Stickler's syndrome.

Affected individuals had a complete review of their past medical history with emphasis placed on those problems related to Stickler's syndrome. A thorough physical examination was performed by specialists in each service. Genetic counselling was provided when appropriate and individuals were given ample time to discuss and review medical information which was pertinent to their general health and well being.

Radiologic studies included a skeletal survey, skull films for cephalometric evaluation and panoramic x-rays of the dentition. A 24 hour urine collection was evaluated for levels of hydroxyproline. Erythrocyte sedimentation rate, complete blood count and rheumatoid factor blood tests were also obtained.

Patients underwent a speech, hearing and nasal airway (rhinomanometry) evaluation as part of the otolaryngology examination. Each subject had a complete eye examination which included measurements of visual acuity, tonometry, refraction, keratometry, gonioscopy, direct and indirect ophthalmoscopy. The axial length of the eye was determined by A scan echography. Fundus photography and fluorescein angiography was performed and many patients also had electrooculography (EOG) and electroretinography (ERG).

RESULTS

Individuals in the study ranged in age from newborn to the seventh decade. Seven isolated cases were found. In 40 individuals, a family history was established.

Orthopedic Evaluation

Excluding children less than 10 years of age, all patients complained of some joint problems. These complaints ranged from minimal knee discomfort after exercise to generalized joint discomfort. Morning stiffness lasting 45 minutes to an hour was a common complaint. Although a few patients complained of joint swelling, none were found to have evidence of active synovitis. The joints primarily affected were the knees, the ankles, the hips, the wrists and the small joints of the hands. The spine and the shoulder were also affected. The physical examination was generally unremarkable, except for the finding of increased laxity at the elbows and the knees. Very few patients had joint laxity greater than one would see in the general population. None of the patients studied could be considered below normal in height, although several adults were short in stature. Within the same kindred there were also individuals with disproportionately long limbs (Marfanoid habitus).

The most striking findings were the roentgenographic studies which showed evidence of generalized epiphyseal dysplasia (Figures 1 & 2). Distortion of the distal radial carpal angle and generalized dysplastic changes of the distal femur, the proximal tibia, the distal radius and the distal tibia were common. Several patients had degenerative changes involving the patella femoral joint, as well as the carpometacarpal joint of the thumb. Schmorl's nodes were evident in numerous vertebra and several individuals had wedging of the vertebral bodies and osteophyte formation anteriorly. Every patient examined had some evidence of epiphyseal dysplasia.

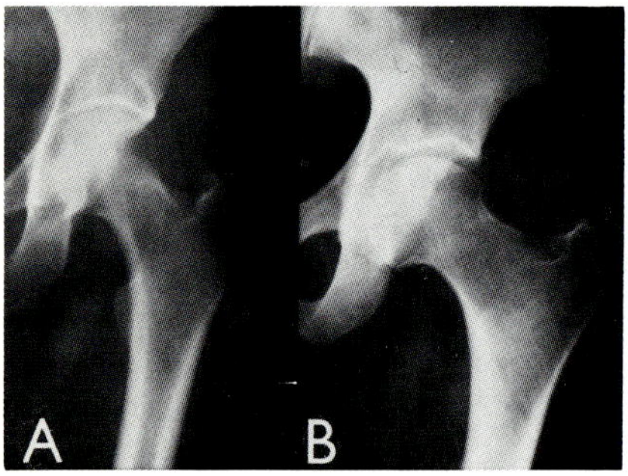

Figure 1 A. Normal pelvis B. Stickler's Syndrome Anterior posterior radiograph of pelvis revealing stunting of the growth of the femoral epiphysis as well as stunting of the growth of the greater and lesser trochanter. There is some irregularity of the joint surface.

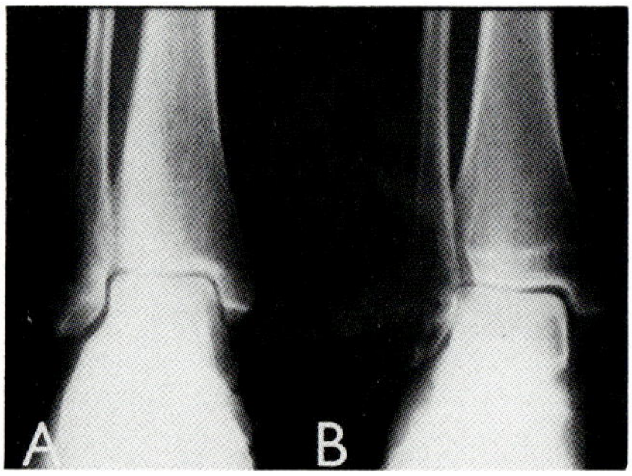

Figure 2 A. Normal ankle B. Stickler's Syndrome Anterior posterior radiograph of the ankle shows some stunting of the growth of the distal tibia with an abnormal slant to the distal tibia and shortening of the tip of the medial malleolus.

Urinary hydroxyproline excretion levels were obtained after patients were placed on a gelatin free diet. All the patients examined were found to have normal levels when corrected for age (Figure 3).

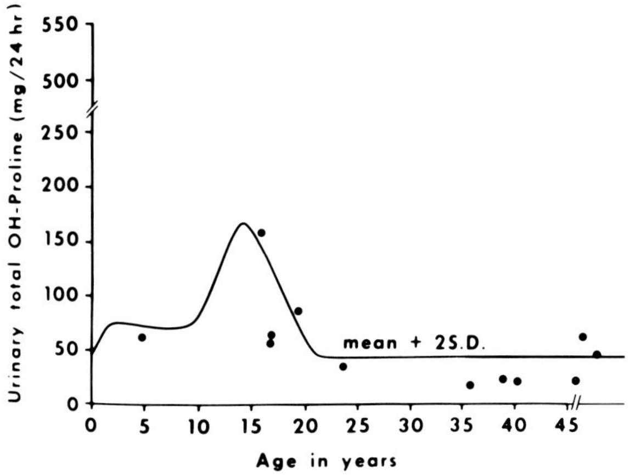

Figure 3. Age-related urine hydroxyproline excretion levels.

Otolaryngology Evaluation

Only 1 of 16 patients was found to have a sensorineural hearing loss of 20 decibels or more by audiometric testing.

Eight of 16 patients had a submucous cleft of the palate. Two additional patients had a complete cleft of the secondary palate. Only 2 of 16 patients were found to have a normal soft palate on clinical examination. Abnormal palates were characterized as being short, cleft, poorly mobile, or by having a bifid uvula. All of these anomalies may interfere with normal speech. Nevertheless, only 3 of 16 patients had "cleft palate speech", that is, hypernasality secondary to frank or marginal velopharyngeal competence. Only one patient was observed to have micrognathia, cleft palate and glossoptosis typical of the Robin malformation sequence (Pierre Robin anomaly).

Dental Examination

Panoramic x-rays revealed no extraordinary problems with the dentition, except for loss of teeth. Seven of 16 patients had dentures. Two had upper dentures only, 5 had both upper and lower dentures. These figures appear to be higher than for the normal population.

Clinically, many of the patients appeared to have mid-facial flattening (Figure 4). Surprisingly, all members of this study, in spite of their clinical appearance, had excellent facial bone development which was supported by study casts and lateral cephalometric radiographs (Figure 5).

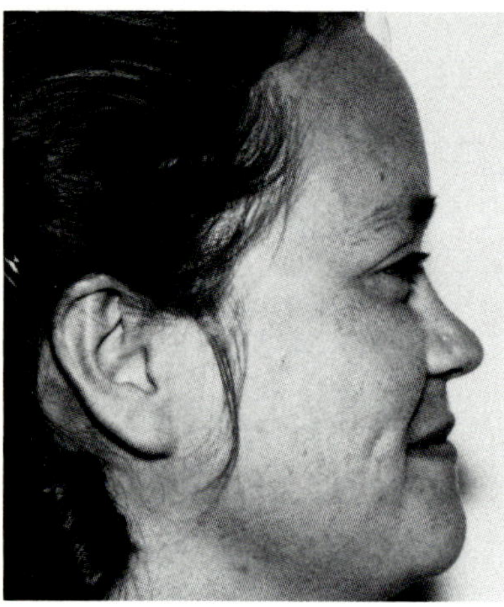

Figure 4. Profile of Stickler Syndrome patient with mid-facial flattening.

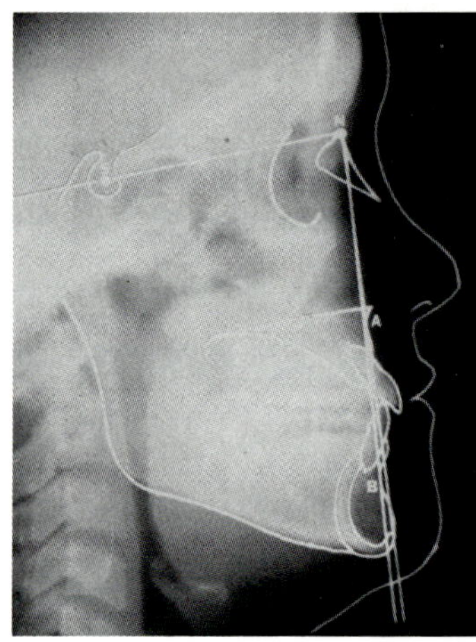

Figure 5. Lateral cephalometric evaluation of same patient reveals satisfactory facial bone development.

Ocular Examination

Myopia. Axial myopia was present in all patients and ranged from -2.75 diopters (D) spherical equivalent to -16.50 D spherical equivalent. Astigmatism greater than 2 D was found in only one patient among those who had not had surgery for repair of a retinal detachment or cataract extraction. Axial length measurements by A scan ultrasonography varied from 25.7 to 31.5 mm in length with an average of 28.1 mm (phthisical globes and eyes that had had scleral buckling procedures were excluded).

Intraocular pressure. Ocular hypertension occurred in more than one third of otherwise normal eyes. Normal pressures were maintained in several eyes on timolol alone, even though the pressures had been in the mid-30's and above without treatment. Few patients had glaucomatous field loss. No chamber angle anomalies were noted by gonioscopy.

Cataracts. Two types of cataracts were observed: peripheral cortical opacities (Figure 6) and presenile nuclear sclerosis. The cortical opacities were usually isolated, comma shaped and stationary since early in life. The ten cortical opacities seen in this group of patients were all outside the visual axis. Five presenile cataracts occurred before the age of 45. These cataracts tended to progress rapidly and to result in severe visual loss within two years of their onset.

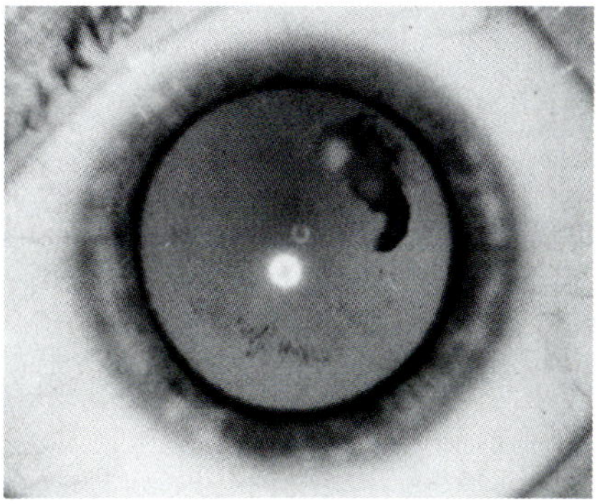

Figure 6. Peripheral cortical lenticular opacity.

Vitreous. Biomicroscopically most patients had marked liquefaction of the vitreous. In some individuals, the vitreous was so optically clear that it could not be seen on slit-lamp examination; however, most patients were found to have pockets of vitreous syneresis and membranes. Some vitreous membranes were attached to the peripheral fundus and were associated with chorioretinal abnormalities (Figure 7). Rarely membranes were attached near the posterior pole. Only occasionally membranes appeared to exert traction on the retina.

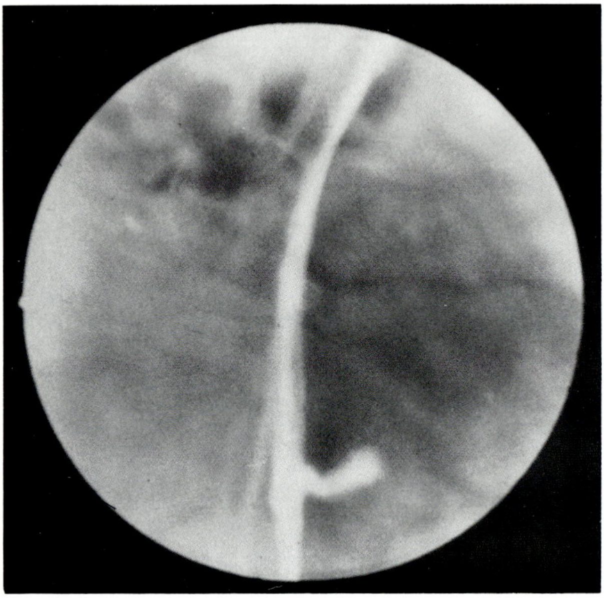

Figure 7. Dense vitreous membrane inserting in peripheral retina above chorioretinal pigmentation.

Retina. The ophthalmoscopic appearance of the posterior pole was largely dependent on the degree of myopia. In mildly myopic individuals the optic nerve head, the vessels and the macula appeared normal. In more myopic individuals a myopic conus was common and the retinal vessels appeared straight and taut (Figure 8). In severe myopia the myopic conus and straightening of the retinal blood vessels was often pronounced (Figure 9). Most patients were found to have hypopigmentation of the fundus. Staphyloma were not seen, nor were any patients found to have lacquer cracks, a Fuchs' spot or evidence of a subretinal neovascular membrane in the macula.

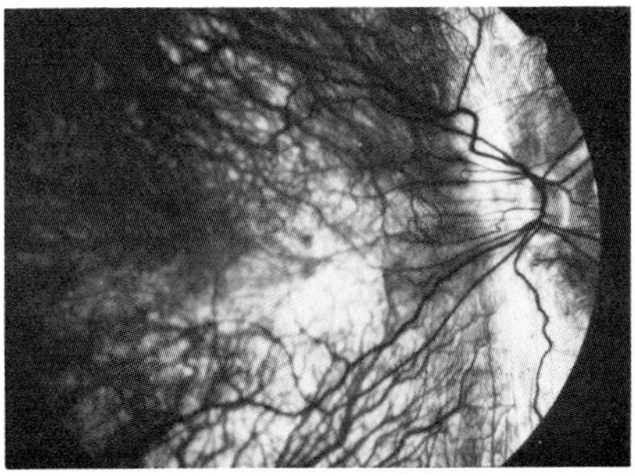

Figure 8. Moderate myopia with straightening of retinal vessels and hypopigmentation of the fundus.

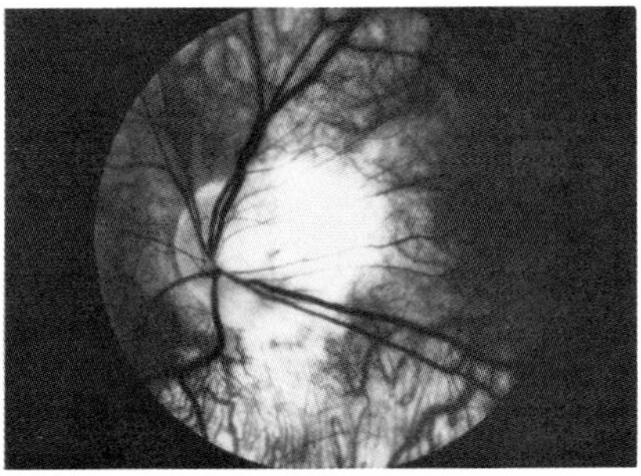

Figure 9. Large myopic conus with straightening of retinal vessels in severe myopia.

Perivascular retinal pigmentation (Figure 10) and chorioretinal hypopigmentation (Figure 11) were common, but were highly variable in appearance. Neither of these changes were directly related to the refractive error. Lattice-like degeneration and atrophic retinal holes with and without subretinal fluid, were also common. Sheathing and marked vascular attenuation occurred in patients.

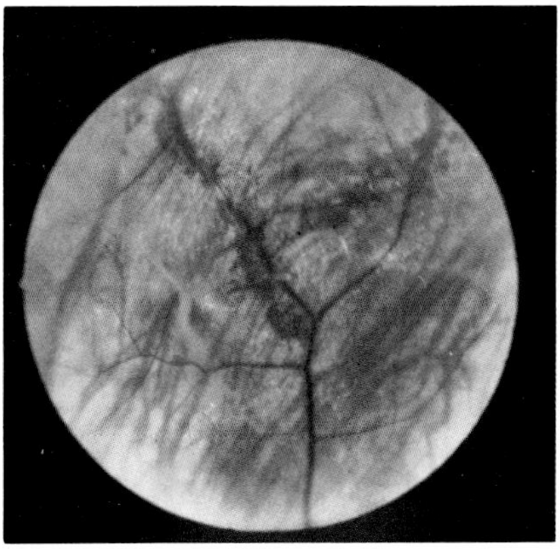

Figure 10. Typical perivascular pigmentation of peripheral retinal vessels and vitreous membranes.

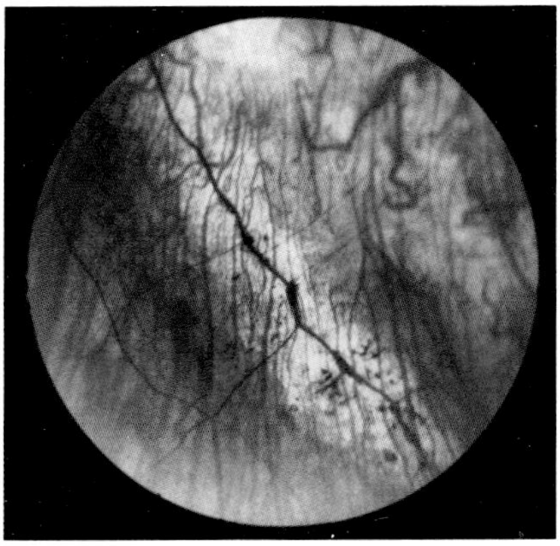

Figure 11. Radial perivascular pigmentation and parallel chorioretinal hypopigmentation.

Among the 32 eyes in this group of patients, 9 developed retinal detachments. Two developed an irreparable giant retinal tear and one had a peripheral retinal dialysis following mild blunt trauma.

Electrophysiology. The amplitude of the scotopic b-wave was abnormally low in several individuals (Figure 12).

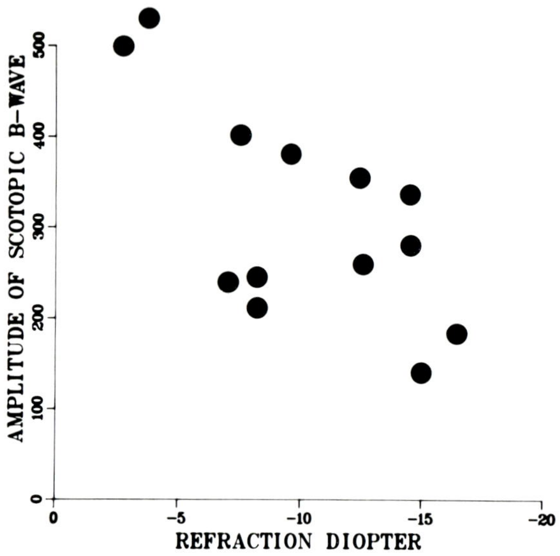

Figure 12. The decrease in the amplitude of the scotopic b-wave correlates with the degree of myopia measured in diopters and in millimeters of axial length determined by echography.

COMMENT

On the basis of our preliminary findings and a review of the literature, we think that Wagner's disease and Stickler's syndrome are distinct entities. Furthermore, we think that the condition originally described by Wagner is extremely rare and that most of the papers published in the past two decades which purport to describe Wagner's hyaloideoretinal degeneration actually concern patients with Stickler's syndrome. We are unsure if we have ever seen a case of Wagner's disease, although some isolated or sporadic cases of Stickler's syndrome would be difficult, if not impossible, to distinguish from Wagner's disease.

Part of the confusion associated with Stickler's syndrome is due to the fact that this autosomal dominant disorder is characterized by marked variability in expressivity and incomplete penetrance. As a result, a definite diagnosis can be extremely difficult, particularly in isolated cases. Seven of the 47 individuals from our larger study were considered to be isolated cases. These presumably represent new mutations or sporadic cases. We have not undertaken a study of the siblings or parents of these individuals yet. Examination of some of these families may reveal additional members who have escaped medical attention because they are only slightly affected. Others may turn out to be truly isolated cases.

Wagner's original pedigree appears to be unique. None of the patients in his pedigree developed retinal detachments and none had common extraocular anomalies. Of the 18 affected individuals in Wagner's original pedigree, clinical details were presented for only 12 (Wagner 1938). Wagner emphasized that all the patients were slightly to moderately myopic. The refractive error was -4.00 D or less, except for three eyes with nuclear sclerotic cataracts which were -11.00 D or greater. No systemic abnormalities were described in any of the patients. Particular mention was made of the unremarkable physical and laboratory findings in three of the case reports. Characteristic lens changes were present in all of the patients by the end of the first decade. Initially, multiple, fluffy dot opacities appeared in the cortex, usually posteriorly. Often the dots formed stripes or a stellate pattern. With time, the density of the opacities increased to involve the entire cortex. The nucleus ultimately opacified so that by age 35 to 40, cataract surgery was indicated. At the time of the initial examination, the vitreous cavity was optically empty except for a few dots, vertical threads, or peripheral preretinal membranes. Patchy peripapillary and posterior pole choroidal atrophy were common. Retinal arterioles were often narrowed. Vessel sheathing and accumulation of pigment along vessels were noted in several patients. Constricted visual fields were present in five patients. Retinal detachment was not reported in any of the patients.

Böhringer et. al. (Böhringer 1960) in 1960 presented the results of their investigation of 18 descendents of the "Wagner family". Ten new individuals were identified and 8 of the patients originally described by Wagner were reexamined. Ricci (Ricci 1960; Ricci 1961) reevaluated 5 patients described by Böhringer et. al. and 3 other patients originally reported by Wagner. It is noteworthy that more than 20 years after Wagner's original paper none of the patients in Wagner's pedigree had developed a retinal detachment, nor were any found with systemic abnormalities like those seen in Stickler's syndrome. On this basis alone, we think it is highly unlikely that Wagner's disease and Stickler's syndrome are the same. All the patients in our study had ocular and extraocular manifestations of Stickler's syndrome and all gave a positive family history of retinal detachment.

The question as to whether Wagner's disease and Stickler's syndrome are separate entities is made more complicated by the confusion that exists in the literature. As Herrmann et. al. (Herrmann 1975) previously noted, many clinical reports contain descriptions of patients with Stickler's syndrome, although the authors thought they were dealing with Wagner's disease (Brown 1978; Frandsen 1966; Hirose 1973; Knobloch 1972; Knobloch 1975). Other investigators (Hagler 1968; Van Balen 1970) were either unaware of Stickler's studies or thought that they were describing a new disease.

The recurring theme in all these reports includes characteristic extraocular signs of high myopia and retinal detachment. Hirose et. al. (Hirose 1973) reported that 17 of 33 eyes that developed retinal detachment could not be surgically reattached. Most authors also found a higher degree of myopia than the -4.00 D maximum seen in the "Wagner family".

Inadequate, or no mention was made of systemic findings in many reports (Alexander 1965; Brown 1978; Jansen 1962); very significant abnormalities were noted in several others. Frandsen (Frandsen 1966) observed that 4 of his patients had a peculiar physiognomy which was characterized by flat faces and a receding chin. One patient had a cleft palate. Three had severe valgus deformities of the knees. Hirose et. al. (Hirose 1973) mentioned cleft palate in four of the patients in their study. Two additional patients had the

Robin anomaly. In one family, a neonatal death occurred secondary to tongue retraction and asphyxiation. Although Knobloch (Knobloch 1975) included a thorough discussion of Stickler's syndrome, as well as references to the fact that none of the members of the "Wagner family" developed retinal detachment or had more than a moderate degree of myopia, he concluded that the patients he evaluated had Wagner's disease. This is remarkable since 15 of 32 patients had myopia of -7.00 D or greater, 21 of 40 developed a retinal detachment, 17 of 40 had some degree of cleft palate, and 24 of 40 had roentgenographic evidence of spondyloepiphyseal dysplasia.

Stickler et. al. (Stickler 1965; Stickler 1967) were not the first authors to describe the constellation of signs which constitute hereditary arthro-ophthalmopathy. Patients with similar findings were previously reported by several investigators (Alexander 1965; Delaney 1963; Friedmann 1961; Smith 1960). Individuals with "Marshall's syndrome" may also have hereditary arthro-ophthalmopathy although this is uncertain (Cohen 1974).

The ocular and systemic manifestations of Stickler's syndrome have been described by several investigators since Stickler's authoritative study (Cohen 1971; Hall 1975; Herrmann 1975; Opitz 1972; Popkin 1974; Schreiner 1973; Turner 1974; Young 1979; Nielsen 1981). A review of these studies raises several questions which the present investigation adresses. The characteristic mid-facial flattening seen in many patients with Stickler's syndrome has been repeatedly attributed to maxillary hypoplasia, although previous studies failed to utilize objective means for determining this. Photographs of only two skull films appear among the many papers in the literature (Herrmann 1975; Sprangler 1974). Lateral cephalometric radiographs and study casts of our patients showed that all had normal facial development even though clinically their faces appeared abnormally flat in profile. It is possible that some individuals do suffer from craniofacial disproportion; however, until this is demonstrated scientifically we must attribute the apparent flattening of the mid-face in patients with Stickler's syndrome to a developmental anomaly involving soft tissues, rather than to bony hypoplasia.

Smith et. al. (Smith 1960) reviewed the ocular findings of 4 individuals with the Robin anomaly who incidentally had Stickler's syndrome. The following year, in a comprehensive review of 39 patients with micrognathia, cleft palate and glossoptosis, it was determined that a majority of patients with the Robin anomaly have no other developmental abnormalities (Smith 1961). Nevertheless, many authors continue to believe that there is a close association between Stickler's syndrome and the Robin anomaly. One group has warned that as many as "one-half of patients with Pierre Robin anomaly may have Stickler's syndrome" (Herrmann 1975). Among the 16 individuals evaluated in our study, only one was found with the Robin anomaly. Other patients with this anomaly exist in our larger study; however, we feel that among the patients seen in the Cleft Palate Clinic with the Robin anomaly, only a small number have Stickler's syndrome.

A sensorineural hearing loss of greater than 20 decibels was found in only one patient. A primary neurosensory deficit may occur from alterations in the pigment epithelium of the ear which is analogous to the retinal pigment epithelium and may be similarly affected. A conductive hearing loss may also arise secondary to chronic otitis media which often develops during childhood as a result of eustachian tube dysfunction. This orofacial abnormality is frequently observed in patients with palate anomalies like those found in Stickler's syndrome. The overall incidence of hearing loss among patients with Stickler's syndrome is probably less than 10%.

Dental anomalies have previously been alluded to Herrmann 1975) and include maleruption, natal teeth, noneruption and enamel hypoplasia. We have not encountered these or any other dental anomalies, but are impressed with the large number of patients who, at a young age, already have dentures. Panoramic x-rays revealed no abnormalities within the mandibular or maxillary bones. No extraordinary dental abnormalities were found among the patients who still had teeth.

Radiologic studies of the long bones and joints in particular, revealed many more abnormalities than were anticipated clinically. Every patient, regardless of how asymptomatic, had x-ray evidence of varying degrees of spondyloepiphyseal dysplasia. Radiologists are seldom aware of the significance of these changes, and frequently fail to report them. Nevertheless, they are evident and are probably progressive.

Urinary hydroxyproline excretion levels fell within normal limits in all patients tested. The fact that previous authors (Popkin 1974) found abnormal levels of this amino acid may be due to dietary factors. All of our patients were placed on a gelatin free diet prior to evaluation. The presence of excessive amounts of this amino acid in the urine is a nonspecific finding, although it has been used as an indicator of the rate of turnover of soluble bone collagen in a variety of diseases.

Several points deserve mention with regard to the ocular examination. Myopia is highly variable. Affected siblings varied from -2.50 D to -16.50 D. Although the myopic conus and straightening of the retinal vessels correlated with the degree of myopia, there appeared to be no correlation with the amount of perivascular pigmentation, chorioretinal pigmentation and "degeneration" or with the appearance of the vitreous. Retinal detachments occurred in mildly and severely myopic individuals alike and were equally difficult to reattach. Staphyloma and other signs of degenerative myopia, such as subretinal neovascular membranes, were not seen even in severe cases. Astigmatism greater than 2 D was uncommon.

Abnormalities in the ERG were related to the severity of myopia. Patients with Stickler's syndrome and mild to moderate myopia had a normal ERG. Those with severe myopia showed a marked decrease in the amplitude of the scotopic b-wave. This relationship between the ERG and myopia has been demonstrated in other myopic populations (Prijot 1966).

Two types of cataracts were noted. The peripheral cortical lens opacities are probably congenital and stationary. The nuclear sclerotic cataract may occur in the third or fourth decade and usually progresses to maturity within two to three years. The development of cataracts is highly variable and presents surgical problems. Vitreous loss can easily occur during intracapsular cataract extraction, especially if the sclera is not supported by a metal ring. Extracapsular cataract extraction may make postoperative evaluation of the retina difficult, or impossible.

In the past, a large number of patients with Stickler's syndrome developed aphakic retinal detachments soon after surgery. The efficacy of prophylactic cryopexy and/or photocoagulation has not been proved. We have only treated symptomatic retinal tears or breaks that have developed subretinal fluid around them. Unfortunately even individuals with minimal peripheral retinal "degeneration" develop retinal detachments. We think that retinal detachment in Stickler's syndrome probably results from abnormal adhesion between the neurosensory retina and the retinal pigmented epithelium rather than from vitreous traction. It is likely that a structural anomaly exists both within "connective tissue" elements of the vitreous and the mucoproteins located between the sensory retina and the retinal pigment epithelium.

Ocular hypertension and glaucoma were relatively common, although the intraocular pressure could usually be controlled medically. In contrast to other studies (Nielsen 1981) we found no anterior chamber angle anomalies in any of our patients.

In the past few years there has been a resurgence of interest in Stickler's syndrome. Maumenee (Maumenee 1979) identified one case among a total of 39 patients with vitreoretinal degeneration and various connective tissue diseases. She provided a classification of syndromes with vitreoretinal degeneration and discussed the significance of alterations of the vitreous as a sign of connective tissue diseases. More recently, Liberfarb et. al. (Liberfarb 1979; Liberfarb 1981) evaluated a large number of patients, many of whom were previously diagnosed as having "Wagner's syndrome" (Hirose 1973) and concluded that Wagner's disease and Stickler's syndrome were the same disorder. They designated this condition, the Wagner-Stickler syndrome. For the reasons outlined above, we feel that these diseases are separate, that Wagner's syndrome affects only the eyes and that Stickler's syndrome has characteristic ocular and nonocular features which distinguish it from other diseases.

Differential diagnosis

Stickler's syndrome is one of many vitreoretinal disorders. Although it is an autosomal dominant condition with ocular and extraocular manifestations, isolated cases can be difficult to diagnose, expecially when there are few systemic abnormalities. In addition to Wagner's disease and high myopia (Table 1), several other primary ocular diseases must be ruled out.

	High Myopia	Wagner's Disease	Stickler's Syndrome
High myopia	+	-	+
Mode of inheritance	AD, AR	AD	AD
Systemic abnormalities	-	-	+
Relative frequency	common	very rare	common
Retinal detachment	+	-	+++
Early cortical lens opacities	-	+	+
Presenile nuclear sclerosis	-	+	+
Vitreoretinal degeneration			
vitreous liquefaction	+	+++	+++
preretinal membranes	-	+++	+++
lattice degeneration	+++	-	+
perivascular pigment clumps	-	+	+

Table 1. AD Autosomal Dominant AR Autosomal Recessive

Ocular diseases. Goldmann-Favré's syndrome, an autosomal recessive disorder is characterized by night blindness which occurs in childhood, an extinguished ERG, macular retinoschisis and peripheral pigmentary degeneration of the retina (Ricci 1960).

There is a striking resemblance between the perivascular pigmentation of Stickler's syndrome and the ophthalmoscopic appearance of patients with pigmentary paravenous chorioretinal degeneration (Hirose 1974); however, in the latter condition the vitreous is normal, there is minimal myopia and retinal detachments have not been described. The condition referred to as radial perivascular chorioretinal degeneration and retinal detachment (Hagler 1968) is probably an example of Stickler's syndrome. Progressive vitreoretinal degeneration, mild myopia and cataracts are all features of the autosomal dominant condition called snowflake degeneration (Hirose 1974). Discrete yellow-white spots occur in the peripheral fundus and there is absence of central or peripheral retinoschisis.

X-linked juvenile retinoschosis typically occurs in males only. The vitreous membranes are similar to those seen in Stickler's syndrome, but they are also associated with peripheral retinoschisis and characteristic macular changes.

Moderate to severe myopia, liquefaction of the vitreous and peripheral pigmentary changes in some patients with retrolental fibroplasia may resemble the ocular signs seen in Stickler's syndrome. A negative family history together with a history of prematurity and supplemental oxygen therapy help to establish the diagnosis.

Ocular and systemic diseases. Maumenee (Maumenee 1979) lists six types of vitreoretinal degeneration associated with systemic connective tissue disorders. In addition to hereditary arthro-ophthalmopathy with Marfanoid habitus (Stickler's syndrome), she includes hereditary arthro-ophthalmopathy with Weill-Marchesani-like habitus, short stature, type undetermined, Kniest syndrome, diastrophic variant and spondyloepiphyseal dysplasia congenita. Anomalies of the palate, ligaments and epiphyseal dysplasia occur in all these conditions. With the exception of Stickler's syndrome, all these patients are below normal in height and some exhibit severe skeletal deformities and "dwarfism". Aside from the fact that these patients have vitreoretinal degeneration and a connective tissue disorder they have little in common.

The ocular features of a condition described by Cotlier and Reinglass (Cotlier 1975) are distinctive enough to distinguish it from Stickler's syndrome since they include, in addition to hyaloideoretinal degeneration, coloboma of the lens and abnormalities of the anterior chamber angle.

SUMMARY

Stickler's syndrome, hereditary progressive arthro-ophthalmopathy, is an autosomal dominant disorder with marked variability in expressivity and incomplete penetrance. Clinically it can be recognized by characteristic ocular and systemic manifestations. The ocular findings include mild to severe axial myopia. Concomitantly, there is a decrease in the amplitude of the scotopic b-wave of the ERG. Cortical lenticular opacities and presenile nuclear sclerosis are common. Optically empty pockets exist within the vitreous. These pockets may be associated with dense vitreous membranes which attach especially to the peripheral fundus. Retinal vascular and chorioretinal pigmentary alterations occur in the peripheral fundus, but are highly variable and unrelated to the degree of myopia in these individuals. Retinal detachments are common and technically difficult to repair by standard scleral buckling procedures and/or in combination with vitrectomy.

Radiologically almost all patients have mild to marked evidence of epiphyseal dysplasia. Affected siblings may have Marfanoid features or appear short in stature. Although the mid-face is flattened in many individuals, lateral cephalometric x-rays fail to demonstrate any disproportion of the skull or facial bones. Anomalies of the palate including submucous cleft, cleft palate or bifid uvula are frequent. The Robin anomaly may occur together with Stickler's syndrome, but probably is not as common as previously described. Hearing loss may also exist and results from either a primary neurosensory deficit or is related to otitis media which occurs in childhood.

Stickler's syndrome differs from Wagner's disease, a very rare autosomal dominant disorder that involves exclusively the eyes, and is not associated with an increased incidence of retinal detachment.

ACKNOWLEDGEMENTS

We are indebted to Terri Fanning for her help in arranging the patient schedules and for typing the manuscript. Without the assistance of the Clinical Research Center and the help of many technicians this study would not have been possible.

REFERENCES

Alexander RL, Shea M (1965). Wagner's disease. Arch Ophthalmol 74:310-318.

Blair NP, Albert DM, Liberfarb RM, Hirose T (1979). Hereditary progressive arthro-ophthalmopathy of Stickler. Am J Ophthalmol 88:876-888.

Böhringer HR, Dieterle P, Landolt E (1960). Zur klinik und pathologie der degeneratio hyaloideo-retinalis hereditaria (Wagner). Ophthalmologica 139:330-338.

Brown GC, Tasman WS (1978). Vitrectomy and Wagner's vitreoretinal degeneration. Am J Ophthalmol 86:485-488.

Cohen MM, Knobloch WH, Gorlin RJ (1971). A dominantly inherited syndrome of hyaloideoretinal degeneration, cleft palate and maxillary hypoplasia. Birth Defects 7:83-86.

Cohen MM (1974). The demise of the Marshall syndrome. Letter to the editor. J Pediatr 85:878.

Cotlier E, Reinglass H (1975). Marfan-like syndrome with lens involvement. Hyaloideoretinal degeneration with anterior chamber angle, facial, dental, and skeletal anomalies. Arch Ophthalmol 93:93-106.

Delaney WV, Podedworny W, Havener WH (1963). Inherited retinal detachment. Arch Ophthalmol 69:44-50.

Frandsen E (1966). Hereditary hyaloideo-retinal degeneration (Wagner) in a Danish family. Acta Ophthalmologica 44:223-232.

Friedmann AI, Epstein E (1961). Familial retinal detachment. Am J Ophthalmol 51:33-35.

Hagler WS, Crosswell HH (1968). Radial perivascular chorioretinal degeneration and retinal detachment. Trans Am Acad Ophthalmol Otolaryngol 72:203-216.

Hall JG, Herrod H (1975). The Stickler syndrome presenting as a dominantly inherited cleft palate and blindness. J Med Genet 12:397-400,

Herrmann J, France TD, Spranger JW, Opitz JM, Wiffler C (1975). The Stickler syndrome (hereditary arthroophthalmopathy). Birth Defects 11:76-103.

Hirose T, Lee KY, Schepens CL (1973). Wagner's hereditary vitreoretinal degeneration and retinal detachment. Arch Ophthalmol 89:176-185.

Hirose T, Lee KY, Schepens CL (1974). Snowflake degeneration in hereditary vitreoretinal degeneration. Am J Ophthalmol 77:143-153.

Hirose T, Miyake Y (1979). Pigmentary paravenous chorioretinal degeneration: Fundus appearance and retinal functions. Ann of Ophthalmol 11:709-718.

Jansen LMAA (1962). Degeneratio hyaloideo-retinalis hereditaria. Ophthalmologica 144:458-464.

Knobloch WH, Layer JM (1972). Clefting syndromes associated with retinal detachment. Am J Ophthalmol 73:517-530.

Knobloch WH (1975). Inherited hyaloideoretinopathy and skeletal dysplasia. Trans Am Ophthalmol Soc 73:417-451.
Liberfarb RM, Hirose T, Holmes LB (1979). The Wagner-Stickler syndrome - A genetic study. Birth Defects 15(5B): 145-154.
Liberfarb RM, Hirose T, Holmes LB (1981). The Wagner-Stickler syndrome: A study of 22 families. J Pediatr 99:394-399.
Marshall D (1958). Ectodermal dysplasia. Report of kindred with ocular abnormalities and hearing defect. Am J Ophthalmol 45:143-156.
Maumenee IH (1979). Vitreoretinal degeneration as a sign of generalized connective tissue diseases. Am J Ophthalmol 88:432-449.
Nielsen CE (1981). Stickler's syndrome. Acta Ophthalmologica 59:286-295.
Opitz JM, France T, Herrmann J, Spranger JW (1972). The Stickler syndrome. Letter to the editor. N Engl J Med 286:546-547.
Popkin JS, Polomeno RC (1974). Stickler's syndrome (hereditary progressive arthro-ophthalmopathy). Can Med Assoc J 111:1071-1076.
Prijot E, Colmant I, Marechal-Courtois C (1966). Electroretinography and myopia. In Francois J (ed): "The Clinical Value of Electroretinography," Symposium in Ghent, August 1-4, 1966. Basel/New York: S. Karger, p. 440.
Ricci A (1960). Clinique et transmission génétique des différentes formes de dégénérescences vitréo-rétiniennes. Ophthalmologica 139:338-343.
Ricci A (1961). Dégénérescence hyaloidéo-rétinienne de Wagner. Bull Soc Ophtalmol Fr 9:646-662.
Schreiner RL, McAlister WH, Marshall RE, Shearer WT (1973). Stickler syndrome in a pedigree of Pierre Robin syndrome. Am J Dis Child 126:86-90.
Smith JL, Cavanaugh JA, Stowe FC (1960). Ocular manifestations of the Pierre Robin syndrome. Arch Ophthalmol 63:984-992.
Smith JL, Stowe FR (1961). The Pierre Robin syndrome (glossoptosis, micrognathia, cleft palate). A review of 39 cases with emphasis on associated ocular lesions. Pediatrics 27:128-133.
Spranger JW, Longer LO, Wiedemann HR (1974). Hereditary arthro-ophthalmopathy. In "Bone Dysplasias. An Atlas of Constitutional Disorders of Skeletal Development," Phildelphia: Saunders, p 16.

Stickler GB, Belau PG, Farrell FJ, Jones JD, Pugh DG, Steinberg AG, Ward LE (1965). Hereditary progressive arthro-ophthalmopathy. Mayo Clin Proc 40:433-447.

Stickler GB, Pugh DG (1967). Hereditary progressive arthro-ophthalmopathy II. Additional observations on vertebral abnormalities, a hearing defect, and a report of a similar case. Mayo Clin Proc 42:495-500.

Turner G (1974). The Stickler syndrome in a family with the Pierre Robin syndrome and severe myopia. Aust Paediatr J 10:103-108.

Van Balen ATM, Falger ELF (1970). Hereditary hyaloideoretinal degeneration and palatoschisis. Arch Ophthalmol 83:152-162.

Wagner H (1938). Ein bisher unbekanntes Erbleiden des Auges (degeneratio hyaloideo-retinalis hereditaria), beobachtet im Kanton Zurich. Klin Monatsbl Augenheilkd 100:840-857.

Young NJA, Hitchings RA, Sehmi K, Bird AC (1979). Stickler's syndrome and neovascular glaucoma. Br J Ophthalmol 63:826-831.

AUTOSOMAL DOMINANT IRIDOGONIODYSGENESIS
A Genetic and Clinical Study

W. G. Pearce, M.D., H. T. Wyatt, M.D.
T. A. S. Boyd, M.D., R. S. Ombres, M.D.
A. B. Salter
Dept. of Ophthalmology
The University of Alberta
Edmonton, Alberta, Canada
T6G 2G3

INTRODUCTION

During the past 50 years there has been a considerable increase in knowledge of the condition, originally described by Berg in 1932 as an autosomal dominant disorder, characterised by iris hypoplasia and juvenile glaucoma.[1-5,8-10] However, it remained to Weatherill and Hart[11] in England, who classified the angle appearance in 17 affected individuals, and Jerndal[6-7] in Sweden, who updated Berg's original pedigree to a total of 25 affected members to provide the studies upon which rests our present understanding of the disorder.

During the earlier years when interest first developed in this disorder patients were screened for evidence of systemic involvement that occurs in certain glaucoma syndromes. No evidence was found of cutaneous or skeletal manifestations of neurofibromatosis nor of the dental and maxillary malformations of Rieger Syndrome. Similarly the lenticular and skeletal abnormalities of both Marfans and Weill-Marchesani syndromes were absent.

MATERIAL

Family A (Fig. 1) were originally from the Maritime region of Canada and have been followed in the Glaucoma Unit of the University of Alberta for twenty years. Family B (Fig. 2), only recently came under our care having immigrated from South Wales in the United Kingdom.

Birth Defects: Original Article Series, Volume 18, Number 6, pages 561–569

AUTOSOMAL DOMINANT IRIDOGONIODYSGENESIS

Fig 1

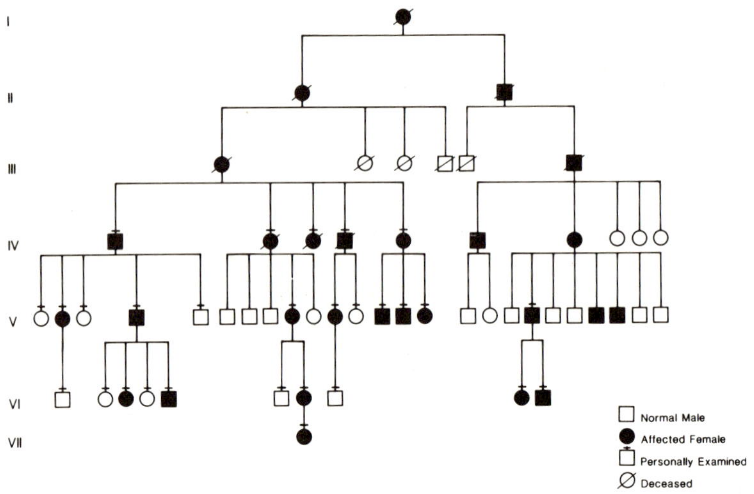

AUTOSOMAL DOMINANT IRIDOGONIODYSGENESIS

Fig 2

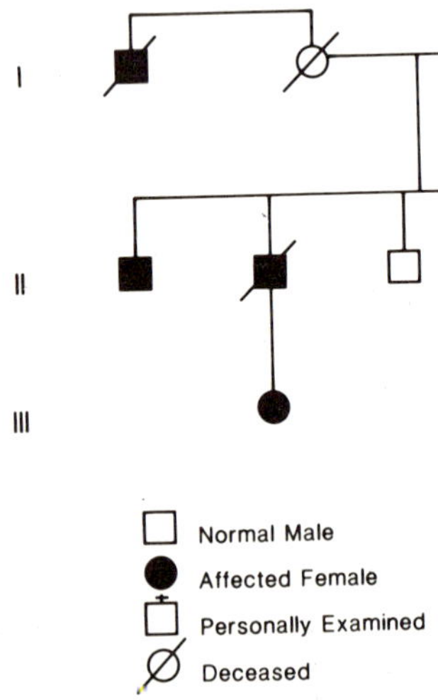

Individuals not personally examined, but indicated as affected on the pedigree, have been described by other members of the family as having the unusual appearing irides and associated glaucoma.

GENETIC FEATURES

Personal examination confirmed the transmission of this disorder through several generations in Family A with 19 affected individuals and in Family B with 3 affected individuals. In Family A, the genetic mechanism of inheritance through personally examined parents (9), all of whose children (21) have been examined, clearly supported the criteria of regular autosomal dominant inheritance. This included:

1) Affected children (12) always found to have an affected parent (9).

2) Number of affected children (12) not significantly different from number of unaffected children (9).

3) Number of affected males (7) not significantly different from number of affected females (5).

4) Transmission through three or more (4) generations.

Although not indicated on the pedigree, several children, the offspring of unaffected siblings of affected patients, have been examined and in no case were exceptions found to criteria, 1-ie, affected children whose parents were unaffected.

CLINICAL FEATURES

I Abnormal Angle Differentiation

In general, the appearance of the angle on gonioscopy was similar to that described by Weatherill and Hart[11]

i) More severly abnormal angles showed thickened, yellow, "woolly", excess tissue occupying the site of the trabecular meshwork (10 pts.). On rotating the gonioscope through 360 degrees, the amount of this tissue present was variable.

ii) Less severely abnormal angles showed the iris to be inserted anteriorly into the region of the trabecular meshwork without excess tissue present (9 pts.).

Additional features of the angle included:

iii) A grey membrane overlying the iris root. Strands of this membrane passed both anteriorly over the iris meshwork and centrally over the surface of the iris where it became thinner and broken up towards the pupil.

iv) Anomalous angle vascularity. This consisted of circumferential angle vessel(s) lying on the surface of or within the trabecular tissue. From this vessel branches passed centrally on the grey membrane towards the pupil.

II Iris Stroma Hypoplasia

Marked attenuation of the iris stroma was regularly noted. This permitted direct observation of the sphincter pupillae and iris pigment epithelium. The normal iris crypts and collarette were absent. Fine vessels, encased in strands from the grey membrane were consistently present running toward the pupil margin. The remaining strands of iris stroma appeared either blue-grey or brown depending on the amount of melanin present in the stroma.

III Elevated Intra-Ocular Pressure

The intra-ocular pressure as measured by applanation tonometry was usually found to be greater than 21 mm Hg. (vide Infra).

MANAGEMENT OF PRESSURE REGULATION DEFECT

Elevated intra-ocular pressures were usually detected at a young age and were characterized as much by lability as by sustained high pressures. Figure 3 shows the pressure ranges

Fig 3

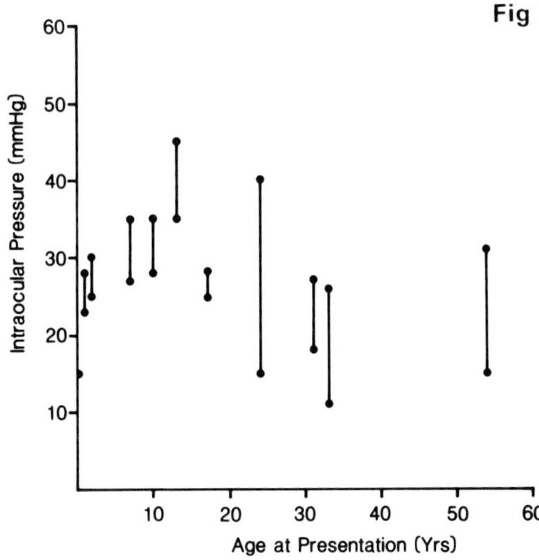

detected in one eye during the early examinations for 10 members. Each range represents at least two and sometimes multiple diurnal measurements.

There was a poor response of pressure to medical treatment in these patients. Table 1 indicates the mean pressure of six subjects without treatment and with maximal treatment. Little difference was found between the two treatment modes. Even with the use of Diamox and Timoptic, the response was poor.

Table 1

Response to Medical R_x for 6 Subjects

Mean of:	No. R_x	Max. R_x
Subject means	26 mm Hg	24 mm Hg
Subject SD's	4.3	4.7

As the intra-ocular pressure was often alarmingly high and responded only poorly to medical treatment, early surgery was frequently recommended. Since the pressure problem appeared to be based on a recognizable angle deformity, goniotomy was the perferred procedure - Table 2. This operation resulted in failure to control the pressure in 15 of the 17 occasions it was performed. Complications occurred in 12 cases.

Table 2

Surgical Procedures and Results

	Goniotomy	Scheie	Cleisis
Eyes	8	6	8
Operations	17	6	8
Pressure Control			
Satisfactory	2	6	8
Fail	15	0	0
Complications	12	6	1

Eight operations were followed by hyphema, and in one case a blackball hyphema led to loss of the eye. Four operations were complicated by loss of the anterior chamber or had other anterior chamber problems.

Scheie's procedure of thermosclerotomy was performed on six eyes. In terms of pressure control, this was successful but complications were serious. Three procedures had significant hyphema and three developed flat anterior chambers. Finally, iridencleisis was performed on 8 eyes achieving excellent pressure control in 6 and partial control in 2 cases. Suprisingly this procedure was essentially free from complications.

Since surgery may be complicated and may fail, and since medical treatment is usually ineffective in lowering pressure, how long should a conservative approach be tried? Of 15 patients with raised pressures, only 2 showed disc damage at the time of presentation and they were 45 and 51 years old (Family A, IV:2 and IV:5). It would appear therefore that the optic nerve heads are resistant to damage even into middle age, and that inspite of poor response to medical treatment, there should be no hurry towards a surgical solution. Close monitoring of pressures, the optic nerve heads and visual fields are indicated throughout life and surgery is resorted to only if evidence of disc damage appears.

GENETIC VARIATION

The cardinal features of abnormal trabecular tissue, iris stroma hypoplasia and elevated intraocular pressure, were present in the majority of the cases. Some variation towards normal was noted in a few instances. (Table 3)

Table 3

Genetic Variation in 22 Patients

	Abnormal	Normal
Gonioscopy	19	3
Iris Hypoplasia	21	1
IOP > 21 mm Hg	19	3

I Gonioscopy

In three instances (Family A, V:1, V:15, VII:1) the angle structures were acceptable as being within normal variation, ie, had the patients not been members of this family, they could not have been identified on gonioscopy alone as being affected. It should be added that in several cases the appearance of the trabecular region while definitely abnormal on careful assessment was not grossly dysplastic. In these instances, where subtle changes predominated, a cursory examination could well have overlooked the findings. All three of the above patients showed iris stroma hypoplasia and ocular hypertension.

II Iris Stroma Hypoplasia

One patient (Family A, IV:4 was recorded as showing no iris hypoplasia when seen in 1963. The patient died in 1968. Abnormal trabecular structures were noted to be present but intra-ocular pressures were normal.

III Elevated Intra-Ocular Pressure

Three patients (Family A, IV:4, V:11, and Family B, III:7) had normal intra-ocular pressures (21 mm Hg. or less). Abnormal trabecular tissue was present in all three but one did not show the characteristic iris hypoplasia (Family 2, IV:4).

When combined with data of Weatherill and Hart[11] and Jerndal[6] the presence of a normal intra-ocular pressure was the most frequently encountered variation (Table 4). It has been termed incomplete glaucoma by Jerndal.[6] This feature has been more commonly noted in the younger affected members[11] and it seems likely that pressure elevation will develop at a later date in at least some of the cases.

Table 4

Genetic Variation in Affected Patients - Combined Data

	Abnormal	Normal	Total
Gonioscopy	68	3	71
Iris Hypoplasia	72	5	77
IOP < 21 mm Hg	64	11	75

* Pooled figures of Weatherill and Hart, Jerndal, and Pearce et al.

What is interpreted as normal iris stroma and normal trabecular region on gonioscopy has been less frequently reported. It could be expected that the expression of the abnormal gene in some individuals may be modified by various factors such as the normal allele. This might well result in such a minimal variation from normal that the iris stroma or trabecular appearance would be acceptable as being within a normal range of variation and would not be identified as definite evidence of the abnormal gene. In no cases, however, were both the iris stroma and trabecular region described as normal in the same patient. Despite the occasional findings of an iris stroma and trabecular region, not dissimilar from normal variation, the disorder exhibits a remarkable pattern of symmetrical involvement of the two eyes and a degree of structural changes that has been shown to be consistent over multiple generations in many different families originating from widely dispersed countries.

KEY WORDS: Heredity - Autosomal Dominant, Iridogoniodysgenesis, Juvenile Glaucoma

REFERENCES

1. Allen L, Ackermann WG (1942). Hereditary glaucoma in a pedigree of three generations. Arch Ophthal 27:139.
2. Berg F (1932). Erbliches jugendliches glaukom. Acta Ophthal (Kbh) 10:568.
3. Courtney RH, Hill E (1931). Hereditary juvenile glaucoma. J Amer Med Assoc 47:1602.
4. François J, Deweer JP, Van den Burge J (1950). Glaucome chronique simple à hérédité dominant. Bull Soc belge Ophtal 96:665.
5. Hambresin L, Schepens CL (1946). Glaucome familial. Bull Soc franç Ophtal 59:219.
6. Jerndal J (1970). Goniodysgenesis and hereditary juvenile glaucoma. Acta Ophthal (Supp) 107.
7. Jerndal J (1972). Dominant goniodysgenesis with late congenital glaucoma. Amer J Ophthal 74:28.
8. Martin JP, Zorab EC (1974). Familial glaucoma. Brit J Ophthal 58:536.
9. McCulloch C, MacRae D (1950). Hereditary juvenile glaucoma. Trans Canad Ophthal Soc 79.
10. Stokes WH (1940). Hereditary primary glaucoma. Arch Ophthal 24:885.
11. Weatherill JR, Hart CT (1969). Familial hypoplasia of the iris stroma associated with glaucoma. Brit J Ophthal 53:433.

RADIAL APLASIA, CHROMOSOMAL ABERRATION, AND ANTERIOR CHAMBER CLEAVAGE MANIFESTATIONS IN TWO SIBLINGS

D. BenEzra, H. Abulafia, G. Maftzir, S. Yatziv, J. Paez and A. Zelikovitch
Departments of Ophthalmology and Pediatrics, Hadassah University Hospital
Jerusalem, Israel

SUMMARY

Two siblings of a Christian Lebanese family are described suffering from varying degrees of bony hypoplasia-aplasia; microphthalmia, with manifestations of the anterior chamber cleavage syndrome; and unusual sister chromatid disjunction at the centromeric region during prophase and metaphase. The unrelated parents as well as a third sibling were phenotypically normal. Because of the unique combination of clinical signs in these two siblings, we suggest the name: Hypomelia, Microphthalmos and Sister Chromatid Disjunction Syndrome.

INTRODUCTION

Limb malformations accompanied by craniofacial abnormalities have been described under various eponyms: pseudothalidomide or SC-phocomelia syndrome (Assemany et al, 1971; Herrman and Opitz, 1977), Roberts syndrome (Roberts, 1919; Freeman et al, 1974) or hypomelia-hypotrichosis-facial hemangioma syndrome (Hall and Greenberg, 1972). We describe herein two brothers of a family with three sons that presented an unusual and previously undescribed complex of phenomena.

CASE REPORTS

Birth Defects: Original Article Series, Volume 18, Number 6, pages 571–575

Family background

Case 1: S.H., an alert and intelligent five-year-old boy at the time of initial examination, is shown in Figure 1. His weight, length and head circumference were below the third percentile. However, well balanced physical proportions resulted in an acceptable appearance. External examination of the face revealed a moderate micrognatia and aplasia of the alae nasi. X-ray of the skeleton disclosed the following findings: absence of radius and a gross shortening of the ulna in both upper limbs and a relative short-

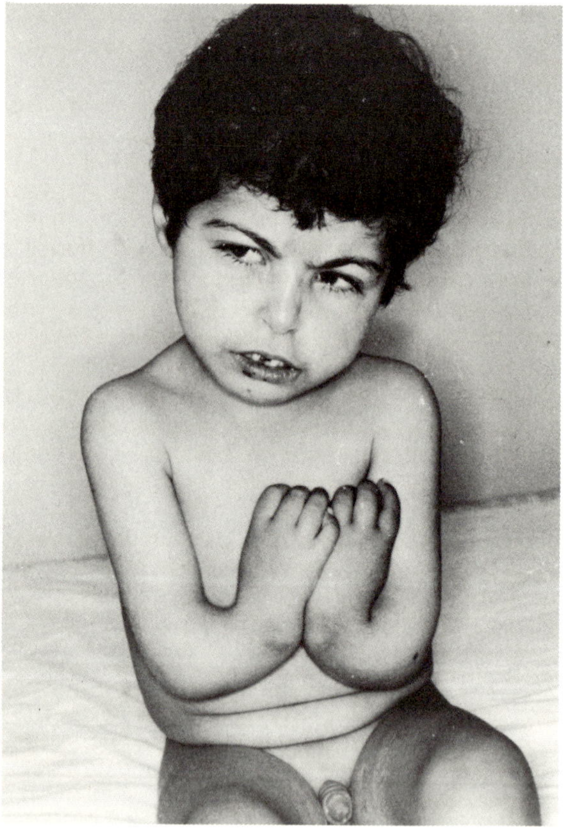

Figure 1. Five year-old male sibling of Lebanese family

ening of the tibia and fibula with a delayed maturation of the cuboid bones in the lower limbs. Ophthalmic examination revealed a bilateral microphthalmia with leukoma cornea centralis, a pendular nystagmus and a strabismus and head posture compatible with a paresis of the right superiod oblique muscle. The corneal periphery was clear and an accentuated Schwalbe line with a moderate posterior embryotoxon could be visualized. The lens, vitreous and fundus appeared normal. Chromosomal studies performed on peripheral blood lymphocytes disclosed a normal karyotype of 46 XY chromosomes along with an unusual repulsive phenomenon between the two sister chromatids at the centromenic region during prophase and metaphase.

Case 2: S.M., the third born, a four-week-old baby on initial examination, is shown in Figure 2. His weight, head circumference and length were below the third percentile. There was an extensive facial hemangioma, a total cleft palate, a slight aplasia of the alae nasi and micrognatia. X-ray of the skeleton disclosed in the upper limbs the following: marked shortening of the humerus, a total aplasia of both the radius and ulna, four metacarpal bones and ectrodactyly of the thumb. In the lower limbs, there was a deformity and hypoplasia of the tibial bone, a complete absence of the fibula and a maldevelopment of the tarsal and metatarsal bones. Ophthalmic examination revealed a bilateral microphthalmia with leukoma and thinning of the central cornea and vascularization of the periphery. Internal ocular structures could not be observed; however, ultrasound disclosed that the lens was adherent to the cornea, a feature compatible with the diagnosis of Peter's anomaly. Chromosomal studies revealed a similar pattern as observed in his older sibling.

DISCUSSION

We have presented two siblings who suffer most probably from an autosomal recessive gene abnormality although, from this family data, a possible recessive X-linked pattern of transmission cannot be ruled out.

The expressivity of the gene abnormality encompasses many organs and systems. However, three phenomena are the most consistent and striking features of this gene expression: the skeletal manifestations that varied markedly between the

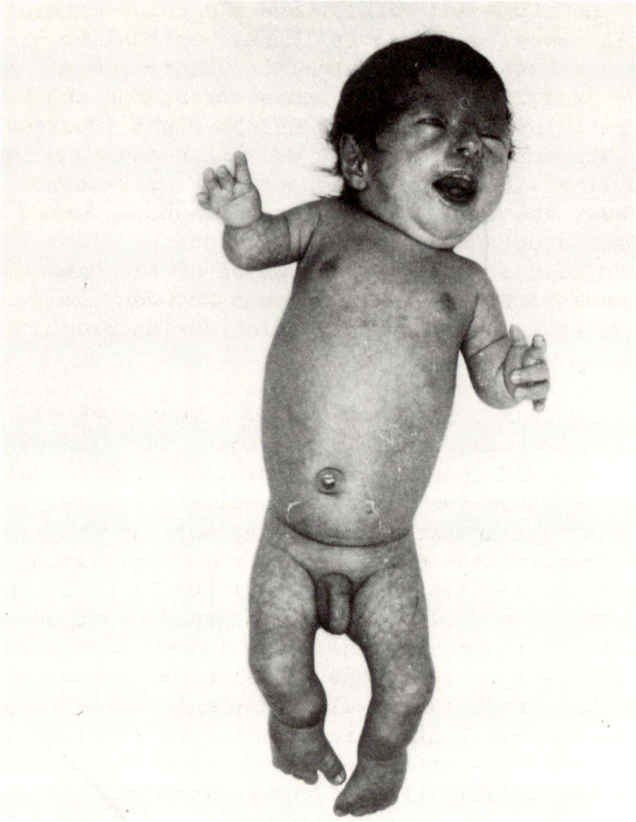

Figure 2. Four week-old male sibling of Lebanese family

two siblings; the constant microphthalmia with various manifestations of the anterior chamber cleavage syndrome; and the constant sister chromatic disjunction phenomenon observed during prophase and metaphase. As such a complex of phenomena has not been described previously, we suggest the eponym of: Hypomelia, Microphthalmos and Sister Chromatid Disjunction Syndrome.

REFERENCES

Assemany SR, Kajii T and Gardner LI (1971). Syndrome of

phocomelia with mandibular hypoplasia. Helv Paediat Acta 26:403

Herrman J and Opitz JM (1977). The SC-phocomelia and the Roberts syndrome: Nosologic aspects. Europ J Pediat 125: 117

Roberts JB (1919). A child with double cleft of lip and palate, protrusion of the intermaxillary portion of the upper jaw and imperfect development of the bones of the four extremities. Ann Surg 70:252

Freeman MVR, Williams DW, Schimke RN and Temtamy SA (1974). The Roberts syndrome. Clin Genetics 5:1

Hall BD and Greenberg MH (1972). Hypomelia-hypotrichosis-facial hemangioma syndrome. Ann J Dis Child 123:602

HEREDITARY SNOWFLAKE VITREORETINAL DEGENERATION

M. GHEILER MD, A. POLLACK MD, D. UCHENIK MD,
V. GODEL MD,* and M. OLIVER MD.
Department of Ophthalmology, Kaplan Hospital,
Rehovot and *Department of Ophthalmology,
Ichilov Hospital, Tel Aviv, Israel.

Snowflake vitreoretinal degeneration was first described as a familial disease by Hirose et al. (1974). The disease is characterized by progressive retinal changes, including a peripheral area of extensive white-with-pressure interspersed with small yellow-white spots like snowflakes, sheathing of retinal vessels and increased pigmentation. A swirling fibrillar vitreous degeneration, equally progressive in nature, accompanies these fundal changes. A high incidence of retinal detachment with poor surgical results was also reported. As far as we are aware, no further family reports have appeared in the literature. In this report of a family with snowflake degeneration, we emphasize the clinical characteristics and the phenotypic variability of this entity.

FAMILY DATA

A Jewish family (Figure) of Algerian origin came to our attention when the proband, a 34-year-old male (II-6) was referred to us for a cataract extraction. We subsequently examined thirty-six members of the family spanning three generations, and a total of 15 affected members were identified.

The first generation comprised seven brothers, offspring of nonconsanguinous parents. Of these the proband's father (I-5) and another sib (I-1) were deceased, and we were informed that both of them, as well as a third sib (I-4), had been blind from a young age. Another sib (I-3) was also blind following unsuccessful operation for retinal detachment.

Birth Defects: Original Article Series, Volume 18, Number 6, pages 577–580

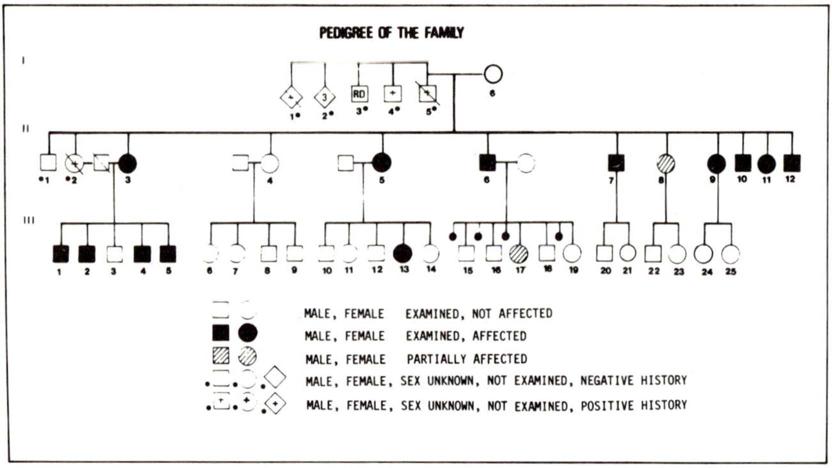

The second generation comprised twelve family members, of whom nine presented with ocular findings characteristic of this type of vitreoretinal degeneration. Three were myopic (II-3, II-6, II-7) and two (II-3, II-6) had cataracts which required extraction at ages 39 years and 34 years respectively. All the affected members had vitreous anomalies, including fibrillar degeneration, gel liquefaction and marked thickening of the cortical vitreous. In one of them (II-5) an optically empty vitreous cavity was found. Eight of the affected members had retinal changes that varied from areas of white-with-pressure interspersed with very small yellow-white dots like snowflakes to sheathing of vessels and accumulation of retinal pigment. An unusual observation was a vascular abnormality located in the upper temporal periphery of the retina of four patients (II-3, II-5, II-6, II-7). Neovascular tufts were seen adjacent to areas with snowflake degeneration and vascular sheathing. In five cases (II-3, II-5, II-6, II-7, II-9) retinal holes were found. In two patients (II-3, II-6) rhegmatogenous retinal detachment developed, with poor surgical results. One case (II-8) presented with only vitreous anomalies without any retinal involvement.

In the third generation, there were six affected patients (III-1, III-2, III-4, III-5, III-13, III-17). Their average age was lower than that of the second generation patients, and they presented with milder findings. Two (III-2, III-4) were myopic and two (III-2, III-4) had small opacities of the lens. All six affected members showed vitreous changes such as fine swirling strands and some degree of thickening of the posterior cortical vitreous. One patient (III-2) showed an optically empty vitreous cavity. Five patients had retinal abnormalities that included peripheral areas of white-with-pressure and snowflake degeneration.

Of the six patients examined electrophysiologically, two (II-3, II-6) had impaired electroretinograms, in which after full dark adaptation the amplitude of both negative and positive waves reached about half of the value of the normal response.

COMMENT

The range of ocular findings in this family resembles that seen in snowflake vitreoretinal degeneration as described by Hirose et al. (1974) (1). Two additional findings were seen in our patients. The first was an optically empty vitreous cavity, which appeared in two patients (II-5, III-2). The second finding was abnormal retinal vessels, most probably of neovascular origin, located in the temporal retinal periphery adjacent to the vascular sheathing. This was observed in four patients (II-3, II-5, II-6, II-7).

Affected members were found in all three generations studied. The disease was transmitted only by affected parents; normal parents had normal offspring. Both sexes were affected, and there were no cases of consanguinity among the parents. All these findings point to a very high and almost certain probability of an autosomal dominant type of inheritance. The variability of expression in the family, with some members being affected severely and others only mildly, and with some having both vitreal and retinal involvement and others having only vitreal abnormality, offers additional support for the assumption of dominant transmission.

Although snowflake vitreoretinal degeneration has a characteristic appearance, clinically it poses a diagnostic problem because of its similarity to and overlap with other well-known types of vitreoretinal degeneration. Hirose et al. (1974) differentiated between snowflake degeneration and other vitreoretinal disorders on the basis of the retinal findings and/or the inheritance pattern. Of greater importance is the distinction between this disorder and Wagner's disease. In the early stage of Wagner's disease the pathological process begins in the deep retinal layers and the choroid, with atrophy of the choriocapillaris and pigment epithelium. In snowflake degeneration, on the other hand, the earliest change occurs in the superficial retinal layers and the cortical vitreous. In addition, most of the affected members in our study did not show the membranous degeneration of the vitreous typical of Wagner's disease, but exhibited fibrillar degeneration of the vitreous which was described by Hirose et al. as a sign of snowflake degeneration.

SUMMARY

Hereditary snowflake vitreoretinal degeneration is described in members of three generations of a family. Abnormal retinal findings included: extensive areas of white-with-pressure, snowflake degeneration, pigmentation and sheathing of vessels. Fibrillar vitreous degeneration accompanied these changes. A finding not previously described was the presence of abnormal retinal vessels with a peculiar neovascular pattern. The findings point to a pattern of autosomal dominant inheritance.

REFERENCES

Hirose T, Lee KY, Schepens CL (1974). Snowflake degeneration in hereditary vitreoretinal degeneration. Am J Ophthalmol 77:143.

Hirose T, Lee KY, Schepens CL (1973). Wagner's hereditary vitreoretinal degeneration and retinal detachment. Arch Ophthalmol 89:176.

VITREORETINAL DEGENERATION IN FACIAL CLEFTING SYNDROME

V.Godel MD PhD, L.Regenbogen MD,
V.Feiler-Ofry MD, M.Lazar MD.
Departments of Ophthalmology, Ichilov
Hospital and Sheba Medical Center,
Tel Aviv University Medical School.

Since vitreoretinal degeneration was reported as an ocular sign in connective tissue diseases, several authors have reaffirmed this relationship, with facial clefts being the most frequent associated anomaly (Frandsen 1966; Cohen et al 1971; Knobloch & Layer 1972). The description of a broad spectrum of associated systemic defects made some authors split this disorder complex into several syndromes. However, more recent tendency has been to accept what seemed to be clinically distinct pictures as the same pathological entity (Hall & Herrod 1975; Blair et al 1979).

In the present report 3 families with vitreoretinal degeneration and facial clefting are described (Fig 1) delineating the phenotypic spectrum of this complex disorder.

CASE REPORTS

Case 1 (III-1,Family 1). This 16 year-old boy was found to have a mild myopia, vitreous syneresis with fibrillar condensations and veil-like vitreous membranes attached to the retina. The retina itself presented small, irregularly shaped pigmentary changes located perivascularly, without any underlying choroidal atrophy. Similar ocular findings were found in the proband's father (II-1).

Birth Defects: Original Article Series, Volume 18, Number 6, pages 581–586

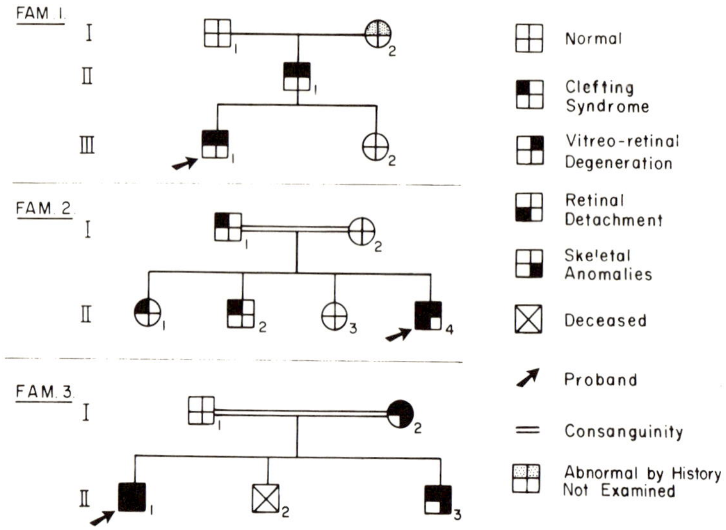

Fig 1. Family pedigrees.

Both the proband and his father presented rudimentary remaining defects of corrected cleft lips and noses. The proband's grandmother (I-2), was not examined by us, but we were informed that she was myopic and had had surgically corrected facial clefts. Although general physical examination disclosed normal findings, both the proband and his father presented mild generalized epiphyseal dysplasia at radiography.

Case 2 (II-4,Family 2). This 5 year-old boy was admitted urgently with a history of visual loss in his only good eye. His medical history revealed a surgical correction for midfacial defects. The ocular examination revealed a bullous rhegmatogenous retinal detachment in his right myopic eye. Multiple retinal tears and holes were present in the detached retina. Translucent strands and vitreal liquefaction gave the impression of an optically empty vitreous cavity. In the left fundus a proliferative whitish fibrous tissue emanating from the optic disc toward the temporal periphery was found and interpreted as retinal dysplasia.

Surgical repair had been attempted, but despite several operations the child became inoperably blind. Significant findings of maxillary hypoplasia with the nasal defect and hypertelorism gave him a characteristic physiognomy of a flattened midface. The father of the proband and two other sibs were found to present facial clefts and vitreoretinal anomalies.

Case 3 (II-1,Family 3). This 26 year-old male was hospitalized following a right retinal detachment. His eye examination revealed a high myopia, an optically empty vitreous cavity and total retinal detachment in the right eye. Five retinal breaks were diagnosed located both nasally and temporally in this eye. The left eye had a visual acuity of 20/40 with -10.0 D. Posterior cortical cataracts were present in both eyes. The fundus of the left eye also presented an optically empty posterior vitreous cavity with a few preretinal membranes. Lattice degenerations were found at the equatorial level.

Three circling buckling operations were done in the right eye to obtain successful anatomic reattachment. In the left eye a big tear in the upper nasal quadrant was photocoagulated during the follow up, but despite this treatment the patient later developed a left temporal retinal detachment caused by two new tears. Retinal reattachment of this eye was obtained only after 4 consecutive surgical procedures.

From his medical history it appeared that the patient had had a surgical correction of complete cleft palate and cleft lip in infancy. A maxillary hypoplasia caused a flattened midface. Physical examination disclosed thoracic kyphosis, bilateral pes planus and adductus and calcanea valgus. The finger, wrist and ankle joints were hyperextensible. A lumbar hyperlordosis, a flattened L-5 vertebra, bilateral triangular navicular bones, medial deviation of the tarsal bones of the left foot and a broad pelvic bone with feminine form were found at radiologic examinations. An audiologic examination showed a high frequency sensorineural hearing defect with increased compliance of the middle ear. The mother (I-2) and a brother (II-3) presented various similar anomalies.

DISCUSSION

Our patients presented a broad spectrum of ocular, facial and skeletal anomalies. The vitreoretinal changes were most conspicuous consisting of an apparently optically empty vitreous cavity with fibrillar condensations and membrane formation. The retinal findings varied from peculiar perivascular retinal pigmentations to retinal breaks and detachments of recurring type. The variability of the associated anomalies confined to the face and skeleton invalidated the concept of a homogemous group of signs characterizing this anomaly.

Circumstantial evidence from familial cases suggests that this anomaly complex is causally and pathogenetically related through a concomitant developmental deviation of genic origin. The diversity of organ involvement encountered in our cases suggest that this developmental defect exerts its effect by its action within groups of developing areas and causes anomalies within these groups. Since not every patient developed retinal detachment, it is possible that what is inherited is a tendency to vitreoretinal maldevelopment which predisposes to retinal breaks rather than retinal detachment itself.

The most likely mode of inheritance in all of our families would seem to be autosomal dominant. The pedigrees showed affected members in successive generations. The marriages fall into the category of an affected person marrying a normal one. The existence of male-to-male transmission and the remarkable variability in gene expression were also characteristic of a dominantly inherited trait. The consanguineous marriages in two of these families did not seem to influence the appearance of homozygosity.

We have, as yet, no simple way of deciding whether the allele or even the locus involved in our pedigrees are the same. The possibility that we are dealing with separate mutations involving type II collage chains, which are long and have multiple sites at which mutations can occur, must be taken into consideration (Maumenee 1979).

The radiologic evidence of mild generalized epiphyseal dysplasia in our first family support previous views that patients with vitreoretinal degeneration of Wagner's type present systemic involvements like in Stickler syndrome, when closely examined (Knobloch 1976).

We think that all these findings of similar clinical manifestations and identical pattern of inheritance, adds to the arguments that all the various types of vitreoretinal degenerations are closely related entities.

SUMMARY

Three families with vitreoretinal degeneration and median cleft face syndrome are described. Associated findings of skeletal anomalies, hearing loss and peculiar physiognomy are reported. Pedigree analyses suggest autosomal dominant inheritance. In view of the similarity between these patients and the clinical overlap existing between themit is assumed that they are all a closely related disease spectrum.

REFERENCES

Blair NP, Albert DM, Lieberfarb RM, Hirose T (1979). Hereditary progressive arthro-ophthalmopathy of Stickler. Am J Ophth 88:876.

Cohen MM, Knobloch WH, Gorlin RJ(1971). A dominantly inherited syndrome of hyaloideo-retinal degeneration, cleft palate and maxillary hypoplasia (Cervenka syndrome).Birth Def 7:83.

Frandsen E(1966). Hereditary hyaloideo-retinal degeneration (Wagner) in a Danish family. Acta Ophth 44:223.

Hall JG, Herrod H(1975). The Stickler syndrome presenting as a dominantly inherited cleft palate and blindness. J Med Gen 12:397.

Knobloch WH, Layer JM(1972). Clefting syndromes associated with retinal detachment. Am J Ophth 73:517.

Knobloch WH(1976). Inherited hyaloideoretinopathy and skeletal dysplasia. Tr Am Ophth Soc 73:413.

Maumenee IH(1979). Vitreoretinal degeneration as a sign of generalized connective tissue diseases. Am J Ophth 88:432.

Reprint requests: Victor Godel MD,PhD, Department of Ophthalmology, Ichilov Hospital, Tel Aviv 64239, Israel.

THE HETEROZYGOTE FEMALE IN X-LINKED RECESSIVE PRIMARY RETINAL DYSPLASIA

VICTOR GODEL MD PhD, RICHARD M. GOODMAN MD

Departments of Ophthalmology, Ichilov Hospital, Genetics, Sheba Medical Center, Tel Aviv University Medical School.

The term retinal dysplasia applies to any abnormal differentiation of the retina and proliferation of one or more of its elements, either neural cells to form rosettes and folds, or the glial cells to produce gliosis. Ophthalmoscopically it varies from congenital retinal folds to highly disorganized tumor-like protrusions in the vitreous cavity. This disorder appears as mainly congenital but may be also due to external insults. A genetic basis as one possible etiology of retinal dysplasia has been suggested and autosomal recessive (Warburg 1974) or sex-linked recessive (Weve 1938) mechanisms were incriminated.

In this paper we wish to report on 3 families with primary retinal dysplasia presumably transmitted as X-linked recessive traits, paying particular attention to the individual presentation of the carrier mothers.

CASE REPORTS

Family 1 (Fig 1). This family was investigated after it was discovered that 5 male cousins had severe visual impairment, head posture, nystagmus and strabismus. They were offspring of 5 sisters descending from a consanguineous mating (first cousins). Their ophthalmoscopic findings varied in shape and extension, ranging from retinal

Birth Defects: Original Article Series, Volume 18, Number 6, pages 587–591

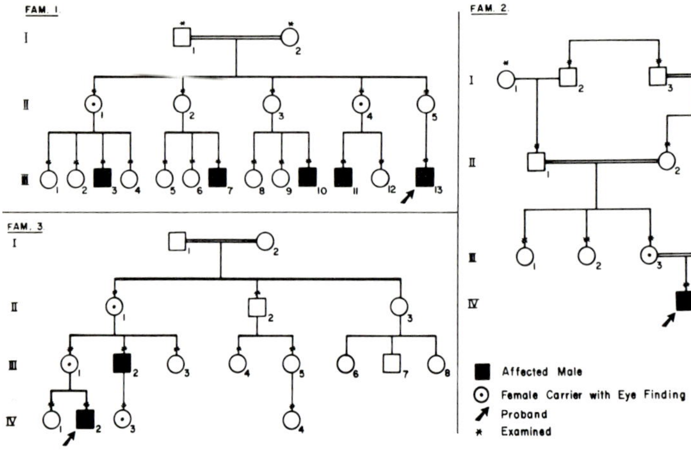

Fig 1. Family pedigrees

folds to dysplastic tissue covering the posterior pole or gliosis with tumor-like protrusion in the vitreous. Of the five mothers, who were presumed heterozygous carriers, two showed retinal changes. A paramacular small retinal fold-like structure in one and a dysplastic tissue in the upper temporal periphery in the other, were found. Both these mothers had gray bluish colored irides with attenuation of the iris stroma, a finding which was at variance with the dark pigmented irides of the other family members. As the pedigree study indicated X-linked recessive transmission, linkage studies were performed but both the Xg blood group and G6PD showed no measurable linkages.

Family 2 (Fig 1). This family was ascertained through a 2 year-old male child with serious visual impairment. The family study revealed the following consanguinity in the kindred: the father of the boy was the uncle of the mother and both parents of the child were offspring of marriages between first cousins. The ophthalmoscopic examination of the proband showed a vascularized retinal fold in the right eye and a pseudoglioma in the left. In the right fundus of the mother a veil-like retinal fold was found.

Family 3 (Fig 1). In this family the proband a 1-year-old boy presented a typical congenital retinal fold in his left eye and a retrolental whitish mass in the right. Family study revealed a 36 year old maternal uncle having a unilateral tumor-like protrusion in a microphthalmic left eye. Another striking feature found in this family was the bright gray colored irides of the mother of the proband, his maternal grandmother and a cousin. Apart from the distinctive color (the other family members had dark brown pigmented irides), the irides lacked the usual stromal pattern all over.

DISCUSSION

The male children in our families exhibited similar diseases of the retina, familial in nature. Clinically the disorder presented itself in a surprisingly wide range of severity or degree from simple congenital retinal folds to central stalks with retinal tissue extending from the optic disc or whitish retrolental masses protruding in the vitreous cavity.

The pedigree analysis offered strong evidence of the possibility of an abnormality affecting the X-chromosome recessively. Three of the obligatory heterozygous females, belonging to 2 families exhibited mild retinal fold changes (Table 1), adding credence to the X-linked recessive nature of this disorder. The hemizygous males showed full expression of the disease and the heterozygous females being mosaic for the X-chromosome, have only minimal features of the disease.

Table 1. Ocular findings in female carriers for X-linked recessive retinal dysplasia.

Carriers	Age yrs.	Gray iris	Retinal fold
Family 1			
II-1	32	+	+
II-4	29	+	+
Family 2			
III-3	21	-	+
Family 3			
II-1	53	+	-
III-1	30	+	-
IV-3	7	+	-

The finding of gray or grayish-blue irides in 5 presumed female carriers representing 2 of the 3 families was unusual (Table 1). All the other family members had brown or dark irides. No pigmentary changes of any nature were noted in these presumed female carriers. Since iris color is normally determined by the intensity of pigment deposition in the iris stroma and not by its structure, it is postulated that the gray color of the irides in these females is due not to direct alteration in pigmentation, but rather a dysplasia of the stroma of the irides with an inability to properly bind the pigment. Evidence for such a hypothesis is based on the hypoplastic stromal pattern with altered textural appearance lacking the normal surface markings. As these iris changes appeared in the heterozygous females of primary retinal dysplasia but not in the affected males, it is difficult to support with certainty that these findings are typical manifestations of the carrier state for this disorder. However, it is conceivable that there is genetic heterogeneity in this condition, and that in some genetic forms of retinal dysplasia the pathology extends beyond the retina to involve the iris. It is hoped that an awareness of this particular iris finding by ophthalmologist will stimulate further observation in an attempt to determine whether such ocular findings may represent a specific component of the X-linked primary retinal dysplasia.

SUMMARY

Three families with primary retinal dysplasia are reported. The ophthalmoscopical findings vary from congenital retinal folds to highly disorganized tumor-like protrusions in the vitreous cavity. The family pedigrees along with the clinical features support an X-linked recessive mode of transmission for this condition. Female carriers for this gene may show retinal fold changes. In addition some of these presumed female carriers also demonstrated changes in the stroma of their irides resulting in a gray to grayish-blue color.

REFERENCES

Warburg M (1974) Norrie's disease and falciform detachment of the retina. In: Genetic and Metabolic Eye Disease, ed. Goldberg. Boston, Little, Brown and Co, pp 441.

Weve HJM (1938) Ablatio falciformis congenita (retinal fold). Brit J Ophth 22:456.

Keywords: Heterozygote carrier, Primary retinal dysplasia, Pseudoglioma, Retinal fold, X-linked recessive inheritance.

Reprint requests: Victor Godel MD PhD, Department of Ophthalmology, Ichilov Hospital, Tel Aviv 64239, Israel.

Syndromes Involving the Eye and Epidemiology of Blindness

FRANCOIS' DYSCEPHALIC SYNDROME

Jules Francois

Ophthalmological Clinic of the University of Ghent
Ghent, Belgium

Hallerman (1948) and Streiff (1950) described a patient with a bird's head and congenital cataract, but did not mention the associated systemic anomalies. On the basis of 22 cases from the literature and of 2 personal cases, we defined (Francois, 1958a and 1958b) a syndrome which is now called "Francois' dyscephalic syndrome" or the "Francois-Hallerman-Streiff syndrome". More than 150 cases are known at the present time. The syndrome is characterized by seven principal signs (Table 1).

TABLE 1. FREQUENCY OF THE PRINCIPAL SIGNS IN FRANCOIS' SYNDROME (AFTER BARRUCAND ET AL, 1978, 100 CASES AND CARLES-MERMET, 1979, 150 CASES)

Anomaly	%
Dyscephaly	98 - 99
Cataract	81 - 90
Microphthalmia	78 - 83
Dental anomalies	80 - 85
Hypotrichosis	80 - 82
Skin atrophy	68 - 70
Dwarfism	45 - 68

Birth Defects: Original Article Series, Volume 18, Number 6, pages 595–619

The dyscrania consists mainly of a brachycephaly with frontal bossing, with or without microcephaly. Scaphocephaly, oxycephaly (Guyard et al, 1962) or dolichocephaly (Watrin, 1964) with or without platybasia (Carones, 1961) are rarely found. Hydrocephaly is rather frequent. Calcifications of the brain falx, sutural anomalies such as open sutures and fontanelles or, on the contrary, premature synostosis (Larmande et al, 1962; Zolog et al, 1967; Barrucand et al, 1978), occipital bossing and hypoplasia of the orbit have also been mentioned.

The mandibulo-facial dysmorphia is characterized by an aplasia or hypoplasia of the mandible and by a thin, tapering nose, incurved as a parrot's bill. The fronto-nasal angle is deep. There is also a typical double cutaneous chin with a central dimple. Hence the physiognomy is distinctive (bird's head) and gives all affected subjects a "family" resemblance to one another.

The obvious hypoplasia of the mandible involves more particularly its horizontal branch and thus produces an opening of the mandibular angle. A slight hypoplasia of the superiod maxillary or of the malar bone may also be seen.

2. Dental Anomalies

Dental anomalies are found in 80-85% of the cases. The teeth are absent or malformed and irregularly set with hialodonty. There is a hypoplasia of the enamel. Caries are frequent and multiple. Supernumerary teeth may be seen. Other stomatological abnormalities are frequent and include micro- or macrostomia (van Balen, 1961; Barrucand et al, 1978), glossoptosis or mordex apertus. In 1/3 of the cases there is an arched palate.

3. Proportioned Dwarfism

Proportioned dwarfism is seen in 45-68% of the cases

4. Hypotrichosis

Hypotrichosis is found in 80-82% of the cases. It is particularly obvious in the region of the scalp (Fig. 2),

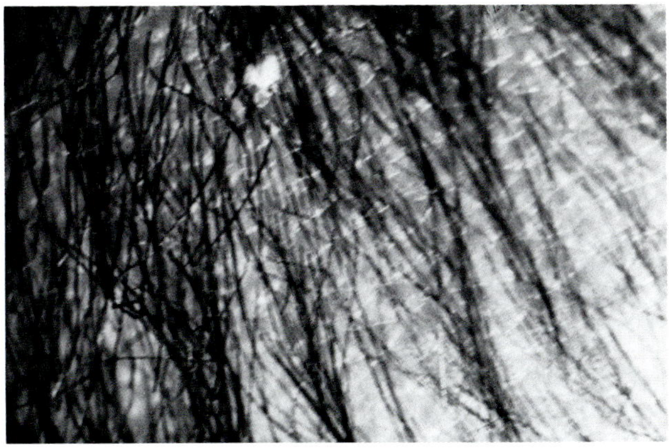

Figure 2. Hypotrichosis of the scalp

the eyelashes and eyebrows, but may also affect the beard as well as the axillary and pubic hair. Alopecic areas are found at the forehead, the temples and along the sutures. Moreover, the hair is fine, sparse and generally light in color.

5. Skin Atrophy

Skin atrophy is seen clinically in 68-70% of the cases. It appears to be localized to the face and more particularly on the nose, where the skin is thin, white, dry, smooth, soft and riddled with telangiectases. Moreover, there may be a hypoplasia of the sebaceous and sweat glands. There is neither a disturbance of the pigmentation nor an atrophy of the subcutaneous adipose tissue.

Other skin anomalies that have been mentioned include: vitiligo (Lamy et al, 1965; Zolog et al, 1967), livedo (Francois, 1958; Ardouin et al, 1962; Francois and Pierard, 1971; Roth, 1971), nevi and freckles (Manzitti and Alezzandrini, 1965), and ichtyosis (Francois and Victoria-Troncoso, 1981) (Figs. 3 and 4).

We were the first to study the skin histologically in two cases (Francois and Pierard, 1971) and to show that the involvement is not localized to the face, but is in fact

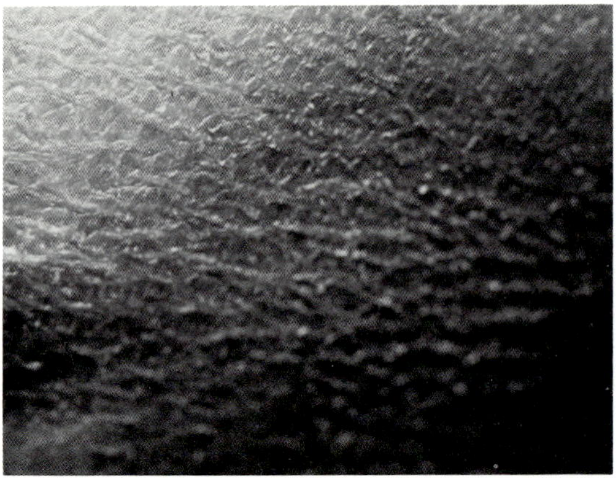

Figure 3. Ichtyosiform alterations of the skin

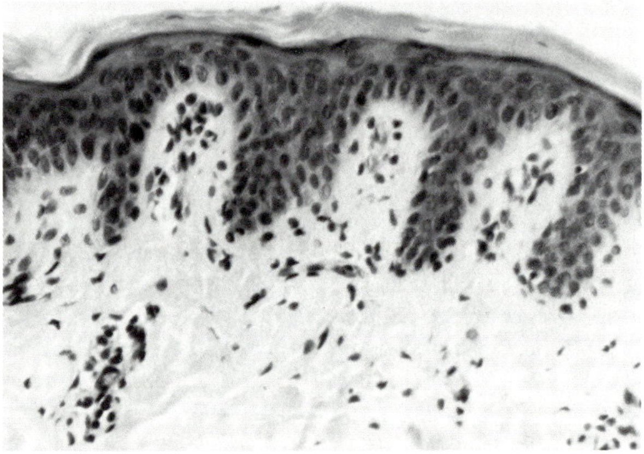

Figure 4. Hyperkeratosis of the epidermis (hematoxylin-eosin-safran staining, x 350)

generalized. An alteration of the connective tissue was observed not only at the sites where the tegument was objectively impaired, but also some distance away, in regions where no clinically detectable anomaly was present. In the apparently healthy skin, it consisted of absence of cohesion of the collagen fibers (Fig. 5), which were tangled and oriented

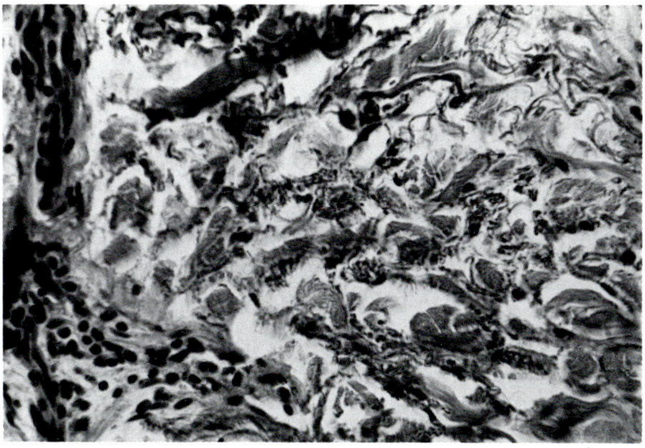

Figure 5. Apparently normal skin of the forearm. Absence of cohesion of the collagen fibers, fragmentation of the elastic fibers (Verhoeff's staining, x 350)

in all directions, and of fragmentation of the elastic fibers into short segments (Figs. 6 and 7). The skin was clinically

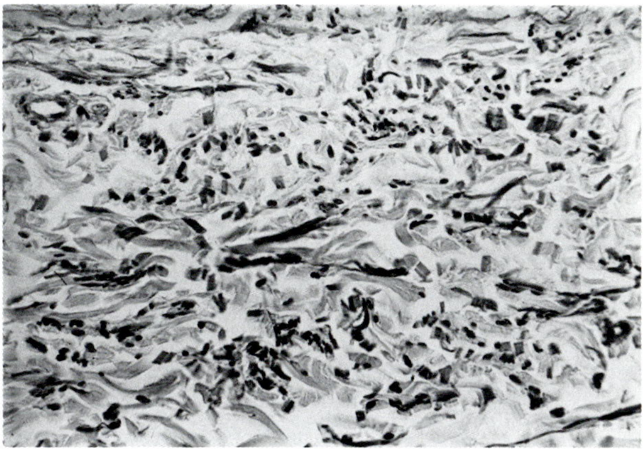

Figure 6. Apparently normal skin of the forearm. Fragmentation of the elastic fibers (Verhoeff's staining, x 350)

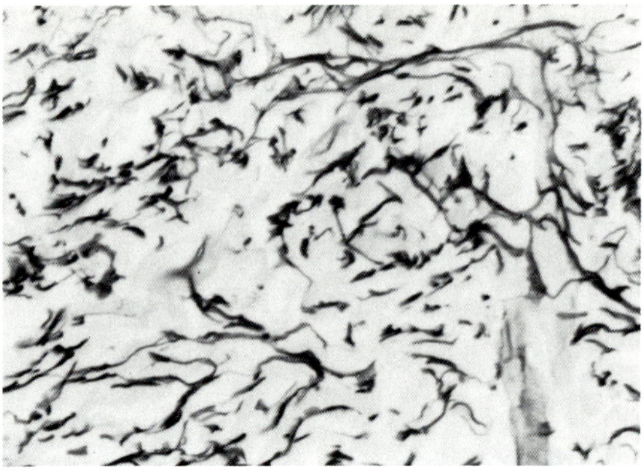

Figure 7. Swollen and fragmented elastic fibers in the dermis (elastic staining, x 350)

modified in the various zones. They were reflected in the upper and middle dermal layers by the same lack of cohesion of collagen and especially by the variability in the aspects of the elastic fibers. Some were fragmented, moniliform, or tangled in tight clusters (Fig. 8); others were swollen and

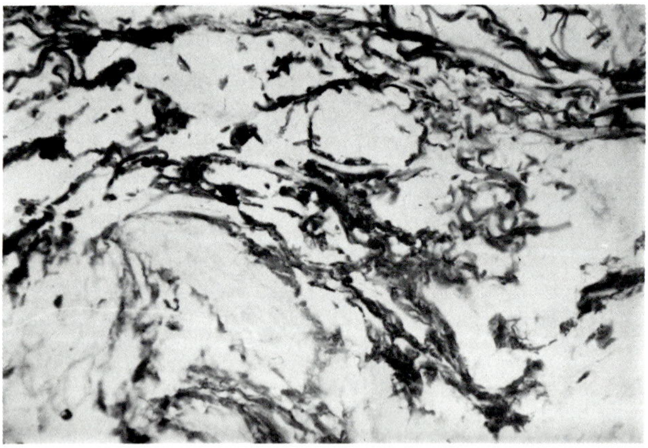

Figure 8. Atrophy of the skin in the temporal region. Alterations resembling those seen in senile elastosis. Scarce elastic network. The elastic fibers form tangled clusters (Orecin staining, x 350)

showed irregular or imprecise contours and uneven staining affinities. In the deep dermal layer the elastic fibers were rare, often narrow, or even thin and sometimes took little stain. These histologic changes in the connective tissue explained the sensation of softness given by palpation of the facial skin of the patients.

It was concluded from these findings that the Francois' dyscephalic syndrome is related in some way to congenital abnormalities in elastin. They are nevertheless of quite a different nature from those observed in pseudoxanthoma elasticum. While the changes in the latter become manifest quite clearly on routine staining by a violet hue with hematoxylin and eosin and by an orange-red hue with Masson's trichome, this is not true in the dyscephalic syndrome, where the elastin is not brought out with these stains. With specific staining methods the appearances also differ appreciably from those seen in pseudoxanthoma. Moreover, no calcium was seen on staining with von Kossa.

Histochemical examinations made in a third case of Francois' dyscephalic syndrome (Francois and Victoria-Troncoso, 1981) showed that there was a global diminution of the glycosaminoglycans (glycoproteins); moreover the polysaccharide chains were weakly sulfated. Furthermore, although in our last case, the collagen fibers appeared to have normal staining characteristics, some of them had nevertheless lost all birefringence.

Finally, and still in our last case, there was a loss of elastin in certain places and accumulation of elastin in the form of irregularly distributed fragments in other places. It is now known that the glycoproteins are the "organizers" of the collagen fibers as well as of the elastic fibers. They are at the basis of the morphology of any connective tissue.

In our syndrome, there is a disturbance in glycoprotein metabolism possibly caused either by an insufficiency in their biosynthesis with inadequate sulfation, or a deficiency of transferase enzymes, which promote the synthesis of the glycoconjugates and also play a role in the linking of structural glycoproteins to collagen and above all to elastin.

Barrucand et al (1978) examined the skin of the leg in one of their cases and confirmed our findings. They found an absence of the dermo-epidermic basement membrane. The elastic fibers were thickened and also fragmented in places, tending to be disposed parallel to the epithelial surface. The collagen seemed to be nearly normal.

6. Bilateral Microphthalmos (Table 3) (Fig. 9).

TABLE 3. FREQUENCY OF THE OCULAR ANOMALIES IN FRANCOIS' SYNDROME (ACCORDING TO BARRUCAND ET AL, 1978, 100 CASES, AND CARLES-MERMET, 1979, 150 CASES)

Anomaly	%
Congenital cataract	81 - 90
Microphthalmia	78 - 83
Nystagmus	32 - 45
Strabismus	33 - 37
Blue scleras	22 - 31
Sparse eyelashes and eyebrows	29
Anomalies of the fundus	18 - 22
Anomalies of the conjunctiva	11
Anomalies of the cornea	9 - 14
Antimongoloid palpebral fissures	12 - 13
Intraocular hypertension	7 - 11
Atrophy of the iris	10 - 14
Degeneration of the vitreous	8
Anomalies of the eyelids	6
Coloboma of the iris	5
Persistance of the pupillary membrane	5
Enophthalmia	2,5 - 4
Hypotelorism	2,5
Epicanthus	2 - 4
Coloboma of the disc	1
Coloboma of the choroid	1
Ptosis	1 - 3
Hypoplasia of the lacrimal puncta	2
Epibulbar tumor	1

Microphthalmia, which is always bilateral, is observed in 78-83% of the cases. The diameter of the cornea varies from 5 to 10 mm (Manzitti and Alezzandrini, 1965).

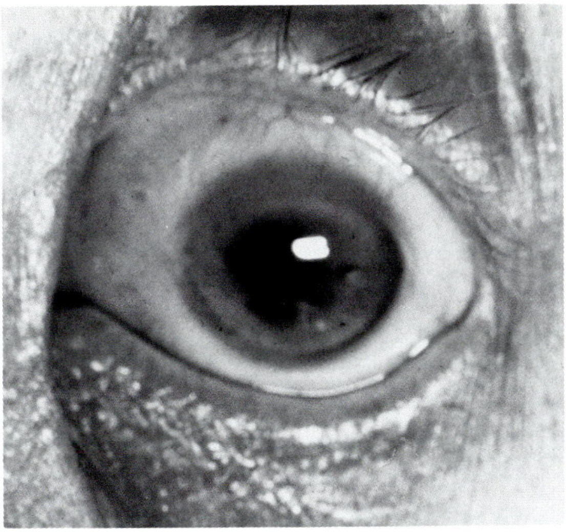

Figure 9. Microphthalmos

7. Congenital Cataracts

Congenital cataracts are seen in 81-90% of the cases. They are always bilateral and usually complete. They consist of liquefied lens masses, as shown by discision which produces a white milky liquid. Spontaneous resorption of the lens is not rare (Forsius and De La Chapelle, 1964; Wolter and Jones, 1965; Sugar et al, 1972; Okajima et al, 1978). This resorption may produce a uveitis (Wolter and Jones, 1965). The results of the operation are poor. In exceptional cases the lens is absent (Konstas et a, 1965; Srivastava et al, 1966) or there is no cataract (Lamy et al, 1965; Verger et al, 1966; Woilliez et al, 1968).

8. Other Ocular Anomalies

Strabismus and nystagmus are present in one third of the cases. Glaucoma is not exceptional. We observed it in 2 cases out of 6, although in the literature the frequency is only 11%. Glaucoma has been mentioned by Hopkins and

Horan (1970), Sugar et al (1972) and Aracena and Sangueza (1977). It may be due to a chronic iridocyclitis following leakage of lens matter.

Some ocular anomalies are very rare: anterior lenticonus (Scoppetta et al, 1979), blue sclera (Okajima et al, 1978), anomalies of the iris, Fuchs' heterochromia (Cambaggi, 1958), persistance of the pupillary membrane (Srivastava et al, 1966), anomalies of the cornea or the conjunctiva, enophthalmos, epicanthus ptosis (Guyard et al, 1962; Woilliez et al, 1968; Russel and Steel, 1970), hypoplasia of the lacrimal puncta, antimongoloid slant of the palpebral fissures.

COMMENTS

The presence of elastic alterations in the skin must make one consider the possibility of alterations in Bruch's membrane (of which one layer is elastic), just as in the Groenblad-Strandberg syndrome where angioid streaks are found. In fact these fundus changes have been observed in the Francois' syndrome by us (Fig. 10) and by others (Calmettes et al, 1960; Carones, 1961; Guyard et al, 1962; Francois, 1963; Gernet, 1964; Blodi and Braley, 1966; Ide and Webb, 1969). Histopathologic examination revealed numerous drusen of the Bruch's membrane (Blodi and Braley, 1966).

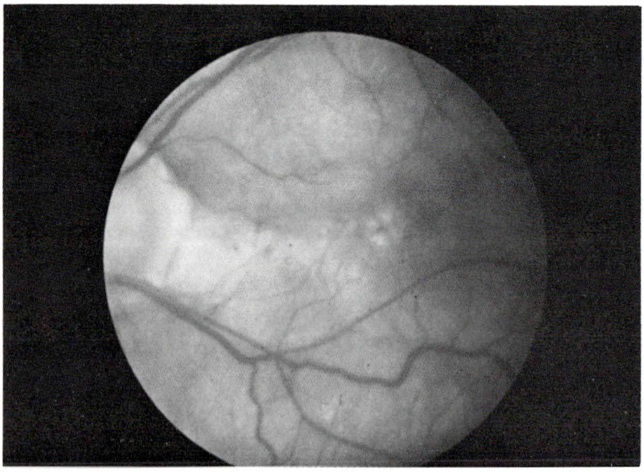

Figure 10. Peripapillary atrophy and drusen-like lesions in the macular region

Although in Francois' syndrome, the fundus often cannot be explored because of microphthalmos and primary or secondary cataract, various fundus abnormalities have been reported. These include peripapillary atrophy (Hallerman, 1948; Nizetic, 1954; Falls and Schull, 1960; van Balen, 1961; Francois and Pierard, 1971), speckled aspect of the fundus (Hallerman, 1948; Nizetic, 1954; Falls and Schull, 1960; van Balen, 1961; Koo et al, 1967; El Massri, 1967; Borghi et al, 1968), diffuse atrophy of the pigment epithelium with macular cracks of red brick color (Calmettes et al, 1960), foci of chorioretinal atrophy (Streiff, 1950; Koo et al, 1967), macular degeneration (Nizetic, 1954; Francois and Pierard, 1971), disseminated brownish dusty pigmentation (Streiff, 1950; Koo et al, 1967; Francois and Pierard, 1971), pigmentary changes of the fundus (Rudobielski and Rudzinska, 1972) or optic atrophy.

In one case we saw a coloboma at the entrance of the optic nerve in the right eye (Francois, 1959) and on the left, peripapillary lesions resembling foci of cicatricial chorioretinitis. In another case, we observed anomalies of the macular region, which covered an area of four disk diameters. Two parts equal in width could be distinguished. The first, parapapillary, was irregularly depigmented and showed a marbled and yellowish aspect. The second part, temporal, was heavily pigmented and was occupied by dusty, tiny, brownish pigments distributed homogeneously. While progressively diminishing in number towards the periphery, they accumulated on the central side, where they suddenly stopped tracing a vertical irregularly undulated line. Carones (1961) saw a similar lesion. The temporal half of the posterior pole showed brownish, dusty pigmentation covering a half-moon space from where it progressively fell off towards the periphery.

Gernet (1964) reported horizontal retinal folds in the macular region of both eyes, their prominence being at the most one diopter. Ide and Webb (1969), observed similar horizontal folds in a depigmented macular area. These folds may well represent changes in the Bruch's membrane as we observed in a Groenblad-Strandberg case. Finally, Guyard et al (1962) saw a coloboma of the choroid in the right eye and in the left eye, outside the disk, glial hyperplasia resembling proliferative retinitis with pigmented patches of cicatricial chorioretinitis. In addition there were cracks in the choroid similar to angioid streaks.

causing death from coronaritis or ictus at the age of about 15 years.

PATHOGENESIS

The Francois' syndrome is most probably due to a disturbance in development during the 5th or 6th week of embryonic life. This disturbance affects the various derivatives of the first branchial arch and involves particularly the ventral part of the cephalic extremity. It can be caused by a disturbance in the domain of the rhomboencephalic organizer and may extend to certain ecto- and mesodermic outlines.

HEREDITY

All cytogenetic studies have been normal (Falls et al, 1960; Bueno, 1961; Guerineau and Plassart, 1965; Hoefnagel and Benirschke, 1965; Lamy et al, 1965; Gaudier et al, 1968; Woilliez et al, 1968; Dublineau, 1970; Pierard and Francois, 1970; Rosenberg and Monnet, 1972; Barrucand et al, 1978), and out of 134 cases, only two abnormal karyotypes were found. Carones (1961) observed a chromosome no. 4 which was too small, and Jalbert et al (1968) also found a deletion of the short arm of chromosome no. 4.

Dermatoglyphs have been examined in 4 cases and found to be normal in two (Dublineau, 1970; Barrucand et al, 1978) and abnormal in the other two (Woilliez et al, 1969). There is no single argument in favor of an exogenous factor or of an embryopathy.

Francois' syndrome seems at the present time to be undoubtedly genetic in nature, the more so when taking into account the fact the patients have no descendants. Indeed the morphological resemblance of the patient is so extraordinary that they all seem to be brother and sisters, a fact which favors a genetic explanation. There is no sex predominance. Barrucand et al (1978) found 42 males for 46 females. Consanguinity of the parents is high. It was observed in 11 cases (7%) (Jambert et al, 1958; Guyard et al, 1962; Ponte, 1962; Manzitti and Alezzandrini, 1963; Gernet, 1964; Bueno, 1966; Spoerl and Romano, 1973; Jorgenson et al, 1975; Barrucand et al, 1978; Ardouin et al, 1962.

Guyard et al (1962) observed consanguinity among the grandparents. A concordance in monozygotic twins has been seen by Waardenburg (1958) and Van Balen (1961). At the present time we know of at least 10 familial cases. Several cases in the same sibship have been observed by Norbis (1952: 2 sisters), Larmande (1959), Ponte (1962: 2 brothers); Bueno (1966: 2 sisters and 1 brother), Hall et al (1974: 2 brothers) Salomon (cited by Carles-Mermet, 1979: 2 sisters).

On the other hand, Guyard et al (1962) observed the syndrome in a father and his daughter. Koliopoulos and Palimeris (1975) described 5 cases in 3 generations with transmission from father to son (Fig. 11). Boschetti (1975) reported a family in which the mother and her 2 sons were affected (Fig. 12).

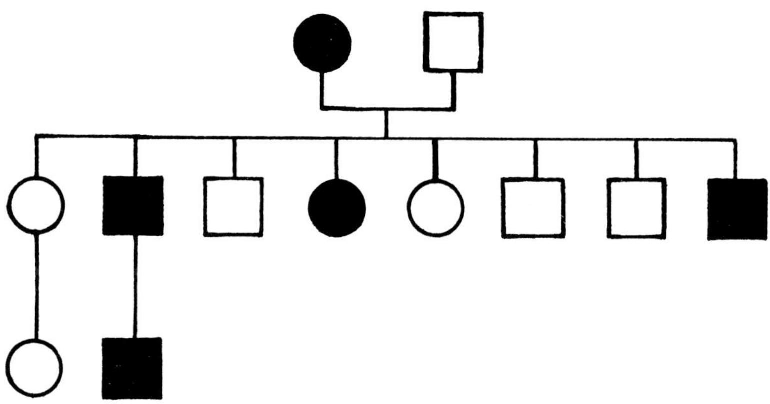

Figure 11. Francois' dyscephalic syndrome: 4 cases in 3 generations (after Koliopoulos and Palimeris, 1975).

It is still impossible to conclude in favor of either an autosomal recessive transmission or an autosomal dominant one, the more so since only a few affected subjects have descendants. In favor of recessive heredity, we should mention the high frequency of consanguinity (7%) and the exclusive existence of the syndrome inside the same sibship. The families of Guyard et al (1962), Kolipoulos and Palimeris (1975) and Boschetti (1975) with 2 or 3 affected generations

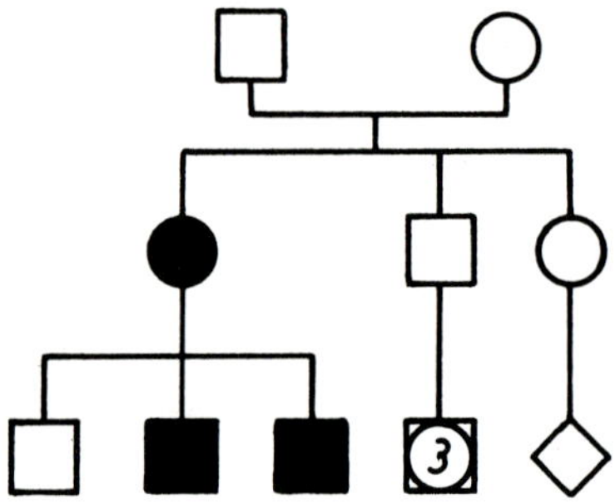

Figure 12. Francois' dyscephalic syndrome in 2 generations (after Boschetti, 1975)

favor dominant heredity, which seems plausible. Opitz et al (1969) have raised the possibility of multifactorial heredity, but the great resemblance of all the affected subjects argues against this hypothesis.

SUMMARY

Francois' dyscephalic syndrome is characterized by a dyscephaly with bird's head, dental anomalies, proportioned dwarfism, hypotrichosis, and skin atrophy, which is generalized and involves particularly the elastic tissue. There is bilateral microphthalmos as well as congenital cataracts and fundus changes, which may indicate an involvement of the Bruch's membrane. The syndrome is genetic, but it is still impossible to conclude in favor of either autosomal recessive or autosomal dominant transmission.

REFERENCES

Afaunov AL (1971). The Hallermann-Streiff syndrome. Vestn Oftal 84:85

Akiyama K, Sugai M and Akiyama H (1971). A case of Hallermann-Streiff syndrome. Rinsho Ganka 25:2065

Apollonio A and Zoldan T (1964). Su alcuni casi di malformazioni cranio-faccia in assoziazione ad altre alterazioni sensoriali. Boll Oculist 43: 76

Aracena T and Sanqueza P (1977). Hallermann-Streiff-Francois syndrome. J Pediat Ophthal 14:373
Ardouin M, Urvoy M and Bezier J (1962). Dyscephalie avec "tete d'oiseau", cataracte bilaterale et keratite en bandelette. Bull Soc Ophtal, France 62:438
Barrucand D, Benradi C and Schmitt J (1978). Syndrome de Francois. A propos de deux cas. Rev Oto-Neuro-Ophtal 50:305
Battin J and Azanka X (1970). Syndrome de Francois, Bordeaux Med 3:2469
Battin J, Hehunstre JP and Corcelle L. Syndrome de Francois. A propos de cinq cas. J Genet Hum 24:261
Bengisu N, Basar D and Idil MK (1967). A case of oculo-mandibulo-facial dyscephaly (the Francois' syndrome). VII Turk Oftal Kong Bult, p. 274
Benradi Ch (1976). Contribution a l'etude du syndrome de Francois. These Med, Rabat, no. 75, 179 p. (bibliog.).
Blodi FC and Braley AE (1966). Die Augenveranderungen im Francois-Hallermann-Streiff Syndrome. Proc XXth Int Congr Ophthal, Munchen, p. 981
Bonamour G and Leopold Ph (1960). Syndrome dyscephale avec tete d'oiseau. Bull Soc Ophtal, France, 60:84
Borghi A, Brancato R, Maiello M and Montali E (1968). Discefalia mandibulo-oculo-faciale "nuova syndrome" di Francois (Dismorfia di Hallermann-Streiff, Discefalia di Ullrich e Fremerey-Dohna). Rass Neurol Veg 22:202
Boschetti (1975). Personal communication
Bueno Sanchez M (1966). Sindrome de Hallerman-Streiff-Francois. A proposito de una presentacion familiar. Bol Soc Vasco-Navarra Pediat 1:21
Calmettes L, Deodati P, Cadenat H and Bechac G (1960). La dysmorphie mandibulo-faciale type Francois (a propos d'un cas). Revue Oto-Neuro-Ophtal 32:275
Cambiaggi A (1958). Sindrome di Hallermann-Streiff con eterocromia di Fuchs. Boll Oculistica 37:365
Carles-Mermet B (1979). Dyscephalie a tete d'oiseau (signes oculaires et etiologie). A propos de 4 observations et revue de la literature. Thesis, Lyon
Carones AB (1961). Syndrome dyscephalique de Francois. Ophthalmologica, Basel 142:510
Caspersen I and Warburg M (1968). Le syndrome de Hallermann-Streiff-Francois. Acta Ophthal 46:385
Cernea P and Constantin F (1974). Dyscephalie, conjonctivite muco-synechiante, et malformations des extremites. Arch Ophtal, Paris, 34:349

Cernea P and Constantin F (1961). Dyscephalie, conjonctivite muco-synechiante, et malformation faciales (type Francheschetti-Goldenhar). Bull Soc Ophtal, France, 61:30

Cordier J, Tridon P, Thiriet M, Babut M and Raspiller A (1968). Syndrome oculo-vertebral de Wevers. Rev Oto-Neuro-Ophtal 40:204

Crevits L, Thiery E and Vander Eecken H (1979). Oculomandibular dyscephaly (Hallermann-Streiff-Francois Syndrome) associated with epilepsy. J Neurol 215:225

De Mulet EM and Guarnieri JC (1971). Cranio-facial malformations. Calssification and aetiopathogenic considerations. Arch Chil Oftal 28:337

Dinwiddie R, Gewitz M and Taylor JFN. Cardiac defects in the Hallermann-Streiff syndrome. J Pediat 92:77

Donders PC (1977). Hallermann-Streiff syndrome. Docum Ophthal, Den Haag 44:161

Dublineau Ph (1970). Le syndrome de Jules Francois. A propos d'une observation. Thesis, Angers

El Massri A. Dyscephaly with congenital cataract. Brit J Ophthal 51:352

Falls HF and Schull WH (1960). Hallermann-Streiff syndrome. A dyscephaly with congenital cataracts and hypotrichosis. Arch Ophthal 63:409

Forsius HR and De La Chapelle A (1964). Dyscephalia oculomandibulo-facialis. Two cases in which the chromosomes were studied. Ann Paediat Fenn 10:388

Francheschetti A (1968). Dysostoses cranio-faciales. Congenital anomalies of the eye. C.V. Mosby Bibl., St. Louis 5:77

Francois J (1958). A new syndrome. Dyscephalia with bird face and dental anomalies, nanism, hypotrichosis, cutaneous atrophy, microphthalmia and congenital cataract. Arch Ophthal, Chicago, 60:842

Francois J (1958a). Un nouveau syndrome. Dyscephalie avec tete d'oiseau et anomalies dentaires, nanisme, hypotrichose, atrophie cutanee, microphtalmie et cataracte congenitale. Boll Oculistica 25:161

Francois J (1958b). Un nouveau syndrome. Bull Universite, Gand, 2:161

Francois J (1961). XVI Jackson Memorial Lecture. Syndromes with congenital cataract. Amer J Ophthal 52:207

Francois J (1963). Congenital cataracts. Thomas, Springfield, p. 278

Francois J (1967). Un nouveau syndrome. Bull Soc Belge Ophtal 117:597

Francois J (1979). Consideration sur l'importance de l'heredite en Ophtalmologie. J Fr Ophtalmol 2:569
Francois J, Berger R, Saraux M et al (1972). Les aberrations chromosomiques en ophtalmologie. Masson ed., 594 p, Paris
Francois J and Haustrate L (1954). Anomalies colobomateuses du globe oculaire et syndromes du ler arc. Ann Oculist 187:340
Francois J and Pierard J (1971). The Francois dyscephalic syndrome and skin manifestations. Amer J Ophthalmol 71:1241
Francois J and Victoria-Troncoso V (1980). The cornea in normal condition and in Groenouw's macular dystrophy. Junk, The Hague
Francois J and Victoria-Troncoso V (in press). Francois' dyscephalic syndrome and skin manifestations. Ophthalmologica
Franklin L (1972). The Hutchinson-Gifford-Progeria syndrome. J Pediat 4:697
Gaudier B, Francois P, Ponte C, Nuyts JP and Bombart E. Encephalopathies infantiles et dysmorphies complexes: Le syndrome de Hallermann-Streiff-Francois. Lille Med 13:698
Gellis SS and Feingold M (1966). Picture of the month: Hallermann-Streiff syndrome. Am J Dis Child 111:635
Gernet H (1964). Ueber Mikrophthalmus, Maculaveranderungen und Refraktion bei einem Fall von Dysostosis mandibulofacialis Hallermann-Streiff (Dysjephalie-Syndrom Francois). Klin Mbl Augenheilk 144:887
Gorlin RJ and Pindborg JJ (1964). Syndromes of the Head and Neck. Mc Graw-Hill, New York
Gorlin RJ, Pindborg JJ and McKusick VA (1976). Syndromes of the Head and Neck. 2 Ed. Mc Graw-Hill, New York
Guerineau P and Plassart H (1965). Syndrome dyscephalique de Francois (a propos d'un cas chez un nourisson de race maure). Arch Fr Ped 22:882
Guerineau P and Plassart H (1965). Syndrome dyscephalique de Francois. A propos d'un cas chez un nourrisson de race maure. Pr Med 73:2514
Guyard M, Perdriel G and Ceruti F (1962). Sur deux cas de syndrome dyscephalique a tete d'oiseau. Bull Soc Ophtal France 62:443
Hall D, Berg O, Rudolph S and Epstein J (1974). Pseudoprogeria. Hallermann-Streiff syndrome. Birth Defects. Orig. Art. Series 10:137
Hallermann W (1948). Vogelsicht und Cataracta congenita. Klin Mbl Augenheilk 113:315

Hoefnagel D and Benirschke K (1965). Dyscephalia mandibulo-oculo-facialis. Hallermann-Streiff syndrome. Arch Dis. Child 40:57

Hopf HC, Pilz H and Althaus HH (1976). Dyskephalie-Katarakt-Hypotrichose-Syndrom (Synonyma: DCH: Ullrich-Fremerey-Dohna; Hallermann-Streiff, Francois). Beubachtung mit extrapyramidaler Storung und Demenz. J Neurol 212:171

Hopkins DJ and Horan EC (1970). Glaucoma in the Hallermann-Streiff syndrome. Brit J Ophthal 54:416

Ide CH and Webb RW (1969). Hallermann-Streiff syndrome. Amer J Ophthal 67:151

Jalbert P, Gilbert Y, Leopold P and Mouriquand D (1958). Syndrome de Hallermann-Streiff-Francois. A propos d'une nouvelle observation associee a une anomalie caryotypique. Pediatrie 23:703

Jancar J (1966). Hallermann-Streiff-Francois syndrome (dyscephalia mandibulo-oculo-facialis). J Ment Def Res 10:255

Jorgenson RJ (1979). Oculo-mandibulo-facial syndrome. In: Bergsma D. Birth Defects Compendium. The National Foundation, Alan R. Liss, New York, p. 797

Jorgenson RJ, Pearlman A and Norton W (1975). Hallermann-Streiff syndrome. Birth Defects, Orig. Art. Ser. 11:391

Judge G and Chakanovski JE (1971). The Hallermann-Streiff syndrome. J Ment Defic Res 15:115

Juglio N (1967). Su di un case di sindrome di Hallermann e Streiff (Nuovo sindrome di Francois). Ann Ottal 93:655

Kermarreg J (1968). Syndrome de Hallermann-Streiff-Francois. These Med., Bordeaux

Koliopoulos J and Palimeris G (1975). A typical Hallermann-Streiff-Francois syndrome in three successive generations. J Pediat Ophthal 12:235

Kondo T, Kunishi M, Takagi M and Hirata A (1970). Ocular symptoms in three cases of congenital anomalies. Folia Ophthal Jap 21:146

Konstas P, Barsolas B, Stangos N and Tsitros A (1964). Syndrome de Francois. Arch Ophth Hetair Boreil hellad 13:159

Koo BS, Rhee SU and Kim JH (1967). A case of the Hallermann-Streiff syndrome. J Korean Ophthal Soc 8:55

Kurlander GJ, Lavy NW and Campbell, JA (1966). Roentgen differentiation of the oculo-dento-digital syndrome and Hallermann-Streiff syndrome in infancy. Radiology 86:77

Lamy M, Jemmet J, Maroteaux P and Assan N (1965). La dyscephalie (syndrome Hallermann-Streiff-Francois). Arch Fr Ped 22:929

Larmande P (1959). Personal communication.

Larmande A, Gillot F, Balaut J, Cohen JP and Schaeffer JC (1962). Dyscephalie a tete d'oiseau (Syndrome d'Hallermann-Streiff-Francois). Pediatrie 49:313

Macciotta A, Zanolla L and Bertoni G (196). Contributo alla conoscenza della discefalia mandibulo-oculo-faciale. Ann Ital Pediat 20:209

Manzitti E and Alezzandrini AA (1963). Syndrome dyscephalique de Francois. Ann Oculistique, Paris 196:456

Massri A (1967). Dyscephaly with congenital cataract. Brit J Ophthal 51:352

Maugery G, Rambaud G, Franche U and Villon J (1972). Fistula carotido caverneuse spontanee chez un sujet jeune dans un contexte plurimalformatif. Bull Soc Ophthal, France, 72:499

Meloni T and Spano G (1971). The Hallermann-Streiff-Francois syndrome. Ann Ottal 97:441

Mendez RF (1970). Sindrome de Hallermann-Streiff. An Soc Mex Oftal 43:119

Neimann N, Cordier J, Manciaux M and Barrucand D (1960). Syndrome de Franceschetti associe au syndrome de Goldenhar et a des malformations vertebrales. Ann Pediat 36:2642

Niwa I and Itoi M (1966). A case of mandibulo-facial dysmorphia. The Hallermann-Streiff syndrome. Rinsho Ganka 20:65

Nizetic D (1954). Dysmorphie mandibulo-faciale et status dysraphicus. Ophthalmologica (Basel) 127:1

Norbis A (1952). El ojo en las dismorfias mesodermicas. Arch Oftal, Buenos Aires, 27:302

Nuyts J and Bombard E (1968). La dyscephalie a tete d'oiseau. Med Infant 75:425

Okajima Y, Nishimura Y and Oshima K (1978). Two cases of the first and second branchial arch syndrome with ocular abnormalities. Jap Clin Ophthal 32:377

Opitz JM, Herrmann J and Dicker H (1969). The study of malformation syndromes in man. Birth Defects, Orig. Art. Series, Vol. V, p. 1

Paufique L, Diderlaurent A, Cotton JP and Maugery J (1967). Trois nouveaux cas de syndrome de Francois (dyscephalie avec tete d'oiseau) Bull Soc Opht France 67:315

Paufique M, Didier A, Laurent M et coll (1967). Trois nouveaux cas de syndrome de Francois. Bull Soc Ophthal, France, 67:315

Pierard J and Francois J (1970). Constatations histologiques sur le syndrome dyscephalique de Francois. Bull Soc Fr Dermat Syphil 77:725

Ponte F (1962). Further contribution to the study of the syndrome of Hallermann-Streiff. Ophthalmologica (Basel), 143:399

Raspiller A (1968). Les malformations associees oculo-rachidiennes. These Med Nancy, no. 81, p. 17

Roca R (1963). Discefalia con cabeza de pajaro (sindrome de Francois-Hallermann-Streiff). Boll Soc Val de Ped 5:17

Rosenberg D and Monnet P (1972). Syndrome de Hallermann-Streiff-Francois. Med Infant 79:227

Roth L (1962). A propos du syndrome de Hallermann-Streiff. Bull Soc Opht France 62:500

Roth L (1971). Contribution a l'etude de la dysostose mandibulo-faciale. These Med, Strasbourg, no. 76, 81 p.

Rucobielski R and Rudzinska A (1972). A case of Hallermann-Streiff syndrome. Klin Oczna 42:1087

Russel M and Steeler M (1970). Hallermann-Streiff syndrome. Clinical and pronostic considerations. Amer J Dis Child 120:462

Saadat M, Behbakht G and Ziai M (1972). Hallermann-Streiff syndrome. Report of two cases seen in Iran. Pahlavi Med J 3:333

Sakaue E. Hallermann-Streiff's syndrome. J Clin Ophth Tokyo, 16:653

Salado-Marin F (1967). The Francois syndrome. Arch Soc Oftal Hisp-Amer 27:473

Sanchez MB (1966). Sindrome de Hallermann-Streiff-Francois. A proposito de una presentation familiar. Bol Soc Vasco-Navarra Pediat 1:21

Schondel A (1943). Two cases of progeria complicated by microphthalmos. Arch Paediat (Uppsala), 30:286

Scoppetta C, Albanese A and Caltagirone C (1979). Oligophrenia with the Hallermann-Streiff syndrome. J Neurol 220:214

Sharp EC and Kopel HM (1970). Cranio-facial and oral manifestations in oculo-mandibulo-dyscephaly (Hallermann-Streiff syndrome). Oral Surg 30:488

Sohi BK, Boparai MS and Sohi AS (1978). Mandibulo-oculo-facial dyscephaly. A case report. Indian Pediatrics 15:521

Sokmen A (1969). A case of mandibulo-facial dyscephaly. Turk Oftal Kong Bult p.123

Spoerl GH and Romano PF (1973). Penetrating keratoplasty in a complicated mandibulo-oculo-facial dyscephaly. J Pediat Ophthal 10:61

Srivastava SP, Jain SC and Nema HV (1966). Mandibulo-oculo facial dyscephaly. Brit J Ophthal 50:543

Stankovic I, Biga S and Drincik V (1971). Contribution to the knowledge of the Hallermann-Streiff-Francois syndrome. Acta Ophthal Jugosl 9:5
Steele RW and Bass JW (1970). Hallermann-Streiff syndrome. Amer J Dis Child 120:462
Stone W (1975). Hallermann-Streiff-syndrome and progeria. South Med J 68:1139
Streiff EB (1950). Dysmorphie mandibulo-faciale (tete d'oiseau) et alterations oculaires. Ophthalmologica (Basel) 120:79
Sugar A, Bigger JF and Podos SM (1972). Hallermann-Streiff-Francois syndrome. J Pediat Ophthal 8:234
Tazia A (1962). Un cas du syndrome nouveau de Francois. Soc Maroc Ophtal, June
Torres Marty L and Dolcet L (1964). Sindrome de Francois-Hallermann-Streiff. Arch Soc Oftal Hisp-Amer 24:474
Uemura Y, Morizane H, Shimizu K and Okada R (1970). A clinical and pathologic study of ocular manifestations of the Hallermann-Streiff syndrome. Rinsho Ganka 24:219
Ulrich O and Fremery-Dohna H (1953). Dyscephalie mit Cataracta congenita und Hypotrichosis als typischer Merkmalskomplex. Ophthalmologica (Basel) 12:73
Van Balen ATM (1961). Dyscephaly with microphthalmos, cataract and hypoplasia of the mandible. Ophthalmologica (Basel) 141:53
Verger P, Corcelle L, Guillard JM and Descamp F (1966). Sur deux cas de syndrome de Francois. Ann Pediat 42:203 and Sem Hop Paris 42:683
Volpi U, Ricci B and Masteoiacovo P (1977). Francois' syndrome and glaucoma. Acta Med Rom 15:239
Waardenburg PJ (1958). Personal communication
Walbaum R, Woilliez M, Francois P and Mayolle P (1968). Le syndrome de Hallermann-Streiff-Francois. Deux observations. Pediatrie 23:787
Watrin E (1964). Un nouveau cas du syndrome de Francois. Bull Soc Ophtal France 64:87
Woilliez M, Fontaine G, Walbaum R and Blevaque A (1968). Syndrome de Hallermann-Streiff-Francois. Discussion nosologique a propos de deux cas. Bull Soc Ophtal France 68:594
Wolter JR and Jones DH (1965). Spontaneous cataract absorption in Hallermann-Streiff syndrome. Ophthalmologica 150:401
Younessian S and Ammann F (1964). Deux cas de malformations cranio-faciales. 1. Microphthalmie (nanisme oculo-palpebral) avec dysostose cranio-faciale et status dysraphique. 2. Dysmorphie mandibulo-oculo-faciale (syndrome de Hallermann-Streiff). Ophthalmologica (Basel) 147:108

AUTOSOMAL DOMINANT GOLDENHAR SYNDROME

V.GODEL MD PhD, L.REGENBOGEN MD,
V.GOYA MD, R.M.GOODMAN MD.
Departments of Ophthalmology and Genetics, Ichilov and Sheba Medical Center, Tel Aviv University Medical School.

Since Goldenhar (1952) described the association of epibulbar dermoids, accessory appendages and pretargal fistulas, several authors reaffirmed this relationship. As increasing varieties of vertebral bony abnormalities have been discovered to be associated to this triad, the term oculo-auriculovertebral dysplasia was proposed to be more appropriate (Gorlin et al 1976).

Many suggestions accounted for the occurrence of the syndrome sporadically, excluding any possible genetic contribution to its etiology. However, there are some reports of this disease affecting siblings or members of same pedigrees, indicating familial clustering of cases (Summit 1969).

The purpose of this report is to describe a family with this multifaceted disorder showing autosomal dominant inheritance.

CASE REPORTS

Three consecutive generations were affected in this Jewish-Oriental family (Fig 1).

The proband (II-1), a 30 year-old woman, was found to have typical findings for the syndrome. In the right eye a small conjunctival

Birth Defects: Original Article Series, Volume 18, Number 6, pages 621-628

REFERENCES

Goldenhar M (1952). Associations malformatives de l'oeil et de l'oreille en particulier le syndrome dermoïde épibulbaire, appendices auriculaires, fistula auris congenita et ses relations avec la dysostose mandibulo-faciale. J Génét Hum 1:243.

Gorlin RJ, Pindborg JJ, Cohen MM (1976). Syndromes of the Head and Neck. 2nd ed. McGraw Hill p 546.

Mandelcorn MS, Merin S, Cardarelli J (1971). Goldenhar's syndrome and phocomelia. Am J Ophth 72:618.

Poswillo D (1973). The pathogenesis of the first and second branchial arch syndrome. Oral Surg 35:302.

Summit R (1969). Familial Goldenhar syndrome. Birth Def 5:106.

Keywords: Autosomal dominant, Genetic heterogeneity, Goldenhar syndrome, Oculoauriculovertebral dysplasia.

Reprint requests: Victor Godel MD PhD, Department of Ophthalmology, Ichilov Hospital, Tel Aviv 64239, Israel.

LOWE'S SYNDROME

Ramesh C. Tripathi+, Gerhard W. Cibis *', David J. Harris# and Brenda Tripathi+
+University of Chicago,*University of Kansas, 'Children's Mercy Hospital,#Children's Mercy Hosp. +Chicago,Il.,*Kansas City, Ks.,'Kansas City, Mo., #Kansas City, Mo.

The oculo-cerebro-renal syndrome was originally described by Lowe, Terrey and MacLachlan (1952). Ophthalmologically it is characterized by congenital cataracts, glaucoma, miosis and corneal opacities. Generalized findings include severe mental retardation and renal abnormalities primarily amino-aciduria. Heredity is X-linked recessive. We report the clinical and histopathologic findings in three cases, one of which had corneal keloids. The occurance of corneal opacities in Lowe's syndrome has been noted by a number of authors. Warburg (1975) and more specifically Cotlier (1976) point out that clinically these lesions are not band keratopathy but keloids.

A 5½ year old boy from a documented family with Lowe's (Holmes and Tucker 1972) (Fig. 1) had classical clinical and biochemical manifestations of Lowe's syndrome since birth. Ophthalmological examination showed bilateral congenital cataracts, borderline intraocular pressures, and miotic pupils resistant to mydriatics. At the age of 3 months, he underwent bilateral optical iridectomy. The intraocular pressures remained borderline. However, his systemic condition gradually deteriorated and he died of bilateral pneumonia. Both eyes obtained at autopsy were fixed initially in 2.5 per cent buffered glutaraldehyde and subsequently transferred to 10 per cent buffered formalin.

Gross examination showed normal sized globes with clear corneae and inferior sector iridectomies. The culloted globes showed small, discoid cataractous lenses measuring 5 mm equatorially and less than 1 mm antero-posteriorly

Birth Defects: Original Article Series, Volume 18, Number 6, pages 629–644

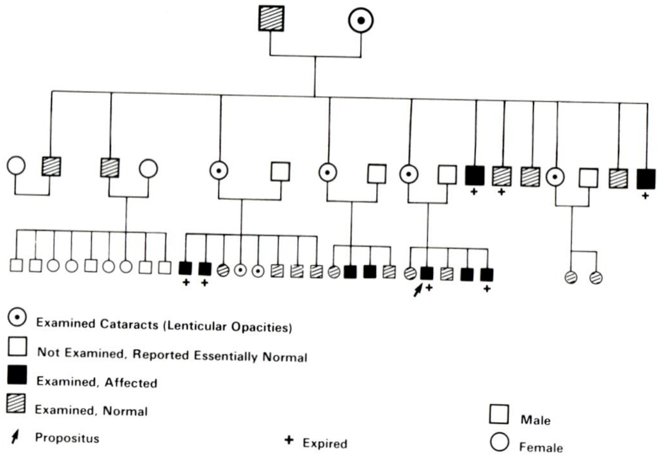

Fig. 1. Family tree of cases 1 and 2. Arrow denotes case 2 the propositus.

(Fig. 2).

Microscopic findings were similar in both eyes. The corneae were unremarkable except for a slight thickening of Descemet's membrane. The angle of the anterior chamber presented an embryonic profile. The iris was inserted anteriorly and partially attached to the base of the trabecular meshwork. The radial and circular ciliary muscle fibers were inconspicuous, and several meridional muscle fibers inserted directly into the trabecular meshwork. The ciliary processes were rudimentary and displaced anteriorly. Many processes arose directly from the posterior aspect of the iris and were supplied by fenestrated capillaries. The dilatator pupillae muscle was segmentally hypoplastic and was absent where the ciliary processes were joined to the iris.

Lange's folds were seen in the peripheral retina, and islands of retinal tissue were present in the pars ciliaris retinae. Cystoid changes were present in the peripheral

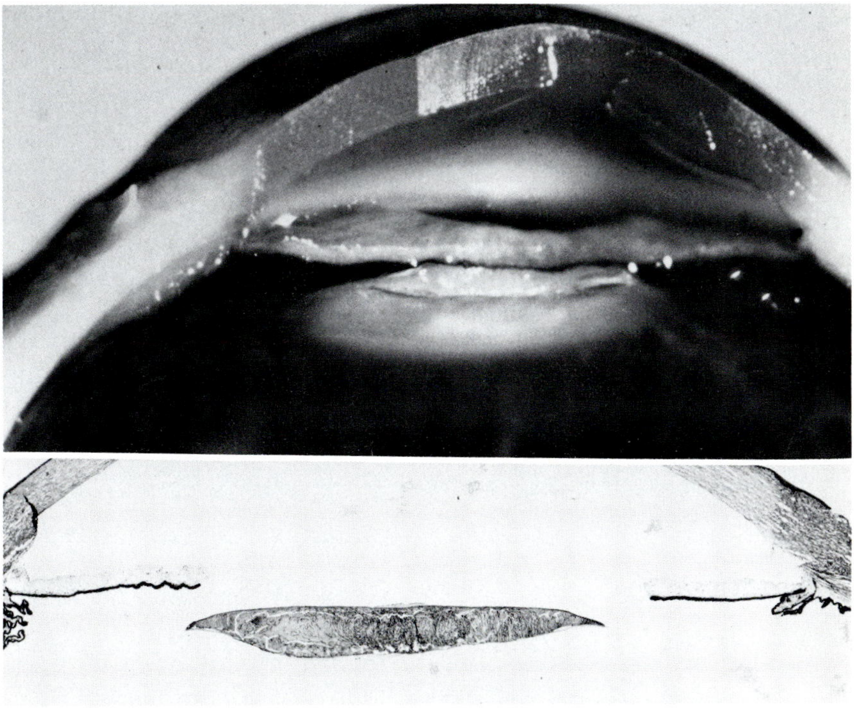

Fig. 2. Culloted globe showing a flattened, discoid lens typical of Lowe's syndrome. The inset shows a sectional view of the lens. Photomicrograph. x 6.

retina, occasionally associated with calcareous nodules in the hyperplastic retinal pigment epithelium. In these regions, the vitreous fibrils coursed through the internal limiting membrane. The zonular fibers were prominent; and the anterior vitreous was condensed.

Both lenses were flattened, totally cataractous, and sharply angulated in the equatorial regions (Fig. 3). The capsule was irregular, conspicuously thickened post-equatorially, and markedly thinned centrally. Anteriorly and

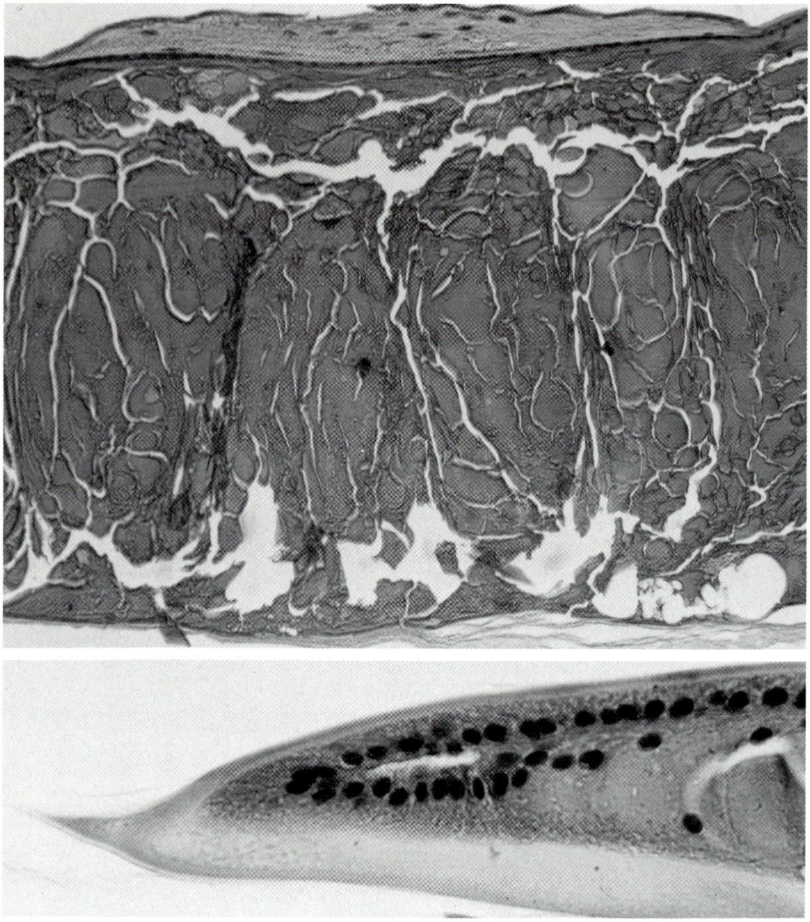

Fig. 3 (a) Central area of cataractous lens lacking demarcation of nucleus and cortex; note also anterior subcapsular cataract. x 145. (b) Sharply angulated lens equator and markedly thickened postequatorial capsule. x 800.

equatorially, capsular excrescences projected into the underlying metaplastic epithelium (Fig. 4). In large localized areas, the lens epithelium was hypertrophic and metaplastic; it continued irregularly over the posterior surface of the lens. The nuclear bow was poorly demarcated. Sheets and islands of aberrant fibrous material were laid down anteriorly and attached to the capsule (Fig. 4).

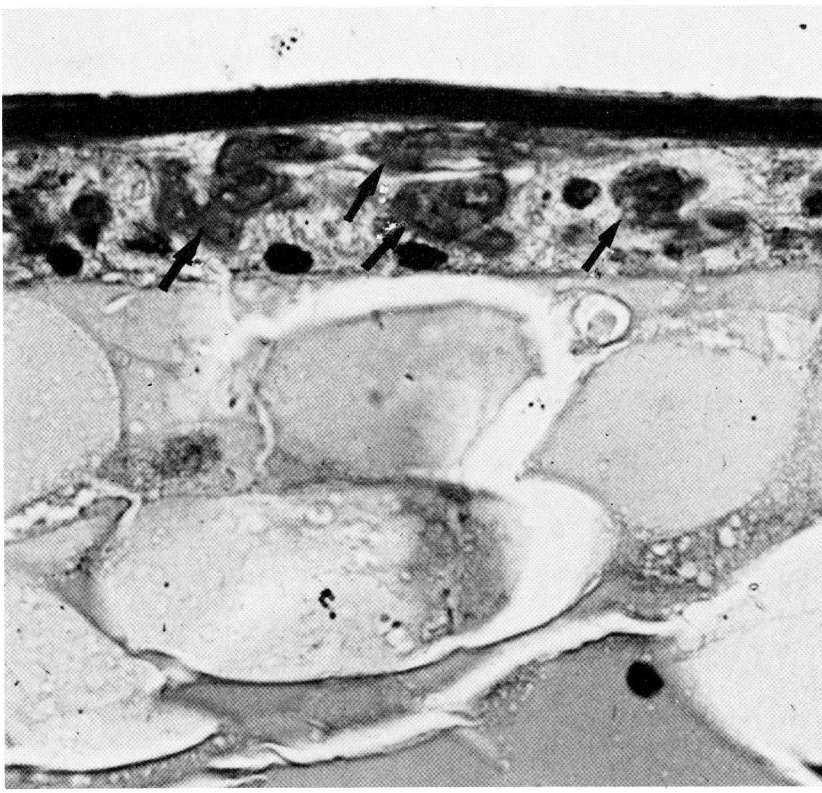

Fig. 4. Anterior region of the lens showing a metaplastic lens epithelium and numerous capsular excrescenses (arrows) which, owing to the plane of section, appear as islands in the epithelium. The underlying cortical cells of the lens show a bladder profile. Photomicrograph. x 800.

Patient 2, an 11 ½-year-old boy, brother of patient one (Fig. 1) had clinical and biochemical signs of Lowe's since birth, although generalized hyperaminoaciduria was not detected until 3½ years of age. At birth, the corneae and anterior chambers were clear in both eyes. Bilateral, congenital nuclear lens opacities were associated with miosed pupils that responded poorly to mydriatics. Bilateral glaucoma was diagnosed at the age of 6 months. One month later, he underwent bilateral goniotomy. Two months later, this procedure was repeated in the left eye. At the age of 14 months, the patient was hospitalized for a left cloudy cornea secondary to glaucoma. No further ocular examinations were recorded until the age of 9½ years when the patient developed a hyphema in the right eye. At that time pannus noted in the inferior segment of both corneae was attributed to incomplete lid closure during sleep. One year later, at age 11 years, one of us (G.W.C.), diagnosed bilateral keloids in the inferior cornea (Fig. 5). The remaining cornea was clear. Six months later the patient died with respiratory infection. Throughtout his life, the patient had been on Dilantin (Parke-Davis) and phenobarbital therapy for seizures as well as vitamin D for rickets associated with Lowe's syndrome.

The eyes, obtained at autopsy, were fixed initially in 2.5 per cent buffered glutaraldehyde and subsequently transferred to 10 per cent buffered formalin. On gross examination, both globes measured 25 x 23 mm with corneal

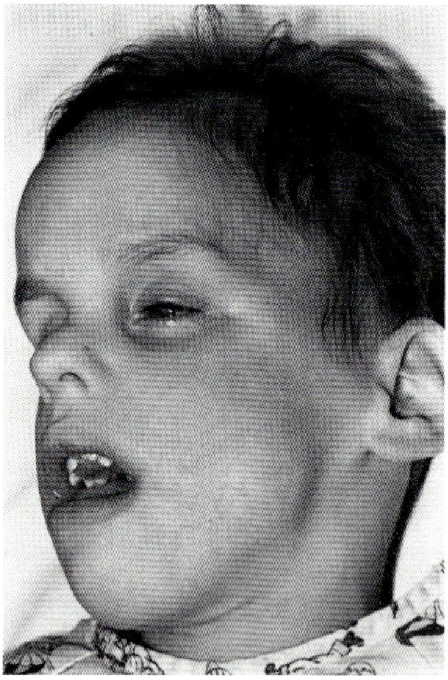

Fig. 5. Clinical photo of patient 2 note corneal keloid.

diameters of 13 x 22 mm. A white, glistening, protuberant, vascularized mass (right - 5 x 5.5 mm, left - 6 x 7 mm) occupied the lower segment of each cornea extending from just above the limbus up to the horizontal corneal axis (Fig. 6 a, 6b, Fig. 7 and Fig. 8). Both culloted globes showed irregular obliteration of the chamber angles and small, discoid, totally cataractous lenses (5 x 2 mm). One lens had a Soemmering's ring presumably **secondary** to surgical rupture of the capsule (Fig. 8). The vitreous cavity was cloudy and condensed bilaterally. A segment of the keloid was post-fixed in osmium tetroxide and embedded in epoxy-resin for electron microscopy. Ultrathin sections stained with uranyl acetate and lead citrate were examined by transmission electron microscopy.

In the region of the keloid, the cornea was enormously thickened. The covering epithelium was markedly hyperplastic, acanthotic, and irregular with hyperkeratosis and parakeratosis, and contained occasional intraepithelial cysts. The basal layer showed variable edematous disorganization, marked irregularity in the cellular arrangement, and many finger-like sinuous downgrowths. Bowman's zone was completely destroyed and replaced by a haphazard growth of fibrovascular tissue infiltrated with moderate numbers of chronic inflammatory cells, mostly lymphocytes and plasma cells. The inflammatory reaction was more marked toward the limbus and in the adjacent edematous conjunctiva. The hypertrophic scar consisted of irregularly arranged and interlacing bundles of collagenous lamellae and fibroblastic cells (Fig. 8). The cellularity and thinness of collagen lamellae were more marked anteriorly. Small vascular channels, more numerous anteriorly, coursed irregularly through the hyperplastic scar. Moderate numbers of lymphocytes, plasma cells, monocytes, and mast cells were seen in the anterior stroma, frequently around the vessels. The chamber angle was irregularly obliterated by goniosynechiae and a cuticular membrane which extended from the peripheral Descemet's membrane onto the anterior iris surface. The trabecular meshwork was partly hyalinized and vascularized. Segments of Schlemm's canal were indiscernible. The iris root was attached anteriorly. Many anteriorly displaced, rudimentary ciliary processes arose directly from the posterior iris surface. The vitreous cavity contained hemorrhagic exudates and organized hemorrhage. Many retinal vessels were sclerosed (Fig. 9). The anterior retina showed mild gliosis.

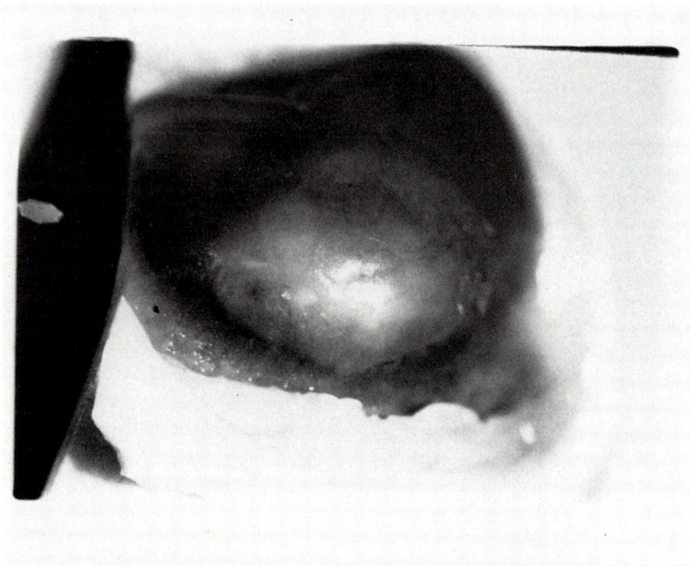

Fig. 6a. Gross appearance of corneal keloid in the fixed specimen.

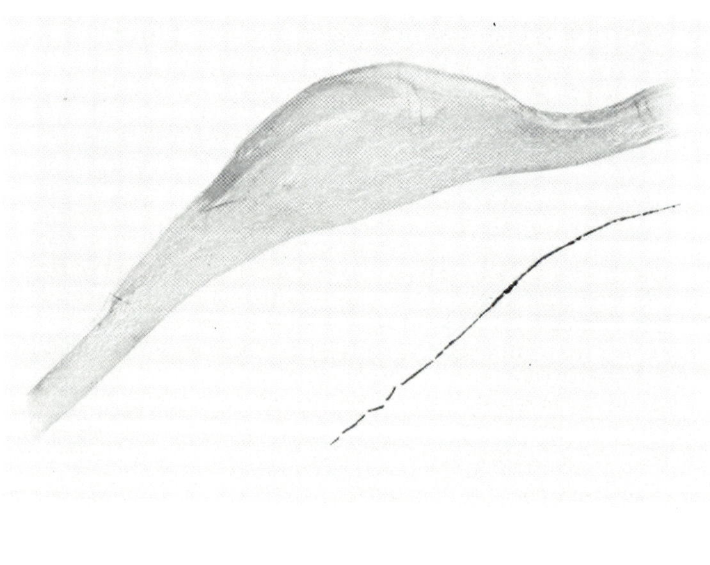

Fig. 6b. Corneal keloid right eye. (H + E x 16).

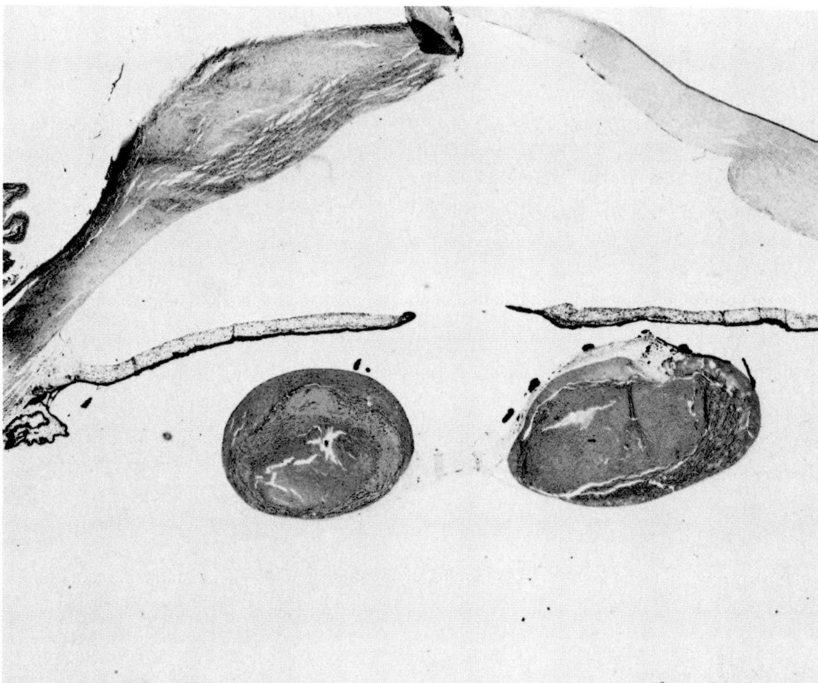

Fig. 7. Sectional view of the Soemmering's ring cataractous lens left eye. Note also the corneal keloid formation on the left side of the micrograph. Photomicrograph. x 16.

A 1 week old male infant unrelated to cases 1 and 2 had miotic pupils which failed to dilate (Fig. 10 and Fig. 11) and congenital cataracts. The patient had frontal bossing suggestive of Lowe's syndrome. The mother had significant lens opacities consistent with the carrier state of Lowe's. Pars plana lensectomy and anterior vitrectomy at 1 week of age yielded lens material which was nucleated (Fig. 12). Calcifications of the lens were also present.

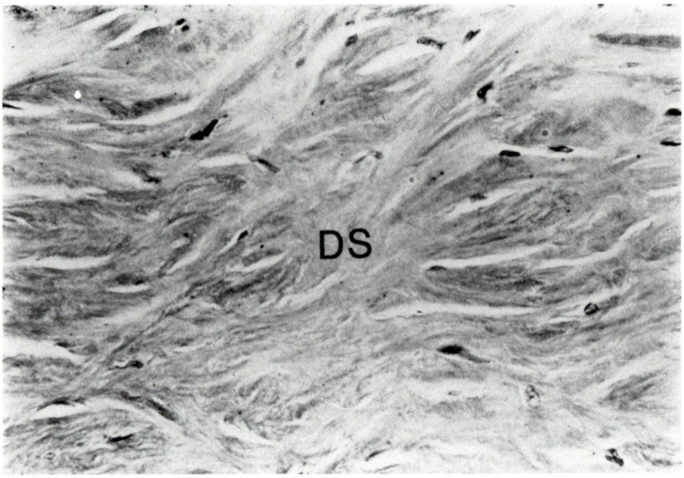

Fig. 8. Photomicrograph of deep regions of keloid which is avascular with irregularly arranged and interlacing bundles of collagenous lamellae and fibroplastic cells. (H+E x 450).

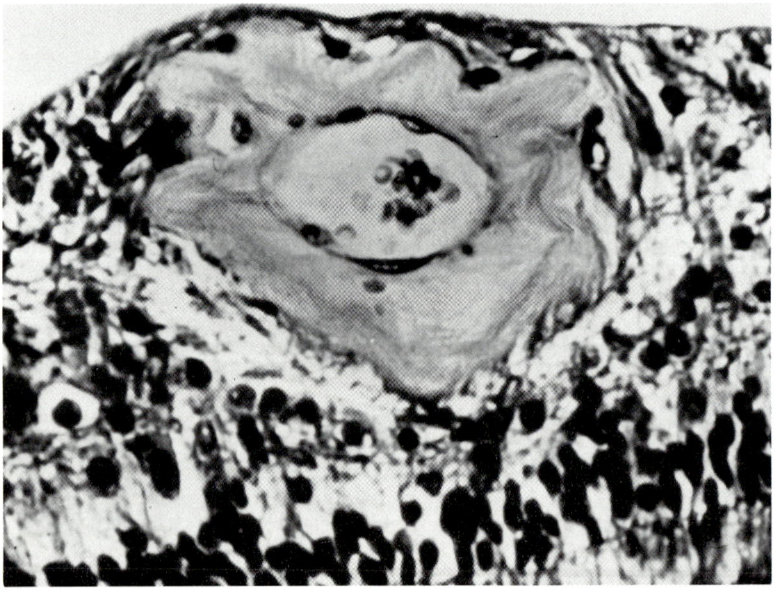

Fig. 9. Sclerosed retinal vessel. (Reticulin stain x 800).

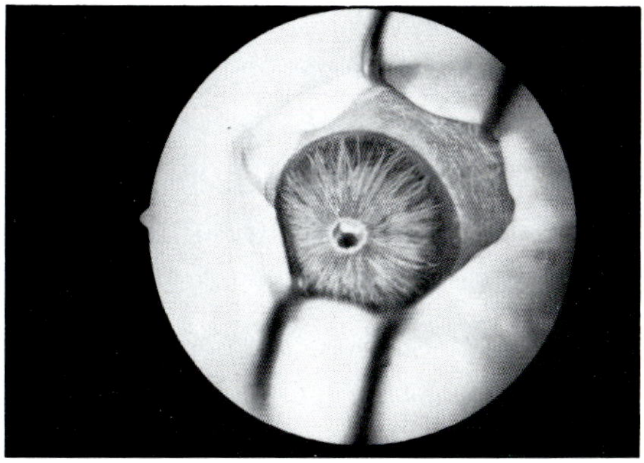

Fig. 10. Early iris fluorescein angiograph of case 3, note miosed pupil and fluorescein leakage at pupillary margin.

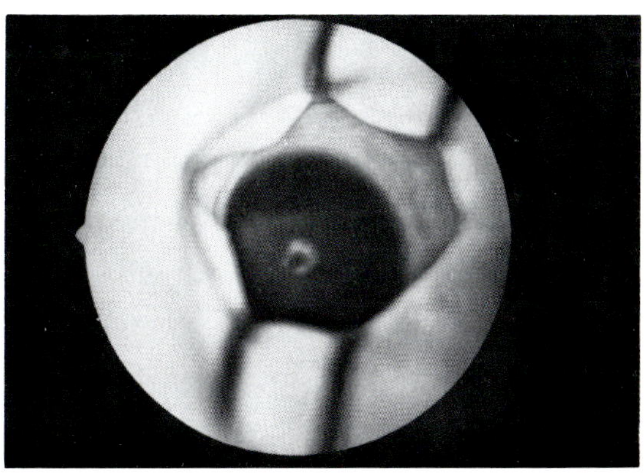

Fig. 11. Four seconds after photo of Fig. 10, there is marked extravasation of fluorescein into the anterior chamber.

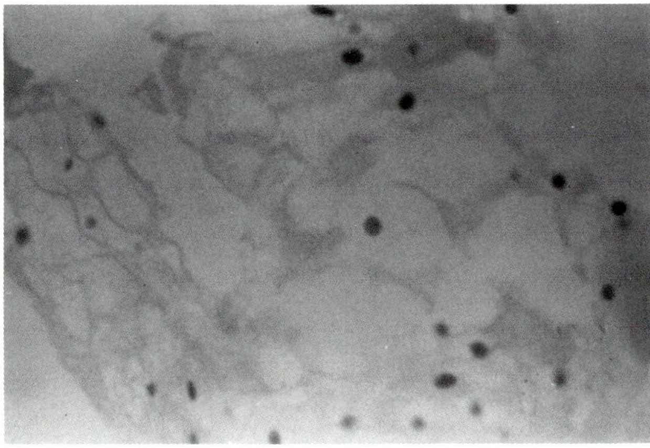

Fig. 12. Nucleated lens material from cataract surgery case 3. (H+E x 800).

Iris was adherrent to the lens capsule in some areas. Pre operative fluorescein angiography showed leakage of iris vessels with rapid extravasation of fluorescein into the anterior chamber (Fig. 10 and Fig. 11). Amino-aciduria was not present at the time of surgery but developed at 3 months of age.

Discussion

There is a striking similarity in the ocular histopathological features among our cases of Lowe's syndrome and those reported in the literature. The common features include a small, discoid, cataractous lens (Fig. 2) with peculiar capsular and epithelial changes,(Fig. 3 and Fig. 4) retained nuclei, (Fig. 12) posterior lenticonus adherent to condensed anterior vitreous, embryonic anterior chamber angle with anteriorly displaced ciliary processes, (Fig. 2 and Fig. 7) and Lange's folds (Francois and Hanssens 1963; Zimmerman and Font 1966; Curtin and others 1967; Lythgoe and Ramsey 1973; Johnson and Hiles 1976).

The cause for glaucoma in Lowe's syndrome is not known. It seems likely, however, that the embryonic anterior chamber angle, similar to that seen in primary congenital glaucoma, plays a role (Zimmerman and Font 1966; Curtin and others 1967; Yanoff and Fine 1975; Johnson and Hiles 1976). The miosis and resistance to mydriatics may be attributable to the segmental hypoplasia of the dilator pupillae muscle and its absence where the ciliary processes attached directly to the posterior iris surface and to posterior synechiae (Case 3). Sclerosis and hyalinization of retinal vessels (Fig. 9) seem to be part of a generalized vascular change seen in our second case. Whereas the proliferating lenticular cells probably contributed to the condensed anterior vitreous fibrils and the posterior polar opacity, this may also be related to a congenital vitreous abnormality (Francois and Hanssens 1963; Zimmerman and Font 1966; Curtin and others 1967; Johnson and Hiles 1976). Occasionally, remains of the hyaloid system have been commented upon (Johnson and Hiles 1976).

The small, discoid, cataractous lens is the most remarkable feature in Lowe's syndrome. The Sommering's ring configuration in one eye of our second patient probably resulted from inadvertent trauma to the lens during the goniotomy procedure. Spontaneous occurrance of Soemmering's ring has been reported in Lowe's (Ginsberg et al 1981). Although distinctive, the proliferation of a metaplastic epithelium and formation of aberrant collagenous and fibrillogranular material do not seem to be unique to Lowe's syndrome as similar changes have been reported in anterior polar and subcapsular cataracts (Lamb 1937; Henkind and Prose 1967; Yanoff and Fine 1975). Such changes have been also observed in a variety of complicated cataracts (R.C.T. - personal observation). The question why the lens capsule, made up predominantly of collagenous material, does not normally organize like the subcapsular fibrous material seems intimately related to the functional properties of the metaplastic epithelium.

The lack of demarcation between nucleus and cortex in patients with Lowe's syndrome is suggestive of a defect very early in the embryogenesis of the lens (Curtin and others 1967). Although the systemic metabolic and biochemical abnormalities in these patients are not detectable until after birth, it is possible that an as yet unidentified enzymatic or biochemical defect is already operative in the eye during the embryogenesis of the lens vesicle, and that the lenticular changes progress further because of an abnormal aqueous environment which may be brought about by the anatomically defective ciliary processes, the fenestrated capillaries in the peripheral iris, and enzymatic disturbances in the blood-aqueous barrier. A biochemical analysis of the aqueous humour and functional evaluation of the blood-aqueous barrier in these cases may prove rewarding. The rapid extravasation of fluorescein into the anterior chamber in case 3 supports such a mechanism.

Corneal keloids are rare lesions usually following significant perforating trauma often with iris incarceration (Smith 1940; Fenton 1964; Tredici 1964; Farkas 1968; O' Grady 1972; and Kirk 1972). In our opinion the histopathology of the corneal scar in Case 2 is most consistent with the dermatologic diagnosis of keloid. Some differences are noteworthy. In the current case, the deeper regions of the corneal keloid were characterized by the maturity and broad span of collagen fibers, reduced numbers of fibroblasts, poor vascularity, occasional inflammatory cells, and reduced amount of ground substance. In comparison, the anterior region of the corneal keloid showed certain features of the "Fibroblastic Stage" of a hypertrophic scar (Mancini 1962; and Quaiffe 1962). These included numerous young fibroblasts, with inclusions, many leaky vessels with perivascular reticulin, many inflammatory cells including mast cells and immature and arborizing collagen fibers. Abundant ground substance was also present. Histologic differences between deeper and superficial regions in corneal keloids were also noted by Smith (1940). Possibly the architectural pecularity of the cornea prevents true whorls and nodule formation characteristic of dermal keloids. Similarly the difference in the clinical appearance of the white corneal keloid verses the pink color of dermal keloid may be due to differences in vascularity and density of collagen stroma.

Case 2 confirms that the corneal lesions seen in Lowe's syndrome are keloids rather than band keratopathy or exposure keratitis. Why such a rare corneal lesion should be so common in Lowe's syndrome must somehow relate to the underlying condition. Minor surgical trauma from goniotomies performed in this case or tears in Descemet's membrane secondary to congenital glaucoma have not been reported to cause corneal keloids. Similarly the phenytoin (Dilantin) therapy thought to simulate collagen formation with gingival hyperplasia as in our patient has not previously been reported to cause corneal keloids. If any of these factors play a role in corneal keloid formation they would appear to be unique to Lowe's syndrome.

Based on the plasma profile of two cases of Lowe's syndrome, Cotlier suggested that increased levels of amino acids, perhaps tyrosine, could cause corneal keloids in Lowe's syndrome. However, in most cases of Lowe's syndrome the plasma level of amino acids are normal and aminoaciduria is considered secondary to the renal defect. Even if plasma levels of amino acids were not elevated, the total delivery could be high because of the leaky nature of the new corneal vessels. It is equally possible though that the new corneal vessels allow passage of other unknown noxious substances that induce excessive fibrous tissue proliferation.

The presence of anteriorly-placed and rudimentary ciliary processes, many attached to the posterior iris surface and supplied by fenestrated capillaries, implies that the blood-aqueous barrier in our patient was defective. This situation, compounded by the degenerate endothelium, can allow seepage of abnormal aqueous into the corneal stroma. The extent of endothelial decompensation may then determine the span and location of the corneal keloid. Alternatively, it may be argued that unknown or inadvertent trauma to the anterior cornea together with corneal exposure during sleep, induced the formation of the hyperplastic scar.

Having recognized the pathology of the corneal lesions in Lowe's syndrome as representing corneal keloids, what suggestions can be made of management? Certainly these are benign and not malignant lesions. The deep stromal involvement defeats lamellar keratoplasty. Penetrating keratoplasty in difficult and young patients would seem equally impractical. Pressure therapy has had variable success in established and developing dermal hypertrophic scars(Larson et al 1971; Robertson et al 1980). The persistance of mast cells in the corneal keloid of this case suggests that suppression of inflammation by topical corticosteroids and control of mast cell degranulation by disodium cromoglycate may be useful.

GLAUCOMA IN

Sturge
blood vesse
almological
The associa
was first d
described a
the above.
patients.

Previo
Syndrome wa
chamber ang
always been
Syndrome
not possibl
of this dia
urements of
lization of

Goniot
tion of cho
chamber ang
1976, the f
trabeculoto
bal base fl
noted. Bec
lack of goo
solely on t
beculectomy
quently, an

Cotlier E
Errors
Natl. F
Ser., V
Farkas T,
66:319-
Fenton R,
loids).
Francois J
Frederique
rubeola
Ginsberg J
of the
Ped Oph
Henkind P,
Holmes GE,
A four
living
Johnson B,
Lamb H (19
Larson DL,
Technic
in the
Lowe C, Te
164.
Lythgoe C,
Mancini RE
tally p
O'Grady RE
73:206-
Robertson
sure th
municat
Smith H (1
38:519-
Tripathi I
ocular
Warburg M
ed. J
Yanoff M,
atlas.
Zimmerman

REPRINT RE
Eye Re
939 Ea

nation has been performed. In the last five years I have examined six children with Sturge-Weber Syndrome and have performed five trabeculectomies on four children. The following is a report of the clinical and histological findings of these patients.

FINDINGS:

Age: When first seen the age range was from four months to eight years.

Sex: Four of the patients were girls and two were boys.

Mental Retardation: Three of the six children were mentally retarded.

Convulsive Disorder: Three of the six children were on anticonvulsive medications. One who was not, had a normal computerized axial tomogram of the head. All who had convulsive disorders were mentally retarded.

Glaucoma: Elevated intraocular pressure was present in five of the six children. Two children who were old enough to cooperate for visual field examination were found to have characteristic abnormalities of open angle glaucoma. Four cases were unilateral and one was bilateral. In each instance, involvement of the upper lid with an hemangioma was associated with glaucoma. Four right eyes and two left eyes had glaucoma. Prominent episcleral vessels were present in every eye with glaucoma (fig one).

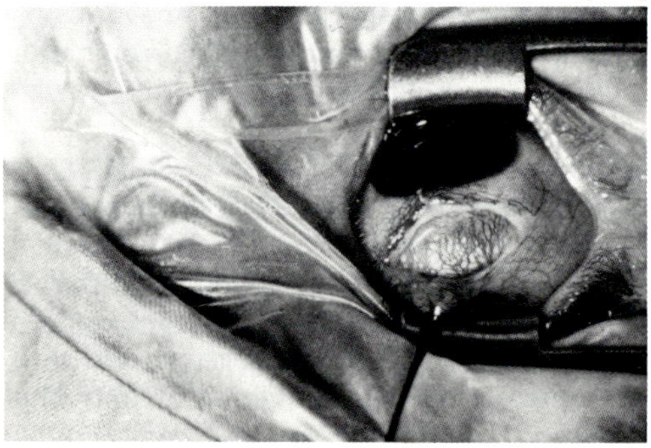

Fig. one Episcleral hemangioma

Gonioscopy showed no specific abnormalities. Although, blood was observed in some patients in Schlemm's canal.

Follow up observations have ranged from seven months to five years.

MANAGEMENT:

One of the six patients was stabilized on medical management for a while, but has recently shown progressive visual field loss and will require surgery. The remaining four patients who had glaucoma, have had surgery. All patients had elevated intraocular pressure and increased cup/disc ratio. In patients who are old enough to cooperate for visual field testing, visual field abnormalities characteristic of open angle glaucoma were found. In three instances, an excisional trabeculectomy was performed and in the fourth a thermal trabeculectomy was performed. All patients have had normalization of intraocular pressure and reduction of the cup/disc ratio. The infants had normalization of the cup/disc ratio while the older children had reduction of the cup/disc ratio, but did not return to normal. In three instances, complications occured. Following the creation of the trabeculectomy fistula site and peripheral iridectomy, ciliary processes and lens zonules prolapsed into the wound in one case and two other times prolapse of the ciliary processes into the fistula site occured. The first time that this occured the zonules broke with the presentation of vitreous into the wound. A vitrectomy was performed behind the lens and post-operatively the patient has done well. In the second case irrigation with a balanced salt solution was sufficient to allow closure of the scleral flap without incarceration of the ciliary processes and post-operative examinations under anesthesia in both of these instances have shown a patent fistula site without incarceration of the ciliary processes. The last such complication occured seven months ago and was managed by using Healon to push the ciliary processes back into their normal position. Post-operative gonioscopy of this child showed a patent fistula and no incarceration of the processes.

PATHOLOGY:

Using light and electron microscopy no evidence of an anterior chamber membrane has been found. However, in every case examined abnormal episcleral vessels were present (Alvarado 1981) (fig two).

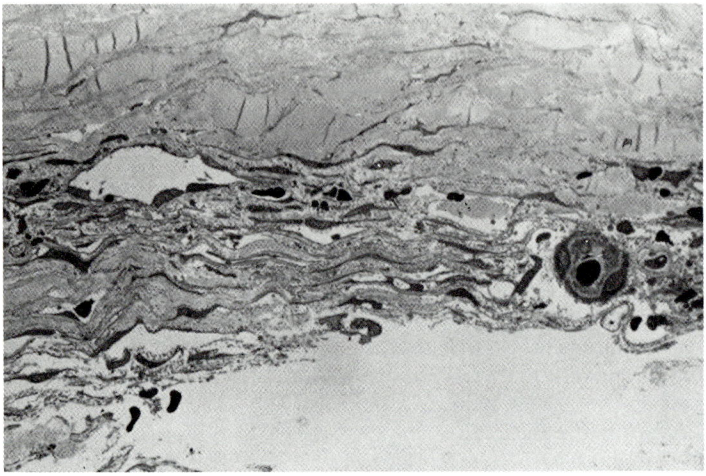

Fig. 2 - Light microscopy of trabecular meshwork

DISCUSSION:

The previous poor prognosis for the management of glaucoma in patients with Sturge-Weber Syndrome is due to the inappropriate surgical procedure being performed. A better understanding of the pathophysiology of this disease has led to a better prognosis. In 1977, Hiles reported success with trabeculectomy in adolescent patients with glaucoma and Sturge-Weber Syndrome. Phelps reported four successful trabeculotomies but did not state the age of the patients (Phelps 1978).

Two of the complications noted in my series occured prior to the report of intraoperative choroidal effusion (Bellows, Chylack, Epstein, Hutchinson 1979). Healon was not generally in use at the time of that report and offers an alternative to posterior sclerostomy.

In conclusion, pathological examination of trabeculectomy specimens supports the hypothesis that glaucoma which occurs in Sturge-Weber Syndrome is on the basis of elevated episcleral venous pressure. Surgery based on this hypothesis has been successful in infants and children.

ACKNOWLEDGEMENTS:

Grateful acknowledgement is given to:
Jorge Alvarado, M.D. for electron microscopy done under research grants #EY-02162A;#EY-02068
Thomas F. Minas, M.D. and Thomas F. Moore, M.D. for patient referrals and to
Georgiana G. Burke for assistance.

REFERENCES:

Alvarado, J (1981) Personal communication
Bellows AR, Chylack Jr LT, Epstein DL, Hutchinson BT (1979) Choroidal effusion during glaucoma surgery in patients with prominent episcleral vessels. Arch Ophthalmol 97(3):493-7.
Chandler PA, Grant WM (1965). "Lectures in Glaucoma." Philadelphia: Lea and Febiger.
Keverline PO, Hiels DA (1977). Trabeculectomy for adolescent onset glaucoma in Struge-Weber Syndrome. J Pediatr Ophthalmol 13:144-48.
Knapp (1927). Trans Am Ophthal Soc 25:154.
Minas TF, Podos SM (1968). Familial glaucoma associated with episcleral venous pressure. Arch Ophthalmol 80: 202-208.
Phelps CD (1978). The pathenogenesis of glaucoma in Sturge-Weber Syndrome. Ophthalmology 85(3): 276-86.
Phelps LP, Armaly MF (1978). Measurement of episcleral venous pressure. Am J Ophthal 85:35.
Schirmer R (1860). Ein fall von tenlangiektasie. Albrecht von Graefes Arch Klen Ophthalmol 7: 119-121.
Shaeffer RN, Weiss DI (1970. "Congenital and Pediatric Glaucoma. " St. Louis: C.V. Mosby, pp 45-47.
Sturge WA (1879). A case of partial epilepsy apparently due to a lesion of the vasomotor centres of the brain. Trans Clin Soc Lond 12: 162-67.
Weiss DI (1973). Dual origin of glaucoma in encephalotrigeminal hemangionatosis. Trans Ophthalmol Soc UK 93:477-491.

EYEGROUND MALFORMATIONS IN THE FETAL ALCOHOL SYNDROME

Kerstin Strömland

Department of Ophthalmology, Sahlgrens Hospital

S-413 45 Göteborg, Sweden

ABSTRACT

The fetal alcohol syndrome (FAS) occurs in children born by alcoholic mothers. The syndrome consists of growth deficiency of prenatal onset, central nervous system effects with retarded mental and motor development and malformations of various organs, the most striking being the facial abnormities. There is a small head circumference and midfacial deformities. Typical eye features are telecanthus, epicanthus, short palpebral fissures, a flat nose bridge, ptosis, microphthalmus and strabismus. 30 children with FAS were examined for defects of the inner parts of the eyes. Malformations of the optic discs and retinal vessels were the most frequent findings, occurring in 16 children. Another five children had borderline findings. Nine had bilateral hypoplasia of the optic discs, eight of them also with changes of the retinal vessels, most often increased tortuousity. Four children showed bilateral optic atrophy. One of them also had highly tortuous retinal vessels. One girl had very tortuous retinal vessels without other findings in her fundi. One boy had pronounced malformations of both eyebulbs and another boy had bilateral changes of his eyeground structures. Various intraocular malformations were observed in 53% of the children with FAS.

Key words

Fetal alcohol syndrome, Fundus malformations, Optic nerve hypoplasia, Optic atrophy, Retinal vessels.

Birth Defects: Original Article Series, Volume 18, Number 6, pages 651–655

INTRODUCTION

The fetal alcohol syndrome - FAS - occurs in children born by alcoholic mothers and consists of growth deficiency, mental and motor retardation and malformations of various parts of the body (Jones et al 1973). It has been estimated that 1 child per 600 births has the full syndrome, while 1 child out of 300 has some alcohol related birth defects. Hence the incidence of FAS is alarmingly high.

The growth deficiency is of prenatal onset and the children generally do not catch up during childhood.

There are several nervous system effects with retarded mental and motor development of different degrees. Cerebral palsy, clumsiness, ataxia, tremolousness occurs and the children have a typical behavior with hyperactivity, poor attention span and difficulties in perception.

The malformations affect different parts of the body, the most striking being the facial anomalies. There is microcephalus, asymmetry of the face and midfacial deformities. Typical eye features are telecanthus, epicanthus, short palpebral fissures, moderate ptosis, a flat broad nose bridge and maxillar hypoplasia. Microphthalmus may occur, usually unilaterally. Strabismus is common.

MATERIALS AND METHODS

This is a report about findings in the fundi of 30 children with FAS (Strömland 1981). 14 are from Helsinki Finland, and 16 from Göteborg Sweden, 7 girls, 23 boys, aged from one month to 16 years. The mothers all had a history of severe alcohol abuse during pregnancy. The diagnosis was made by pediatricians with a special experience in this syndrome.

RESULTS

The most frequent findings were malformations of the optic nerves and the retinal vessels with 16 out of 30 children affected. (Table 1).

TABLE 1

Fundus malformations in 30 children with FAS

Hypoplasia of the optic nerves		9
abnormal retinal vessels	8	
normal retinal vessels	1	
Atrophy of the optic nerves		4
abnormal retinal vessels	1	
normal retinal vessels	3	
Abnormality of the retinal vessels		1
Malformations of the anterior and posterior segments		1
Malformations of the total fundus		1
Total		16

13 children - 43% - had bilateral changes of the optic nerve head, 9 of them had hypoplasia and 4 optic atrophy. One had malformations of her retinal vessels. One child had pronounced malformations of both bulbs, and another had malformations of the posterior parts of the eyes. Hence 53% of the children had eyeground malformations.

Nine children had a pronounced bilateral hypoplasia of the optic nerves. The optic nerve head was extremely small with irregular margins and pallor. In eight children the retinal vasculature was abnormal, most often with an increased tortuosity of the vessels. In one girl the vessels nearly covered all disc tissue resembling a racemosum hemangioma. Fluoresceinangiography showed the discs to be hypoplastic. Refraction varied from -13 diopters to +1 diopters. Vision below 0.3 (20/70) was observed in all eyes with hypoplasia but one. This eye showed a less pronounced hypoplasia with visual acuity 0.8 (20/25).

Four children had optic atrophy in both eyes. One of them showed tortuosity and early branching of the vessels covering most of the tissue of the very pale discs. Vision acuity could not be measured in these children because of low age but none gave the impression of severely reduced vision. Refraction could be measured in two children and was +4 diopters both eyes in one child and -1 diopters both eyes in the other.

Five children had small optic discs with normal colour but with more distinct borders than normally found and without nerve fiber bundles and vessels crowded on the disc margins. Visual acuity was normal or slightly reduced. This could be minimal hypoplasia of the optic nerve.

Hypoplasia of the optic nerve has been reported more frequently during the last years. The etiology remains obscure in most cases. Prenatal infections, anticonvulsant drugs, toxic agents like Quinine, maternal diabetes, some inherited malformation syndromes like septo-optic dysplasia occur together with hypoplasia. Hypoplasia was observed so often in these children with FAS - 30% - that it does not seem to be an accidental occurrence but suggests that alcohol is a cause of underdevelopment of the optic nerve.

One girl had increased tortuosity of her retinal vessels. There was no obvious malformation of other eyeground structures although her discs were thought to be hypoplastic.

One boy with severe motor and mental retardation had glaucoma, malformations of the anterior chamber angle, cataract and pronounced malformation of his entire eyegrounds. There was a pupillary reaction to light in one eye only.

One boy had malformations of his right fundus structures. The disc was deformed and the temporal peripapillary tissue had a white atrophic appearence. The retina was very thin, the macula was not discernible and the retinal vessels were very tortuous. Refraction was -16 diopters and vision was fingercounting only. The fellow eye showed a pale disc of normal size, tortuous vessels and two cilioretinal arteries. Refraction was -8 diopters, visual acuity 0.5 (20/40). The retina was very thin.

We do not know when alcohol affects the foetus or the quantity of alcohol required to produce defects in the foetus but we believe that a daily intake of alcohol during periods of the pregnancy is required to produce defects. The brain and the eye has proved to be especially vulnerable to alcohol.

Various malformations of the optic nerves and retinal vessels were observed in 53% of children with the fetal alcohol syndrome, which means that we have to consider these of great value in diagnosing the syndrome. FAS has a close connection to ophthalmologists because of the abnormalities observed both in the outer and the inner parts of the eyes and the effects of reduced vision in the affected children.

REFERENCES

Jones K, Smith D, Ulleland C, Pytkowicz Streissguth A (1973). Pattern of malformation in offspring of chronic alcoholic mothers. Lancet I:1267-1271.

Strömland K (1981). Eyeground malformations in the fetal alcohol syndrome. Neuropediatrics 12:97-98.

The main purpose of the work was to get as exactly as possible an estimate of the number of blind and partially sighted persons and causes of blindness in a selected area of Norway. In order to get this as acurate as possible, all available sources were made use of such as different sorts of card index of registered blind and partially sighted, radio, newspaper etc. Also an extensive field service was done (Odland 1977).

It was found that 1441 were visually impaired with vision of 6/18 or less, that is 0.38 % of the total population. There were a high frequency of hereditary diseases (29.6 %). A number of 493 had some type of retinal disease. Of these 140 (9.7 %) were caused by a disease with a hereditary factor or possible hereditary factor. The purpose of this paper is to study more in detail what types of hereditary diseases this last group represents and its distribution among the inhabitants.

Senile macular degeneration was the cause of impaired vision in 264 cases. Among these there were 25 who had other members of the family with the same condition. It was mostly scattered single cases and therefore not possible to trace any inheritance. This number is possible too small. Some knew there had been or still were members of the family who developed impaired vision in old age, but did not know anything about the cause.

Retinitis pigmentosa was seen in 71 persons. Among these 35 had other family members with retinitis pigmentosa and these were distributed in 9 families. Five of these had their origin in a community on an island with 9854 inhabitants. Although it was only possible to trace a relationship between 3 of these families, it is reasonable to assume that a relationship between all these pedigrees really existed far back in time. The parents were blood-related in 24 cases, and 2 persons had one of the parents with the same illness. According to Francois (Francois 1961) recessive inheritance is the most common type of transmission, and this was also found in this material. Fig. 2 shows the pedigree which had the highest number of affected members. One notice the high frequency of consanguinity.

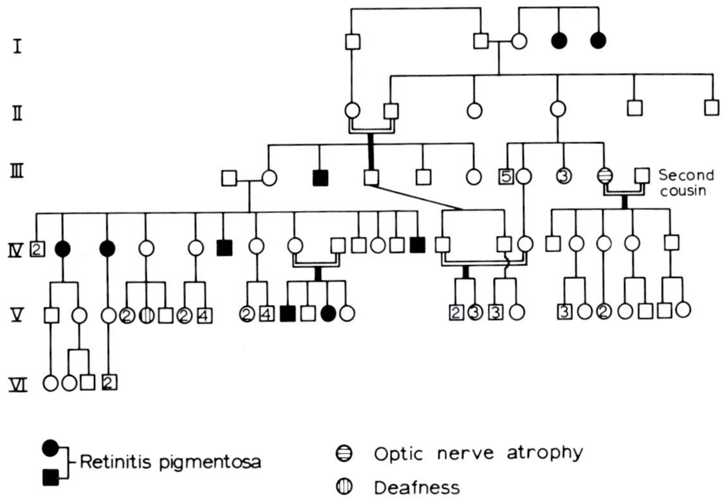

Fig. 2. Pedigree of a family with retinitis pigmentosa.

Three had Laurence-Moon-Biedl syndrome. Two men, 66-years-old, were twins and totally blind. They had both 6 toes. Their retina had a retinitis pigmentosa like picture. The other case was a 25-year-old-woman. She also had typical changes in the retina. She had obesity and was slightly mentally retarded. She had 5 fingers and toes, but a deceased older brother had the same condition,and he had 6 fingers.

Congenital amaurosis (Leber) was diagnosed in 6 cases. This number is probably too small and some persons registered under the heading of retinitis pigmentosa, might have belonged to this group. One family where the parents were blood-related, had 3 boys who were blind from this disease.

There was one family with gyrate choroidal atrophy living on a small island. Fig. 3 shows the pedigree of this family.

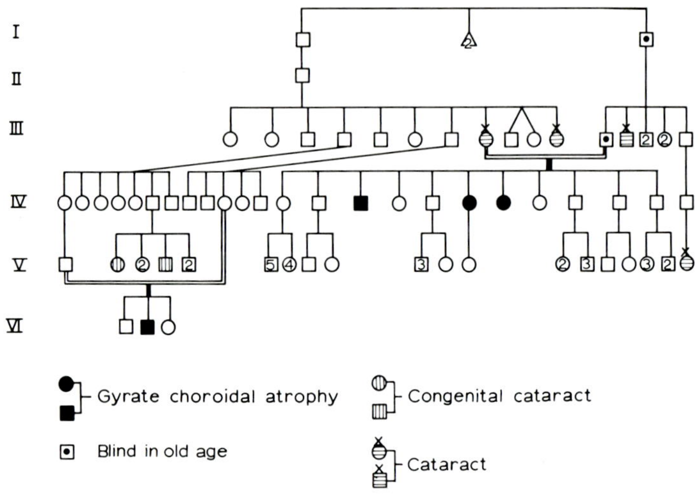

Fig. 3. Pedigree of a family with gyrate choroidal atrophy

One notices that other eye defects are also present such as congenital cataract, other types of cataract and loss of vision in old age. The members in the 4th generation noticed the first symptoms of visual disturbance in school age. The boy in 6th generation had already fundus changes when he was seen at the age of 3 years. One of the women was operated on for cataract without improvement of vision. They all had marked degenerative changes in the retina. The sclera was whitish exposed peripherally and only an island centrally showed some degree of normal colour (Fig. 4). They all had reduced vision to fingercounting in 1 meter or less, and their visual field was reduced to tunnel field. The boy in the 6th generation, when he was seen the first time, had more typical atrophic areas with scallopped margins and polygonal figures. Later when he was seen 15 years old, he had almost the same massive atrophic changes as the others. He had vision 6/24. All the affected members had marked hearing defects as well.

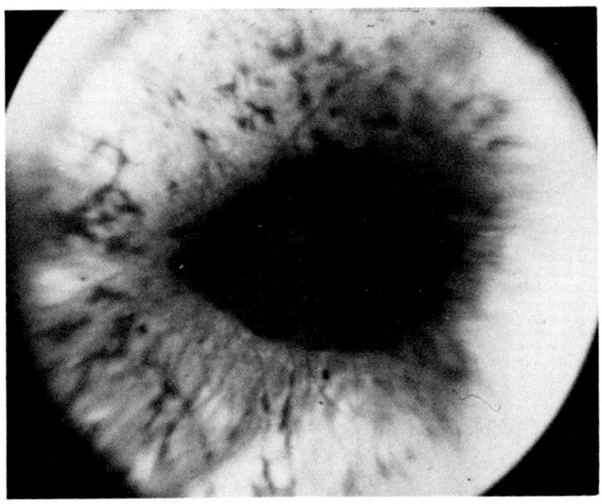

Fig. 4. Fundus at an advanced stage of gyrate choroidal atrophy.

There was also found other types of hereditary retinal degeneration where the macular region was mostly involved, 16 persons altogether. In this group belongs a family with Stargardt's disease, 2 brothers and 1 sister. The disease started at school age, and they were now in the age of 49-56 years. They all had marked degenerative changes localized to the macular region. The vision was reduced to fingercounting in 2 - 3 meters. This family was related to a family where many members were blind because of high myopia.

Another family with a hereditary macular degeneration we see on fig. 5. The members in the 4th generation were all visually impaired. The disease started at the age of 15 years. The 2 oldest women who are now around 25 years have marked macular changes almost with an oedematous appearance. The vision was reduced to fingercounting in 1 - 2 meters. The youngest sister had normal fundus. Her vision was only slightly reduced, but the visual field had concentric limitation. On their father's side there were 2 persons with marked reduced vision from childhood. On the mother's side 1 had glaucoma and 1 was almost blind from choroidal sclerosis.

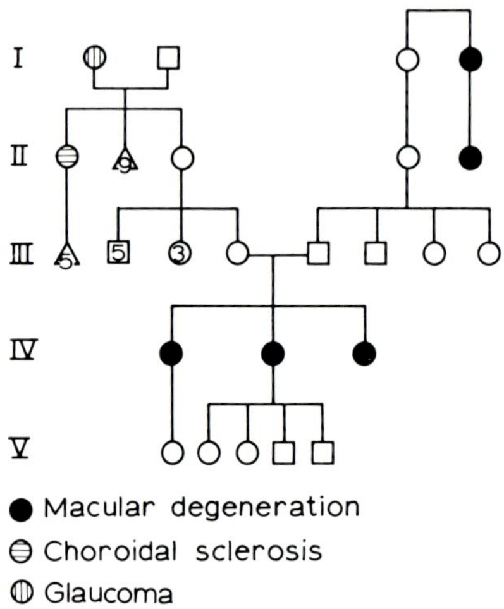

Fig. 5. Pedigree of a family with a hereditary macular degeneration.

There was also a family with marked choroidal sclerosis. The affected members were 2 brothers and 2 sisters and their vision was reduced to finger counting.

Congenital retinoschisis is a relative rare disease. One family with 9 affected members was encountered and the pedigree is shown in fig. 6. This condition has a sex-linked recessive inheritance. The vision in all the members in the 2nd generation had almost been stable the last 20 years varying from finger counting in 4 meters to 6/36 in the youngest person.

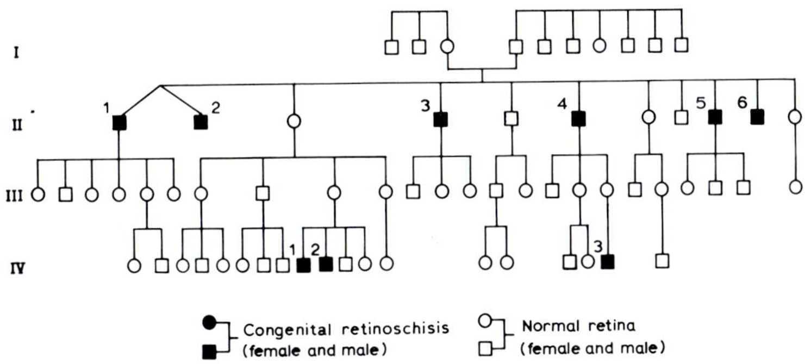

Fig. 6. Pedigree of a family with congenital retinoschisis.

Fig. 7 shows the typical starfigure in the macula in case 2 in 4th generation. Later when degenerative changes takes place, there may be marked

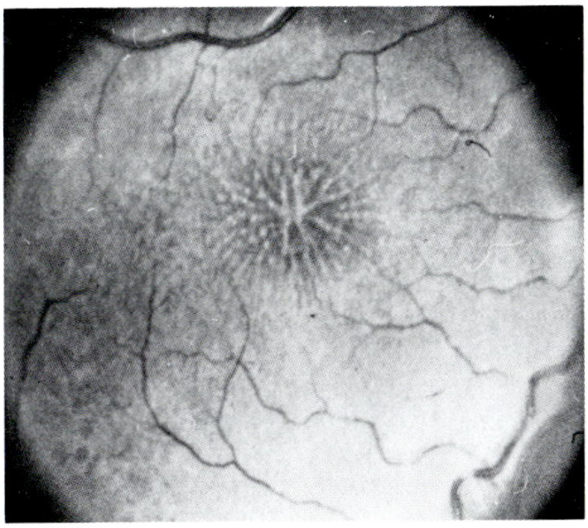

Fig. 7. Typical stellate figure in the macula in a young person with congenital retinoschisis.

atrophy (fig. 8 and 9) and the diagnosis may be difficult to establish. Area of peripheral schisis was only seen in 2 persons. The disease is thoroughly described by Vainio-Mattila et al. (1969).

Fig. 8

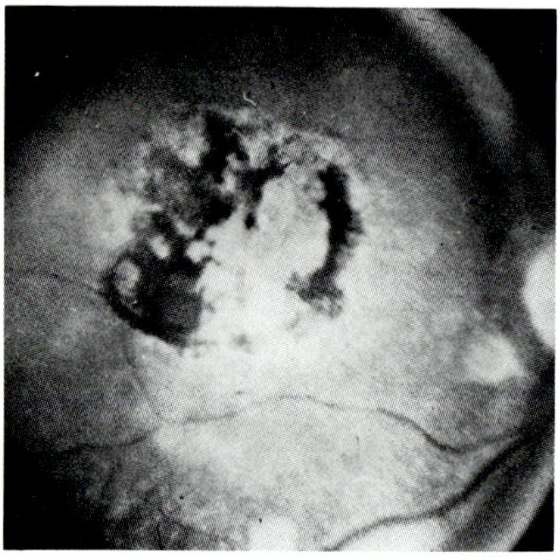

Fig. 9

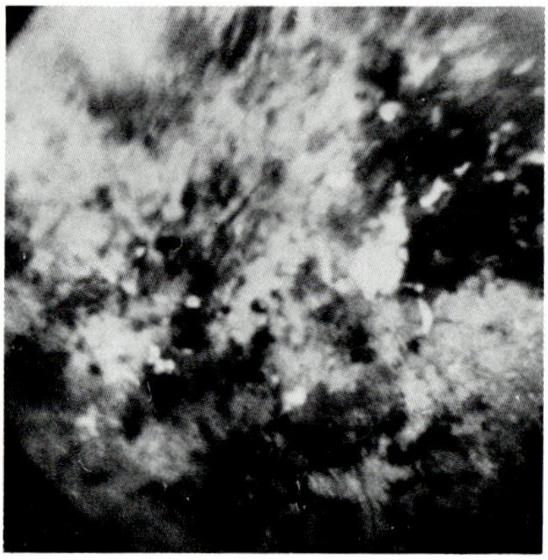

Fig. 8 and 9. Marked atrophic macular scar and more general degenerative changes in 2 patients with congenital retinoschisis.

Five children had Spielmeyer-Vogts disease. Two of them were sisters. They all were in the age of 9-15 years. Relationship between their parents could not be traced. The grandmother of one child was related to a family where 3 children had died from this disease.

One boy was blind of bilateral retinoblastoma.

Retinal detachment was the cause of blindness and partially sightness in 27 persons. In 23 cases the detachment was bilateral. The cause of the detachment was due to a primary retinal degeneration in 5 cases. The pedigree seen in fig. 10 had 4 persons with retinal detachment, and the cause was lattice degeneration. In the other the detachment was caused by trauma, congenital cataract, Marfans syndrome and ectopic lens.

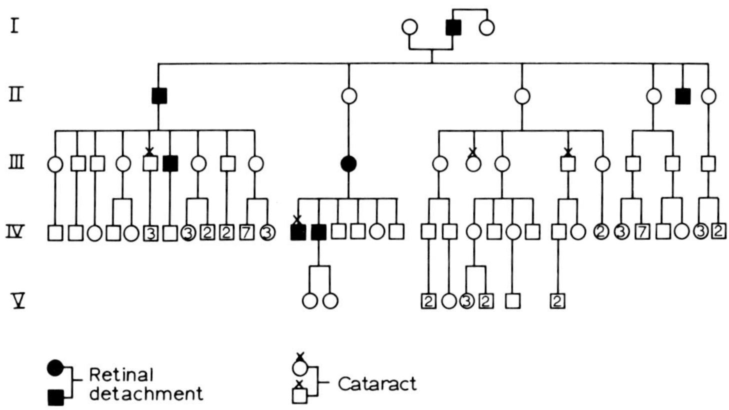

Fig. 10. Pedigree of a family with retinal detachment due to lattice degeneration.

Comments

One quite frequently noticed that in a family with a certain type of hereditary eye disease, other hereditary eye diseases were also seen. The explanation for this phenomenon must be that because of blood-relation, genes must be present among the family members which are responsible for several eye diseases.

When we look at the topographical aspect of Hordaland county where there is a lot of islands and fjords that makes many areas isolated, it is reasonable to believe that inter-marriages do not infrequently occur, and diseases with recessive inheritance may appear. Because of this one might assume that we here have an excess of hereditary eye diseases. But the whole coastline has more or less the same topographical condition. In south and east Norway there are a number of vallyes which are separated by mountain ridges. Because of this there is no reason to believe that we here have a greater representation of hereditary eye diseases compared to the rest of the country. A study of blindness due to retinitis pigmentosa from east Norway shows almost the same frequency as was found here (INAS 1975).

From available statistics it seems that Norway may have a somewhat higher frequency of inherited eye diseases than Sweden (Lindstedt 1969) and England (Sorsby 1966). In Canada, however, there is a statistical record (Mac Donald 1965) where the same criterion of blindness was applied as in this study, and it was found a slightly higher frequency of inherited eye diseases than in Norway.

References

Francois J (1961). "Heredity in Ophthalmology". St. Louis: Mosby, p. 441.

Institutt for anvendt sosialvitenskapelig forskning (INAS 1975): Sosialmedisinsk undersøkelse av blinde i Hedmark, INAS arbeidsrapport nr. 20, Oslo.

Lindstedt E (1969). Causes of blindness in Sweden. Acta Ophthalmol (Kbh), suppl. 104.

MacDonald AE (1966). Causes of blindness in Canada: An analysis of 24605 cases registered with Canadian Institute for the Blind. Canad Med Ass J 92:264.

Odland M (1977). "Svaksyn og blindhet i Bergen og Hordaland". En medisinsk og sosialmedisinsk undersøkelse. Thesis Univ Bergen.

Sorsby A (1966). The incidence and causes of

blindness in England and Wales 1963-1968. Rep Health and Soc Subj (Lond) 128.

Vainio-Mattila B, Eriksson AW and Forsius H (1969). X-chromosomal recessive retinoschisis in the region of Pori. Acta Ophthalmol (Kbh) 47: 1135.

DISTRIBUTION OF COMMON EYE DISEASES IN THE FAMILIES OF NORWEGIAN TWINS

W.E. Nance, L.A. Corey, J.A. Boughman, K. Berg, P. Magnus
Medical College of Virginia, Richmond , Va., U.S.A. and Institute of Medical Genetics, Oslo, Norway

INTRODUCTION

Progress in genetics has depended to a remarkable extent upon the identification and exploitation of research paradigms that are inherently capable of resolving the many known and postulated causes for biologic variation. In human genetics, studies of the families of twins--including the twins, their spouses and offspring--constitute a powerful research design that can provide insight into the causes and consequences of nonrandom mating, and the existence of maternal effects, as well as a more incisive separation of genetic and environmental effects than has heretofore been possible. In this paper, we show how an analysis of the distribution of common eye diseases in the families of twins can lead to the recognition of important new etiologic mechanisms that may contribute to the pathogenesis and frequency of these traits in the population.

MATERIALS AND METHODS

Research Design

Familial aggregation can arise from either genetic or environmental causes which may be distinguished by contrasting the patterns of similarity displayed by individuals who share either a common exposure to various aspects of the environment or different degrees of genetic covariation. The families of twins contain pairs of indi-

Birth Defects: Original Article Series, Volume 18, Number 6, pages 669–678

viduals who possess many different social and biological relationships to each other (Nance and Corey, 1976), and it is the presence of this large array of distinct relationships within each family unit that accounts for the power and efficiency of this research design (Moll and Sing, 1979). For example, although the offspring of identical twins may be considered cousins socially, they are related genetically in the same way as half-siblings and share one quarter of their genes. The offspring of a single twin are, of course, full siblings to each other and share one half of their genes. Finally the identical twin parents share all of their genes, while the spouses of twins are usually genetically unrelated. Husbands and wives can resemble one another either because of the common home environment that they share or because of nonrandom mate selection. As described more fully later, assortative mating can have a dramatic influence on the distribution of phenotypes in the offspring generation, and an analysis of the multiple correlations that exist among monozygotic (MZ) or dizygotic (DZ) twins and their spouses permits a detailed resolution of the genetic, environmental and sex-limited causes for nonrandom mate selection (Nance, 1979a; Nance et al., 1981; Eaves and Heath, 1981). A unique feature of the twin family design is its ability to detect maternal effects by contrasting the similarity of the half-sib offspring of female MZ twins with the offspring of male pairs, whose mothers are genetically unrelated. Maternal effects can arise from cytoplasmic differences, from genetic or environmental influences in the intrauterine environment provided by the mother, or from any aspect of postnatal nurture, care or training that is provided by the mother. Some idea of the relative contribution of genetic factors to maternal effects can be gained by a comparison of the correlated maternal effects in MZ and DZ twins, whereas a formal resolution of cytoplasmic influences from other types of maternal effects can be achieved by extending the analysis to the grandchildren of twins (Corey, Nance, and Berg, 1978). Although the twin family design is ideally suited to the analysis of continuously distributed metric traits (Nance, Corey, and Boughman, 1978), it may also be applied to qualitative or discontinuous traits (Golden, 1980) and can readily be extended to multivariate analyses (Cantor, 1981). Procedures have previously been described for the joint analysis of the multiple relationships contained within the families of twins by least squares or maximum likelihood methods (Nance, 1979b; Cantor et al.,

1981). These techniques can be used to test hypotheses about the latent causes of phenotypic variation as well as to estimate genetic and environmental parameters of interest.

Subject Population

In 1978, a clinical survey of a large sample of adult Norwegian twins was initiated. As part of that study, zygosity, health status and reproductive history questionnaires were sent to all living members of twin pairs born between 1915 and 1960 whose current addresses could be located in the Norwegian population registry. The zygosity of the twins was determined from their responses to a series of questions by a decision tree that correctly identified the zygosity of 98 percent of the twins in a control series of 208 pairs in whom zygosity had been independently determined by extensive blood typing (Golden, 1980). The health status questionnaire specifically requested information about the presence or absence of nearsightedness, farsightedness, astigmatism, glaucoma, cataract and squint in the parents, siblings, and offspring of the twins and their spouses, as well as the twins and spouses themselves. The present report is based on a subset of 742 of these twin kinships in which completed questionnaires had been received from both twins and both spouses as of May, 1981. The questionnaire responses of twins generally showed a high degree of concordance with respect to the reported occurrence of eye diseases in family members. Although this finding provides a unique measure of the reliability of the questionnaire, we have as yet made no attempt in these preliminary studies to establish the validity of questionnaire responses either by independent clinical evaluations or by a review of medical records.

RESULTS

As shown in Table 1, the six ocular defects about which we inquired occurred rather frequently in this population sample, with more than half the kinships reporting at least one of these conditions in one or more family members. Of the six conditions, nearsightedness, farsightedness and astigmatism were reported with sufficient fre-

TABLE 1: Common Eye Diseases Reported Among 10,183 Members of the Families of 742 Norwegian Twin Pairs

Condition	Families with affected		Reported prevalence	
	Number	Percent	Adults* (N=7420)	Offspring (N=2763)
Nearsightedness	381	51.3	0.0701	0.0560
Astigmatism	352	47.4	0.0592	0.0398
Farsightedness	257	34.6	0.0447	0.0184
Squint	178	24.0	0.0128	0.0264
Cataracts	167	22.5	0.0245	0.0004
Glaucoma	84	11.3	0.0111	0.0000

*Includes twins, spouses and parents of twins and spouses

quency in both the parents and offspring to warrant further analysis.

Normal refraction results from an interaction of multiple components of the visual system. Previous studies have shown that variation in each of the relevant elements, including the sphericity of the cornea, the depth of the anterior chamber, the optical properties of the lens and the length of the optical axis of the eye, can generally be well described by normal distribution curves (Francois, 1961). Although monogenic syndromes that include myopia, hypermetropia or astigmatism as pleiotropic features are known (McKusick, 1978), it seems plausible, in view of the physiologic basis of refraction, to regard at least the less severe forms of myopia and hypermetropia as polygenic threshold traits.

Table 2 summarizes the reported distribution of these three defects in the twins themselves. The reported concordance rates ranged from 49 to 66 percent in the monozygotic twins and from 14 to 33 percent in the dizygotic pairs. Heritability estimates may be obtained from these data by the method of tetrachoric correlation (Smith, 1971), and ranged from 62 percent for astigmatism to 92 percent for nearsightedness. Although these data clearly imply that both genetic and environmental factors influence these errors of refraction, they do not in themselves permit a distinction between a monogenic and a multifactorial mechanism. For a fully penetrant monogenic trait, the expected concordance of MZ twins would be 100 percent but

TABLE 2: Common Eye Diseases in Norwegian Twins

Condition	No. of pairs		Concordance rate (%)		H^2
	MZ	DZ	MZ	DZ	
Nearsightedness	86	61	66	33	0.92
Farsightedness	30	35	53	14	0.82
Astigmatism	145	78	49	17	0.62

the expected concordance in DZ twins would vary, depending upon the frequency of the trait (and therefore the gene frequency) as well as the mode of inheritance (dominant or recessive). Penrose showed that for a monogenic trait, no combination of assumed penetrance, gene frequencies or inheritance pattern can lead to a predicted concordance rate in MZ twins that is more than four times that observed in DZ pairs. For traits that exhibit an MZ/DZ concordance ratio in excess of four, Penrose assumed that a multifactorial mechanism of genetic determination could safely be inferred (Penrose, 1953). For the traits shown in Table 2, the concordance rates in MZ twins are in every case less than four times those observed among the DZ pairs, and thus do not permit a distinction between a monogenic or a multifactorial mechanism.

In an attempt to gain further insight into the most likely mode of inheritance, we next compared the segregation ratios in full- and half-siblings. If a trait is determined by an autosomal dominant gene at a single locus, the recurrence risk for half-siblings cannot be less than half that of full-siblings regardless of the assumed gene frequency or penetrance of the phenotype. However, for a wide range of heritabilities and population frequencies, the expected risk for half-siblings will be less than half that of full-siblings under a multifactorial model. As shown in Table 3, for nearsightedness and astigmatism, the segregation rates for half-sibs were substantially lower than one half the estimate for full-sibs, thus providing support for the hypothesis of polygenic determination. Although the estimated risk for farsightedness in half-sibs was more than half that for full-sibs, the reported prevalence of this trait in the offspring was low, and the recurrence risk estimates were therefore associated with a large standard error. In Table 4, the distribution of affected individuals in the maternal and paternal half-sib-

TABLE 3: Disease Prevalence and Segregation Ratio in Full- and Half-sibs

Condition	Prevalence (N=2763)	Segregation ratio (p) Full-sibs	Half-sibs
Nearsightedness	0.0561	0.319 ± .041	0.055 ± .017
Farsightedness	0.0185	0.073 ± .039	0.051 ± .025
Astigmatism	0.0398	0.186 ± .039	0.068 ± .020

ships is contrasted where every independent pair of affected half-siblings is counted separatedly. It can be seen that errors of refraction in the half-sibs of affected probands occurred exclusively among the offspring of the female MZ twins. Taken at face value, these findings suggest that genetically influenced maternal effects may be of importance in the etiology of these diseases. The present research design will detect maternal influences that arise either from the rearing behavior of the mother during childhood or from prenatal factors acting during intrauterine life. Before we conclude that the data provide clear evidence for an intrauterine maternal effect on the embryologic development of the eye, it would be important to exclude the possiblity that the findings can be explained by some form of reporting bias. Although refraction errors were reported with the same overall frequency among the offspring of the male and female twins, it is conceivable that female twins are more likely to seek medical care for their children in a similar manner and thus more likely to obtain similar diagnoses in their offspring.

TABLE 4: Comparison of Segregation Ratios (p) in Maternal and Paternal Half-sibs

Half-sib type	Nearsightedness p	Nearsightedness Aff./Tot.	Farsightedness p	Farsightedness Aff./Tot.	Astigmatism p	Astigmatism Aff./Tot.
Paternal	0.00	0/82	0.00	0/25	0.00	0/70
Maternal	0.10	10/100	0.07	4/53	0.12	10/82
χ^2	6.90		1.21		8.92	
P	0.008		0.271		0.003	

As noted previously, nonrandom mating can have a striking influence on the distribution of phenotypes in a population for a continuously distributed trait such as body height or I.Q. The effect of assortative mating is to increase the variance in the offspring generation without altering the population mean. Thus in the case of I.Q. where marital correlations of 0.3-0.4 have frequently been documented, the introduction of random mating would be expected to reduce the frequency of individuals with I.Q.'s above 130 to one third of their former value and the frequency of those with I.Q.'s above 140 to one sixth of the frequency observed in an assortatively mating population. For multifactorial traits, changes in the mating structure of the population could lead to rapid changes in the frequency of the trait. Multifactorial traits are assumed to arise when a continuously distributed underlying disease liability exceeds a critical threshold required for phenotypic expression. Thus by increasing the variance of the underlying liability, assortative mating could increase the frequency of a trait in the population. Conventional wisdom in human genetics holds that genetic factors cannot account for rapid changes in the frequency of a multifactorial trait by themselves since many generations of selection are usually required to alter the gene frequencies in natural populations. However, this facile rationale ignores the rapid changes in the frequency of a multifactorial trait that could arise from a change in the mating structure of a population.

To search for evidence that such effects may have influenced the frequency of common eye diseases, we exam-

TABLE 5: Marital Correlations for Ocular Disease in Parents of 742 Norwegian Twin Pairs and their Spouses

Condition	Birth year of twins 1915-30 (N=477)	1931-45 (N=1191)	1946-- (N=558)	Pooled (N=2226)
Nearsightedness	-0.013	0.248**	0.314**	0.279**
Farsightedness	0.358**	0.455**	0.516**	0.475**
Astigmatism	0.402**	0.167**	0.181**	0.200**
Glaucoma	0.091*	-0.016	0.090*	0.035
Cataracts	-0.015	0.046	0.038	0.029

*p<0.05; **p<0.01

TABLE 6: Effect of Assortative Mating on the Incidence of a Multifactorial Threshold Trait

Liability threshold (in s.d)	Expected population incidence for various marital correlations (r)			
	r = 0.0	r = 0.1	r = 0.3	r = 0.5
1.3	10.0	11.1	13.0	14.8
1.6	5.0	5.8	7.5	9.0
2.3	1.0	1.3	2.1	2.9
3.1	0.1	0.2	0.3	0.6

ined the reported distribution of these conditions in the parents of the twins and their spouses, a total of 2226 husband-wife pairs in all. As shown in Table 5, the reported family histories provided evidence for a significant marital correlation with respect to nearsightedness, farsightedness and astigmatism but not for glaucoma or for cataracts. When the data were partitioned into three age cohorts depending on the birth year of the twins, there was an apparent increase in the intensity of assortative mating with respect to farsightedness and nearsightedness across the three time periods, whereas the reverse was true for astigmatism.

Table 6 illustrates the magnitude of the effect that changes in the intensity of assortative mating can have on the frequency of a multifactorial trait in the population. For a trait with a frequency of 1 percent in a randomly mating population, the introduction of assortative mating with a marital correlation of r = 0.3 would result in more than a 100 percent increase in the frequency of the trait. In our sample, the reported prevalences of farsightedness, nearsightedness and astigmatism among the parents of the twins and their spouses were approximately 7, 12 and 4 percent, respectively. From these frequencies, the previously derived heritability estimates and the observed marital correlations, the contribution of nonrandom mating to the prevalence of the traits may be estimated. The data suggest that 31 percent of all cases of nearsightedness, 62 percent of all cases of farsightedness and 21 percent of all cases of astigmatism may be directly attributable to the mating structure of the population and that with respect to nearsightedness and farsightedness, changes in the intensity of assortative mating during the past century may have been responsible for 31 and 43 percent increases in the frequencies of these traits, respectively.

DISCUSSION

The present analysis serves to illustrate how the use of an appropriate study design for genetic research can lead to important new insights into the causes of common ocular disorders in man. Our findings are consistent with the hypothesis that common errors of refraction are determined by a polygenic mechanism. They raise the possibility that maternal effects may be of importance in the etiology of these conditions, and illustrate the potential effect that changes in the mating structure of a population can have on the incidence of a multifactorial trait. Although the limitations and potential biases of questionnaire data must be borne in mind when our results are evaluated, it is to be hoped that these findings will serve as a stimulus for more definitive studies.

ACKNOWLEDGEMENT

This is paper #141 from the Department of Human Genetics of the Medical College of Virginia, and was supported in part by USPHS Grants HD-10291 and HD-15838. We gratefully acknowledge the assistance of R. Horowitz and T. Mayo with data processing and typing of the manuscript.

REFERENCES

Cantor RM (1981). A multivariate analysis of ridge count data from the offspring of monozygotic twins. Masters Thesis, Medical College of Virginia

Cantor RM, Nance WE, Eaves LJ, Winter PM, Blanchard MM (1981). Analysis of the covariance structure of digital ridge counts in the offspring of monozygotic twins. Submitted for publication.

Corey LA, Nance WE, Berg K (1978). A new tool for birth defects research: The MZ half-sib model and its extension to grandchildren of identical twins. Birth Defects Orig. Art. Ser. XIV-6A:193.

Eaves LJ, Heath AC (1981). Sex limitation and "asymmetric" assortative mating. In Gedda L, Parisi P,

Nance WE (eds): "Twin Research 3 Part B. Intelligence, Personality and Development," New York: Alan R. Liss, p 73.
Francois J (1961). "Heredity in Ophthalmology." St. Louis: Mosby, p 186.
Golden WL (1980). "Reproductive histories in a Norwegian twin population: Evaluation of the maternal effect in early spontaneous abortion." Ph.D. Thesis, Medical College of Virginia.
McKusick VA (1978). "Mendelian Inheritance in Man, 5th Ed." Baltimore: Johns Hopkins Press.
Moll PP, Sing CF (1979). Sampling strategies for the analysis of quantitative traits. In Sing CF, Skolnick M (eds): "Genetic Analysis of Common Diseases," New York: Alan R. Liss, p 307.
Nance WE (1979a). A note on assortative mating and maternal effects. In Sing CF, Skolnick M (eds): "Genetic Analysis of Common Diseases," New York: Alan R. Liss, p 453.
Nance WE (1979b). The role of twin studies in human quantitative genetics. Prog Med Genet (New Ser.) 3:73.
Nance WE, and Corey LA (1976). Genetic models for the analysis of data from the families of identical twins. Genetics 83:811.
Nance WE, Corey LA, Boughman JA (1978). Monozygotic twin kinships: A new design for genetic and epidemiologic research. In Morton NE, Chung CN (eds): "Genetic Epidemiology," New York: Academic Press, p 87.
Nance WE, Corey LA, Rose RJ, Eaves LJ (1981). Relevance of the marriages of twins to the causal analysis of non-random mating. In Gedda L, Parisi P, Nance WE (eds): "Twin Research 3 Part B Intelligence, Personality and Development," New York: Alan R. Liss, p 61.
Penrose LS (1953). The genetical background of common diseases. Acta Genet (Basel) 4:257.
Smith C (1971). Recurrence risks for multifactorial inheritance. Am J Hum Genet 23:578.

Retinoblastoma and Norrie's Disease

RECENT DEVELOPMENTS IN THE GENETICS AND TREATMENT OF RETINOBLASTOMA

A. Linn Murphree[1,2], Charles J. Gomer[1,3], Daniel R. Doiron[1], and William F. Benedict[1,3]

Clayton Ocular Oncology Center[1]
Divisions of Ophthalmology[2] and Hematology-Oncology[3], Childrens Hospital of Los Angeles

Recent linkage studies and tumor karyotypic analysis have improved our understanding of retinoblastoma. The gene for the 13 deletion form of retinoblastoma located in chromosomal region 13q14 is closely linked to esterase D, a clinically useful polymorphic enzyme marker system (Sparkes *et al.*, 1980). In addition, observations on the karyotypic changes in the tumor itself suggest a possible role for chromosomal changes in tumorigenesis (Hashem and Khalifa, 1975; Balaban *et al.*, in press, Benedict *et al.*, in press). At the Clayton Center for Ocular Oncology at Childrens Hospital of Los Angeles, we have not only been engaged in esterase D linkage studies and tumor karyotypic analysis but also are evaluating a new cancer treatment modality, hematoporphyrin derivative photoradiation therapy (HpD PRT), for possible use against retinoblastoma.

ESTERASE D

Esterase D is a polymorphic enzyme whose activity is expressed in almost all human tissues including fetal amniotic fibroblasts (Rivera *et al.*, 1981) but whose biological function is unknown. Its electrophoretic mobility and relative specificity for the methylumbelliferyl substrate distinguish it from other esterases. Two alleles, types 1 and 2, are present at the esterase D locus and are separated by their electrophoretic mobility. The locus for this enzyme was assigned to chromosomes 13 by somatic cell hybridization studies (van Heyningen *et al.*, 1975). Gene dose effect for esterase D, i.e. 50% normal activity, was demonstrated in

Birth Defects: Original Article Series, Volume 18, Number 6, pages 681–687

the 13 deletion form of retinoblastoma (Sparkes et al.,1980).

ESTERASE D AS A SCREENING ASSAY FOR THE 13 DELETION FORM OF RETINOBLASTOMA

We have recently shown that quantitative esterase D analysis is a sensitive and cost effective method to detect patients with the 13 deletion form of retinoblastoma (Murphree et al.,1981). In an esterase D screening study, 106 unselected patients with retinoblastoma had red cell esterase D quantitative analysis. The assay showed normal esterase D activity in all but three specimens. Two of the three patients had been clinically diagnosed as representing the 13 deletion form of retinoblastoma because of associated clinical anomalies. The blood from these patients was sent from out of state and the clinical information was not available at the time a 50% esterase D activity was found in the patient's red cells and a diagnosis of 13 deletion form of retinoblastoma was made. The other patient had bilateral retinoblastoma with no developmental delay or other minor neurologic abnormalities. Repeated esterase D values in the red cells from this patient showed approximately 50% activity.

Subsequently, similar decreased esterase D values were found in cultured fibroblasts and a lymphoblastoid line established from the patient (Benedict et al., submitted for publication). No deletion of 13q14 could be observed in metaphase and prophase chromosomes using high resolution banding techniques. This represents the first known patient with a submicroscopic deletion of 13q14 and thus strengthens the recommendation that the esterase D assay be used as a screening test for all patients with retinoblastoma. In addition, it has been shown for the first time that the gene dose effect for esterase D can be detected in fetal cells obtained at amniocentesis (Rivera et al.,1981). These observations make prenatal diagnosis possible in families with deletions or translocations involving region 13q14.

THE ROLE OF ESTERASE D IN MAPPING THE GENE FOR NON-DELETION DOMINANTLY INHERITED RETINOBLASTOMA

Because esterase D is a polymorphic enzyme, it has potential as a marker system for genes closely linked to it on chromosome 13. If the gene for non-deletion dominantly inherited retinoblastoma consistently could be shown to segregate with one of the two esterase D alleles, the linkage between esterase D and the non-deletion form of retinoblastoma also would be established. Working in collaboration with Dr. Robert Sparkes and his group, we have established such a linkage relationship (manuscript in preparation). In four families with hereditary retinoblastoma, where the affected parent was heterozygous (type 1, 2), it could be shown that offspring who received a 13 chromosome containing the esterase D allele associated with retinoblastoma from the affected parent always developed retinoblastoma. Those children who received the other allele from the affected parent never developed the tumor. No discordant segregation was observed.

The demonstration that the locus for dominantly inherited non-deletion retinoblastoma is on chromosome 13 and is closely linked to esterase D in 13q14 has significant implications for genetic counseling of patients with retinoblastoma. In certain informative families, it will be possible to detect the presence of the abnormal gene for retinoblastoma either prenatally or within the first few months of life before the tumor develops. If the individual at risk has received the parental chromosome 13 with the esterase D allele known to segregate with the tumor, then that individual has an almost certain chance of developing the tumor. If the individual at risk has inherited the other chromosome 13, then there is virtually no chance that he or she will develop the tumor. In this case, unnecessary examinations under anesthesia would be avoided.

Unfortunately, the esterase D marker may be informative in only a small number of families since the following criteria must be met: (1) there is a positive family history of the tumor; (2) it is possible to identify which EsD allele is segregating with the tumor, and;(3) the parent with retinoblastoma is heterozygous for esterase D and the other parent is homozygous for esterase D. Although the applicability may be limited, the mapping of the gene for dominantly inherited retinoblastoma is an extremely powerful tool in genetic counseling for this disorder.

TUMOR KARYOTYPING IN RETINOBLASTOMA

As stated above there is a subgroup of patients with retinoblastoma who have a constitutional deletion of chromosomal region 13q14. Constitutional deletions also are found in other tumors. A deletion of chromosomal region 11p13 has been associated in patients with Wilms' tumor, aniridia, and genitourinary abnormalities (Ricardi et al., 1978). In addition, renal cell carcinoma has been associated with a chromosome 3/8 translocation (Cohen et al., 1979).

Recently there has been considerable interest in whether the specific constitutional defect seen in a small portion of retinoblastoma patients, namely deletion of chromosomal region 13q14, might also be present at the tumor level in a significant number of patients with the non-deletion form of retinoblastoma. In early studies done on tumor specimens a long arm deletion of a D group chromosome was found in 4 of 5 cases (Hashem and Khalifa, 1975). The deleted chromosome could not be positively identified as a 13 since chromosomal banding was not done. Balaban and her colleagues subsequently have identified deletions of chromosomal region 13q14 in the tumors from 5 of 6 patients, all of whose constitutional karyotype was normal (Balaban et al., in press).

During the last three years at the Clayton Center for Ocular Oncology we have made direct chromosomal preparations from all retinoblastomas which were enucleated (Benedict et al., in press). Well spread metaphases were banded using the trypsin-Giemsa banding technique. In several bilateral cases more than one tumor stem line was found, indicating that the tumors arose from at least two independently transformed cells. In contrast, in the unilateral cases, with a single exception, only one stem line was observed. This suggests that in general unilateral tumors arose from one stem cell. The unilateral case having two stem lines may represent one of the 15% of sporadic cases which are hereditary. Thus tumor karyotyping may be useful in primary genetic counseling.

A patient with the deletion form of retinoblastoma and bilateral involvement was particularly interesting in that a missing 13 chromosome was found in each of two tumor stem lines. Since the tumor had no esterase activity it was possible to show that the normal 13 chromosome had been lost in each stem line (Benedict et al., submitted for publication).

These and other studies as outlined above have allowed us the possibility to suggest an expanded and unifying theory of tumorigenesis for both the deletion and non-deletion forms of retinoblastoma (Murphree and Benedict, manuscript in preparation).

HEMATOPORPHYRIN DERIVATIVE PHOTORADIATION THERAPY

Hematoporphyrin derivative (HpD) photoradiation therapy (PRT) has been shown to effectively destroy human tumors (Dougherty _et al_., 1978). We became interested in the possibility that this new treatment modality might be adapted for use against intraocular tumors, especially retinoblastoma. Hematoporphyrin derivative (HpD), a photosensitive dye preferentially accumulates in tumor tissue and when exposed to visible red light (630 nm) initiates the photodynamic production of cytotoxic singlet oxygen (Weishaupt _et al_., 1976). Tumor necrosis is rapid. We have shown that HpD PRT is effective in killing human retinoblastoma when heterotransplanted to the eye of the "nude" athymic mouse (Benedict _et al_., 1980). Tissue distribution performed with the same model demonstrated that ^{3}H-HpD accumulated to a greater degree in eyes with retinoblastoma when compared to eyes with no tumor (Gomer _et al_., 1982). This differential drug distribution (tumor vs. normal tissue) accounts for the selectiveness of HpD PRT. Studies designed to examine acute normal ocular toxicity showed that retinal damage occurred in the rabbit following exposures to light alone at levels of 400 mW/cm^2 for a 1.0 cm^2 or larger area. In addition, discrete and well demarcated areas of retinal damage corresponding only to the treatment field were induced by HpD PRT (1 to 5 mg HpD per Kg and a 15 minute exposure to 630 nm light at 40 to 100 mW/cm^2 given 48 hours after administration of the drug). Treatment parameters previously shown not to produce acute retinal damage outside the treatment field were found to be effective in destroying Greene melanoma growing in the anterior chamber of the pigmented rabbit.

We hope that HpD PRT may eventually be useful as an adjunctive treatment modality against retinoblastoma and choroidal melanoma. Clinical trials with HpD PRT for intraocular tumors are currently underway at Childrens Hospital of Los Angeles.

Balaban G, Gilbert F, Nichols W, Meadows AT, Shields J (in press). Abnormalities of chromosome 13 in retinoblastoma from individuals with normal constitutional karyotypes. Canc Genet and Cytogenet.

Benedict WF, Lingua RW, Doiron DR, Dawson JA, Murphree AL (1980). Tumor regression of human retinoblastoma in the nude mouse following photoradiation therapy: A preliminary report. Med Pediatr Oncol 8:397.

Benedict WF, Murphree AL, Banerjee A (in press). Chromosomal changes in unilateral vs. bilateral retinoblastoma: Important differences and implications to etiology. Proc AACR.

Benedict WF, Murphree AL, Banerjee A, Spinna C, Sparkes MC, Sparkes RS (submitted). Deletion retinoblastoma beyond cytogenetic detection: Loss of the normal 13 chromosome in tumor stem lines and implications to retinoblastoma formation.

Cohen AJ, Li F, Berg S, Marchetto D, Tsai S, Jacobs S, Brown R (1979). Hereditary renal-cell carcinoma associated with a chromosomal translocation. New Engl J Med 301:592.

Dougherty TJ, Kaufman JE, Goldfarb A, Weishaupt KR, Boyle D, Mittleman A (1978). Photoradiation therapy for the treatment of malignant tumors. Cancer Res 38:2628.

Gomer CJ, Rucker N, Mark C, Benedict WF, Murphree AL (1982). Tissue distribution of ^{3}H-hematoporphyrin derivative in athymic "nude" mice heterotransplanted with human retinoblastoma. Invest Ophthalmol Vis Sci 22:118.

Hashem N, Khalifa S (1975). Retinoblastoma: A model of hereditary fragile chromosomal regions. Hum Hered 25:35.

Murphree AL, Benedict WF (submitted). A general theory of tumorigenesis for human retinoblastoma.

Murphree AL, Lingua RW, Sparkes RS, Sparkes MC, Benedict WF (1981). Esterase D: A screening assay for 13 deletion retinoblastoma. Abst. VI Int. Cong. Hum. Genetics, Jerusalem.

Riccardi VM, Sujansky E, Smith AC, Francke U (1978). Chromosomal imbalance in the aniridia-Wilms' tumor association: 11p institial deletion. Ped 61:604.

Rivera H, Turleau C, deGrouchy J, Junien C, Despoisse S, Zucker JM (1981). Retinoblastoma - del (13q14): Report of two patients, one with a trisomic sibling due to maternal insertion. Gene-dosage effect for esterase D. Hum Genet 59:211.

Sparkes RS, Sparkes MC, Wilson MG, Towner JW, Benedict WF, Murphree AL, Yunis JJ (1980). Regional assignment of genes for human esterase D and retinoblastoma to chromosome band 13q14. Science 208:1042.

van Heyningen R, Bobrow M, Bodmer WF, Gardiner SF, Povey S, Hopkinson DA (1975). Chromosome assignment of some human enzyme loci: Mitochondrial malate dehydrogenase to 7, mannose phosphate isomerase and pyruvate kinase to 15 and probably esterase D to 13. Ann Hum Genet Lond 38:295.

Weishaupt KR, Gomer CJ, Dougherty TJ (1976). Identification of singlet oxygen as the cytotoxic agent in photo-inactivation of a murine tumor. Cancer Res 39:146.

MULTIPLE MANIFESTATIONS OF THE RETINOBLASTOMA GENE

Brenda L. Gallie and Robert A. Phillips

Departments of Ophthalmology and Medical Biophysics, University of Toronto and the Ontario Cancer Institute, 500 Sherbourne Street, Toronto, Canada M4X 1K9.

Clinical observations have established that a specific genetic mutation is associated with predisposition to retinoblastoma (RB). Cytogenetic studies have shown an association of RB with deletions in chromosome 13 (Yunis and Ramsay, 1978). Studies in families with RB indicate a close linkage of the RB locus and the enzyme, esterase D (Sparkes, R; Payne, R, personal communications). From these data the RB locus has been assigned to the q14 band on chromosome 13. However, the mechanism by which alteration in the gene(s) at this locus leads to RB remains unknown.

Knudson (1971) provided a clue to the induction process when he described a novel way to analyse the age-incidence data for RB. In contrast to tumors in adults, the incidence of RB decreases with age, almost all cases being diagnosed before 4 years of age. For a defined cohort of bilateral and unilateral RB patients, Knudson plotted the age of the population (t, months) versus the proportion not yet diagnosed (S). Figure 1 shows similar analysis for patients seen in the Toronto clinic; the shapes of the curves are essentially identical to those previously reported by Knudson. This analysis illustrates several points about RB. First, different shapes of curves for bilateral and unilateral RB suggest different inductive processes for the heritable and non-heritable forms of the disease. Second, the curve for the bilateral cases fits a simple exponential, ($\log S = -t/31.3$), implying that a single event in addition to the germline mutation is required to produce tumors. Finally, the concave shape of the curve for the unilateral cases ($\log S = -3.5 \times 10^{-4} t^2$) suggests that induction of a tumor

Birth Defects: Original Article Series, Volume 18, Number 6, pages 689–701

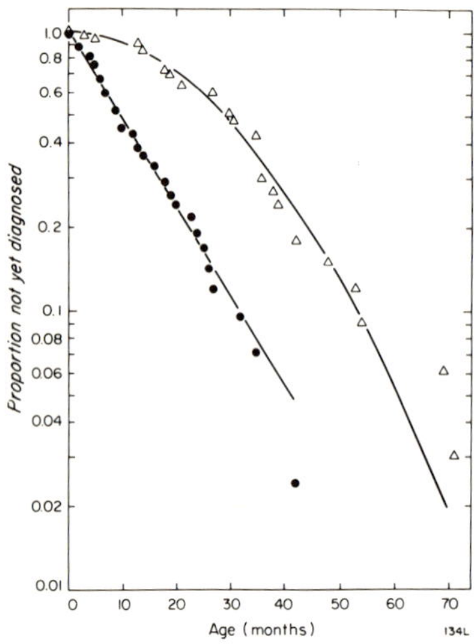

Figure 1.
Semi-logarithmic plot of proportion of cases not yet diagnosed versus age for bilateral ( ) and unilateral ( ) RB cases.

requires multiple events; the curve shown in figure 1 can be fit by a 2-hit curve.

From these data, Knudson formulated a model for the generation of RB tumors in which two events, or mutations, were required to convert a normal cell into a malignant cell. In the heritable cases, where the first event is considered to be a germ-line mutation, only one subsequent event in any cell at risk results in malignancy. Therefore, it is not surprising that patients with the heritable form of the disease develop multiple primary tumors on both retinas. In the non-heritable phenocopy, both events are somatic and must occur in the same cell. Although this simple model accounts for several features of RB, it does not make any predictions about the nature of the events, the genes involved, or the mechanism by which the changes lead to a malignant phenotype.

Presented below are data from three seemingly unrelated studies that describe various aspects of the inductive process: 1) growth properties of fibroblasts known to have the RB gene show that this gene has a small but statistically significant effect on growth of non-retinal cells under sub-optimal growth conditions (low serum). 2) evidence for a benign manifestation of the RB gene in the retina is provided by observations on non-progressive retinal tumors, retinomas. 3) karyotypic rearrangements in the tumors rarely involve chromosome 13q14 but every tumor studied contains abnormalities of chromosome 1q or 6p.

EFFECT OF THE RB GENE IN NON-RETINAL CELLS (FIBROBLASTS)

In addition to multiple RB tumors, children with the RB gene have a 15-30% chance of developing a second, non-ocular malignancy in the second and third decade, most commonly osteogenic sarcoma (Abramson et al, 1976). This observation suggests that the RB gene is expressed in other tissues besides embryonic retina.

Skin fibroblasts from patients with another malignancy associated with an autosomal dominant mutation, adenomatosis of the colon and rectum, have been reported to grow better than normal fibroblasts in low concentrations of fetal calf serum (FCS)(Pfeffer et al, 1976). We have presented data showing that the initial growth rate and the plating efficiency of fibroblasts from bilateral RB patients in low concentrations of FCS are significantly greater than those from normal donors (Kossakowska et al, 1982). In order to look for similar abnormalities in cells known to carry the RB gene, fibroblasts were obtained from biopsies of sub-epidermal skin or conjunctiva of bilateral RB patients and controls. To measure growth rate fibroblasts were harvested by trypsinization between the second and sixth passage, and grown in tissue culture medium supplemented with various concentrations of FCS. At intervals the cells were removed by trypsinization and counted in a hemocytometer. Initial experiments showed that the ability of fibroblasts to grow in low concentrations of serum depends on the age of the donor. Fibroblasts from donors less than one year of age grew well in 1% FCS and fibroblasts from donors over five years of age grew poorly, whether the donor carried the RB gene or not. However fibroblasts from donors between one and five years of age grew poorly when the donor was a normal control, a unilateral RB patient, or an unaffected sibling of an RB patient. Fibroblasts from bilaterally affected RB patients grew slightly better. Therefore the remainder of our studies on growth properties of fibroblasts were performed on fibroblasts obtained from patients and controls between one and five years of age.

The relative growth of fibroblasts in 0.5% FCS, expressed as a ratio of the number of cells present on day 5 compared to the number of cells used to initiate the culture (N_5/N_0) was very similar on separate biopsies from five individuals, illustrating the reproducibility of the measurement. The importance of genetic factors in this measurement is shown by results on two identical twins with bilateral RB: relative growth of fibroblasts was 1.80 and 1.78 on biopsies at age 19 months, and 1.57 and 1.58 on biopsies at age 25 months.

For twelve bilateral RB patients and twelve controls of comparable age N_5/N_0 in 15% FCS is not significantly different. However, there is a significant difference ($P \leq 0.025$) in 0.5% FCS, the N_5/N_0 of fibroblasts from the bilateral RB patients being 1.4 ± 0.08 (mean ± S.E.) compared to N_5/N_0 of 1.16 ± 0.04 for controls.

Cloning efficiency, or the percentage of cells added that adhere to the plastic dish and grow to form colonies containing more than 50 cells, was measured in growth medium containing 15% or 1% serum. Cloning efficiency of fibroblasts is significantly better from bilateral RB patients than from normal controls both in 15% FCS (35.6% ± 2.9 versus 27.7% ± 4.4) (mean ± S.E.) ($P \leq 0.025$) and in 1% FCS (1.65%, 1.24-2.15 versus 0.49%, 0.29-0.82) (geometric mean, range of 1 S.E.) ($P \leq 0.05$).

Two autosomal recessive syndromes, ataxia telangiectasia and xeroderma pigmentosa, associated with increased risk of cancer, have defective mechanisms to repair specific DNA damage. For example, in cells from patients with xeroderma pigmentosa, UV damage is not adequately repaired, and fibroblasts from patients with ataxia telangiectasia can not effectively repair x-ray induced damage. Abnormal radiation sensitivity has been reported for bilateral RB patients, based on radiation survival curves for skin fibroblasts (Weichselbaum et al, 1978). Studies by the same group have also shown however that a locus which affects sensitivity to ionizing radiation is closely linked to the RB gene on chromosome 13, but that the "radiosensitivity gene" is not identical to the RB gene, the two genes being separable in patients with various 13q deletions (Nove et al, 1979).

We determined radiation sensitivity of skin fibroblasts from patients with normal peripheral blood karyotype (Kossakowska et al, 1982). When plotted as log survival versus radiation dose, all curves had a small shoulder at low doses followed by an exponential decrease in survival with increase in dose. The inverse of the slope in the exponential portion of the curve is the dose required to reduce survival of the fibroblasts to 37%, the D_o. The D_o of eight control fibroblast strains was 118 ± 3 rads (mean ± S.E.); the D_o of 10 fibroblast strains from bilateral RB patients was 115 ± 4 (mean ± S.E.). Thus, we observed no consistent abnormality in radiation sensitivity of fibroblasts from bilateral RB patients. In three families there was also no difference in the radiation response of RB patients compared to other siblings. Several other groups have now also reported normal sensitivity to ionizing radiation in hereditary RB (Morten et al, 1981; Cleaver et al, 1982). It is unlikely that tumor production by the RB gene involves a deficiency in the ability to repair radiation-induced DNA damage.

BENIGN MANIFESTATION OF THE RB GENE IN RETINA

Some families with heritable RB fail to show the usual pattern of high penetrance and in these families many of the proven carriers are carefully examined with full pupillary dilatation and the indirect ophthalmoscope, retinal lesions are occasionally detected which resemble RB tumors but do not show malignant progression. We have proposed that these lesions be called "retinomas" (Gallie, Phillips et al, 1982). Three characteristics are distinctive for retinoma: a translucent, greyish retinal mass protrudes into vitreous; "cottage-cheese" calcification is present in 75%; and retinal pigment epithelial migration and proliferation is present in 60% (figure 2). Ischemic necrosis is very common in large RB tumors, but the retinomas have an intact blood supply easily demonstrated on fluorescein angiography.

Among 32 cases studied, 11 had unilateral or bilateral retinomas, but no proof of the presence of the RB gene. The other 21 cases were known to carry the RB gene by either family studies (7 cases) or because the other eye had been affected by RB (4 cases) or both (10 cases). The retinomas in our patients were diagnosed at much older ages than RB (mean 16 years, range 3 - 40 years). All have been observed

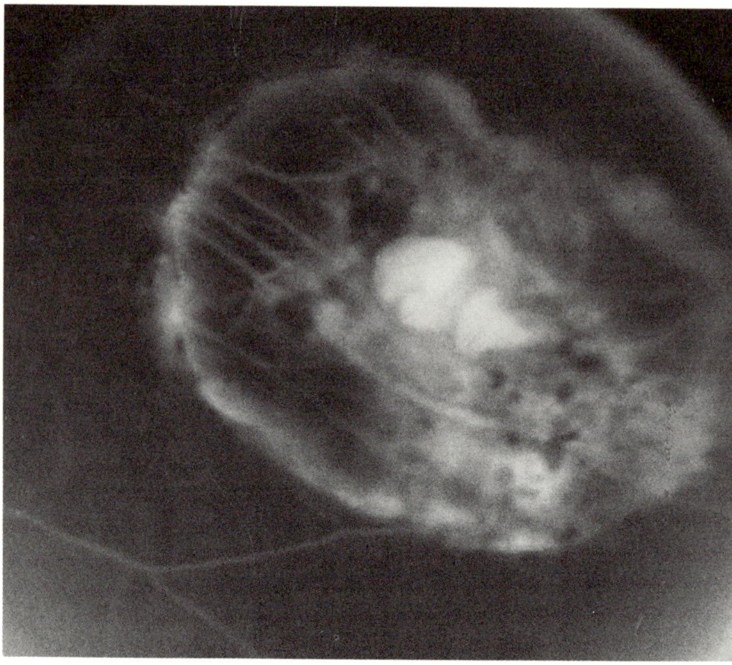

Figure 2. Fluorescein angiography demonstrating the three characteristics of retinoma (translucent mass, calcification, and pigment epithelial disturbance) with intact blood supply.

for several years beyond initial diagnosis, the longest having been followed for 20 years without significant change.

Prior to our analysis of this group of patients, lesions identical to retinoma were reported in the literature and usually were considered to represent "spontaneous regression of RB". We have found no evidence for any immunological reactivity in these cases against RB tumor (Gallie et al, 1979) and no correlation with HLA type (Gallie, Dupont et al, 1977).

Smith (1974) reported the pathological examination of two eyes whose clinical description fitted retinoma. Both lesions consisted of viable, non-proliferating small, round cells similar to RB. No Flexner-Wintersteiner rosette differentiation was observed in either eye. About one half of eyes containing RB tumors that respond successfully to radiation therapy do not show complete resolution of tumor or calcific scarring, but remain indefinitely as translucent masses. Histological examination by Zimmermann (personal communication) of such a "regression" from the eye of a successfully treated child who subsequently died of other causes, showed a pattern of intact, non-proliferating, small, round cells similar to the two cases reported by Smith.

We propose that retinoma represents benign manifestation of the RB gene. The fact that new retinal tumors do not appear in adults with the RB gene implies that the cell of origin of RB, the retinoblast, differentiates into a cell that cannot be transformed, presumably because cell division has ceased. When the transforming event occurs in a partially differentiated cell prior to terminal differentiation, it causes limited abnormal proliferation, resulting in a retinoma. Perhaps retinomas occur frequently in RB and are the retinal lesions remaining after successful radiation or chemotherapy.

KARYOTYPIC REARRANGEMENTS IN RB TUMORS

Chromosome rearrangement in tumors may have specific relevance to the tissue of origin and function of the tumor cells, as illustrated by the translocation of chromosome 8 to chromosomes 14, 2 or 22 in Burkitt's lymphoma, and the correlation of the translocation with the immunoglobulin genes expressed by the tumor cells (Klein, 1981). Since the RB gene is probably located at chromosome 13q14, it is of interest to look in tumors for chromosome abnormalities involving this region. An attractive hypothesis, first elaborated by Knudson (1971) for the genesis of retinal tumors, is that a retinoblast becomes malignant when both alleles at 13q14 are mutated.

The following karyotypic data are based in part on analysis of fresh specimens, but most detailed analyses were prepared on tumors proliferating either in athymic nude mice (Gallie, Albert et al, 1977), or in vitro (Gallie, Holmes, 1982). Therefore we have analysed stem-lines of the tumor best suited to grow in culture or in nude mice. Detailed karyotypes of some of these tumors are published elsewhere (Gardner et al, 1982).

All tumors have a near diploid chromosome number but

every tumor has at least two detectable chromosome abnormalities. The mean number of abnormalities was 6 for 15 RB tumors that had been maintained in culture for only a few months. A heavily irradiated (9000 rad) metastatic RB showed 17 chromosomal rearrangements including many inversions. Two of the tumors that have now been maintained in culture for more than two years have shown a significant increase in the number of rearrangements from 6 to 12 and from 8 to 17. A third line, however, maintained in culture for a similar length of time, has remained stable with only 3 chromosomal rearrangements.

Chromosome Involved	Unilateral (8)	# of tumors Bilateral (9)	Total (17)
1	5	8	13
triplication 1q	5	6	11
16	4	6	10
"iso 6 p"	4	5	9
17	5	4	9
7	4	4	8
4	3	4	7
2,5,13			5
3,9,10,12,14,20,22			4
1,15,19			3
8,11,18,22			2
X, 6(other than iso 6p)			1
triplication of 1q and/or iso 6p			17 (100%)

Table 1. Frequency of chromosome abnormalities in retinoblastoma tumors.

The frequency of involvement of various chromosomes in abnormalities of 17 RB tumors (8 unilateral, 9 bilateral) is shown in table 1. Chromosome 13 was abnormal in only 5 out of of 17 tumors and in only 1 did the rearrangement result in deletion of the region 13q14. If a retinal cell must be altered in both alleles at this locus in order to become malignant, this process must involve a point mutation, not detectable by chromosome analysis. Chromosome 1 was most frequently abnormal, (13 out of 17 tumors) and in 11 tumors the result was triplication for region 1q25-32. Triplication of the same chromosomal segment has been reported in many other malignancies (Rowley, 1973; Kovacs, 1978). Chromosome 16 was abnormal in 10 out of the 17 tumors, but in each the region and the type of rearrangement was different.

In our initial publication of chromosome abnormalities in RB tumors (Gardner et al, 1982) the second most common marker chromosome was identified as an iso17q. Like triplication of 1q, this is an abnormality that has been observed in other malignant cells, especially hematological (Lobb et al, 1972). Careful scrutiny of this abnormal chromosome, however has led us to the conclusion that the marker in the RB tumors is not an iso17q, but an iso6p. Data supporting this conclusion will be published elsewhere (Gallie et al, in preparation). It is possible that other reports of iso17q are actually iso6p. The iso6p marker is present in 9 of 17 RB tumors.

Of a total of 19 RB tumors examined, all have either triplication of 1q or the iso6p chromosome, or both abnormalities, when first examined. Since RB tumors are removed when they are still very small compared to other human malignancies, the chromosome abnormalities found in these RB tumors probably represent an early stage in karyotype evolution. Therefore, the presence of the markers in all tumors suggests that changes at loci on chromosomes 1 and 6 are involved in the evolution of the malignant phenotype in RB tumors. However, it is not clear whether these loci are involved in the primary transformation of RB or are secondary events associated with progression of already malignant cells.

DISCUSSION OF THE RESULTS IN RELATION TO KNUDSON'S TWO STAGE MODEL OF CARCINOGENESIS

The results presented above are best discussed in the context of the two-hit model of Knudson and its recent application to all human cancer (Moolgavkar and Knudson, 1981). The model as it applies to RB is shown schematically in figure 3.

In this model it is assumed that the retinoblasts, R, in the retina are stem cells. Each R will self renew to make more R with a probability, p, or will differentiate with a probability 1-p into mature retinal cells (D) such as photoreceptors. The differentiation into D probably goes

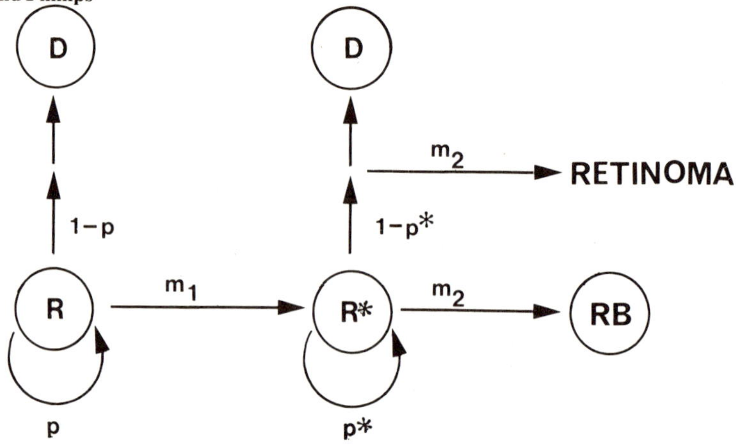

Figure 3. Two-hit model for generation of retinoblastoma

through several stages and may involve cell proliferation. Conversion of an R to a malignant RB requires two mutations, m_1 and m_2 . Following the first mutation, the R can be visualized as being "activated" and ready to become malignant; in the model this stage is shown as R*. Because the unaffected retina in RB patients appears normal, it is assumed that R* can differentiate normally. However, R* may have an altered probability for self renewal, p*, even though it can produce normal D. It is also clear from epidemiological studies that neither R nor R* survive for the lifetime of the individual. Sometime in early childhood all R and R* differentiate into D, reducing the risk of RB to zero.

As discussed by Moolgavkar and Knudson (1981), this model readily explains the incidence data for the heritable and non-heritable cases of RB. The risk of developing RB depends primarily on the number of R*. Although normal individuals may acquire by somatic mutation a few R*, the relatively short lifespan of R* will usually result in their differentiation into D before m_2 causes RB. In contrast, in patients with heritable RB, m_1 is present in all cells and all R will be at the R* stage. Thus, it is not surprising that such individuals have a high risk of developing RB and commonly have multiple tumors affecting both eyes. The chance of a normal individual having one R* in each eye, also acquire m_2 and develop RB is so unlikely that all patients with bilateral tumors must be classed as gene carriers. However, a significant proportion (25%) of individuals carrying m_1 in their germline only develop tumors in one eye.

Several individuals have been reported who had a visible deletion of the long arm of chromosome 13 and also developed RB (Yunis et al, 1978). This observation must mean that m_1 results in a deletion of gene function. If the other allele at 13q14 continues to function, then R* may have only half as much gene product as R. Our chromosome data do not support the idea presented by others that m_2 involves localized changes in the remaining normal allele at 13q14. Since malignancy in general is so closely associated with gross chromosomal abnormalities, m_2 may involve large rearrangements of the genome (Cairns, 1981), and may well involve recombinations between non-homologous regions in different parts of the genome, such as 1q or 6p. Hopefully, experiments using DNA-mediated transfer of the malignant phenotype may reveal the precise nature of m_1 and/or m_2 in RB.

As mentioned above it is possible that R* may have a different self renewal probability than R. It is possible that the increased growth potential of fibroblasts from patients with heritable RB reflects an increased self renewal probability. To identify carriers of the RB gene, ie, m_1 , it is important to search for effects of m_1 in readily available somatic cells. The fibroblast data suggest that such an approach is feasible.

Knudson and Meadows (1980) have suggested that benign retinoma-like lesions in other heritable cancers such as Wilm's tumor and neuroblastoma represent alteration by m_1 of the normal differentiation pathway. We feel that this explanation is unlikely for RB. If m_1 alone were sufficient to cause retinomas, retinomas should be observed in high frequency in all patients with heritable RB. Instead retinomas occur infrequently. Therefore, we suggest that the development of retinomas requires a second mutation. As a working model we propose that the second mutation, m_2 , is the same one that converts R* to RB, but retinoma results when m_2 occurs in a partially differentiated cell. Although proliferation increases, differentiation continues and the cells ultimately lose their proliferative potential. The end result is a small hypoplastic nodule containing only abnormally differentiated cells.

Retinoma and RB would occasionally occur in the same eye. Retinoma would be unaffected by therapy due to lack of proliferation and would only be clinically evident after the malignant cells were destroyed. Although retinomas are rare, ophthalmologists should monitor their patients carefully for such lesions because their presence can be highly significant in providing accurate genetic counselling.

This work was supported by grants from the Medical Research Council of Canada, the Ontario Cancer Treatment and Research Foundation, and the Hospital for Sick Children Foundation.

Abramson DH, Ellsworth RM, Zimmermann LE (1976). Non-ocular cancer in retinoblastoma survivors. Trans Am Acad Ophthalmol 81:454.

Cairns J (1981). The origin of human cancers. Nature 289:353.

Cleaver JE, Char D, Charles WC, Rand N (1982). Repair and replication of DNA in hereditary (bilateral) retinoblastoma cells after x-irradiation. Cancer Res 42:1343.

Gallie BL, Albert DM, Wong JJY, Buyukmikci N, Puliafita CA (1977). Heterotransplantation of retinoblastoma into the athymic "nude" mouse. Invest Ophthalmol 16:256.

Gallie BL, Dupont B, Whitsett C, Kitchen FD, Ellsworth RM, Good RA (1977). Histocompatibility typing in spontaneous regression of retinoblastoma. In Murphy GP (ed): "HLA and Malignancy," New York: Alan R. Liss, P.220.

Gallie BL, Holmes W, Phillips RA (1982). Reproducible growth in tissue culture of fresh retinoblastoma tumor specimens. Cancer Res 42:301.

Gallie BL, Phillips RA, Ellsworth RM, Abramson DH (1982). Retinoma: Spontaneous regression of retinoblastoma or benign manifestation of the mutation? Brit J Cancer, in press.

Gallie BL, Wong JJY, Ellsworth RM, Dupont B, Good RA (1979). Immunological mechanisms in spontaneous regression of retinoblastoma. In Silverstein AM, and O'Connor GR, (eds): "Immunology and Immunopathology of the Eye," New York: Masson, P.190.

Gardner HA, Gallie BL, Knight LA, Phillips RA (1982). Multiple karyotypic changes in retinoblastoma tumor cells: presence of normal chromosome 13 in most tumors. J Cell Genet and Cytogenet (in press).

Klein G (1981). Role of genetic transposition in carcinogenesis. Nature 294:313.

Knudson AG (1971). Mutation and cancer: A statistical study of retinoblastoma. Proc Natl Acad Sci USA 68:820.

Knudson AG, Meadows AT (1980). Regression of neuroblastoma IV-S: a genetic hypothesis. N Engl J Med. 302:1254.

Kossakowska AE, Gallie BL, Phillips RA (1982). Fibroblasts from retinoblastoma patients: enhanced growth in fetal calf serum and a normal response to ionizing radiation. J Cell Physiol, in press.

Kovacs G (1978). Letter to editor. The Lancet i:55.

Lobb DS, Reeves BR, Lawler JD (1972). Identification of isochromosome 17 in myeloid leukemia. Lancet i:849.

Moolgavkar SH, Knudson AG (1981). Mutation and cancer: A model for human carcinogenesis. J Nat Cancer Instit 66: 1037.

Morten JEN, Harnden DG, Taylor AMR (1981). Chromosome damage in G_0 X-irradiated lymphocytes from patients with hereditary retinoblastoma. Cancer Res 41:3635.

Nove J, Little JB, Weichselbaum RR, Nichols WW, Hoffman E (1979). Retinoblastoma, chromosome 13 and in vitro cellular radiosensitivity. Cytogenet Cell Genet 24:176.

Pfeffer L, Lipkin M, Stuttman O, Kopelovich L (1976). Growth abnormalities of cultured human skin fibroblasts derived from individuals with hereditary adenomatosis of the colon and rectum. J Cell Physiol 89:29.

Rowley JD (1973). A new consistent chromosomal abnormality in chronic myelogenous leukemia identified by quinacrine fluorescence and giemsa staining. Nature 243:290.

Smith JLS (1974). Histology and spontaneous regression of retinoblastoma. Trans Ophthalmol Soc U.K. 94:953.

Weichselbaum RR, Nove J, Little JB (1978). X-ray sensitivity of diploid fibroblasts from patients with hereditary or sporadic retinoblastoma. Proc Natl Acad Sci USA 75:3962.

Yunis J, Ramsay N (1978). Retinoblastoma and subband deletion of chromosome 13, Am J Dis Child 132:161.

CHROMOSOME ERRORS IN RETINOBLASTOMA

Rufus O. Howard, M. D.,Ph.D.

From the Department of Ophthalmology and Visual Sciences, Yale University of Medicine, New Haven, Connecticut, and the Department of Surgery, University of Connecticut Medical School, Farmington, Connecticut

The most common malignant intraocular tumor in children, retinoblastoma, occurs in individuals 1) as an apparent sporadic event in the majority of patients, 2) with a clinical pattern consistent with autosomal dominant inheritance less often, and 3) in a few individuals with chromosome aberration. In this report, the chromosome errors associated with retinoblastoma will be reviewed.

Chromosomes in Peripheral Tissues

Thirteen studies provide information to make an estimate of the incidence of chromosome error associated with retinoblastoma. Wilson studied 50 retinoblastoma patients with a banding technique and identified one 13q- individual and a second with XXY[97]. Ejima found 4 with 13q- from 44 retinoblastoma patients[16]. Motegi studied 42 retinoblastoma patients and found one 13q14- and two mosaic 13q14 deletions[57]. Waldbaum identified one 13q- among 33 retinoblastoma patients[89]. Welch identified one 13q- out of 12 retinoblastoma patients[93]; Davison one 13q- out of 8[12];Thompson one Dq- out of 5[85]; and Lele one Dq- (later shown to be 13q-[40]) out of 6 retinoblastoma patients[51]. No chromosome errors were identified in surveys of retinoblastoma by Ladda[50],

Birth Defects: Original Article Series, Volume 18, Number 6, pages 703–727

Wiener [94], Pruett[73], Hossfeld[37], and Morgan[56]. Thus, 14 out of 259 retinoblastoma patients have had a recognizable chromosome error. If the incidence of retinoblastoma is taken as 1/20,000, then the incidence of retinoblastoma associated with chromosome error may be estimated as 14/259 X 1/20,000 = 1/370,000. This estimate will be refined with additional studies.

Fifty-two or fifty-three children have been described with retinoblastoma and a chromosome error. The chromosome errors described include deletion of chromosome 13, duplication of chromosomes 13 and 21, and duplication of sex chromosomes (Table I). If a clinical finding such as retinoblastoma is to be considered an integral part of a chromosome aberration, the clinical finding must occur more often associated with the chromosome error than in the general population. Thus, in patients with trisomy 21, the incidence of retinoblastoma would be expected to be 1/20,000 X 1/700 = 1/14,000,000 (the incidence of retinoblastoma x the incidence of trisomy 21). In Table I the incidence of retinoblastoma plus a chromosome error has been calculated for each of the different chromosome abnormalities. With small numbers of patients, it is difficult to be sure that mathematical significance is or is not present. The individual case reports of patients with retinoblastoma and 21 trisomy mosaicism, 13 trisomy, trisomy 21 plus XXX, and XXXXY: and the two case reports of trisomy 21 plus XXY, and the seven case reports of trisomy 21 and retinoblastoma, if considered only on the basis of mathematic significance, probably should be considered sporadic cases, with the co-existence of retinoblastoma and the chromosome error occurring no more often than in the general population. However, there

TABLE I

RETINOBLASTOMA AND CHROMOSOME ABNORMALITY

Pts. with Retinoblastoma and Chromosome Error	Number patients	Estimated Incidence of Retinoblastoma and Chromosome Error
46, 13q-	37	1/20,000 x rare *
47, 13+ [32,33]	1 (?2)	1/20,000 x 1/(4 - 10,000) [8]
47, 21+ [2,19,33,43,55,81]	7	1/20,000 x 1/700 [26]
46/47, 21+ [6]	1	1/20,000 x 1/2600 [27]
47, XXY [20,74,97]	3	1/20,000 x 1/850 [28]
48, 21+, XXX [13]	1	1/20,000 x 1/500,000 [13]
48, 21+, XXY [20]	1	1/20,000 x 1/700 x 1/772 [31]
49, XXXXY [82]	1	1/20,000 x rare *

* Not identified in 31,000 newborn children [22]

is a non-random involvement of only chromosomes 13, 21, and X (including 2 cases of 13 - X translocation) with retinoblastoma. In addition, the calculated incidence of retinoblastoma plus chromosome error is extremely low for some of the abnormalities. The calculated incidence of trisomy 21 plus XXX, plus retinoblastoma is 1/12.5 billion[13]! In spite of the few case reports, it is our interpretation that the concurrence of retinoblastoma and chromosome error are not random, sporadic events.

The 37 patients with partial deletion of the long arm of chromosome 13 (13q-) represent a significant association of chromosome error with retinoblastoma.

13q- Retinoblastoma

A better understanding of the association of 13q- and retinoblastoma is provided by examining the 37 case reports. In six early unbanded chromosome studies, the abnormality was described only as Dq-. When banding techniques were developed, it was possible to identify deletion of the long arm of chromosome 13 in the later case reports. As the number of case reports increased, it became apparent that a common segment of chromosome, 13q14, was missing in the patients with retinoblastoma (Table II).

The band 13q14 was not missing from individuals identified with partial deletion of chromosome 13q and no retinoblastoma (Table III). Most case reports of retinoblastoma and 13q deletion have been described in Caucasians, but reports have recognized affected Blacks, Mexicans, Korean and Japanese individuals.

TABLE II

RETINOBLASTOMA AND 13q DELETION

Patient No.	Reference	Sex	Tumor Unilateral/Bilateral	Age at Diagnosis (months)	Chromosome Analysis 13 deletion
1	Lele et al [51]	F (English)	B	10	q14-q22
2	Thompson & Lyons [85]	M	U	18 (died 3 yrs)	D-/Dq-
3	van Kempen [88]	M (Netherlands)	B	6	Dq-
4	Wilson et al [95,96]	F	B	18	13q-
5	Taylor [83]	F (English)	B	3	Dq-/Dr
6	Gey [23]	M (German)	B	20 (died 2.5 yrs)	Dq-
7	Grace et al [24]	F (English)	B	birth (died 6 mo)	13r
8	Orye et al [64]	F (Belgian)	B	12	13q14-q22
9	Howard et al [39]	F	U	84	13q12-q14
10	O'Grady et al [63]	F (Brazilian)	B	30 (died 33 mo)	Dq-
11	O'Grady et al	F	U	11	Dq-
12	Francke & Kung [18]	F (Mexican)	B	8	13q12-q14
13	Knudson et al [46]	F	U	27	13q14-q22
14	Noel et al [61]	F (French)		birth	
15	Wilson et al [97]	M	U	4	13q12-q14
16	Cross et al [9,59]	F (Mexican)	B	4	
17	Yunis & Ramsey [100]	M (Korean)	B	5	13q14-q21

18	Yunis & Ramsay[89]	F	U	3	13q14.3 (subband deletion)
19	Walbaum et al[40]	F (French)	B	24	13q12-q14
20	Howard et al[90]	M	B	13	13q14-q22(5% mosaic deletio
21	Warburton[90]	F	B	5	13q13-q21
22	Warburton[29]	F	B	3	13q13-q22
23	deGrouchy[68]	M (French)	B	9 (died)	13q13-q21
24	Ozawa et al[75]	F (Japanese)	B	6	13q13-q31
25	Riccardi et al[75]	M (Mexican)	B	birth (died 3.5 mo)	13q12.5-q22.1
26	Riccardi et al[75]	M	B	?	13q-
27	Riccardi et al[12]	F	B	?	13q-
28	Davison[78]	M (English)	U	?	t(1:13) (p22;q12)
29	Sparkes et al[71]	F	U	48	13q14-q22
30	Petit & Fryns[101]	F (French)	U	5	13q12-q22
31	Yunis et al[34]	M	U	3 (died)	13q12-q14
32	Hida et al[93]	F (Japanese)	B	3	t(x;13) (p22;q13)
33	Welch et al	M (Canadian)	?	?	13q12-q14
34	Motegi et al	M (Japanese)	B	3	13q14.1-q14.3 (51% Mosaic deletion
35	Motegi et al	F (Japanese)	B	18	13q14.1-q14.3 (27% mosaic deletion
36	Motegi et al*	M (Japanese)	B	10	13q14.1-q21.2
37	Akazana	M	B		q12-q22

* Cited by Motegi

TABLE III

13q DELETION AND NO RETINOBLASTOMA

Patient No.	Reference	Sex	Chromosome 13 Deletion
1	Noel et al case 2b[61]	(French)	q14 (Distal) -qter (also trisomic for 5p13-pter)
2	Noel et al case 3	M	q32 or 34-qter
3	Noel et al case 4	F	q22-q31
4	Ikeuchi et al[42]	M (Japanese)	q22-qter
5	Cuschieri et al[10]	F (Malta)	q21-qter
6	Suzuki et al[80]	F (Japanese)	pter-q12 (also 18q-)
7	Fonatsch & Flatz[17]		pter-q12
8	Howard-Peebles et al[41]	F	pter-q12 (also trisomic for 9pter-q22)
9	Breg[3]		q21-q32
10	Aronson et al[1]	F	pter-q14
11	Weisswichert & Stogmann[92]	F	q21.2-q31.2
12	Pai et al[69]	F	q21-q31
13	Toomey & Mohandus[86]		q21-q31
14	Martin & Elias[98]		q22
15	Niikawa & Tamara et al[60]		
16	Nichols et al[58]	M	q22-q32
17	Krishna & Murthy[48]		q32-qter
18	Emanuel & Zackai[15]		q33

19	Chemke & Fisher[7]		q (distal)
20	Nomoto et al[62]		
21	Gross et al[25]	M	q-
22	Kucerova[49]	F	q22
23	Lungarotti et al (case 1)[4,53]	F	q21-q31
24	Lungarotti et al (case 2)	F	q12-q21
25	Carakushansky[5]		
26	Carakushansky		
26	Wilson et al[98]	F	q22-q31

The clinical features of 13q- retinoblastoma are variable and seem to show some difference from other patients with retinoblastoma. Twenty-one patients were female, and 15 were male. Most have exhibited mild to severe mental retardation, but others appeared to be of normal intelligence, especially those with a very small number of abnormal cells (mosaics)[40,57] and the patient with a minute subband deletion[100]. Details from case histories are limited in many reports, but physical development was retarded in at least 15 individuals. Other abnormalities have included low set ears[39,101], high arch palate[39,83,85,88,97], micrognathia [75,83,85], hypotonia[75,83,100], abnormal nipples[38,63,100], cardiomegaly[63,75,101], jejunal atresia[100], inguinal hernia [85,100], clinodactyly[39,57,63,75,100], abnormal fingers or thumb[18,63,83,85,100], transverse palmar crease[63,78,83,85], polydactyly[63], club foot[24,83], hirsutism[18,63,75,85], genital abnormalities[23,24,75,85,88], skeletal defects[24,38,63,85,88], muscular defects[18,23,39,75,78], and absent anus[24]. It is rather surprising that 7/37 (19%) of these patients have died.

The retinoblastoma tumor has been unilateral in 10 patients and bilateral in 24. The tumor has been diagnosed as early as birth or as late as 7 years of age with an average of 13.6 months. Microphthalmia has been noted at least 5 times[18,39,51,83,85]. Coloboma of the iris and/or choroid was reported for three patients[29,63,85]. Four patients demonstrated esotropia[23,39,65,85] and one patient had exotropia[100], and two unspecified strabismus[57]. The tumor was associated with elevated intraocular pressure and buphthalmus twice in patients with large tumor masses[18,63]. Reports indicate 17 left eyes and 7 right eyes were enucleated. In one individual, the ERG had normal photopic but decreased scotopic response[35].

Some possible problems in cytogenetic interpretation in this group of patients also have been apparent. 1) One retinoblastoma patient initially had a banded chromosome evaluation and was considered to be normal; however, when the banded study was repeated, and a large number of cells were counted, it was found that the patient was mosaic for 13q14 deletion, with only approximately 5% of the cells showing the abnormality[40]. While a small number of abnormal cells can probably never be excluded, a large number of cells should be examined and possibly different cells (leukocytes, fibroblasts, etc.) should be evaluated to exclude mosaicism. 2) Another patient with retinoblastoma was considered to have no deletion using conventional banding techniques. However, when re-examined using extended chromosomes (at prophase or prometaphase), the patient had a subband deletion of 13q14[100]. Two additional patients have been identified with the same subband deletion[57]. It would be possible to miss a small deletion in another retinoblastoma patient without employing such a chromosome technique.

While the majority of studies suggest deletion of chromosome band 13q14 is unique for retinoblastoma, four reports cast some doubt on this unique interpretation. 3) Two individuals have been recognized with an apparent intact translocation of band 13q14 to the X chromosome[9,34,59]. While this would seem to be an exception to the loss of this band in retinoblastoma, it is possible that gene activity is altered by transfer to a different site. A gene transferred to the X chromosome of a female would be expected to have at least a partially reduced activity as a consequence of the Lyon hypothesis. Moreover, a gene transferred to a different chromosome might not be activated by the usual stimuli. The assay of esterase D activity in this patient would be very informative. 4) Deletion of band 13q14 was identified in two other individuals who did not have retinoblastoma. One was a child who died at birth, so he may not have survived long enough to have developed retinoblastoma[61]. A second patient was an 18 year old girl with normal fundi[53]. While the levels of esterase D would be very helpful for both patients, they could represent true exceptions to the deletion of 13q14 always being associated with retinoblastoma.

Chromosome Markers in Retinoblastoma

No histopathological differences have been recognized between sporadic, autosomal dominant and 13q14 deletion retinoblastoma. Numerous attempts have been made to differentiate between the different "kinds" of retinoblastomas, and possibly identify those patients at risk for developing retinoblastomas.

Esterase D

The enzyme esterase D (E.C.3.1.1.1.) is found in most human tissues. It is characterized by its electrophoretic mobility and its specificity to hydrolyze 4- methyl umbelliferyl esters[36]. Assay of the enzyme activity is measured conveniently on erythrocytes. Early studies showed variable localization for esterase D on 13. Recent studies have localized the gene locus to the chromosome band 13q14 on the basis of finding the enzyme activity reduced to approximately 1/2 normal in individuals with deletion of chromosome band 13q14, including a unique person with subband deletion 13q14, and while normal esterase activity in otherswith deletion of 13q, but not including band q14[79]. This interpretation has been confirmed recently when a gene dosage effect has been shown for 13q14 deletion and duplication[14]. It is interesting that one individual with retinoblastoma and 13q14 deletion had normal erythrocyte esterase D activity, while fibroblasts from the same individual exhibited reduced esterase D activity[79]. Both esterase D phenotypes (ED^1 and ED^2) have occurred in 13q14- retinoblastoma. No reduction of esterase D activity was found in erythrocytes from individuals with autosomal dominant or sporadic retinoblastoma. It would be most important to know if esterase D activity is reduced in the retinoblastoma cells of these patients.

The level of esterase D activity would probably be of limited value in a mosaic individual with a low percent of 13q14- cells. In such an individual, the esterase D assay would not permit positive identification or exclusion of those at risk for retinoblastoma. In spite of this limitation, esterase D is currently the best chemical marker for retinoblastoma in individuals with 13q14 deletion.

Since most individuals with 13q14 deletion have had retinoblastoma, the localization of esterase D to the same or adjacent site allows one to infer a direct causual relationship of the enzyme deficiency to the development of retinoblastoma. The enzyme defect would be expected in all retinoblastoma cells, while the tumor develops only in a single cell or a few separate sites. It is possible that esterase D has as one function the inactivation by hydrolysis of an esterified intranuclear "key", which is able, with difficulty, to activate an embryonal cellular pathway for rapid growth, thus resulting in the tumor. This suggested model for retinoblastoma could be tested experimentally by introducing into retinal cells (intranuclear), an inhibitor for esterase D, in an effort to induce tumor formation, or by introducing (or inducing) esterase D activity in tumor cells to inhibit or stop tumor growth.

Fluorescent Marker Pale, medium and intense fluorescent markers occur with variable frequency on the short arm of chromosome 13. Four families with autosomal dominant retinoblastoma have been studied for segregation of fluorescent markers with retinoblastoma[45]. In one family there was an apparent segregation of a fluorescent marker with retinoblastoma, thereby infering that the gene for autosomal dominant retinoblastoma was located on chromosome 13. However, in three families, a discordant segregation of chromosome 13 fluorescent marker and retinoblastoma was observed. An explanation for this finding was that there had been a meiotic crossing over between the site of the fluorescent marker on the short arm of the chromosome 13 and the site of the retinoblastoma gene, which was probably on the long arm; another explanation would be that the site for the dominant retinoblastoma gene was located on another chromosome.

Tissue Culture It has been claimed that unilateral and bilateral retinoblastoma cells, when placed in tissue culture, exhibit different growth characteristics. Specifically, contact inhibition is said to occur with unilateral (sporadic) retinoblastoma, but not with bilateral (dominant) retinoblastoma cells[72]. However, the variability described by the authors infer that this is not a definite marker at the present stage of development. This test does not seem to have been tried with 13q14- retinoblastoma cells.

Increased Chromosome Fragility Turleau et al have found an increase in sister chromatid exchanges in fibroblasts from patients with 13q14- and retinoblastoma when compared to controls[87]. Weichselbaum et al have subjected fibroblasts from patients to x-radiation[91]. Fibroblasts from patients with dominant and 13q14 retinoblastoma were considered to be more susceptible to lethal radiation than sporadic or control fibroblasts. Cziezel has reported increased aneuploidy, chromatid type aberrations and stable chromosome changes in retinoblastoma patients[11]. Knight et al could not confirm increased chromosome fragility[44].

Chromosomes in Retinoblastoma Cells

Tumor cells are usually characterized by abnormal metaphase chromosomes. In contrast to 22 pairs of autosomes and 2 sex chromosomes, whole or partial chromosome duplication or deletion occurs in retinoblastoma cells, in addition to marker chromosomes. In 1963, Yoneda reported 36 to 60 metaphase chromosomes in retinoblastoma cells[99]. However, no abnormality was recognized in one subsequent study[76]. A later report by Kobayashi described polynuclear and polypoid tumor cells, with chromosome deletion, and duplication, and tetraploidy in retinoblastoma cells[47]. Mark examined retinoblastoma cells in an effort to demonstrate Dq-[54], which had been shown by Lele in peripheral leucocytes of one patient[51]. He did not identify Dq-, in tumor cells or retinoblastoma cells in tissue culture, but found marker chromosomes, duplication and deletion of whole chromosomes, with a total chromosome number varying from 45 to 49, and tetraploidy in other cells.

In subsequent studies, Dq- has been identified in retinoblastoma cells by Oyre[66], Hashem[30] and Hittner[35]. 14q+ was associated with other chromosome duplication and deletion in another report[38]. The extra chromosomal material on 14q appeared to be translocated from another chromosome, possibly 11.

In some experimental studies on the rat, it has been possible to produce a sarcoma by Rous sarcoma virus which is indistinguishable histologically from a sarcoma produced by 7, 12 dimethyl benzyl-anthracene[52]. The chromosomes of these tumors had non random patterns of aberration which were characteristic for the causative agent. If a similar difference should exist in human retinoblastoma cells, it might be possible to differentiate between sporadic, autosomal dominant and 13q deletion retinoblastoma. Thus far, no difference has been shown in the chromosomes of retinoblastoma from sporadic, autosomal dominant or 13q presentations.

BIBLIOGRAPHY

1. Aronson, M., Zackai, E., Mellman, W., et al, A (13) terminal deletion, 46 chromosomes, Repository Identification No. GM-250, Cytogenetic Cell. Genet., 15:57-58, 1975.

2. Bentley, D., A case of Down's syndrome complicated by retinoblastoma and celiac disease, Pediatrics, 56:131-133, 1975.

3. Breg, W. R., Unpublished case report.

4. Calabro, A., Delezione Interstiziale del 13(q21-q31) Pathologica, 71:359, 1979.

5. Carakushansky, G., Monossomia parcial do cromossomo 13: Estudo de dois casos., Revista Da Associacao Medica Brasileira (Sao Paulo) 25 (11): 392-394, 1979.

6. Cernea, P., Teodorescu, F., Angheloni, T., Retinoblastome: A mosaicisme chromosomien 46XX/47XX, G+, Ann. Oculist (Paris) 206:607-611, 1973.

7. Chemke, J., Fishel, E., Zalish, M. et al, Multiple skeletal anomalies in the "13q-" syndrome, Eur. J. Ped., 128:27-31, 1978.

8. Conen, P.E., and Erkman, B., Frequency and occurrence of chromosomal syndrome, I. D- trisomy, Am. J. Hum. Genet., 18:374-386, 1966.

9. Cross, H.E., Hansen, R.C., Morrow, G., et al, Retinoblastoma in a patient with 13qXp translocation, Am. J. Ophth. 84:548-554, 1977.

10. Cuschieri, A., Agius, P.V., Scheres, JMJC, Partial deletion of the long arm of chromosome no. 13, Hum. Genet. 36:341-344, 1977.

11. Czeizel, A., Czosz, L., Gardonyi, J., et al, Chromosome studies in twelve patients with retinoblastoma, Humangenetik 22:159-166, 1974.

12. Davison, E.V., Gibbons, B., Aherne, G.E.S., Roberts, D. F., Chromosomes in retinoblastoma patients,

Clin. Genet., 15:505-508, 1979.

13. Day, R.W., Wright, S.W., Koons, A., et al, XXX,21-trisomy and retinoblastoma, Lancet ii, 154-155, 1963.

14. Despoisse, S., Junien, C., Turleau, C., et al, Gene dosage studies for Esterase D, Human Gene Mapping VI, Oslo Conf., 1981, Cytogenet. Cell. Genet. (in press).

15. Emanuel, B.S., Zackai, E.H., Moreau, L., et al, Interstitial deletion 13q33 resulting from maternal insertional translocation, Clin. Genet. 16:340-346, 1979.

16. Ejima, Y., Sasaki, M.S., and Takebe, H., Chromosome rearrangements in retinoblastoma with or without 13q-, Human Gene Mapping, Oslo Conf., 1981, Cytogenet. Cell. Genet. (in press).

17. Fonatsch, C., Flatz, S.D., De novo (11:13) translocation, Humangenetik, 28:87-91, 1975.

18. Francke, U., Kung, F., Sporadic bilateral retinoblastoma and 13q- chromosomal deletion., Med. Ped. Oncology, 2:379-385, 1976.

19. Francois, J., Berger, R., and Saraux, H., Les aberrations chromosomiques en Ophtalmologie, Masson et Cie, Paris, 1972, p. 359.

20. Francois, J., Berger, R., and Saraux, H., op. cit. p. 355.

21. Francois, T., DeBie, S., Matton-Van Leuven, M.T., Genesis and Genetics of Retinoblastoma, Jap. J. Ophth. 22:301-306, 1978.

22. Friedrich, U., and Nielsen, J., Chromosome studies in 5,049 consecutive newborn children, Clin. Genet., 4:333-343, 1973.

23. Gey, W., Dq-, multiple missbildungen und retinoblastom, Humangenetik 10:362-365, 1970.

24. Grace, E., Drennan, J., Colver, D., et al, The 13q-deletion syndrome, J. Med. Genet., 8:351-357, 1971.

25. Gross, K.P., Schwanitz, G., Ein Neues Syndrom durch Chromosomenstuckverlust (13q-), Klin. Padiat., 185:468-473, 1973.

26. Grouchy, J. de, Turleau, C., Clinical Atlas of Human Chromosomes, John Wiley, NY, 1977, p. 189.

27. Grouchy, J. de, Turleau, C., op. cit. p. 193.

28. Grouchy, J. de, Turleau, C., op. cit. p. 243.

29. Grouchy, J. de, Turleau, C., Cabanis, M., et al, Retinoblastome et deletion intercalaire du chromsome 13, Arch. Fr. Pediatr., 37:(8)531-535, 1980.

30. Hashem, N., Khalifa, S., Retinoblastoma: A model of hereditary fragile chromosome regions, Hum. Hered. 25:35-49, 1975.

31. Hecht, F., Nievaard, J.E., Duncanson, N., et al, Double Aneuploidy: The frequency of XXY in males with Down's syndrome, Am. J. Hum. Genet., 21:352-359, 1969.

32. Herrmann, J., Gilbert, E.F., Opitz, J.M., Dysplasia, malformations, and cancer, especially with respect to the Wiedemann-Beckwith Syndrome. In Warren W. Nichols, Ed., Institute for Medical Research Workshop on Regulation of Cell Proliferation and Differentiation (Proc. Workshop on Regulation of Cell Proliferation and Differentiation, p. 1-55, 1975).

33. Herrmann, J., Delayed mutation as a cause of retinoblastoma: application to genetic counseling, Birth Defects, Orig. Art. Ser. XII No. 1, 79-90, 1976.

34. Hida, T., Kinoshita, Y., Matsumoto, R., et al, Bilateral retinoblastoma with 13qXp translocation, J. Ped. Ophthal. and Strab., 17:144-146, 1980.

35. Hittner, H.M., Riccardi, V.M., Kretzer, F.L., et al, Two step mutation theory for retinoblastoma: ultra structure support, Doc. Ophthal., 48(2): 345-362, 1979.

36. Hopkinson, D.A., Mestriner, M.A., Cortner, J., et al, Esterase D: A new human polymorphism., Ann. Hum. Genet. 37:119-137, 1973.

37. Hossfeld, K.D., Heopping, W., Vogel, M., Chromosome patterns in retinoblastoma in Fifth International Congress Human Genetics, Excepta Medica, 1976.

38. Hossfeld, D.K., Chromosome 14q+, in a retinoblastoma, Inter. J. Cancer, 21(6), 720-723, 1978.

39. Howard R.O., Breg, W.R., Albert, D.M., et al, Retinoblastoma and chromosome abnormality, Arch. Ophth. 92:490-493, 1974.

40. Howard R.O., Warburton, D., Breg, W.R., et al, Retinoblastoma and partial deletion of the long arm of chromosome 13, Tr. Am. Ophth. Soc. 76:172-183, 1978.

41. Howard-Peebles, P.N., Yarbrough, K., Stoddard, G., et al, Translocation 9q/13q resulting in duplication (trisomy 9pter-9q22) and deficiency (monosomy 13pter-13q12), Clin. Genet., 11:46-52, 1977.

42. Ikeuchi, T., Sonta, S., Sasaki, M., et al, Chromosome banding patterns in an infant with 13q- syndrome, Humangenetik, 21:309-314, 1974.

43. Jackson, E.W., Turner, J.H., Klauber, M.R., et al, Down's syndrome: Variation of leukemia occurrence in institutionalized populations, J. Chron. Dis., 21:247-253, 1968.

44. Knight, L.A., Gardner, H.A., and Gallie, B.L., Absence of chromosome breakage in patients with retinoblastoma, Hum. Genet. 51:73-78, 1979.

45. Knight, L.A., Gardner, H.A., and Gallie, B.L., Familial retinoblastoma: Segretation of chromosome 13 in four families, Am. J. Hum. Genet., 32:194-201, 1980.

46. Knudson, A.G., Meadows, A.T., Nichols, W.W., et al, Chromosomal deletion and retinoblastoma, New Eng. J. Med. 295:1120-1123, 1976.

47. Kobayashi, M., Shimada, K., Oda, I., Chromosomal aberrations in retinoblastoma: report of seven cases, Jap. J. Ophthal., 12(2), 96-102, 1968.

48. Krishna Murthy, D.S., Patel, Z.M., A
Trisomy 18q: 46XX, 13q+, t(13,18),
newborn associated with multiple con
due to paternal reciprocal transloca
+der (13), t(13, 18), (q32, q11), Cl
238, 1980.

49. Kucerova, M., Polivkova, Z., Pokorn
long arm of chromosome 13, Humangene
1975.

50. Ladda, R., Atkins, L., Littlefield,
Retinoblastoma: Chromosome Banding
heritable tumor, Lancet ii,506, 197

51. Lele, K.P., Penrose, L.S., Stallard
deletion in a case of retinoblastom
27:171--174, 1963.

52. Levan, A., Chromosome Patterns in
in, Chromosome Identification: Te
tion in biology and medicine, Ed.
L. Zech, Academic Press, NY, 1973.

53. Lungarotti, M.S., Mariotti, G., Pr
etti, G., Delezione Interstiziale
46,XX,del 13(q12-q21): Descrizion
Genet. 52:269-274, 1979.

54. Mark, J., Chromosomal analysis of
toma, Acta. Ophthal. 48:124-135,

55. Miller, R.W., Neoplasia and Down'
Acad. Sci., 171:637-644, 1970.

56. Morgan, S.S., and Bair, H.L., Her
toma: Report of a family with re
ing in three successive generatic
65:43-47, 1968.

57. Motegi, T., Lymphocyte Chromosome
with Retinoblastoma: Effort to
mosaicism, Hum. Genet. 38:168-17

interstitial deletion of the long a
somy 8, Johns Hopkins Med. J., 145:

70. Palmer, C.G., Stephenson, S., Weave
Clinical findings of both partial t
monosomy 13 in a child with 2 diffe
population, Abstracts, p. 190, Birt
ence, Chicago, 1979.

71. Petit, P.Fryns, J.P. Interstitial d
associated with retinoblastoma and
tions, Ann. Genet. 22:106-107, 1979

72. Prop, F.J.A., Prop-Arnold, G.C.B.,
H., An attempt to discriminate betw
hereditary retinoblastoma by means
p. 97-104 in, P.P. Dendy, Ed. Human
term culture: Technique and clinic

73. Pruett, R.C., Atkins, L., Chromosom
ients with retinoblastoma, Arch. Op
1969.

74. Rethore, M.O., Saraux, H., Prieur,
48, XXY, +21, et retinoblastome, Ar
29:533-538, 1972.

75. Riccardi, V.M., Hittner, H.M., Fran
Partial triplication and deletion o
family presenting with retinoblasto
15:332-345, 1979.

76. Schappert-Kimmijser, J., Hemmes, G.
heredity of retinoblastoma, Ophthal
213, 1966.

77. Schwanitz, G., Reither, M., Grosse,
monosomy 13 as the result of a bala
3/13 pat., Humangenetik, 28:93-96,

78. Sparkes, R.S., Muller, H., Klisak,
with 13q-chromosomal deletion assoc
paracentric inversion of 13q, Scien
1979.

79. Sparkes, R.S., Sparkes, M.C., Wilson, M.G., et al, Regional assignment of genes for human esterase D and retinoblastoma to chromosome band 13q14, Science, 208-1042-1044, 1980.

80. Suzuki, Y., Ono, K., Oka, S., et al, A case of (13q:18q) translocation with proximal 13q monosomy, Hum. Genet. 38:337-341, 1977.

81. Taktikos, A., Association of retinoblastoma with mental defect and other pathological manifestation, Brit., J. Ophthal. 48:495-498, 1964.

82. Tan, K.E.W.P., Van Biervliet, J.P.G.M., Van Hemel, J.O., Retinoblastoma combined with severe chromosomal disorders, Ophthalmologica, 176:280, 1978.

83. Taylor, A.I., Dq-, Dr, and retinoblastoma, Humangenetik, 10:209-217, 1970.

84. Telfer, M.A., Clark, C.E., Cowell, H.R., et al, Long arm deletion of chromosome 13 with exclusion of esterase D from 13q32-13qter, Clin. Genet. 17:428-432, 1980.

85. Thompson, H., Lyons, R.B., Retinoblastoma and multiple congenital anomalies associated with complex mosaicism with deletion of D-chromosome and probably D/C translocation, Hum. Chrom. Newsletter 15:21, 1965.

86. Toomey, K.C., Mohandas, T., Sparkes, R.S., et al, Segregation of an insertional chromosome rearrangement in 3 generations, J. Med. Genet. 15:382-387, 1978.

87. Turleau, C., Cabanis, M.O., Grouchy, J.de, Augmentation des echanges de chromatides dans les fibroblasts d'un enfant atteint de del (13) retinoblastome, Ann. Genet. 23(3):169-170, 1980.

88. Van Kempen, C., A case of retinoblastoma combined with severe mental retardation and a few other congenital anomalies associated with complex aberrations of the karyotype, Maandrschr Kindergeneeskd, 34:92-95, 1966.

89. Walbaum, R., Francois, P., et al, Un cas de retinoblastome bilateral avec monosomie 13 partielle (q12-q14), Hum. Genet. 44(2):219-226, 1978.

90. Warburton, D., Personal communication.

91. Weischselbaum, R.R., Nove, J., Little, J.B., X-ray sensitivity of diploid fibroblasts from patients with hereditary or sporadic retinoblastoma, Proc. Natl. Acad. Sci., 75:3962-3964, 1978.

92. Weisswichert, P., Stogmann, W., Interstitieller Stuckverlust am Chromosom Nr. 13: Ein neues Syndrom? Klin. Padiat. 191:318-324, 1979.

93. Welch, J.P., Flander, D.C., Main, M., Evidence for chromosomal instability in retinoblastoma patients and band assignment of the occasionally associated chromosome 13 deletion, Am. J. Hum. Genet., 29:113a, 1977.

94. Wiener, S., Reese, A.B., Hyman, G.A., Chromosome studies in retinoblastoma Arch. Ophth. 69:311-313, 1963.

95. Wilson, M.G., Melnyk, J., Towner, J.W., Retinoblastoma and deletion D(14) syndrome, J. Med. Genet. 6:322-327, 1969.

96. Wilson, M.G., Towner, J.W., Fujimoto, A., Retinoblastoma and D chromosome deletions, Am. J. Hum. Genet. 25:57-61, 1973.

97. Wilson, M.G., Ebbin, A.J., Towner, J.W., et al, Chromosomal anomalies in patients with retinoblastoma, Clin. Genet. 12:1-8, 1977.

98. Wilson, L., Hodes, B.L., Martin, A.O., et al, Cytogenetic Analysis of a case of "13q- Syndrome" (46,XX del 13) using banding techniques, J. Ped. Ophthal. and Strab., 17:63-67, 1980.

99. Yoneda, D., Herkk, W. Van, Tissue culture cell strain dereived from retinoblastoma, Am. J. Ophthal. 55:987-992, 1963.

100. Yunis, J.J., Ramsey, N., Retinoblastoma and subband deletion of chromosome 13, Am. J. Dis. Child., 132:161-163, 1978.

101. Yunis, E., Zuniga, R., Ramirez, E., Retinoblastoma, Gross internal malformations and deletion 13q14-q31, Hum. Genet. 56:283-286, 1981.

NORRIE'S DISEASE

S.S. Johnston*, J.E. Hanna+, N.C. Nevin+ and J.H. Bryars*.
* Department of Ophthalmology,
Royal Victoria Hospital, Belfast.
+ Department of Medical Genetics,
The Queen's University of Belfast.

Norrie's disease or congenital progressive oculo-acoustico-cerebral dysplasia, a rare X-linked condition was first described in blind boys from two Danish families by Gordon Norrie in 1927. Warburg (1961) reported seven cases in seven generations of a Danish family and suggested the disorder should be designated Norrie's disease. Since then she has written extensively on the disease. In 1975 she reported a further six cases in four families making a total of 47 families comprising 249 published in the literature. Since then six further families with 25 affected patients have been described (Sauter 1974; Schmitz-Valckenberg 1977; Moreira-Filko and Neustein 1979; Jacklin 1980; Fujita et al 1980). This paper describes a further two families, the first reported from Ireland, with eight affected males.

CASE REPORTS

The first family (Fig. 1) shows five affected males in three generations. The proband (IV,17), born April 26, 1975, is the last of a sibship of two, the older sib being a girl with normal vision. He presented in October 1976 at the Genetic Eye Clinic and examination showed no perception of light in either eye. Both eyes were microphthalmic with corneal scarring and shallow anterior chambers. Each had retrolental membranes and cataract. At this time there was no hearing loss and his development was in keeping with his chronological age and visual handicap. His mother (111,12) had normal visual acuity. A maternal uncle (11,15) has been blind since infancy. The family had lost trace of him so we have been unable to examine him. A contemporary of his who

Birth Defects: Original Article Series, Volume 18, Number 6, pages 729–738

now teaches blind children reports that he was of low average intelligence but his hearing remained clinically good. 11,8 now aged 58 years old has always been blind. Examination in January 1977 showed no perception of light in either eye. The eyes were microphthalmic with bilateral cataract, and pendular nystagmus also was present. His IQ was 70 and his audiogram showed a rightsided neurosensory loss. 11,5 died in early childhood but is reported to have been blind from birth. 111,6 also has been blind since birth and when examined in November, 1976, aged 40 years old, showed no perception of light in either eye. The eyes were microphthalmic with shallow anterior chambers, bilateral band degeneration and pendular nystagmus. His audiogram showed a bilateral neurosensory loss. He has a profound stammer and is of low intelligence, IQ 70. His mother 11,6 has normal corrected visual acuity.

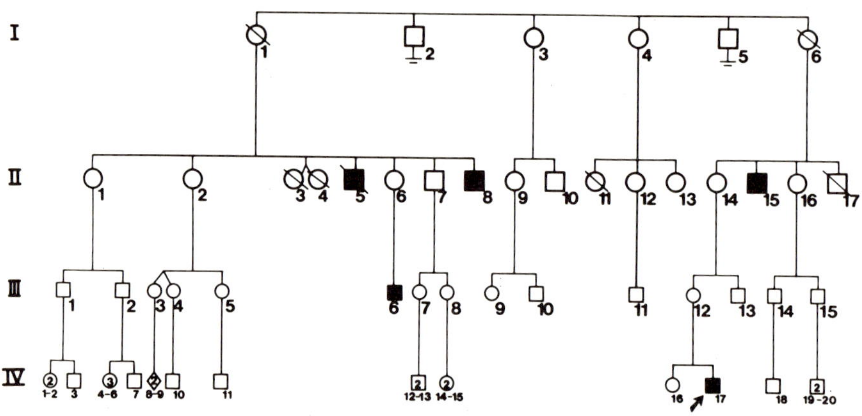

Fig. 1. Pedigree of first family

The second family (Fig. 2) has three affected males in two generations. The proband (V,6) was born in May 1970, the youngest in a sibship of three boys, the other two having normal vision. When one month old, his mother noticed that his right eye looked different from the left. Examination under anaesthetic revealed that the right eye was microphthalmic with a hazy cornea. The left cornea was clear. The right anterior chamber was virtually absent with anterior synechiae and elongated ciliary processes were present. The left anterior chamber had normal depth and the pupil reacted normally. The right pupil was irregular and fixed. There was a yellowish/white mass behind the lens and ectropion uveae was present. Provisional diagnosis of primary hyperplastic vitreous was made with a differential diagnosis of retinoblastoma or toxoplasmosis. A repeat E.U.A. in November 1970 showed no change but in May 1971, progressive deterioration was evident with bilateral corneal oedema, both pupils were irregular and miosed and both anterior chambers were shallow.

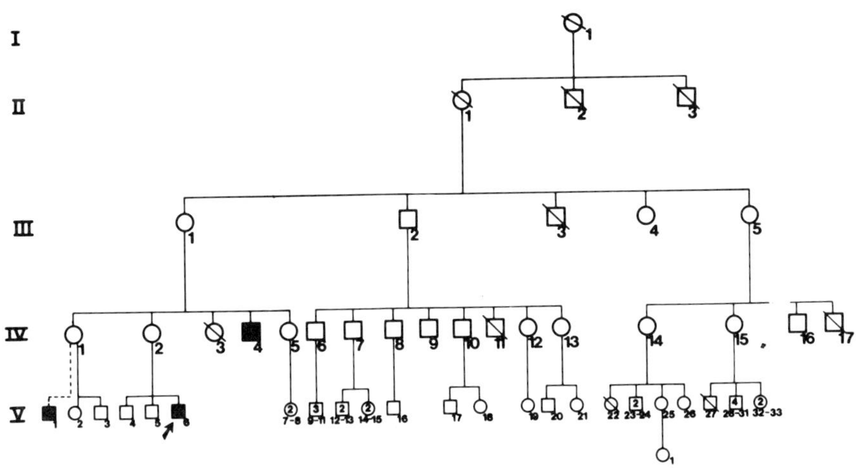

Fig. 2. Pedigree of second family

The iris was atrophic and vascularised and what was thought to be a mature cataract was seen in either eye. The patient was seen at the Medical Genetic Clinic and it was then that a family history of other affected male relatives came to light. At present his hearing is normal but although he commenced his education in a special school for the blind, his mental retardation was such that he will probably be reascertained as severely subnormal.

A maternal first cousin (V,1) was adopted shortly after birth. With much difficulty he was traced and at the age of three months was unable to see. The left eye was smaller than the right and both eyes rolled continuously. As a diagnosis of retinoblastoma had been made the left eye was enucleated. The specimen was sent to Professor Norman Ashton of the Institute of Ophthalmology, London, and his findings were as follows - "The posterior segment showed a retrolental fibro-cellular mass of disorganised and detached retinal tissue with areas of encysted haemorrhage and blood pigment, widely, dilated thin walled vessels and rosette granules, and the subretinal space contained a large number of macrophages with pigment granules and the subretinal fluid was haemorrhagic. In the anterior segment a mild inflammatory reaction of the iris and posterior synechiae are present while the filtration angle is not well developed and the lens is cataractous. The optic nerve is hypercellular". In 1962 in the absence of any known family history the diagnosis was made of haemorrhagic, retinal detachment. When the family history was established in 1971, Professor Ashton reviewed the pathology and diagnosed Norrie's disease. This case was presented by him in 1971 at the European Pathology Society meeting. This boy had an unsuccessful trial at a special school for the blind and in June 1968, was ascertained as severely subnormal. His hearing appeared clinically normal. A maternal uncle (lV,4) who was blind from birth died aged two and a half years following an accident. We have been unable to trace any of his records.

DISCUSSION

In these two families there are eight affected males, six of whom are still alive. Of these, five are mentally retarded, two severely so, both in one family, and the other is just two years old. In the six living males, two have a definite neurosensory hearing loss. Of the four remaining, three are still of school age and we have been unable to trace the other. Warburg (1966) reports that impairment of hearing is noticeable in one third of affected patients after about the age of 10 years and pyschotic behaviour appears after the first or second year in some 25 percent of patients. The former would appear to be purely of cochlear origin with no involvement of the brain stem as measured by electrocochleography and brain stem evoked responses (Parving, Elberling and Warburg 1978). The hearing loss may appear as early as four months (Blodi et al 1969) and as late as 45 years (Warburg 1966). It would appear that the so-called mental retardation is due partly to psychotic reaction and partly to organic cerebral damage as evidenced by epileptic seizures (Warburg 1975). Other associated abnormal features may be hypogenitalism (Hara et al 1969) and in addition microcephaly (Moreira-Filho and Neustein 1979).

Ocular Findings

Characteristically there is bilateral blindness at or shortly after birth. This presents as falciform folds of the retina, leukocoria, haemorrhagic retinal detachment, shallow anterior chambers, posterior synechiae and elongated ciliary processes. Later there is microphthalmos, nystagmus, band degeneration of the cornea, secondary cataract and phthisis bulbi. A few early cases have been followed clinically to full detachment (Arruga 1950; Warburg 1966 and 1971; and Jacklin 1980). The latter describes in detail the clinical course from vitreous haemorrhage and falciform fold at the age of eight weeks to retrolental detachment at the age of eight months.

Differential Diagnosis

The ocular findings are variable in presentation and the definitive diagnosis cannot be made on these alone but only in conjunction with histopathology, if available, and with a positive family history. The affected individuals in our first family all attended the Genetic Eye Clinic and presented no problem in diagnosis. In our second family an initial differential diagnosis of persistent hyperplastic vitreous, retinoblastoma or toxoplasmosis was made in the proband (V,6) and a definitive diagnosis was not made until the family was seen for genetic counselling, when a history of other affected males came to light. His cousin (V,1) was initially diagnosed as retinoblastoma and even with histopathology a diagnosis of Norrie's disease was not made until the family history was available. The differential diagnosis is best considered aetiologically (Warburg 1979). In infancy, she considers the differential diagnosis in three groups; tumours, acquired anomalies and malformations which may be due to monogenic traits, syndromes or chromosomal abnormalities. Tumours are bilateral retinoblastoma. The acquired anomalies may be inflammatory such as toxoplasmosis, traumatic or non-accidental injury, drugs such as Thalidomide and excess oxygen therapy in premature infants, giving retrolental fibroplasia. Congenital non-attachment of the retina occurs in many malformations. Monogenic disorders such as falciform folds may be dominant, recessive or X-linked. It should be remembered that Norrie's disease may initially present in only one eye and persistent hyperplastic primary vitreous and Coats disease must be considered. Syndromes may be X-linked dominant such as incontinentia pigmenti recessive, of which there are several, or X-linked recessive as in Norrie's disease. The chromosomal abnormality to be considered is Trisomy 13 (Pautau's syndrome). Norrie's disease would appear to be the commonest genetic disorder in which retinal non-attachment has been described.

In adults, all causes of microphthalmia, secondary cataract, band degeneration of the cornea and phthisis bulbi must be taken into account. X-linked microphthalmia and X-linked cataract are listed amongst the hereditary causes.

Histopathology

Including the present case, histological examination has now been reported on 30 eyes (Warburg 1975; Jacklin 1980; Fujita 1980). Case V,I (Fig. 2) shows the typical findings of retinal dysplasia posteriorly with glial and vascular proliferation and haemorrhages. Anteriorly there is a mild inflammatory reaction with posterior synechiae, elongated ciliary processes and cataract. This appearance is non-specific, occurring in many conditions (Hunter and Zimmerman 1965; Warburg 1966 and 1979). Blodi and Hunter (1969) postulated a relationship with Coats disease because of the vascular changes but Apple et al (1974) in describing an early case could not demonstrate any evidence of vascular malformation or primary retinal blood vessel defects. Warburg (1966 and 1974) regards the essential lesion as a genetically determined biochemical defect, causing an arrest in development of the inner layer of the optic cup at the 10 to 17 mm stage. There is associated malformation of the primary and secondary vitreous. Examination of the brain in one case with mental retardation showed atrophy of the visual pathways and lateral geniculate bodies and incomplete stratification of the cortex and abnormalities of the mesencephalon and pons (Warburg 1968).

Hereditary and Linkage Studies

No ocular or otological stigmata have been found in any female carrier apart from one case with a colobomatous-like lesion in one eye and a cataract in the other (Capella et al 1963). Linkage studies have shown no relationship between the Norrie's locus (Nd) and The Xg. blood groups (Warburg et al 1965 and Nance 1969). Nance et al (1969) found a loose linkage between the Nd and G-6PD loci. Moeira-Filho and Neustein (1979) presented a family with a measurable g-linkage associated with classical Norrie's disease. This family in addition had microcephaly and cryptorchidism.

The disease has now been reported from widely spread geographical areas and in different races. In Europe, cases are described from Scandinavia, England, Germany, Switzerland, Holland, Spain, Poland and Cyprus. Families reviewed have emigrated within Europe and from Europe to the Americas and Australia including Danish and English stock. In America, apart from Caucasions, North American Indians in Canada, and Negroes including Cubans and Brazilians are reported. The first cases from Asia were published in Japan (Fujita 1980). It has not been possible to trace our first family beyond four generations. The second family has been traced for eight generations, back to 1759. All have been born and lived within Northern Ireland.

Counselling

A correct diagnosis is necessary not only for genetic counselling but to avoid unneedful enucleation or other surgery. When the diagnosis has been established on the basis of X-linked inheritance, typical ocular findings and possible hearing loss and dementia, then counselling is of course straightforward and necessary to avoid recurrence of similarly affected males in the family. It is now possible to offer carrier females during pregnancy amniocentesis to sex the fetus with a view to termination if the fetus is male.

Treatment

There is no known treatment but Jacklin (1980) carried out lensectomy and vitrectromy in an affected infant. Although it was not possible to reattach the retina, the eye, after two years, had not become phthisical as compared with the unoperated eye. Mann (1977) has successfully treated bilateral detachments in an infant with microphthalmia between nine and thirteen weeks. However the detachments in this case were rhegmatogenous. The management of blind children is difficult but becomes even more so, if psychiatric and hearing problems also occur. Warburg (1975) stresses the importance of protecting the affected children from early parental deprivation and to avoid rearing them in boarding schools for the blind.

REFERENCES

Ashton N (1971). Norrie's disease. Joint Meeting European Pathology Soc and Verhoeff Soc London.

Apple DJ, Fishman GA and Goldberg MF (1974). Ocular histopathology of Norrie's disease. Am J Ophthalmol 78:2:196.

Arruga MH (1950). Une rarete clinique: Decollment de la retine hereditaire et binoculaire. Bull Soc Ophthal Fr 63:160.

Blodi FC and Hunter WS (1969). Norrie's disease in North America. Doc Ophthal 26:434.

Capella JA, Kaufman HE, Lill FJ and Cooper G (1963). Hereditary cataracts and microphthalmia. Am J Ophthal 56:454.

Fujita S, Fujiwara N and Ohba N (1980). Norrie's disease: Report of two cases in two Japanese families. Jpn J Ophthalmol 24:22.

Hara S, Jansen A, Crump, Elliott J and Nance W (1969). Clinical studies of a negro family with Norrie's disease. Quoted in preparation by Nance et al (1969).

Hunter WS and Zimmerman LE (1965). Unilateral retinal dysplasia. Arch Ophthal 74:23.

Jacklin HN (1980). Falciform fold, retinal detachment and Norrie's disease. Am J Ophthalmol 90:76.

Mann E, Kut LJ and Lee CB (1977). Rhegmatogenous retinal detachment in infancy. Arch Ophthalmol 1774.

Moreira-Filho CA and Neustein I (1979). A presumptive new variant of Norrie's disease. J Med Genet 16:125.

Nance WE, Hara S, Hansen A, Elliott J, Lewis M and Chown B (1969). Genetic linkage studies in a negro kindred with Norrie's disease. Am J Genet 21:5:423.

Norrie G (1927). Causes of blindness in children. Acta Ophthal (Kbh) 5:357.

Parving A, Elberling C and Warburg M (1978). Electro-physiological study of Norrie's disease. An X-linked progressive trait with hearing loss. Audiology 17(4):293.

Sauter K (1974). Zespol Norriego. Klin Oczna 44:1281.

Schmitz-Valckenberg P and Scholz W (1977). Das-Norrie-syndrom. Klin Mbl Augenheilk 171:562.

Warburg M (1961). Norrie's disease. A new hereditary bilateral pseudotumor of the retina. Acta Ophthal (Kbh) 39:757.

Warburg M, Hauge M and Sanger R (1965). Norrie's disease and the Xg blood group system; linkage data. Acta Genet (Basel) 15:103.

Warburg M (1966). Norrie's disease. A congenital progressive oculo-acoustico-cerebral degeneration. Acta Ophthal (Kbh) 89(Suppl):1.

Warburg M (1968). Norrie's disease. J Ment Def Res 12:247.

Warburg M (1974). "Norrie's disease and falciform detachment of the retina". In Goldberg M (ed) "Genetic and Metabolic aspects of eye disease". Boston, Little Brown and Co.

Warburg M (1975). Norrie's disease: differential diagnosis and treatment. Acta Ophthal (Kbh) 53:2:217).

Warburg M (1979). Retinal malformations. Aetiological heterogeneity and morphological similarity in congenital retinal non-attachment and falciform folds. Trans Ophthal Soc UK 99:272.

Index

BOOKS PUBLISHED BY ALAN R. LISS, INC.
FOR THE MARCH OF DIMES BIRTH DEFECTS FOUNDATION

BIRTH DEFECTS: ORIGINAL ARTICLE SERIES

1975 — Volume XI

No. 7 **Morphogenesis and Malformation of Face and Brain,** Daniel Bergsma and Jan Langman, *Editors*

1976 — Volume XII

No. 1 **Cancer and Genetics,** Daniel Bergsma, R. Neil Schimke, Robert L. Summitt, and David J. Harris, *Editors*
No. 3 **The Eye and Inborn Errors of Metabolism,** Daniel Bergsma, Anthony J. Bron, and Edward Cotlier, *Editors*
No. 4 **Developmental Disabilities: Psychologic and Social Implications,** Daniel Bergsma and Ann E. Pulver, *Editors*
No. 5 **Cytogenetics, Environment and Malformation Syndromes,** Daniel Bergsma and R. Neil Schimke, *Editors*
No. 6 **Growth Problems and Clinical Advances,** Daniel Bergsma and R. Neil Schimke, *Editors*
No. 8 **Iron Metabolism and Thalassemia,** Daniel Bergsma, Anthony Cerami, Charles M. Peterson, and Joseph H. Graziano, *Editors*

1977 — Volume XIII

No. 1 **Morphogenesis and Malformation of the Limb,** Daniel Bergsma and Widukind Lenz, *Editors*
No. 2 **Morphogenesis and Malformation of the Genital System,** Richard J. Blandau and Daniel Bergsma, *Editors*
No. 3 **Annual Review of Birth Defects, 1976,** Daniel Bergsma and R. Brian Lowry, *Editors*
Proceedings of the 1976 Vancouver Birth Defects Conference. Published in 4 volumes:
- 3A **Numerical Taxonomy of Birth Defects** *and* **Polygenic Disorders**
- 3B **New Syndromes**
- 3C **Natural History of Specific Birth Defects**
- 3D **Embryology and Pathogenesis** *and* **Prenatal Diagnosis**

No. 5 **Urinary System Malformations in Children,** Daniel Bergsma and John W. Duckett, *Editors*
No. 6 **Trends and Teaching in Clinical Genetics,** Daniel Bergsma, Frederick Hecht, Gerald H. Prescott, and Joan H. Marks, *Editors*

1978 — Volume XIV

No. 1 **Genetic Effects on Aging,** Daniel Bergsma and David E. Harrison, *Editors*
No. 2 **The Molecular Basis of Cell-Cell Interactions,** Richard A. Lerner and Daniel Bergsma, *Editors*
No. 3 **The Genetics of Hand Malformations,** *by* Samia A. Temtamy and Victor A. McKusick
No. 5 **Neurochemical and Immunologic Components in Schizophrenia,** Daniel Bergsma and Allan L. Goldstein, *Editors*

No. 6 **Annual Review of Birth Defects 1977,** Robert L. Summitt and Daniel Bergsma, *Editors* Proceedings of the 1977 Memphis Birth Defects Conference. Published in 3 volumes:
- 6A **Cell Surface Factors, Immune Deficiencies. Twin Studies**
- 6B **Recent Advances** *and* **New Syndromes**
- 6C **Sex Differentiation** *and* **Chromosomal Abnormalities**

No. 7 **Morphogenesis and Malformation of the Cardiovascular System,** Glenn C. Rosenquist and Daniel Bergsma, *Editors*

1979 — Volume XV

No. 1 **Sex Chromosome Aneuploidy: Prospective Studies on Children,** Arthur Robinson, Herbert A. Lubs, and Daniel Bergsma, *Editors*

No. 2 **Genetic Counseling: Facts, Values, and Norms,** Alexander M. Capron, Marc Lappe, Robert F. Murray, Jr., Tabitha M. Powledge, Sumner B. Twiss, and Daniel Bergsma, *Editors*

No. 3 **Recent Advances in the Developmental Biology of Central Nervous System Malformations,** Ntinos C. Myrianthopoulos and Daniel Bergsma, *Editors*

No. 4 **Continuous Transcutaneous Blood Gas Monitoring,** A Huch, R. Huch, and J. Lucey, *Editors*

No. 5 **Annual Review of Birth Defects, 1978,** Proceedings of the 1978 San Francisco Birth Defects Conference. Published in 3 volumes:
- 5A **Diagnostic Approaches to the Malformed Fetus, Abortus, Stillborn, and Deceased Newborn,** Mitchell S. Golbus and Bryan D. Hall, *Editors*
- 5B **Penetrance and Variability in Malformation Syndromes,** James J. O'Donnell and Bryan D. Hall, *Editors*
- 5C **Risk, Communication, and Decision Making in Genetic Counseling,** Charles J. Epstein, Cynthia J.R. Curry, Seymour Packman, Sanford Sherman, and Bryan D. Hall, *Editors*

No. 6 **Dermatoglyphics—Fifty Years Later,** Wladimir Wertelecki and Chris C. Plato, *Editors*

No. 7 **Newborn Behavioral Organization: Nursing Research and Implications,** Gene Cranston Anderson and Beverly Raff, *Editors*

No. 8 **Developmental Aspects of Craniofacial Dysmorphology,** Michael Melnick and Ronald Jorgenson, *Editors*

No. 9 **External Ear Malformations: Epidemiology, Genetics, and Natural History,** *by* Michael Melnick and Ntinos C. Myrianthopoulos

1980 — Volume XVI

No. 1 **Enzyme Therapy in Genetic Diseases: 2.** Robert J. Desnick, *Editor*

No. 2 **In Vitro Epithelia and Birth Defects,** B. Shannon Danes, *Editor*

No. 3 **Diet in Pregnancy: A Randomized Controlled Trial of Nutritional Supplements,** *by* David Rush, Zena Stein, and Mervyn Susser

No. 4 **Morphogenesis and Malformation of the Ear,** Robert J. Gorlin, *Editor*

No. 5 **Dentistry in the Interdisciplinary Treatment of Genetic Diseases,** Carlos F. Salinas and Ronald J. Jorgenson, *Editors*

No. 7 **Genetic and Environmental Hearing Loss: Syndromic and Nonsyndromic,** L. Stefan Levin and Connie H. Knight, *Editors*

[redacted]